WHAT SHOULD WE KNOW ABOUT PREVENTED, DIAGNOSTIC, AND INTERVENTIONAL THERAPY IN CORONARY ARTERY DISEASE

Edited by **Branislav G. Baskot**

What Should We Know About Prevented, Diagnostic, and Interventional Therapy in Coronary Artery Disease
http://dx.doi.org/10.5772/45953
Edited by Branislav G. Baskot

Contributors

Omer Toprak, Jasmin Caluk, Maria Anna Staniszewska, Frantisek Kovar, Miloš Kňazeje, Marian Mokan, Ri-Ichiro Kakihara, Amir Farhang Zand Parsa, Darren Walters, Kenei Shimada, Takao Hasegawa, Alfredo Ruggero Galassi, Massimo Cocchi, Maurizio Turiel, Luigi Gianturco, Bruno Dino Bodini, Vincenzo Gianturco, Juan, Yen-Hung Lin, Ananthasubramaniam, Sabha Bhatti, Abdul Hakeem, Mohamed Bamoshmoosh, Teresa Pinheiro, Catarina Ramos, Patrícia Napoleão, Rui Cruz Ferreira, Cristina Fondinho, Mafalda Selas, Miguel Mota Carmo, Ana Viegas-Crespo, Bong Gun Song, Mohd Shah Azarisman, M Oudkerk, Rozemarijn Vliegenthart, Noach E.J.K, Baskot Branislav

Published by InTech

Janeza Trdine 9, 51000 Rijeka, Croatia

Notice

Publishing Process Manager Danijela Duric
Technical Editor InTech DTP team
Cover InTech Design team

Additional hard copies can be obtained from orders@intechopen.com

What Should We Know About Prevented, Diagnostic, and Interventional Therapy in Coronary Artery Disease, Edited by Branislav G. Baskot
p. cm.
ISBN 978-953-51-1043-9

For EU product safety concerns:
IN TECH d.o.o., Prolaz Marije Krucifikse Kozulić 3, 51000 Rijeka, Croatia,
info@intechopen.com or visit our website at intechopen.com.

Meet the editor

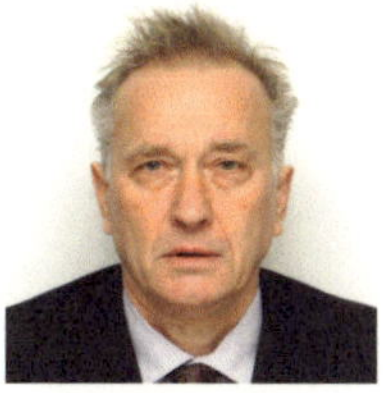

Branislav Baskot MD PhD Ass Prof; was born 1958 in Ruma, Serbia. Medicine Faculty finishes in Sarajevo BiH, specialization of Nuclear Medicine finish 1994 on Military Medical Academy Belgrade Serbia. The main occupation in the field of Nuclear medicine was nuclear cardiology. Doctoral degree 2005; "Determination of culprit lesion before and after percutaneous coronary intervention by myocardial perfusion imaging". In the 2003 finished Master's Degree; "Myocardial perfusion imaging with 99mTc-Tetrofosmin in the diagnosis ischemic heart disease".

Contents

Preface

The mortality from ischemic heart disease has decreased in recent years. The better understanding of risk factors associated with development of coronary artery disease (CAD) has significantly contributed to this decline. Preventive measures such as aggressive therapy of arterial hypertension, diabetes mellitus, and lipid disorders and by campaigning against the smoking are important components of this medical success. Furthermore, improvements in medical and interventional therapy have reduced the complications associated with acute myocardial infarction as well as revascularization.

This book brings together contributions from around the world, investigators who are clinical versus imaging science in their orientation, and representatives from academic medical centers and the imaging industry. Each article is written to be accessible to those with a basic knowledge of coronary imaging but also to be stimulating and educational to those who are experts and investigators in medical imaging.

This book covers where advances have been dramatic in the past two decades and shows the major contributions of the imaging scientists and engineers from both academia and industry. Patients with know or suspected coronary artery disease who are asymptomatic or who have stable symptoms are often evaluated noninvasive. Functional test, such as stress electrocardiography, stress echocardiography, and stress nuclear perfusion imaging, detect and quantity the presence of ischemia based on electrical, mechanical, or perfusion abnormalities, indirectly, but nuclear perfusion imaging directly, establishing the burden of coronary artery disease. Nuclear cardiology imaging (MPI) is well establishment imaging techniques and is already integral part of the management of CAD, and is included in a number of professional guidelines. Coronary angiography, considered the "gold standard" for the diagnosis of CAD, often does not provide information about the functional significance of coronary stenosis, especially in borderline lesions. Andres Gruentzig said; *when coronary angiography founded coronary narrowing, I would like to have some kind of diagnostic procedure who gives me functional significance that lesion.* Nuclear cardiology imaging is very important diagnostic tool for the diagnosis culprit lesions, and indicating for cardiovascular intervention (PCI or ACBP). *The predominant theme* is that MPI finding can serve as the gatekeeper for more costly and more risky invasive strategies in the evaluation and treatment of patients with coronary artery disease.

This book includes a series of articles that provide a state-of-the-art summary of the current clinical applications of cardiac CT, reviews data that support the accuracy and the prognostic use of CT coronary angiography and reports of the newest technologic advances and promising future applications of these imaging modalities. Its also provide other diagnostic approach like functional test, which finding helps to make decision about invasive strategies with best benefit for patients. Finally, the next decades should see even greater advances in the field, and such breakthroughs will be instrumental in further enhancing the information that can be derived from functional testing for the assessment of myocardial blood flow, cardiac function, and myocardial viability.

Readers of *Coronary Angiography* will enjoy in this section and will find the information and expert opinions very useful to their clinical practice.

Branislav G. Baskot MD PhD Ass Prof
Department of Nuclear Medicine Imaging "Dr Baskot"

Section 1

Something About Prevence of Coronary Heart Disease

Chapter 1

Reduced Consumption of Olive Oil: A Risk for Ischemic Heart Disease?

Massimo Cocchi and Giovanni Lercker

Additional information is available at the end of the chapter

http://dx.doi.org/10.5772/54035

1. Introduction

Comparing the nutritional content of food to individual health status, there are several considerations that can be informative and raise troubling concerns. For many decades, researchers have investigated the relationships between health status and consumption of extra virgin olive oil. Extra virgin olive oil (and oleic acid) is considered important for the prevention and coronary heart disease. While the biomolecular aspects involving G protein need further research, oleic acid levels in platelets may be a discriminating factor, together with linoleic and arachidonic acid, for coronary heart disease. There is still a huge debate regarding the effects of oleic acid alone or in combination with antioxidants.

Coronary Heart Disease (CHD) is the main cause of death and morbidity in industrialized countries. The incidence of myocardial infarction, however, is highly variable, with lower rates in Mediterranean countries compared to those in northern Europe, USA, or Australia [1]. Paradoxically, the low incidence of myocardial infarction occurs in spite of a high prevalence of classical cardiovascular risk factors [2].

Olive oil is the primary source of fat in the Mediterranean diet. The beneficial effects of olive oil on CHD have now been recognized, and are often attributed to the high levels of monounsaturated fatty acids (MUFA) [3]. Indeed, in November 2004, the US Federal Drug Administration (FDA) allowed a claim on olive oil labels concerning "the benefits on the risk of coronary heart disease of eating about two tablespoons (23 g) of olive oil daily, due to the MUFA in olive oil" [4].

2. A crucial element for a healthy heart: oleic acid and platelets

Oleic acid, and especially that obtained from pressing olives, is a crucial element in the prevention of ischemic cardiovascular disease, as has been demonstrated by a series of international scientific activity. Fatty acids other than n-3 Polyunsaturated Fatty Acids (PUFAs) can interact with the metabolism of eicosanoids and potentially influence platelet function. For example, there is evidence that diets rich in unsaturated fatty acids, such as linoleic acid and oleic acid, can also decrease thromboembolic risk by replacing arachidonic acid in platelet phospholipids, decreasing, at least in vitro, the production of thromboxane A_2 [TXA2] and platelet aggregation. However, there is little conclusive evidence that platelet function in vivo is affected by diet [5].

Oleic acid has been found to be a potent inhibitor of platelet aggregating factor (PAF) and serotonin secretion. Consequently, in order to understand the molecular mechanisms of oleic acid action, the effects of this fatty acid on several biochemical events associated with platelet aggregation induced by PAF have been investigated. In particular, it has been found that oleic acid causes a decrease in the levels of phosphatidyl inositide phosphate (PIP) and PIP2, which is associated with an inhibition of platelet aggregation induced by PAF. These results suggest that inhibition of the PAF response by oleic acid may be at least one of the steps involved in signal transduction [6].

Several literature reports have further suggested that olive oil may inhibit platelet function. This possible effect is of interest for two reasons. First, it may contribute to the apparent anti-atherogenic effects of olive oil, and second, it may invalidate the use of olive oil as an inert placebo in studies of platelet function. After exposure to olive oil, platelet aggregation and TXA2 release decreased, and the content of platelet membrane oleic acid increased significantly; platelet membrane arachidonic acid content was found to significantly decrease. This suggests that excess of oleic acid impairs the incorporation of arachidonic acid into platelet phospholipids.

Olive oil also has an inhibitory effect on various aspects of platelet function, which might be associated with decreased risk for heart disease, although fish intake also plays a protective role [7].

The beneficial effects of olive oil can be attributed to its high content of oleic acid (70-80%). The consumption of olive oil increases the levels of oleic acid in cell membranes, which helps to regulate the structure of membrane lipids through the control of signal-mediated G-protein, causing a reduction in blood pressure [8].

In rats, cardiovascular tissues treated with 2-OHOA (hydroxy oleic acid) show activation of cAMP in response to activation of Gsα protein, which can be attributed to increased expression of Gsα proteins. As a result, there is significant reduction in systolic blood pressure [9]. The involvement of Gs alpha protein is also of interest considering the hypothesis forwarded by Cocchi, Tonello, Rasenick and Hameroff in psychiatric disorders as depression, suicide etc. (private meeting, 2008). In light of the below model, the role of Gsα protein in ischemic heart disease merits further investigation.

http://dx.doi.org/10.5772/54035

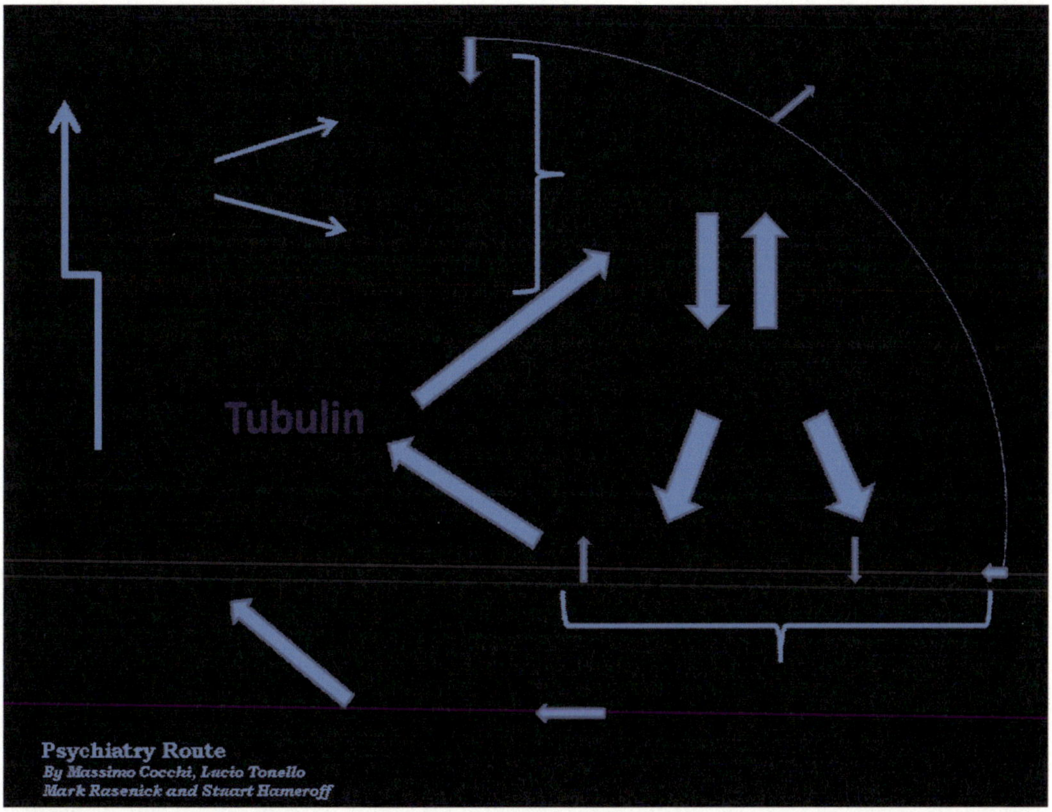

Figure 1. Description of selected biochemical and biomolecular events potentially involved in psychiatric disorders.

In figure 1, the molecular depression hypothesis described by Cocchi et al. [10], Donati et al. [11] and Hameroff and Penrose [12] is shown. Because of the possible similarity of the platelet to neurons, membrane viscosity can modify Gsα protein status. The Gsα protein is associated with tubulin. Depending on local membrane lipid composition, tubulin may serve as a positive or negative regulator of phosphatidylinositol bisphosphate hydrolysis (PIP2) similar to G proteins. Tubulin is known to form high-affinity complexes with certain G proteins. The formation of these complexes allows tubulin to activate Gsα protein and creates a system whereby elements of the cytoskeleton can influence G-protein signaling. Rapid changes in membrane lipid composition or the cytoskeleton can modify neuronal signaling through such a mechanism.

Protein kinase C (PKC) activation (Figure 2) is preceded by a number of steps, originating from the binding of an extracellular ligand that activates a G-protein on the cytosolic side of the plasma membrane. This G-protein, using guanosine triphosphate (GTP) as an energy source, then activates protein kinase C (PKC) via the phosphatidylinositol bisphosphate (PIP2) intermediate, which is shown as the diacylglycerol DAG/IP3 complex. Several studies have shown that a reduced functionality of the serotonin (5-HT) transporter in some psychiatric disorders, such as obsessive-compulsive disorder (OCD), may be related to alterations in its regulation at an intracellular level. PKC has also been reported to provoke a decrease in the number of 5-HT transporter proteins. The increased activity of PKC in OCD may be the result of increased activity of the phosphatidylinositol pathway.

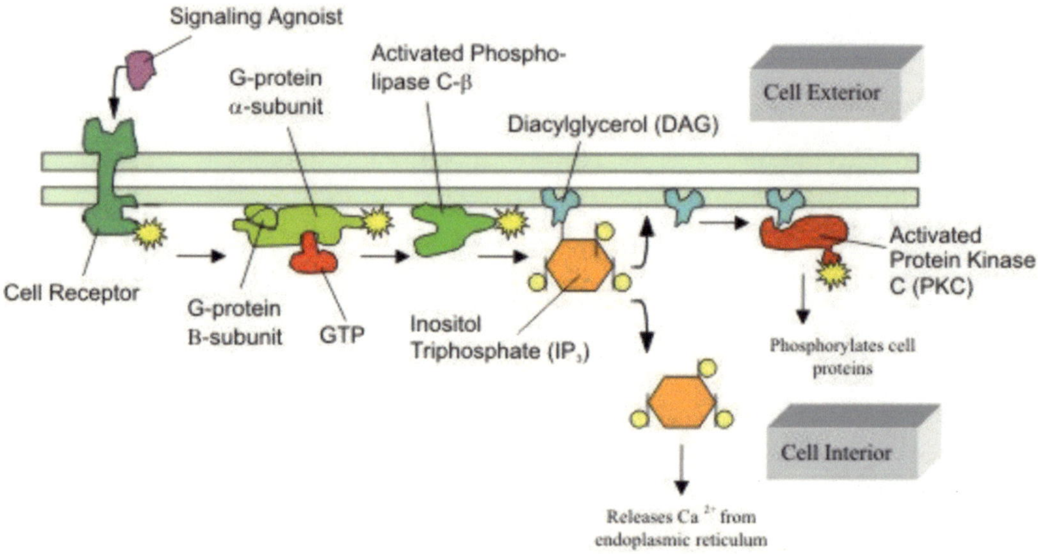

Figure 2. Description of PKC activation. Adapted from Alberts et al. [13].

The exclusive use of olive oil during food preparation seems to offer significant protection against ischemic heart disease, in spite of poor clinical conditions, lifestyle and other characteristics of individuals [14]. In addition, several historical papers have reported on the positive effects of olive oil on CHD.

In 1985, Mattson and Grundy [15] reported that olive oil reduces HDL cholesterol, which plays a protective, anti-atherogenic function, favoring the elimination of LDL-cholesterol. In 1986, Sirtori et al. [16] have shown that in addition to its effects on cholesterol and atherosclerosis, olive oil has preventive action on thrombosis and platelet aggregation. High intake of olive oil is not harmful, and reduces the levels of LDL-cholesterol, but not HDL [17 - 25].

3. Oleic acid and Atherogenesis

Atherosclerosis is considered to be an inflammatory disease [26], and endothelial dysfunction occurs early in the development of the pathology. Traditional risk factors for atherosclerosis promote endothelium activation, which induces adhesion and trans-endothelial migration of monocytes [26]. Several inflammatory mediators are released by the endothelium such as the eicosanoids derived from n-6 PUFA arachidonic acid. These include prostaglandin E2 (PGE2), leukotriene B4, a chemoattractant and neutrophile activator, thromboxane, a potent vasoconstrictor, and platelet-aggregating factor [27].

http://dx.doi.org/10.5772/54035

Monocytes and macrophages are critical cells present in all stages of atherosclerosis. In addition to promoting LDL oxidation through free radical production, they also secrete proinflammatory cytokines such as IL-1 and Tumor Necrosis Factor (TNF), which stimulate the expression of adhesion molecules such as intercellular cell adhesion molecule-1 (ICAM-1), vascular-cell adhesion molecule-1 (VCAM-1), and E-selectin [25]. Circulating monocytes are attracted by these molecules and adhere to the endothelium, from which they transmigrate to the subendothelial space. Once within the endothelium, monocytes differentiate into macrophages, which in turn scavenge oxidized LDL, thus becoming foam cells and lead to plaque formation.

The proinflammatory response releases a principal messenger from macrophages, namely cytokine IL6. After engagement of its receptor on the liver, IL6 promotes the secretion of C Reactive Protein (CRP), a prototypic marker of inflammation [28, 29]. Serum IL6 and CRP have been shown to be predictive of CHD. Altered levels of serum CRP, IL6, and ICAM-1 have been associated with progression of atherosclerosis, and IL6 has been shown to be a good predictor of progressive peripheral atherosclerosis [30, 31].

The inflammatory protection of diets rich in oleic acid has been attributed to a decrease in the content of LDL linoleic acid [32]. The low susceptibility of oleic acid to oxidation, and the scavenging capacity of minor compounds in olive oil, can decrease the activation of proinflammatory transcription factors, such as nuclear factor-kappa B (NFkB), through a reduction of reactive oxygen spices and peroxyl radicals [33]. In this regard, it has been reported that consumption of meals enriched in olive oil do not activate NFkB in monocytes in contrast to meals rich in butter and walnut-enriched meals [34]. Studies on oleic acid enriched liposomes and vascular endothelium exposed to oleic acid, however, suggest a protective mechanism of oleic acid on free radical generation, oxidative damage to lipids, and inflammatory activity [35, 36].

Recent data suggest that oleic acid is not the only agent responsible for the anti-inflammatory properties of olive oil. In experimental studies, minor components of the unsaponifiable fraction of olive oil, such as alfa-tocopherol, beta-sitosterol, and triterpenes, in addition to phenolic compounds, have all been shown to have both anti-inflammatory and anti-endothelial activation properties [37]. The results of a meta-analysis of 14 studies carried out during 1983–1994 showed that the replacement of SFA by oils enriched in MUFA or PUFA had similar effects on total, LDL, and HDL cholesterol, whereas PUFA-enriched oil had a slight triglyceride-lowering effect [38]. Dubois et al. [39] showed that increasing the amount of fat up to 50 g led to stepwise increases in the postprandial rise of serum triglycerides, while the ingestion of 15 g fat had no effect on postprandial lipemia or lipoproteins in healthy adults. A meal containing 31 g of fat induced considerably less variations in lipemia, chylomicrons, and lipoproteins than a 42 g fat meal [39]. A single dose of 25 mL olive oil was not found to promote postprandial lipemia [40], in contrast to 40 mL and 50 mL doses [41, 42] with no effect on the phenolic content of the olive oil.

Abia et al. [43] reported that virgin olive oil intake resulted in lower postprandial triacylglyceride-rich-lipoprotein (TRL) levels and a faster disappearance of TRL-TG from blood, compared to intake of sunflower oil with a high content of oleic acid. Chylomicrons produced after olive oil [44, 45] or n-3 PUFA [46] ingestion seem to enter the circulation more rapidly, and cleared at a faster rate, in comparison to those produced after intake of fats rich in SFA or PUFA. Although fat intake appears to be the major nutritional determinant of the postprandrial triglyceride response, it is also influenced by other dietary components, including fiber, glucose, starch, and alcohol in a meal [47].

The oxidative modification of LDL plays a key role in development of atherosclerosis and CHD. Oxidation of lipids and lipoproteins present in LDL leads to a change in the lipoprotein conformation by which LDL are more facilitated to enter the monocyte/macrophage system of the arterial wall, and promote the atherosclerotic process [48]. It is currently believed that oxidized LDL are more damaging to the arterial wall than native LDL [49]. Elevated concentrations of circulating oxidized LDL show a positive relationship with the severity of acute coronary events [50, 51]. They are also independently associated with carotid intima-media thickness [52] and are predictors for CHD both in CHD patients [53] and the general population [54]. Several studies have been performed comparing the effects of MUFA-rich diets on the susceptibility of LDL to oxidation with those of PUFA- or carbohydrate-rich diets. Oleate-rich LDL have been shown to be less susceptible to oxidation than linoleate rich LDL [55-61].

4. Depression and Ischemic Heart Disease: a common role for oleic acid?

Because of the particular role of platelets on depressive and thrombogenetic risk, our group has investigated the platelet fatty acid profile in three groups of subjects: healthy (n=60), ischemic (n= 50) and depressive (n= 84). The aim of the study was to understand which fatty acid could be utilized as markers of ischemic cardiovascular pathology and depressive disorder, and to classify subjects using an artificial neural network (ANN). All the ANNs tested gave essentially the same result. However, one type of ANN, known as Self-Organizing Map (SOM), [62, 63, 64], gave additional information by allowing the results to be described in a two-dimensional plane with potentially informative border areas. The central property of the SOM is that it forms a nonlinear projection of a high-dimensional data manifold on a regular, low-dimensional (usually 2D) grid.

A series of repeated and independent SOM simulations, with the input parameters being changed each time, led to the finding that the best discriminating map was that obtained by inclusion of the following three fatty acids: palmitic acid (C16:0), linoleic acid (C18:2 *n*-6) and arachidonic acid (C20:4 *n*-6) for depressive subjects and oleic acid (C18:1), linoleic acid and arachidonic acid for ischemic subjects [10, 65-67] (Figures 3, 4).

5. A case study

A 42-year-old female with a very high familial risk for ischemic cardiovascular disease (one sister 34 years old died of heart attack; another sister, 48 years old, heart attack; uncle, two infarctions; mother, 69 years old, died of heart attack; aunt, 59 years old, died of heart at-

http://dx.doi.org/10.5772/54035

tack), was submitted to a classic complete functional cardiovascular investigation which resulted negative. The subject is a heavy smoker, cholesterol: 230 mg/dl, HDL: 84 mg/dl. Framingham score: 13 (low risk score). Platelet levels of oleic acid, linoleic acid and arachidonic acid were analyzed using the SOM designed for ischemic patients, and the concentrations of those fatty acids were entered in the SOM. The subject detailed information on the study and provided informed consent. The patient's fatty acid triplet, tested in the SOM, gave the following result (Figure 5).

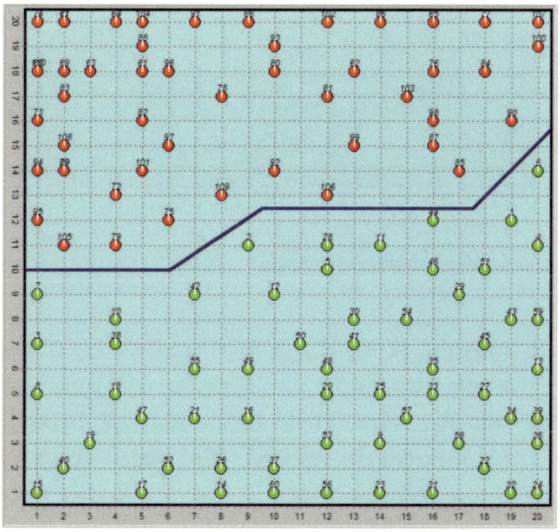

Figure 3. SOM classification of depressive subjects (red) against normal subjects (green). Platelet arachidonic acid ($C_{20:4}$), palmitic acid ($C_{16:0}$), and linoleic acid ($C_{18:2}$) can discriminate depression and have diagnostic power.

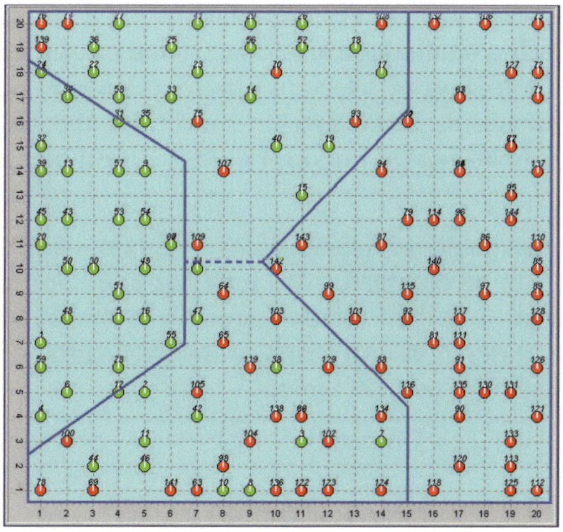

Figure 4. SOM classification of ischemic subjects (red) against normal subjects (green). Platelet oleic acid ($C_{18:1}$), arachidonic acid ($C_{20:4}$), linoleic acid ($C_{18:2}$) can discriminate ischemia and have diagnostic power.

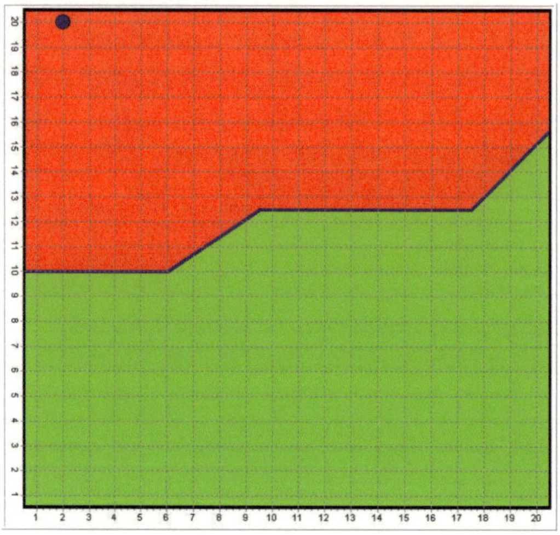

Figure 5. Position of the patient according to the three fatty acids (oleic, linoleic and arachidonic) on the SOM, which classifies ischemic patients.

This result was compared with the SOM classification of normal and pathologic subjects, as shown in figure 4. The patient was asked to submit herself to a Coronary TAC and the images showed "Interventricular Anterior (IVA) branch: small mixed plaque in the proximal tract, 33% of the lumen" (radiological diagnosis). The result suggests the opportunity to select young high risk subjects to evaluate not only the diagnostic power of the SOM, but also the possibility for early diagnosis of plaque formation. A large trial is necessary to validate this result, but based on the classical rules of Evidence Based Medicine, it is very difficult to obtain approval from an ethic's committee.

Medical science has not yet fully understood or accepted the use of the ANN mathematic models in relation to experimental conditions, which are still strongly linked to traditional protocols. The task of finding biomarkers according to the rules dictated by Evidence Based Medicine requires the elimination of selection bias, and leads to selection of a population that may be clinically unrealistic. The characteristics of the above-described method nonetheless allow the analysis to be carried out, and permit to find differences among subsets of the population.

The first fundamental consequence of the use of fatty acids is that an extremely effective and practical diagnostic tool can be obtained, with a strong tolerance to "noise". Secondly, the choice of specific fatty acids and their relative strength in the classification by the SOM allows investigating more in-depth investigation of the problem and helps in understanding the disease from the biochemical point of view.

6. Commonalities between CHD and depression

To demonstrate the powerful grouping capacity of the SOM, we created a new network where all three groups were inserted and grouped simultaneously on the basis of the characteristics of the triplets previously highlighted, which were all different from one another [68] (Figure 6).

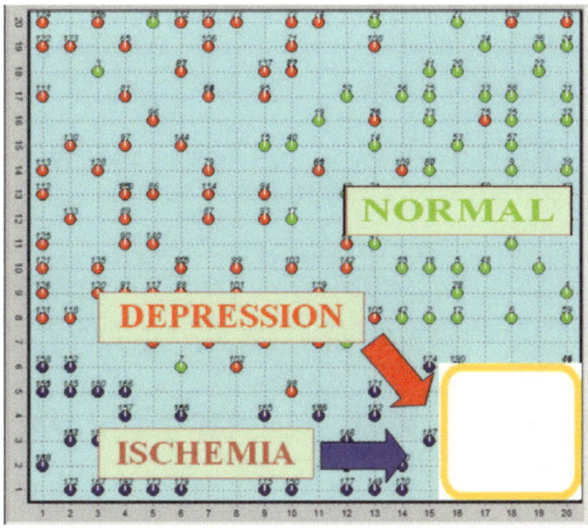

Figure 6. Simultaneous classification, using the SOM, of three groups of subjects (normal, depressive and ischemic). In the right corner of the map, ischemic and depressive subjects are mixed and have, in common, a low level of platelet oleic acid.

As shown by the SOM, it is possible that reduced amounts of oleic acid not only are critical in the biochemical classification of ischemic heart disease, but are also common to a condition that characterizes a relationship between depression and ischemia [69]. It seems possible that levels of C18:1 in platelets dominate in ischemia, and are linked to depression. Furthermore, it can be conjectured that there are two different types of depression, namely classical and ischemia-induced according to the findings of different platelet membrane viscosity and its effect at the biomolecular level. [10-12, 70]. The relationships between depression and ischemic heart disease have been widely studied [71, 72]. Interestingly, Weyers and Colquhoun [73] reported improvements in depressive symptoms in patients with CHD after consumption of olive oil.

7. Do we eat enough extra virgin olive oil?

The question then arises as to whether there is sufficient consumption of olive oil and oleic acid in the Italian population. Knowing that oleic acid can significantly change the composition of platelet fatty acids, which are crucial in the genesis of plaque formation, and can significantly alter the amount of oleic acid in platelet membranes, an experiment on a large group of pigs (80 Duroc x Large White) was performed [74]. Four groups of pigs were studied, 20 animals each, which received four diets containing different lipid fractions, as follows:

Diet 1: corn oil (low linoleic acid.), diet 2: corn oil (medium linoleic acid.), diet 3: sunflower oil (high oleic acid.), diet 4: sunflower oil (high oleic acid) + palm oil (high palmitic acid). The diets fed to animals, to meet the needs for growth, had the following lipid composition (Table 1):

Period (kg)	Diet	EE	C16:0	C18:0	C18:1n9	C18:2n6	C18:3n3
50 - 90	1	2.70	13.13	2.05	31.07	50.90	2.59
50 - 90	2	2.86	14.37	2.04	26.40	54.54	2.42
50 - 90	3	5.30	8.91	2.39	56.47	30.23	1.27
50 - 90	4	5.37	18.67	8.36	39.99	30.86	1.40
90 - 120	1	2.63	12.83	1.72	31.60	51.15	2.38
90 - 120	2	2.57	14.16	1.94	25.76	54.96	2.55
90 - 120	3	5.56	8.81	2.44	57.12	29.73	1.26
90 - 120	4	5.62	20.02	9.26	39.41	29.59	1.12
120 - 160	1	2.83	13.32	1.69	30.46	52.00	2.41
120 - 160	2	2.89	13.75	1.88	25.65	56.29	2.35
120 - 160	3	5.74	8.54	2.10	57.18	30.91	1.07
120 - 160	4	5.76	19.71	9.25	39.16	30.25	1.17

Table 1. Ether extract (% dry Matter) and fatty acid composition of lipid fractions

Fatty Acids		C16:0	C18:0	C18:1n9	C18:2n6	C18:3n3	C20:4
Diet 1	Media s.d.	28.51^{a}	32.00	17.38 ^{B}	9.30	0.63a	12.19 ^{AB}
		1.84	10.70	5.63	3.40	0.36	5.18
Diet 2	Media s.d.	27.73 ^{ab}	29.01	18.0 ^{B}	9.07	0.48ab	15.6 ^{A}
		1.47	8.48	3.17	2.88	0.29	4.52
Diet 3	Media s.d.	27.00^{ab}	27.78	24.93 ^{A}	9.37	0.34^{b}	10.59^{B}
		2.07	8.12	6.78	3.10	0.25	4.48
Diet 4	Media s.d.	26.51^{b}	32.04	19.36 ^{B}	9.32	0.51^{ab}	12.25^{AB}
		2.63	11.07	5.43	3.64	0.32	4.27
P		<0.05	n.s.	<0.01	n.s.	<0.05	<0.01

Table 2. Mean values ± SD of platelet fatty acids in the different treatment groups

The platelet fatty acids (Table 2) were plotted as for ischemic and normal human subjects in the SOM for ischemia (Figure 7).

http://dx.doi.org/10.5772/54035

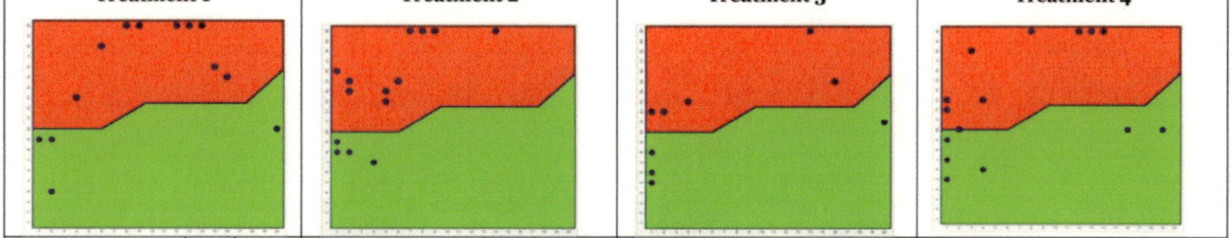

Treatment 1

Summary	N	%
Normal Area	5	25
Ischemic Area	15	75
Border line	0	0
Total	20	100

Treatment 2

Summary	N	%
Normal Area	5	25
Ischemic Area	15	75
Border line	0	0
Total	20	100

Treatment 3

Summary	N	%
Normal Area	8	40
Ischemic Area	12	60
Border line	0	0
Total	20	100

Treatment 4

Summary	N	%
Normal Area	8	30
Ischemic Area	12	65
Border line	0	5
Total	20	100

Figure 7. By increasing the oleic acid content in diets is possible to move pig platelets, in agreement with the fatty acid triplet [66, 67], from the pathologic (red area) to the normal (green area) area.

It is feasible to obtain similar results in humans. If one considers the characteristics described for the pig model of atherosclerosis [75], and applying similar characteristics to humans, it can be assumed that we should consume a quantity of oleic acid, and consequently, extra virgin olive oil, that is at least twice that of current levels. To demonstrate this, we made simple considerations based on the purchase of olive oil in Italy (Data provided by the Istituto di Servizi per il Mercato Agricolo Alimentare (ISMEA).

Based on data provided and taking into account that the value derived from the table should be increased by 40%, since about 40% of purchase data were excluded, the consumption of extra virgin olive oil for each Italian is on average, about 11.76 grams of oleic acid daily, considering that olive oil is on average value about 70% oleic acid. This value is even likely to be less, as much oil is also used for frying, and therefore cannot be included as part of raw consumption. While this quantity is very small, there are also regional differences between the north and south of Italy.

This observation is also related to the observation that current eating behavior does not allow large consumption of olive oil. It should be remembered that meals eaten out of the household, often consisting of a sandwich, make it difficult to consume extra virgin olive oil in larger quantities. While the eating habits of rural areas may still be able to compensate this situation, there is an increasing trend to gradually move away from such traditions.

Recently, we investigated the consumption of olive oil in a restaurant in the Center-North of Italy, (2750 subjects in one month). The average consumption of olive oil was 1.8 g per customer per month, which corresponds to about 1.26 g of oleic acid. Together with the above cited data, this results confirms that olive oil is not consumed in large quantities. Given this, as Ancel Keys pointed out, one wonders if the Mediterranean diet is still a model of health, considering the consumption of extra virgin olive oil.

Systematic name	Trivial name	Shorthand designation	Molecular weight	Melting point (°C)
butanoic	butyric	4:0	88.1	-7.9
pentanoic	valeric	5:0	102,1	-19
hexanoic	caproic	6:0	116.1	-3.4
octanoic	caprylic	8:0	144.2	16.7
nonanoic	pelargonic	9:0	158.2	12.5
decanoic	capric	10:0	172.3	31.6
dodecanoic	lauric	12:0	200.3	44.2
tetradecanoic	myristic	14:0	228.4	53.9
hexadecanoic	palmitic	16:0	256.4	63.1
heptadecanoic	margaric (daturic)	17:0	270.4	61.3
octadecanoic	stearic	18:0	284.4	69.6
eicosanoic	arachidic	20:0	312.5	75.3
docosanoic	behenic	22:0	340.5	79.9
tetracosanoic	lignoceric	24:0	368.6	84.2
cis-9-hexadecenoic	palmitoleic	16:1(n-7)	254.4	0.5
cis-9-octadecenoic	oleic	18:1(n-9)	282.4	16.2
trans-9-octadecenoic	elaidic	tr18:1(n-9)	282.4	43.7
cis-11-octadecenoic	*cis*-vaccenic (asclepic)	18:1(n-7)	282.4	39
cis-9-eicosenoic	gadoleic	20:1(n-11)	310.5	25
cis-13-docosenoic	erucic	22:1(n-9)	338.6	33.4
9,12-octadecadienoic	linoleic	18:2(n-6)	280.4	-5
6,9,12-octadecatrienoic	γ-linolenic	18:3(n-6)	278.4	
9,12,15-octadecatrienoic	α-linolenic	18:3(n-3)	278.4	-11
8,11,14-eiosatrienoic	dihomo-γ-linolenic	20:3(n-6)	306.5	
5,8,11,14-eicosatetraenoic	arachidonic	20:4(n-6)	304.	-50
6,912,15-octadecatetraenoic	stearidonic	18:4(n-3)	276.4	-57
5,8,11,14,17-eicosapentaenoic	EPA	20:5(n-3)	302.5	-54
7,10,13,16,19-docosapentaenoi	DPA	22:5(n-3)	330.6	
4,7,10,13,16,19-docosahexaenoic	DHA	22:6(n-3)	328.6	-44

(see: http://216.239.59.104/search?q=cache:qTHq_xfePkIJ:www.cyberlipid.org/fa/acid0001.htm+Aitzetm%C3%BCller+K&hl=it)

Table 3. Selected chemical and physical characteristics of fatty acids

http://dx.doi.org/10.5772/54035

8. Chemical and technological considerations about oleic acid

Fatty acids have different functions in living organisms, including the structural one, which are determined by the length of their hydrocarbon chain and the presence or absence of double bonds. Hydrocarbon chain length, in the same conditions of unsaturation, is directly proportional to the melting point (as well as the boiling point) (Table 3). The solubility in water (Table 4) and unsaturation, for the same chain length, is inversely proportional to the melting point (see Table 3), with very few exceptions.

Carbon number	Solubility
2	Infinite
4	Infinite
6	9.7
8	0.7
10	0.15
12	0.055
14	0.02
16	0.007
18	0.003

Table 4. Fatty acid solubility in water at 20°C (in grams per liter)

These chemical differences are determined in large part by chemical and physical interactions that exist when molecules are close enough to unsaturate them. In the case of fatty acids, the possibility to join molecules depends only on the hydrocarbon chain (Van der Waals forces), which is facilitated when it is saturated and more difficult when unsaturated (especially at the point of unsaturation). The longer and more linear the chain, the greater the interaction, and the more unsaturated it will be, consequently, the interaction will be lower. When fatty acids are part of a triglyceride or phospholipid, the effect occurs in a similar manner and therefore, in biological membranes, a greater or lesser chance of interaction corresponds to greater or lesser "fluidity" of the membrane, which is proportional to more or less functionality (permeability).

At room temperature, in terms of membrane structure, fatty acids are important, and the ones that are more widespread in nature are those with 18 total carbon atoms, especially unsaturated. Modulation of proper membrane fluidity requires that some fatty acids are relatively "rigid", such as palmitic and stearic acid, with a preference for the former since it has a lower melting point and thus is more effective in bringing about small changes.

One of the most important aspects of biological systems that protect themselves through membranes is the preservation of integrity of the membrane itself, which is subject to contact with chemical reactive oxygen species (ROS), and capable of chemically attacking the unsaturated zone of the molecule. Greater effectiveness is related to a greater level of unsaturation, leading to subsequent breakage of the molecule with increased membrane fragility. For these reasons, the membrane is associated with a series of antioxidants, whose action is linked to their position in the membrane [75]. Oleic acid is the least oxidizable among unsaturated fatty acids (Table 5), and is also not too fluid or too rigid, and is thus suitable for prolonging membrane stability [76, 77].

FATTY ACID	1) AUTOXIDATION	2) AUTOXIDATION	PHOTOSENSITIZED OXIDATION (PHOTOXIDATION)
SATURATED	1	1	
MONOENES	10	100	1.1 (32,000)*
DIENES	100	1200	2.9 (1600)*
TRIENES	200	2500	3.5
TETRAENES**	300		
PENTAENES**	400		
HESAENES**	500		

* In brackets ratio between photoxidation and autoxidation is shown

** Hypothesis based on physical-chemical behavior

Table 5. Oxidation rate of several unsaturated fatty acids [Modified from Gunstone et al. [76]]

The rate of oxidation between various unsaturated fatty acids shown in Table 5 appears increased between oleic acid (monoenes) and linoleic acid (dienes), but upon increasing the unsaturation (trienes), the variation is much less pronounced. In biological systems, the position of the fatty acid in glycerides or phospholipids [77] appears to influence the rate of oxidation, and is slower when inserted in position 2, or in the β position of the molecule. In the case of olive oil, as in all vegetable fats (Table 6), the 2 position is occupied by unsaturated fatty acids, and is more available in that position because it can directly cross the intestinal wall of the 2-monoglycerides, resulting from digestion of glycerides by pancreatic lipase. In particular, on a molar basis, 83% of unsaturated fatty acids, in position 2 of triglycerides in olive oil, is occupied by oleic acid.

For extra virgin olive oil, its total unsaturation makes it particularly stable (Table 7) [79, 80] so that appropriate conservation, which is further prolonged by the presence of numerous and effective natural antioxidants (biophenol), is still present after refining, in contrast to other oils.

Fat or Oil source	Fatty acid position	14:0	16:0	18:0	18:1	18:2	18:3	20:0	22:0
Women milk*	1	3.2	16.1	15.0	46.1	11	0.4		
	2	7.3	58.2	3.3	12.7	7.3	0.6		
	3	7.1	6.2	2.0	49.7	2.0	1.6		
Women milk	1	18.2	20.0	73.9	42.5	33.3	15.4		
	2	41.5	72.3	16.3	11.7	22.1	23.1		
	3	40.3	7.7	9.9	45.8	44.5	61.5		
Cow milk	1	11	36	15	21	1			
	2	20	33	6	14	3			
	3	7	10	4	15	<1			
Pig	1	1	10	30	51	6			
	2	4	72	2	13	3			
	3			7	73	8			
Cow	1	4	41	17	20	4	1		
	2	9	17	9	41	5	1		
	3	1	22	24	37	5	1		
Cocoa butter	1		34	50	12	1			
	2		2	2	87	9			
	3		37	53	9				
Groundnut	1		14	5	59	18		1	-
	2		1	<1	58	39		-	-
	3		11	5	57	10		4	6
Corn	1		18	3	27	50	1		
	2		2	<1	26	70	<1		
	3		13	3	31	51	1		
Soya	1		14	6	23	48	9		
	2		1	1	21	70	7		
	3		13	6	28	45	8		
Olive	1		13	3	72	10	<1		
	2		1	-	83	14	1		
	3		7	4	74	5	1		

Mol % = molar percentage

*Relative GC area % (http://www.cyberlipid.org/index.htm); ** Sørensen A.D.M. et al., 2010 [78]

Table 6. Main fatty acid (mol %) distribution in the three positions of glycerine molecule of the corresponding triacylglycerols (triglycerides) of several fats and oils.

Fattyacids	Caprylic (C8:0)	Capric (C10:0)	Lauric (C12:0)	Mirystic (C14:0)	Palmitic (C16:0)	Stearic (C18:0)	Oleic (C18:1)	Linoleic (C18:2)	Linolenic (C18:3)	Eicosenoic (C20:1)	Total Unsaturation[a] (unstability factor)	Iodine number
Oil from:												
Groundnut				ND-0.1	8.0-14.0	1.0-4.5	35.0-69.0	12.0-43.0	0-0.3	0.7-1.7	200-481	86-107
Rapeseed (0 erucic)				ND-0.2	2.5-7.0	0.8-3.0	51.0-70.0	15.0-30.0	5.0-14.0	0.1-4.3	320-630	105-126
Safflower				ND-0.2	5.3-8.0	1.9-2.9	8.4-21.3	67.8-83.2	ND-0.1	0.1-0.3	700-740	136-148
Safflower (HO)				ND-0.2	3.6-6.0	1.5-2.4	70.0-83.7	9.0-19.9	ND-0.2	0.1-0.5	175-270	80-100
Sunflower			ND-0.1	ND-0.2	5.0-7.6	2.7-6.5	14.0-39.4	48.3-74.0	0-0.3	0-0.3	531-766	118-141
Sunflower (HO)				ND-0.1	2.6-5.0	2.9-6.2	70.0-90.7	2.1-20.0	ND-3.0	0.1-0.5	118-270	78-90
Corn			ND-0.3	ND-0.3	8.6-14.0	ND-3.3	20.0-42.0	34.0-65.6	0-1.2	0.2-0.6	400-481	103-135
Olive (CODEX)					7.5-20.0		55.0-83.0	3.5-21.0	Max 1.0	Max 0.4	163-285	75-94
Soya Bean			ND-0.1	ND-0.2	8.0-13.5	2.5-5.4	17.0-30.0	48.0-59.0	4.5-11.0	0-0.5	600-840	124-139
Grape seed				ND-0.3	5.5-11.0	3.0-6.5	12.0-28.0	58.0-78.0	0-1.0	0-0.3	596-802	128-150
Fat from:												
Cocoa butter					22.6-30.4	30.2-36.0	29.2-36.4	1.3-4.0	ND-0.5		370-380	34-40
Coconut	4.6-10	5.0-8.0	45.1-53.2	16.8-21.0	7.5-10.2	2.0-4.0	5.0-10.0	1.0-2.5	ND-0.2	ND-0.2	24-34	6.3-10.6
Palm			ND-0.5	0.5-2.0	39.3-47.5	3.5-6.0	36.3-44.0	9.0-12.0	ND-0.5	ND-0.4	130-391	50.0-55.0
Palm olein			0.1-0.5	0.5-1.5	38.0-43.5	3.5-5.0	39.8-46.0	10.0-13.5	ND-0.6	ND-04	158-187	56
Palm stearin			0.1-0.5	1.0-2.0	48.0-74.0	3.9-6.0	15.5-36.0	3.0-10.0	ND-0.5	ND-0.4	76-270	33
Palm kernel	2.4-6.2	2.6-5.0	45.0-55.0	14.0-18.0	6.5-10.0	1.0-3.0	12.0-19.0	1.0-3.5	ND-0.2	ND-0.2	33-51	14.1-21.0

[a] Total unsaturation is calculated as the relative percentage of single fatty acid for a different factor, for each unsaturation, the degree is proportional to the oxidative instability. The factors utilized were: 1 for monounsaturated, 10 for diunsaturated and 20 for triunsaturated fatty acids. HO =high oleic. ND = not detectable

Table 7. Main fatty acid composition of fats and oils

Not all olive oils have the same concentration of oleic acid. The International Olive Oil Council (IOOC) has dictated that the content of oleic acid in olive oils can vary from 55% to 83% of total fatty acids [81]. The regulations of the European Community do not indicate the amount of oleic acid in olive oil, but simply indicate the specifications of several other parameters that are useful for detecting fraud and require the distinction between various commercial products obtained from olive processing.

Among these, extra virgin oils are those that must have the highest quality. Extra virgin olive oils with the highest content of oleic acid have always been regarded as those with the highest quality, but only because of their higher stability during storage, as a consequence of the low reactivity of oleic acid compared with polyunsaturated fats. The Food and Drug Administration (FDA) has stated (November 1, 2004) that U.S. consumption of 23 g of olive oil each day (about two tablespoons) helps in prevention of cardiovascular diseases [4].

Today, there are other sources of oil high in oleic acid, such as safflower, sunflower and canola (the new name for rapeseed oil low in erucic acid), and therefore based solely on the content of oleic acid, these sources would also be optimal in this regard. However, the reputation of olive oil as a healthy product is most likely due to the presence of the numerous "minor elements" contained within [82, 83]. Among these minor components, several compounds are worthy of mention including biophenols, which consists of phenols and polyphenols with high antioxidant and antiradical activity, some triterpene alcohols, phytosterols, squalene, and tocopherols. These latter are considered important because of the content of vitamin E, and for their ability to facilitate the assimilation of polyunsaturated fatty acids: 1 mg allows the assimilation of 1 g of polyunsaturated fatty acids [84].

The discovery of health effects from the minor components in olive oil has led to a large gap in the nutritional properties of edible oils. In fact, oils from seeds, subject to refining, loose many minor components and do not have the health properties that the corresponding matrix has. The technology for olive processing influences the quality and organoleptic characteristics of the final product, which is not always considered by industrial operators as much of the scientific knowledge is particularly new. The olive oil is encapsulated in small drops (10-30 micrometers) within vacuoles with a polysaccharide wall: oil droplets, during processing, are released in crushing and come into contact with the other components of olives during grinding of the paste. It is the prolonged contact with the oil-pasta that allows joining of small droplets such that they can then leave the dough during the separation process that emulsifies all the minor components in oil.

Therefore, time and temperature of processing can also affect the final product, and even if the starting characteristics of the olives are similar they can yield very different products. Moreover, during the same oil-paste stage, enzyme activities are capable of forming the fragrance of the oil through a series of biochemical steps that, in part, may reduce the antioxidant ability of biophenol components and their effects on health. Therefore, choices made during the processing of olives should take these effects into consideration.

There are several hundred olive cultivars grown in Italy, which can produce many oils that have a very different composition, although all can be considered of excellent quality. In particular, the richness in antioxidants (especially biophenols) can affect characteristics of the oil in terms of taste, storage stability, and health properties. Even if much scientific knowledge has been learned about olive production and processing technology, there are still many questions that must be answered in order to improve the quality, especially those related to health, of the oils obtained by processing olives

9. Conclusion

The ability to transform, by the action of delta9-desaturase, stearic acid to oleic acid, and vice versa makes oleic acid very useful for the modulation of the fluidity (and functionality)

of cell membranes. Recalling that the fatty acid composition of platelets can be correlated with depression and also with ischemia [85], we can consider the oil obtained from olive processing such as the lipid substrate better balanced with respect to the fatty acid unsaturations, for the platelet membrane composition of normal individuals.

We must remember that the presence of high concentrations of oleic acid from olive oil is one of the stabilizing factors against oxidative modification, in both cases, for the oil itself and for cell membranes. Furthermore, the oil from olives when is classified as extra virgin, possesses a wealth of biophenols, powerful antioxidants predominantly of antiradical type, which further increase the stability of the oil and, more or less directly, even of the membrane lipids.

Olive oil, and, particularly an extra virgin olive oil-rich diet, decreases prothrombotic activity, and modify platelet adhesion, coagulation, and fibrinolysis. The wide range of antiatherogenic effects associated with olive oil consumption can help to justify the low rate of cardiovascular mortality found in southern European Mediterranean countries, in comparison with other western countries, despite a high prevalence of CHD risk factors. Experimental evidence confirms a critical role of reduced levels of oleic acid in platelets in ischemic subjects with a diagnostic discriminant capacity from normal subjects [85]. At present, although traditional cardiovascular risk factors are under revision, a new field of research in platelets, and in particular oleic acid and its relationship with linoleic and arachidonic acid, should be pursued. The mechanisms by which olive oil exerts its beneficial effects merit further investigation, and additional studies are required to document the benefits of olive oil consumption on primary endpoints for cardiovascular disease. In this regard, consumption of extra virgin olive oil and daily intake of oleic acid should, however, be promoted.

Author details

Massimo Cocchi[1,2] and Giovanni Lercker[3]

1 "Paolo Sotgiu" Institute for research in Quantitative & Quantum Psychiatry & Cardiology, L.U.de.S University, Lugano, Switzerland

2 Department of Medical Veterinary Sciences, University of Bologna, Italy

3 DISA, University of Bologna, Italy

References

[1] Tunstall-Pedoe, H. Kuulasmaa, K. Mahonen, M. Tolonen, H. Ruokokoski, E. Amouyel, P. Contribution of trends in survival and coronary-event rates to changes in coronary heart disease mortality: 10-year results from 37 WHO MONICA project

populations. Monitoring trends and determinants in cardiovascular disease. Lancet, 1999, 353: 1547–57.

[2] Masia, R. Pena, A Marrugat, J. Sala, J. Vila, J. Pavesi, Covas, M. Aubo, Elosua, C. R. High prevalence of cardiovascular risk factors in Gerona, Spain, a province with low myocardial infarction incidence. REGICOR Investigators. J Epidemiol Community Health, 1998, 52: 707–15.

[3] Covas, MI. Olive oil and the cardiovascular system. Pharmacological Research, 2007, 55: 175–186.

[4] US Food and Drug Administration. Press Release P04-100. November 1, 2004. http://www.fda.gov/bbs/topics/news/2004/NEW01129.htlm. Accessed on October 28, 2006.

[5] Kris-Etherton, P M.; Mustad V. Derr J.A. Effects of dietary stearic acid on plasma lipids and thrombosis, Nutrition Today. 1993, 28: 30-38.

[6] Nunez, J Randon, C Gandhi, A Siafaka-Kapadai, MS Olson and DJ Hanahan: The inhibition of platelet-activating factor-induced platelet activation by oleic acid is associated with a decrease in polyphosphoinositide metabolism, Journal of Biological Chemisty, Volume 265, n° 30, October 25, pp18330-18338, 1990.

[7] Barradas, M.A. Christofides, J.A. Jeremy, J.Y. Mikhailidis, D.P. Fry, D.E. Dandona, P. The Effect of Olive Oil Supplementation on Human Platelet Function, Serum Cholesterol-Related Variables and Plasma Fibrinogen Concentrations: A Pilot Study, Nutrition Research, 1990, 10: 403-411.

[8] Teres, S. Barcelo-Coblijn, G. Benet, M. Alvarez, R. A, Bressani, R. Halver, J. E. Escriba, P. V. Oleic acid content is responsible for the reduction in blood pressure induced by olive oil. PNAS. 2008, 105: 13811-13816.

[9] Alemany R. Terés S., Baamonde C., Benet M., Vögler O., Escribá P. V. 2-Hydroxyoleic Acid. A New Hypotensive Molecule, Hypertension. 2004, 43: 249-54.

[10] Cocchi, M., Tonello, L. Tsaluchidu, S. Puri, B.K. The use of artificial neural networks to study fatty acids in neuropsychiatric disorders. BMC Psychiatry. 2008, 8(Suppl. 1):S3. doi: 10.1186/1471-244X-8-S1-S3.

[11] Donati, R.J. Dwivedi, Y. Roberts, R.C. Conley, R.R. Pandey, G.N. Rasenick, M.M. Postmortem Brain Tissue of Depressed Suicides Reveals Increased Gs Localization in Lipid Raft Domains Where It Is Less Likely to Activate Adenylyl Cyclase. J. Neurosci. 2008, 28:3042-3050.

[12] Hameroff, S.R. Penrose, R. Orchestrated reduction of quantum coherence in brain microtubules: A model for consciousness. In: SR Hameroff, A Kaszniak and AC Scott (eds.) Toward a Science of Consciousness - The First Tucson Discussions and Debates. MIT Press, Cambridge, UK. 1996, 507-540.

[13] Hameroff, S.R. The "conscious pilot"-dendritic synchrony moves through the brain to mediate consciousness. J. Biol. Phys. 2009, Published online: doi: 10.1007/s10867-009-9148-x.

[14] Alberts B., Bray D., Lewis J., Raff M., Roberts K., Watson JD. Molecular Biology of the cell. Garland Publishing, 1994.

[15] Mattson, F.H. Grundy, S. M. Comparison of effects of dietary saturated, monounsaturated, and polyunsaturated fatty acids on plasma lipids and lipoproteins in man. J Lipid Res. 1985, 26:194-202.

[16] Sirtori, C. R. Tremoli, E. Gatti, E. Montanari, G. Sirtori, M. Colli, S. Gianfranceschi, G. Maderna, P. Dentone, C. Z. Testolin, G. Galli, C. (). Controlled evaluation of fat intake in the Mediterranean diet: comparative activities of olive oil and corn oil on plasma lipids and platelets in high-risk patients. Am. J. Clin. Nutr. 1986, 44: 635-642.

[17] Carmena, R. Ascaso, J.F. Camejo, G. Varela, G. Hurt-Camejo, E. Ordovas, J.M. Martinez-Valls, J. Bergstöm, M. Wallin, B. Effect of olive oil and sunflower oils on low density lipoprotein level, composition, size, oxidation and interaction with arterial proteoglycans. Atherosclerosis, 1996, 125: 243-255.

[18] Mata, P. Alvarez-Sala, L. A. Rubio, M. J. Nun O. J. De Oya, M. Effects of long-term monounsaturated- vs polyunsaturated-enriched diets on lipoproteins in healthy men and women. Am. J. Clin. Nutr. 1992, 55: 846–850.

[19] Nicolaïew, N. Lemort, N. Adorni, L. Berra, B. Montorfano, G. Rapelli, S. Cortesi, N. Jacotot, B. Comparison between Extra Virgin Olive Oil and Oleic Acid Rich Sunflower Oil: Effects on Postprandial Lipemia and LDL Susceptibility to Oxidation. Ann. Nutr. Metab. 1998, 42: 251-260.

[20] Mensink, R. De Groot, M. Vanden Broeke, L. Severigen-Nobels, A. Demacker, P. Katan, M. Effect of monounsaturated fatty acids vs. complex carbohydrates on serum lipoproteins and apolipoproteins in healthy men and women. Metabolism. 1989, 38: 172-178.

[21] Carmena, R. Ros, E. Gómez Gerique, J. A. Masana, L. Ascaso, J. F. Betancort, P. Ecomen daciones para la prevención de la arteriosclerosis en España. Documento Oficial de la Sociedad Española de Arteriosclerosis (Recommendations for atherosclerosis prevention in Spain). In: Official document by The Spanish Atherosclerosis Society Clin Invest Arterios clerosis 1, 1989, 1–9.

[22] Grundy, S. M. Comparison of monounsaturated fatty acids and carbohydrates. N Eng J Med. 1986, 314: 745-748.

[23] Grundy, S. M. Flosentin, L. Nix, D. Whelan, M. F. Comparison of monounsaturated fatty acids and carbohydrates for reducing raised levels of plasma cholesterol in man. Am J Clin Nutr. 1988, 47: 965-969.

[24] Mattson, F.H. Grundy, S.M. Comparison of effects of dietary saturated, monounsaturated, and polyunsaturated fatty acids on plasma lipids and lipoproteins in man J Lipid Res. 1985, 26: 194-202.

[25] Keys, A. Coronary heart diseases in seven countries. Circulation, 1970, 41 sppl 1: 163–211.

[26] Ross, R. Atherosclerosis: an inflammatory disease. N Eng J Med. 1999, 340: 115–26.

[27] Dogne, J.M. de Leval, X. Hanson, J. Frederich, M. Lambermont, B. Ghuysen, A. Casini, A. Masereel, B. Ruan, K. H., Pirotte, B. Kolh, P. New developments on thromboxane and prostacyclin modulators. Part I. Thromboxane modulators. Curr Med Chem. 2004, 11: 1223–41.

[28] Jialal, I. Devaraj, S. Venugopal, S.K. C-reactive protein: risk marker or mediator in atherothrombosis? Hypertension, 2004, 44: 6–11.

[29] Jialal, I. Devaraj, S. Inflammation and atherosclerosis: the value of the high sensitivity C-reactive protein assay as a risk marker. Am J Clin Pathol. 2001, 116(Sup):S108–15.

[30] Kritchevsky, S.B. Cesari, M. Pahor, M. Inflammatory markers and cardiovascular health in older adults. Cardiovasc Res. 2005, 66: 265–75.

[31] Tzoulaki, I. Murray G.D., Lee, A.J. Rumley, A. Lowe, G.D. Fowkes, F.G. C-reactive protein, interleukin-6, and soluble adhesion molecules as predictors of progressive peripheral atherosclerosis in the general population: Edinburgh Artery Study. Circulation 2005, 112: 976–83.

[32] Tsimikas, S. Philis-Tsimikas, A. Alexopoulos, S. Sigari, F. Lee, C. Reaven, P.D. LDL isolated from Greek subjects on a typical diet or from American subjects on an oleate-supplemented diet induces less monocyte chemotaxis and adhesion when exposed to oxidative stress. Arterioscler Thromb.Vasc Biol. 1999, 19: 122–30.

[33] Thanos, D. Maniatis, T. NFkB: a lesson in family values. Cell, 1995, 80: 529–32.

[34] Bellido, C. Lopez-Miranda, J. Blanco-Colio, L.M. Pérez-Martínez, P. Muriana F.J. Martín-Ventura, J.L. Marín, C. Gomez, P. Fuentes, F. Egido, J. Pérez-Jiménez, F. Butter and walnuts, but not olive oil, elicit postprandial activation of nuclear transcription factor kappaB in peripheral blood mononuclear cells. Am J Clin Nutr. 2004, 80: 1487–91.

[35] Lee, C. Barnett, J. Reaven, P.D. Liposomes enriched in oleic acid are less susceptible to oxidation and have less proinflammatory activity when exposed to oxidizing conditions. J Lipid Res. 1998, 39: 1239–47.

[36] Massaro, M. basta, G. Lazzerini, G. Carluccio, M. A. Bosetti, F. Solaini, G. Visioli, F. Paolicchi, A. De Caterina, R. Quenching of intracellular ROS generation as a mechanism for oleate-induced reduction of endothelial activation and early atherogenesis. Thromb Haemost. 2002, 88: 335–44.

[37] Perona, J.S. Cabello-Moruno, R. Ruız-Gutierrez, V. The role of virgin olive oil components in the modulation of endotelial function. J Nutr Biochem, 2006, 17: 429–45.

[38] Gardner, C.D. Kraemer, H.C. Monounsaturated versus polyunsaturated dietary fat and serum lipids. A meta-analysis. Arterioscler Thromb Vasc Biol. 1995, 15: 1917–27.

[39] Dubois, C. Armand, M. Azais-Braesco, V. Portugal, H. Pauli, A.M. Bernard, P.M. Latge, C. Lafont, H. Borel, P. Lairon, D. Effects of moderate amounts of emulsified dietary fat on postprandial lipemia and lipoproteins in normolipidemic adults. Am J Clin Nutr. 1994, 60: 374–82.

[40] Weinbrenner, T. Fitò, M. Farre-Albaladejo, M. Saez, G. Rijken, P. Tormos, C. Coolen, S. de la Torre, R. Covas M.I. Bioavailability of phenolic compounds from olive oil and oxidative/ antioxidant status at postprandial state in healthy humans. Drugs Exp Clin Res. 2004, 30: 207–14.

[41] Fitò, M. Gimeno, E. Covas M.I. Mirò, E. Lòpez-Sabater, M.C. Farrè, M. de la Torre, Jmarrugat, R. Postprandial and short-term dietary intervention effects of virgin olive oil ingestion on the oxidative/antioxidative status. Lipids 2002, 37: 245–51.

[42] Covas, M.I. de la Torre, K. Farrè-Albaladejo, M. Kaikkonen, J. Fitò, M. Lopez-Sabater, C. Pujadas-Bastardes, M.A. Joglar, J. Weinbrenner, T. Lamuela-Raventós, R.M., de la Torre, R. Postprandial LDL phenolic content and LDL oxidation is modulated by olive oil phenolic compound in humans. Free Rad Biol Med. 2006, 40: 608–16.

[43] Abia, R. Pacheco, Y.M. Perona, J.S. Montero, E. Muriana, F.J. Ruiz-Gutierrez, V. The metabolic availability of dietary triacylglycerols from two high oleic oils during the postprandial period does not depend on the amount of oleic acid ingested by healthy men. J Nutr. 2001, 131: 59–65.

[44] Roche, H.M. Zampelas, A. Knapper, J.M. Webb, D. Brooks, C. Jackson, K.G. Wright, J. W. Gould, B. J. Kafatos, A. Gibney, M.J. Williams, C.M. Effect of long-term olive oil dietary intervention on postprandial triacylglycerol and factor VII metabolism. Am J Clin Nutr 1998, 68: 552– 60.

[45] Williams, C.M. Dietary interventions affecting chylomicron and chylomicron remnant clearance. Atherosclerosis 1998, 141(Suppl 1):S87–92.

[46] Rivellese, A.A. Iovine, C. Ciano, O. Costagliola, L. Galasso, R. Riccardi, G. Vaccaro, O. Nutrient determinants of postprandial triglyceride response in a population-based sample of type II diabetic patients. Eur J Clin Nutr. 2006, 60: 1168–73.

[47] Witztum, J.L. Steinberg, D. Role of oxidized low density lipoprotein in atherogenesis. J Clin Invest. 1991, 88: 1785–92.

[48] Navab, M. Berliner, J.A. Watson, A.D. Hama, S.Y. Territo, M.C. Lusis, A.J. Shih, D.M. Van Lenten, B.J. Frank, J.S. Demer, L.L. Edwards, P.A. Fogelman, A.M. The Ying and Tang of oxidation in the development of the fatty streak. Arterioscler Thromb Vasc Biol. 1996, 16: 831–42.

[49] Holvoet, P. Mertens, A. Verhamme, P. Bogaerts, K. Beyens, G. Verhaeghe, R. Collen, D. Muls, E. Van de Werf, F. Circulating oxidized LDL is a useful marker for identifying patients with coronary artery disease. Arterioscler Thromb Vasc Biol. 2001, 21: 844–8.

[50] Weinbrenner, T. Cladellas, M. Covas, M.I. Fitò, M. Tomas, M. Senti, M. Bruguera, J. Marrugat, J. High oxidative stress in patients with stable coronary heart disease. Atherosclerosis, 2003, 168: 99–106.

[51] Liu, M.L. Ylitalo, K. Salonen, R. Salonen, J.T. Taskinen, M.R. Circulating oxidized low-density lipoprotein and its association with carotid intima-media thickness in asymptomatic members of familial combined hyperlipidemia families. Arterioscler ThrombVasc Biol. 2004, 24: 1492–7.

[52] Toshima, S. Hasegawa, A. Kurabayashi, M. Itabe, H. Takano, T. Sugano, J. Shimamura, K. Kimura, Michishita, J.I. Suzuki, T. Nagai, R. Circulating oxidized low density lipoprotein levels. A biochemical risk marker for coronary heart disease. Arterioscler Thromb Vasc Biol 2000, 20: 2243–7.

[53] Meisinger, C. Baumert, J. Khuseyinova, N. Loewel, H. Koenig, W. Plasma oxidized low-density lipoprotein, a strong predictor for acute coronary heart disease events un apparently healthy, middle-aged men from the general population. Circulation, 2005, 112: 651–7.

[54] Parthasarathy, S. Khoo, J.C. Miller, E. Barnett, J. Witztum, J.L. Steinberg, D. Low density lipoprotein rich in oleic acid is protected against oxidative modification: implications for dietary prevention of atherosclerosis. Proc Natl Acad Sci USA. 1990, 87: 3894–8.

[55] Berry, E.M. Eisenberg, S. Harats, D. Friedlander, Y. Norman, Y. Kaufmann, N.A. Norman, Y. Stein, Y. Effects of diets rich in monounsaturated fatty acids on plasma lipoproteins – the Jerusalem Nutrition Study: high MUFAs vs high PUFAs. Am J Clin Nutr.1991, 53: 899–907.

[56] Reaven, P. Parthasarathy, S. Grasse, B.J. Miller, E. Steinberg, D. Witztum, J.L. Effects of oleate-rich and linoleate-rich diets on the susceptibility of low density lipoprotein to oxidative modification in mildly hypercholesterolemic subjects. J Clin Invest. 1993, 91: 668–76.

[57] Bonanome, A. Pagnan, A. Biffanti, S. Opportuno, A. Sorgato, F. Dorella, M. Maiorino, M. Ursini, F. Effect of dietary monounsaturated and polyunsaturated fatty acids on the susceptibility of plasma low density lipoproteins to oxidativemodification. Arterioscler Thromb. 1992, 12: 529–33.

[58] Abbey, M. Belling, G.B. Noakes, M. Hirata, F. Nestel, P.J. Oxidation of lowdensity lipoproteins: intraindividual variability and the effect of dietary linoleate supplementation. Am J Clin Nutr. 1993, 57: 391–8.

[59] Baroni, S.S. Amelio, M. Sangiorgi, Z. Gaddi, A. Battino, M. Solid monounsaturated diet lowers LDL unsaturation trait and oxidisability in hypercholesterolemic (type IIb) patients. Free Radic Res. 1999, 30: 275–85.

[60] Mata, P. Varela, O. Alonso, R. Lahoz, C. de Oya, M. Badimon, L. Monounsaturated and polyunsaturated n-6 fatty acid-enriched diets modify LDL oxidation and decrease human coronary smooth muscle cell DNA synthesis. Arterioscler Thromb Vasc Biol. 1997, 17: 2088–95.

[61] Kohonen, T. Self-Organized formation of topologically correct feature maps. Biol. Cybern. 1982, 43: 59-69.

[62] Kohonen, T. Self-Organizing Maps. 3rd ed. Springer, 2001, Berlin, Germany.

[63] Kohonen, T. Kaski, S. Somervuo, P. Lagus, K. Oja, M. Paatero, V. Self-organizing map, Neurocomputing, 1998. 21: 113-122.

[64] Cocchi, M. Tonello, L. Bosi, S. Cremonesi, A. Castriota, F. Puri, B. Tsaluchidu, S. Platelet oleic acid as Ischemic Cardiovascular Disease marker. BMJ. 2007, Electronic letter to the editor.

[65] Cocchi, M. Tonello, L. Cappello, G. Bosi, S. Cremonesi, A. Castriota, F. Mercante, M. Tarozzi, G. Bochicchio, D. Della Casa, G. Caramia, G. Membrane platelet fatty acids: a model of biochemical characterisation of the ischemic cardiovascular disease, through an artificial neural network interpretation, Progr Nutr. 2008, 10, 1: 48-52.

[66] Cocchi, M. Tonello, L. Lercker, G. Platelet Stearic Acid in different population groups: biochemical and functional hypothesis. Nutr. clín. diet. hosp. 2009, 29: 34-45.

[67] Tonello, L. Cappello, G. Cocchi, M. "Nutritional Effects on Cardiovascular System", 3rd International Conference on Gravity and Cardiovascular System, 2006. INRC and CSV Italian Air Force (Pratica di Mare Air Force Base, November 13-15).

[68] Cocchi, M. Tonello, L. Platelets, Fatty Acids, Depression and Cardiovascular Ischemic Pathology, Progr Nutr. 2007, 9, 2: 94-104.

[69] Tiemeier, H. van Dijck, W. Hofman, A. Witteman, J.C.M. Stijnen, T. Breteler, M.M.B. Relationship between Atherosclerosis and Late-Life Depression. Arch Gen Psychiatry, 2004, 61: 369-376.

[70] Musselman, D.L. Evans, D.L. Nemeroff, C.B. The relationship of depression to cardiovascular disease epidemiology, biology, and treatment. Archives of General Psychiatry, 1998, 55: 580-592.

[71] Weyers, J. Colquhoun, D. For the OLIVE Study Group. A Mediterranean Diet (Med) Vs A Low Fat (Lf) Diet Improves Depression Independent of Cholesterol In Coronary Heart Disease Patients (CHD) June 29, 2000: Poster Abstracts.

[72] Cocchi, M. Mordenti, A.L. Merendi, F. Sardi, L. Tonello, L. Bochicchio, D. Faeti, V. Della Casa, G. Pig platelet fatty acids composition in different lipid treatments. LXI National Meeting SISVet (Salsomaggiore Terme, PR, Italy, Sep 26-29, 2007).

[73] Nichols, T.C. du Laney, T. Zheng, B. Bellinger Dwight, A. Nickols, G.A. Engleman, W. Clemmons, D.R. Reduction in Atherosclerotic Lesion Size in Pigs by aVb3 Inhibitors Is Associated With Inhibition of Insulin-Like Growth Factor-I–Mediated Signaling Circulation Research, 1999, 85: 1040-1045.

[74] Afri, M. Ehrenberg, B. Talmon, Y. Schmidt, J. Cohen, Y. Frimer, A.A. Active oxygen chemistry within the liposomial bilayer. Part III: Locating vitamin E, ubiquinol and ubiquinone and their derivatives in the lipid layer. Chem Phys Lipids, 2004, 3: 107-121.

[75] Gunstone, F.D. Harwood, J.L. Padley, F.B. The lipid handbook, Chapman & Hall Eds. London-New York, 1986, 453-457.

[76] Belitz H-D, Grosch W, Schieberle, P. Food Chemistry, Springer Verlag Ed., Berlin, Heidelberg, New York, London, Paris, Tokyo, 1987, 175.

[77] Wijesundera, C. Ceccato, C. Watkins, P. Fagan, P. Thienthong, N. Perlmutter, P. Docosahesaenoic acid is more stable to oxidation when located at the sn-2 position of triacylglycerol compared to sn-1(3). J Am Chem Soc. 2008, 85: 543-548.

[78] Sørensen A.D.M., Xu X., Zhang L., Kristensen J.B., Jacobsen C. (2010) Human Milk Fat Substitute from Butterfat: Production by Enzymatic Interesterification and Evaluation of Oxidative Stability. J. Am. Oil Chem. Soc., 87,185–194.

[79] La Rivista Italiana Delle Sostanze Grasse, 2002, Caratteristiche degli Oli e Grassi Vegetali. Suppl. n. 1-2.

[80] Bockish, M. Fats and Oils Handbook, 1998, AOCS Press, Champaign, Illinois, USA.

[81] International Olive Oil Council, IOOC Norms Refined olive oil, olive oil, olive-pomace-oil Purity criteria, www.oliveoilquotation.com/data/files/IOOC.

[82] Lercker, G. "I componenti minori delle sostanza grasse". Proceedings: IV Congresso Nazionale Acidi Grassi Polinsaturi Omega 3, CLA e Antiossidanti. Progr. Nutr. 2003, 5: 93-115.

[83] Regolamento (CEE) n. 2568/91 della Commissione dell'11 luglio 1991, relativo alle caratteristiche degli oli d'oliva e degli oli di sansa d'oliva nonché ai metodi ad essi attinenti, (G.U.C.E. L. 248 del 5 settembre 1991).

[84] Hove, E. L. Harris, P. L. Covitamin studies. V. The interrelation of a-tocopherol and essential unsaturated fat acids. J. Nutrition. 1946, 31: 699-713.

[85] Cocchi, M. Tonello, L. Bio molecular considerations in Major Depression and Ischemic Cardiovascular Disease. Central Nervous System Agents in Medicinal Chemistry. 2010, 10: 97-107.

Chapter 2

Relationship Between Ox–LDL, Immune Cells, Atheroma Dimensions and Angiographic Measurements Assessed by Coronary Angiography and Intravascular Ultrasound

Catarina Ramos, Patrícia Napoleão,
Rui Cruz Ferreira, Cristina Fondinho, Mafalda Selas,
Miguel Mota Carmo, Ana Maria Crespo and
Teresa Pinheiro

Additional information is available at the end of the chapter

http://dx.doi.org/10.5772/54084

1. Introduction

In this chapter we report on the relationship between angiographic findings, measured by coronary angiography (CA) and intravascular ultrasound virtual histology (IVUS-VH) modalities, and indicators of vascular inflammation in the context of coronary artery disease (CAD). We sought to explore *in vivo* the relationship between patient demographics, anthropometric measures, risk factors, soluble biomarkers and plaque composition or its morphological characteristics.

The interplay of inflammatory cells, cytokines and indicators of cell death may concur to the plaque phenotype in the context of coronary artery disease. Therefore, the lymphocyte populations expressing CD4 and CD8, the circulating levels of oxidized low density lipoprotein (ox-LDL), which may be primarily originated in the atheroma, the levels of tumour necrosis factor alpha (TNF- α) and of soluble Fas ligand (sFasL), which may reflect the inflammatory response and vascular apoptosis, were studied.

These biomarkers would provide useful tools to improve medical diagnosis of the clinical atheroma. Noninvasive identification of high-risk/vulnerable coronary atherosclerotic plaques is one of the ultimate goals of coronary imaging and would dramatically improve risk stratification of both symptomatic and asymptomatic patients [1]. Therefore, correlations between plaque composition, bio-indicators and the severity of cardiac events may provide unique information about plaque type to enhance the precision of clinical and laboratory variables used to assess patients at risk of CAD.

1.1. Coronary artery disease

Coronary artery disease is still the main cause of death worldwide and coronary atherothrombosis is the leading cause of death in the United States and Europe [2,3]. A large number of individuals who die suddenly of CAD due to atherosclerosis have no previous symptoms [4].

Atherosclerosis is a chronic pathological process of the vasculature characterized by focal arterial wall inflammation that leads to plaque build-up, intraluminal narrowing, and atherothrombotic stenosis or occlusion with distal organ damage [5,6]. The atherosclerotic lesion is a thickening of the artery intima that consists of inflammatory and smooth muscle cells [7], as well as connective-tissue, lipids and debris [8]. The atheroma formation is initiated by an accumulation of lipid-laden cells beneath the endothelium, denominated fatty streak [9,10]. As atherosclerosis progresses from a benign phenotype, the atheroma becomes fibrotic, with a large necrotic core. Also, the plaque becomes more inflamed, resulting in an infiltration of macrophages and T-lymphocytes to the metabolically active fibrous cap [3]. Disintegration of foam cells and production of matrix metalloproteinases by activated leukocytes have detrimental consequences leading to the destabilization of lipid rich cores and the thinning of the fibrous cap [8]. This leads to a rupture-prone thin-cap fibroatheroma. The plaque rupture may cause arterial thrombosis, which results in a clinical spectrum of presentations ranging from sudden cardiac death, due to coronary occlusion, to an asymptomatic event with plaque progression [3]. In fact, the rupture of vulnerable atherosclerotic plaque is the cause of most acute coronary syndromes, e.g. myocardial infarction and unstable angina [8,11].

Atherosclerotic plaque stability is related to histological composition however biomarkers for the disease severity are still lacking today [12-14]. Multiple evidences link risk factors for atherosclerosis and its complications with altered histology, including the operation of both innate and adaptive immunity and the balance of stimulatory and inhibitory pathways that regulate their participation in atheroma formation and complication [15].

The early involvement of monocytes and macrophages in atherosclerosis is initiated with endothelial cell activation. Several protein mediators, specifically cytokines and chemokines, and LDL oxidative modification [16], direct monocyte migration to the intima and promote their maturation into macrophages, which are retained in the lesion [17,18]. These pro-inflammatory monocytes propagate the innate response by expressing high levels of pro-inflammatory cytokines and other macrophages mediators including metalloproteinases [6,19,20]. Dendritic cells that populate atherosclerotic plaques can present antigens to T-cells, which mount a cellular immune response [21]. These immune cells are also involved in thrombosis. Coagulation proteins elicit the expression of pro-inflammatory cytokines and mediators that interact with toll-like receptors of immune cells. These events promote endothelial cell apoptosis [22,23].

The ox-LDL has been described as a relevant pro-atherogenic autoantigen and its inflammatory and immunogenic activity has been implicated in atherosclerosis development and CAD [14,24]. Experimental data showed that ox-LDL is formed in the arterial wall where it is internalized by macrophages to form foam cells, contributing to the plaque progression [14]. The co-localization of ox-LDL with lymphocytes and monocyte-derived cells in the human atherosclerotic lesions reinforce the pro-atherogenic and immunogenic properties of ox-LDL, which was verified *in vitro* [24]. Eventually, ox-LDL formed in the arterial wall is released in the circulation [13], being their circulating levels strongly associated with angiographically documented coronary artery disease [25]. The proximity of ox-LDL and inflammatory cells, such as lymphocyte populations, in the atherosclerotic plaque may accelerate macrophage activity and therefore promote atherogenesis [26]. The T-cells expressing CD4 surface marker recognize antigens presented by dendritic cells and macrophages. The T-cell expressing CD8 when activated are capable of killing smooth muscle cells and macrophages. Both CD4 and CD8 T cells share the capacity to recognize protein antigens bound to histocompatibility molecules on cell surfaces [27].

Thus, the *in vivo* identification of plaque vulnerability whether by characterizing its components or by providing measures of plaque-related oxidative and inflammation markers may improve diagnostic and eventually allow the detection of vulnerable atheroma before rupture.

1.2. Coronary angiography

Since its implementation over 30 years ago, invasive coronary angiography has become the standard clinical method for describing the coronary arteries and the "gold standard" for diagnosing CAD. The use of contrast-enhanced coronary angiography has been introduced for stenosis detection and for assessing blood flow in the epicardial arteries. The approach based on edge-detection algorithms has also been proposed as an emerging tool for the detection, characterization, and quantification of coronary atherosclerotic plaques [11].

The increased understanding of atherosclerosis has highlighted inherent limitations of coronary angiography as a technique for the assessment of coronary atherosclerotic plaques. Angiography provides a 2-dimensional view of the arterial lumen, but with no visualization of the vessel wall. Atherosclerosis primarily affects the arterial wall and since only the lumen is displayed, angiography does not provide extensive information about the plaque [28,29] and may obscure the true plaque burden, leading to an underestimation of plaque severity [3]. Also, the atherosclerotic plaque initially grows in an outwardly manner, expanding to the vessel wall, a process denominated positive remodeling. Therefore, as a result of positive remodeling, angiography frequently fails to detect the early stages of atherosclerosis. Although positively remodeled lesions do not restrict blood flow, they may be unstable and may contribute to the onset of acute coronary syndromes [30]. Furthermore, because putative sites of stenosis are compared with an apparently normal arterial segment, angiography often fails to detect diffuse disease in which a large portion of the artery is impacted by atherosclerotic disease. Both positive remodeling and diffuse disease are common in atherosclerotic progression and may be determinants of clinical outcome.

Also, the assessment of angiograms is solely visual and, consequently, subject to significant variation in image interpretation (observer bias) which may lead to a significant underestimation of lesion severity [30].

Assessing the atheroma dimensions by coronary angiography (CA) has been more recently surpassed by new methods for cardiovascular imaging using ultrasound [28,29,31] and multislice CT [32-34], which allow a more accurate and complete imaging of atherosclerotic coronary vessels.

1.3. Intravascular ultrasound

Intravascular ultrasound (IVUS), a catheter-based technique that provides high resolution cross-sectional images of the coronary vessel in vivo, is a tomographic technique that permits two-dimensional visualization of the arterial wall and allows further characterization of its individual layers. Thus, IVUS is a unique imaging modality for the direct examination of vessel dimensions and arterial wall characteristics in live subjects.

The coronary artery is inspected by a catheter incorporating a miniature ultrasound transducer, which emits high-frequency ultrasound, usually in the range of 20 to 50 MHz providing an axial resolution of about 100–200 μm. Lateral resolution of the ultrasonic waves is less specific and may vary depending on imaging depth and beam width, averaging around 250 μm [35].

Given their proximity to the plaque, intravascular catheters have the inherent advantage of a high signal-to-noise ratio [3]. The information obtained through IVUS imaging depicts the morphological characteristics of the atheromatous plaque and is used to illustrate the geometrical configuration of its layers and architecture. Most clinical centers use a pullback system to withdraw the catheter at a constant rate of 0.5 mm/s following its initial deployment distal to the area of interest. As the transducer is moved through the artery, ultrasonic reflections are electronically converted to cross-sectional images [31]. This IVUS modality is called "virtual histology" IVUS (IVUS-VH) and allows the identification of the composition of atherosclerotic plaques by discriminating varying echolucent regions within the atheroma [12]. Four plaque components, fibrotic, fibro-fatty, calcification and necrotic core, can be identified as they exhibit a defined radiofrequency spectrum, which can be analyzed and mathematically transformed into a color-coded representation of the plaque composition [36].

Therefore, IVUS imaging delivers precise geometric measurements of the coronary wall and lumen and enables the identification of different types of plaques according to their content in lipid, fibrin calcium and necrotic tissues [12,32,37,38]. The evaluation of lipid deposits contents commonly associated to vulnerable plaques and positive remodeling has been used to assess lesion severity [39]. In addition, three-dimensional IVUS image reconstruction is possible and is essential for proper assessment of the longitudinal distribution of the plaque [36], because multiple plaque morphologies varying from a fibrotic stable plaque to sites containing large lipids/necrotic cores can be found in a single arterial segment.

Because of its methodology, IVUS is not subject to the same limitations as angiography. Not only is IVUS more sensitive than angiography for the detection of stenosis, it can also identify diffuse disease and positive remodeling of the vessel wall. Furthermore, since IVUS allows the identification of morphologic characteristics of vulnerable plaques, it may be helpful in the characterization of atherosclerotic plaque formation [31,40] and in the detection of plaques with a high risk of spontaneous rupture [31]. However, coronary angiography is still regarded by many as the principal imaging technique for guiding coronary interventions. Recently, the correlation of coronary artery geometric measurements using both CA and IVUS has been reported [41-43], calling the attention for the value of IVUS alone or in conjugation with VH as precise measurements of plaque geometric parameters and tissue histological characteristics can be obtained with this modality.

2. Methods

2.1. Study design and participants

Individual data and blood samples were obtained from patients enrolled in a prospective study performed at the Cardiology Service of Santa Marta Hospital (CHLC, Lisbon, Portugal). The study was designed to investigate the association of circulating levels of ox-LDL, TNF-α, sFasL and T-lymphocytes with angiographic data and atherosclerotic plaque morphological and biological characteristics.

Patients, men and women aged between 56 and 71 years old with suspected and known coronary artery disease were included in the study. A total of 35 subjects were eligible to participate: 4 patients with ST-elevation myocardial infarction (STEMI), 7 patients with non-ST elevation myocardial infarction (NSTEMI), 11 stable angina (SA) patients, 10 unstable angina (UA) patients and 3 silent ischemia patients (SI). All patients underwent standard diagnostic procedures and treated accordingly. Acute coronary syndrome patients were enrolled in the first 24 hours of hospital admission, although the time period from the onset of chest pain to the intervention was less than 9 hours for the majority of them. Demographic information and history, including traditional risk factors for CAD were obtained at study entry. Evaluations included cardiac testing and imaging, cardiac characteristics and procedures, such as angioplasty and stenting. Coronary angiography and IVUS-VH data was recorded. One prespecified study lesion was identified in each patient. An anatomical segment containing the entirety of the study lesion was then selected, which could be easily identified based on standard anatomical landmarks on two modalities (CA and IVUS-VH). All patients received standard care therapy after discharge including dual antiplatelet therapy after angioplasty.

Subjects with age above 85, significant co-morbidities as peripheral artery disease or carotid artery disease, known antecedents of malignance or infectious diseases, chronic renal insufficiency, concurrent inflammatory disorders, malignant neoplasm or infection and previous myocardial infarction in the previous 5 years were not enrolled. Also, patients were ineligible if coronary anatomy was inappropriate for IVUS.

The study protocol was approved by the CHLC Ethical Committee board and all patients signed an informed consent accepting their participation before study enrollment.

2.2. Patient characterization

All subjects were characterized demographically, clinically and biochemically (Table I).

Diabetes was diagnosed on the basis of fasting plasma glucose concentration ≥7.0 mmol/l (126 mg/dl) or 2h plasma glucose ≥11.1 mmol/l (200 mg/dl) or confirmed as clinically known and treated diabetes mellitus. Subjects were diagnosed hypertensive if they were documented to have systolic blood pressure ≥140 mmHg and/or diastolic blood pressure ≥90 mmHg or were already on anti-hypertensive therapy. Dyslipidaemia was identified in subjects who had total serum cholesterol level ≥190 mg/dl and/or serum triglycerides ≥180 mg/dl or were on lipid-lowering medication. Smoking was defined as the inhaled use of cigarettes, cigars or pipes in any quantity. Subjects who smoked within the previous year were also defined as smokers.

Patients characterization		
Demographics	Male sex (n, %)	23, 66
	Age (y)	63 (56 – 71)
	Weight (kg)	75 (67 – 80)
	Height (m)	1.7 (1.6 – 1.7)
	BMI (kg/m^2)	27.3 (23.7 – 29)
Risk factors / Co-morbidities	Smoking (n, %)	6, 34
	Hypercholesterolemia (n, %)	25, 71
	Arterial hypertension (n, %)	25, 71
	Diabetes mellitus (n, %)	8, 23
Previous medication	Aspirin (n, %)	18, 51
	ACE Inhibitors (n, %)	16, 46
	Anti-platelets (n, %)	14, 40
	β - blockers (n, %)	15, 43
	Statins (n, %)	25, 7
Biochemical analysis	Total cholesterol (mg/dl)	156 (133 – 188)
	LDL (mg/dl)	104 (82 – 127)
	HDL (mg/dl)	36 (27 – 45)
	Triglycerides (mg/dl)	85 (59 – 127)
	Glucose (mg/dl)	111 (95 – 137)
	Leucocytes (x10^3/µl)	6.8 (5.4 – 8.5)
	Neutrophils (x10^3/µl)	4.4 (3.3 – 5.7)
	Lymphocytes (x10^3/µl)	1.8 (1.3 – 2.7)
	Monocytes (x10^3/µl)	0.5 (0.3 – 0.8)
	Platelets (x10^3/µl)	190 (156 – 235)
	CK (U/l)	84 (47 – 169)
	CRP (mg/l)	5.3 (2.5 – 18.4)
	Pro-BNP (pg/ml)	203 (64 – 916)

Table 1. Patients demographic, clinical and biochemical characterization. Results are presented in median (Q25 – Q75) unless otherwise specified.

2.3. Percutaneous angiography

All patients were clinically evaluated for the extension of coronary artery disease through the characterization of lesion morphology to define the coronary stenosis, the number of diseased vessels, the thrombolysis in myocardial infarction (TIMI) risk score, which refers to the level of coronary blood flow assessed during coronary angiography (ranging from 3 – complete perfusion, to 0 – total occlusion), lesion length and the presence of calcium and/or thrombi in the lesions. The number and type of stents positioned in patients undergoing coronary angiography were also recorded. A coronary stenosis was considered clinically significant (high-grade) as a ≥70% narrowing in the luminal diameter. Multivessel disease was defined when more than one major coronary artery presented high-grade stenosis: left anterior descending artery (LAD); right coronary artery (RCA); left circumflex artery (LCX).

Patients angiographic characterization		
Stenosis (%)		87.5 (70 – 91)
Lesion length (mm)		18.5 (13– 28)
Multivessel (n, %)		6, 19
Diseased vessels (n, %)	0	4, 11
	1	20, 57
	2	7, 20
	3	2, 6
Lesions (n, %)	0	4, 11
	1	17, 49
	2	6, 17
	3	2, 6
	4	4, 11
Culprit vessel (n, %)	LAD / TC	20, 61
	RCA	11, 31
	LCX	2, 6
TIMI score (n, %)	0	1, 3
	3	26, 74
Lesion type (n, %)	A	3, 9
	B	17, 49
	C	2, 6
Lesion morphology (n, %)	Concentric	5, 14
	Eccentric	20, 57

Table 2. Patients angiographic characterization. Results are presented in median (Q25–Q75) unless otherwise specified.

The extent (severity) of CAD was assessed following a graded angiographic system based on previous reports by others [43, 44]. The number of diseased vessels, number of lesions, culprit lesion and TIMI were the contributing parameters. The severity score was calculated on the basis of the sum of individual scores assigned to each parameter assuming normal arteries as grade "0": a) each vessel with ≥70% stenosis lesions contributed as 2, and vessels with <70% stenosis lesions contributed as 1; b) each lesion treated contributed as 1; c) the most severe lesions were graded 3 when occurring in LAD, 2 in RCA and 1 in LCX; d) the TIMI values contributed as 0 = no occlusion to 3 = total occlusion.

2.4. Intravascular ultrasound (IVUS)

The IVUS-VH acquisition was performed using a EagleEye catheter (20 MHz) at pullback speed of 0.5 mm/sec. The IVUS data was recorded for the reconstruction of the radiofrequency backscatter information using In-Vision gold commercial software (Volcano Corporation, USA).

For each lesion, vessel and lumen area data were obtained for every cross-section throughout the region of interest and lesion borders were established using the leading edges of external elastic lamina (EEL) and the luminal contour. Minimal lumen diameter and reference diameter were measured and percentage of diameter stenosis was calculated. The composition of coronary atheroma was assessed using spectral analysis of backscatter RF signals. The percentages of fibrotic, fibro-fatty, calcified and necrotic core were assessed. Atheroma area and volume and were obtained after EEL and lumen diameter (LD) measures were completed at the lumen/plaque boundary and at the media/adventitia boundary in each cross-section forming the region of interest.

Atheroma or plaque area (PA) was determined as the difference between EEL and lumen areas. The plaque burden was calculated as the plaque cross sectional area divided by the EEL area and multiplying by 100. IVUS measurements were recorded at three different regions-of-interest of the selected lesion: larger stenosis region cross-section and distal and proximal cross-sections. Median values and 25% and 75% quartile intervals for the various parameters measured and/or calculated are listed in Table 3.

2.5. Blood sampling and laboratory assays

Peripheral blood was drawn from all patients into blood collection tubes (Vacuette) with appropriate anti-coagulant, and centrifuged at 2500 rpm for 10 minutes. Serum and plasma were collected and stored at -80ºC until analysis, for a period not exceeding 6 months. Samples were thawed only once.

Levels of glucose, creatinine kinase, troponin T, N-terminal pro-brain natriuretic peptide (NT-proBNP) and C-reactive protein (CRP), blood cells count and lipid profile were routinely measured in the hospital. Plasma concentrations of ox-LDL and sFasL and serum concentrations of TNF-α were measured by enzyme-linked immunosorbent assays (ELISA) commercial kits (R&D Systems).

All the assays were performed according to the manufacturer's recommendations. Each sample was measured in duplicate; intra-assay variation among the duplicates for all samples was <10%.

Lymphocyte populations were analyzed by flow cytometry (FASCalibur, BD) in whole blood lysed with lysing solution (BD). The following antibodies were used: PerCP mouse anti-human CD45 (2D1, BD Pharmigen), FITC mouse anti-human CD3 (HIT3a, BD Pharmigen), APC mouse anti-human CD4 (RPA-T4, BD Pharmigen), PE mouse anti-human CD8 (RPA-T8, BD Pharmigen).

Atherosclerotic plaque characterization			
Stenosis (%)		Larger stenosis region	77.6 (65 – 84)
		Proximal region	49 (40 – 58)
		Distal region	48.1 (37 – 59.5)
Fibrotic tissue (%)		Larger stenosis region	58.5 (51 – 75)
		Proximal region	61.7 (48 – 75.5)
		Distal region	59 (43 – 74.5)
Fibro-fatty tissue (%)		Larger stenosis region	9.6 (6.4 – 18)
		Proximal region	13 (5 – 17.5)
		Distal region	9 (4.7 – 20)
Calcified tissue (%)		Larger stenosis region	11 (2.7 – 17)
		Proximal region	6 (0.3 – 14.2)
		Distal region	12.8 (0.5 – 22)
Necrotic core (%)		Larger stenosis region	16.5 (8 – 22)
		Proximal region	17.4 (8 – 24)
		Distal region	16.5 (10 – 24)
Lumen	diameter (mm)	Minimum	2.1 (1.8 – 2.3)
		Maximum	2.4 (2.1 – 3)
		Median	2.2 (1.9 – 2.7)
	area (mm^2)		3.8 (2.9 – 5.1)
External elastic lamina	diameter (mm)	Minimum	4.3 (4 – 4.6)
		Maximum	4.9 (4.5 – 5.1)
		Median	4.6 (4.2 – 4.9)
	area (mm^2)		17.2 (15 – 19)
Plaque area (mm^2)			13 (10 – 15)
Plaque burden (%)			77.4 (65 – 84)

Table 3. Atherosclerotic plaque measurements obtained by IVUS-VH. Results of the plaque morphology and composition are presented in median (Q25 – Q75).

2.6. Statistical analysis

Data were summarized and represented (box-plots) as median and inter-quartiles 25% and 75% (Q25-Q75) for continuous variables and as proportions for categorical variables. Non-continuous variables were analyzed using a 2x2 table and $\chi 2$ test. Continuous variables, such as plaque measures at proximal, distal and larger stenosis region cross-sections of the plaque, transformed into categorical variables based on median values. Differences between classes of variables were compared using a Mann-Whitney test. Associations between variables, angiographic data and IVUS measures were evaluated using non-parametric Spearman correlations.

The calculations were performed using SPSS (v. 19.0, IBM 2010) and linear regressions were made using OriginLab (v. 7.5 SR6, OriginaLab Comp, 2006).

3. Results

The atherosclerotic plaque physical characteristics and composition obtained by IVUS were studied and related with the severity of CAD following CA scores. These parameters were also associated with plaque-related oxidative and inflammation bio-indicators measured in the blood. The inter-relations between the parameters measured are described below.

3.1. Analysis of plaque components along the lesion

The composition of the plaque along its length in terms of fibrotic, fibro-fatty, necrotic and calcified tissues assessed by IVUS-VH can be inferred from data listed in Table 3. Measurements were carried out along the plaque at three plaque regions. Therefore, larger stenosis region, proximal and distal cross-sections were studied.

The variations observed between proximal, distal and larger stenosis region cross-sections did not reach statistical significance, although major variations were also observed in fibro-fatty and calcified tissues. To further analyze the plaque composition, the associations between the fibrotic, fibro-fatty, calcified and necrotic components of the plaque were assessed.

In the overall, high fibrotic and fibro-fatty tissue contents were correlated to low content of calcified tissue and low necrotic core (Fig. 1).

The necrotic core content was positively correlated with calcified tissue ($r=0.675$, $p<0.001$). The correlation values were more representative in the region with larger stenosis, although the associations were observed in proximal and distal cross-sections.

Categorizing the plaque necrotic core and calcified tissue contents by the median value, it was confirmed that these two components were significantly associated with the fibrotic and fibro-fatty tissues. Plaques with large areas of necrotic core (≥16.5%) had low percentage of fibrotic ($p=0.001$) and fibro-fatty ($p=0.002$) tissues and these levels were significantly different from those in plaques with necrotic core <16.5%. Moreover, the percentage of calcium content increased in plaques with necrotic core content ≥16.5% relative to plaques with necrotic core below 16.5% ($p=0.001$) (Fig. 2). These differences were valid and equally significant along the plaque length, i.e. for distal, proximal and larger stenosis region cross-sections.

http://dx.doi.org/10.5772/54084

However, when the plaque components were analyzed relative to the calcified tissue content of plaques (cut-point and median value of 11%) only the plaque fibrotic content could be discriminated in the larger stenosis region (Q25-Q75=58.8-77.5% fibrotic tissue for calcified tissue <11%; Q25-Q75=33.1-58.7% fibrotic tissue for calcified tissue ≥11%; p<0.001).

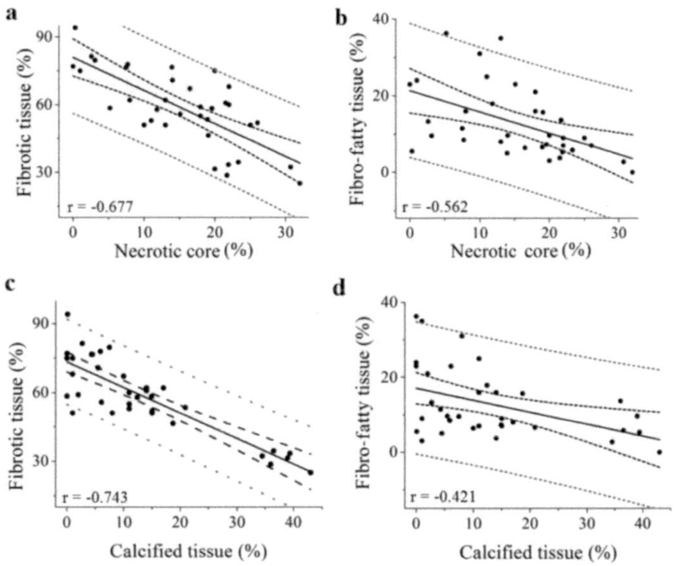

Figure 1. Correlation of necrotic core (a and b) and calcified tissue (c and d) with fibrotic tissue (r=-0.677, p<0.001 and r=-0.743, p<0.001, respectively) and fibro-fatty tissue (r=-0.562, p<0.001, r=-0.421 and p=0.012, respectively) in the larger stenosis region. Solid line represents the linear regression, black dashed lines represent 95% confidence bands and grey dashed lines represent prediction bands.

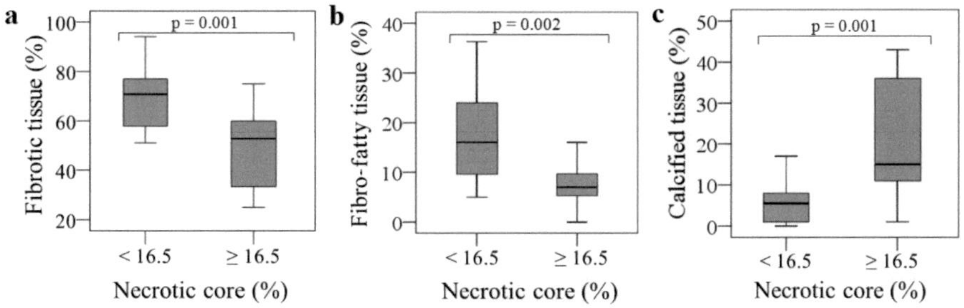

Figure 2. Box-plots of plaque content in fibrotic (a), fibro-fatty (b) and calcified (c) tissues according to the necrotic core levels <16.5% and ≥16.5% in the larger stenosis region.

3.2. Association between plaque components and plaque morphology

Measures of the EEL diameter and area, lumen diameter and area, plaque area and plaque burden were related with the plaque composition in order to assess whether the correlations between these parameters could identify plaque types. It was observed that associations between morphology and components of the plaque varied along the lesion. The relationship between the plaque content in calcified and fibrotic tissues and plaque morphology was only verified in proximal cross-sections of the plaques.

It was observed that the calcified tissue content was positively correlated with the EEL diameter (r=0.525, p=0.001), the EEL area (r=0.478, p=0.004) and plaque area (r=0.442, p=0.008) in proximal cross-sections (see Fig. 3).

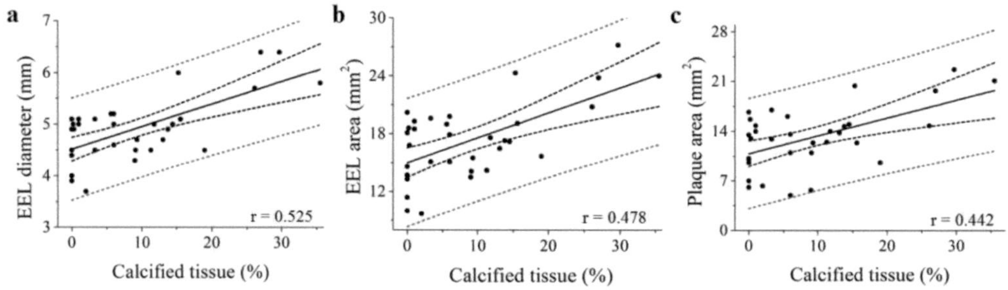

Figure 3. Correlation of calcified tissue content in the proximal region with EEL maximum diameter (a) and plaque area (b). Solid line represents the linear regression, black dashed lines represent 95% confidence bands and grey dashed lines represent prediction bands.

Also in the proximal region of the plaques, the fibrotic content discriminated plaque sizes as expressed by the EEL diameter and area. Both EEL diameter and area were significantly higher for fibrotic tissue percentages below median value (<59%) by report to plaques with fibrotic tissue percentages above median (p=0.041) (Fig. 4).

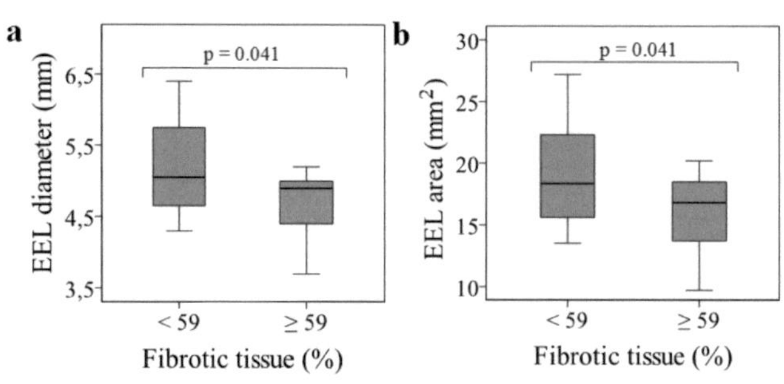

Figure 4. Variations of EEL diameter (a) and area (b) according to fibrotic content <59% and ≥59% in the proximal region.

3.3. Coronary angiography data versus IVUS measures

The IVUS-derived measures of coronary atherosclerotic plaques were evaluated having into account the severity score established with angiographic data. Severity of CAD was found to be unambiguously associated to vessel lumen decrease and increased plaque burden. The severity score was negatively correlated with the plaque geometry IVUS VH-derived measures, such as lumen diameter (r=-0.402, p=0.038) and lumen area (r=-0.419, p=0.03), and positively correlated with plaque burden (r=0.496, p=0.009) as can be depicted in Fig. 5.

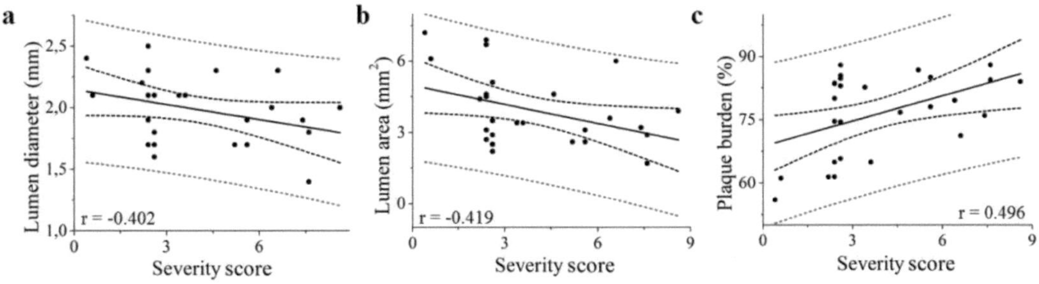

Figure 5. Correlation of angiographic severity with IVUS-derived measures of the atherosclerotic plaque: a) lumen diameter; b) lumen area; and c) plaque burden. Solid line represents the linear regression, black dashed lines represent 95% confidence bands and grey dashed lines represent prediction bands.

3.4. Association of soluble biomarkers and T-cells with IVUS and angiography derived measures

The relationship between the levels of indicators of oxidation and inflammation in the blood circulation with IVUS- and angiography-derived measures of the atherosclerotic plaque was examined with the aim of establishing relevant associations between biomarkers and plaque type.

Indicators of the inflammatory process associated to cell activation and apoptosis, such as TNF-α and sFasL, were determined. Also the concentration of ox-LDL in circulation was assessed as a measure of plaque outflow and inflammation. The variations observed in the concentration levels of these parameters were studied relative to the plaque IVUS-derived measures and angiographic data and severity score.

Several associations were observed between the plaque morphology and components, such as fibrotic, fibro-fatty and necrotic core, with $CD4^+$ and $CD8^+$ T-cell populations and TNF-α, sFasL and ox-LDL concentrations in the blood circulation. Due to the limited number of patients enrolled in this prospective study and to improve statistical results enabling the concurrent evaluation of IVUS and angiographic data, including the severity score, IVUS variables (see variables listed in Table 3) were categorized using the median value as cut-off point.

Following this procedure, and in what concerns soluble biomarkers, it was observed that sFasL, TNF-α and ox-LDL levels in circulation were strongly associated to the median values of lumen and plaque dimensions.

The concentration of TNF-α significantly increased for large plaque areas, as expressed by EEL diameter and area (p=0.05 in both cases), whereas sFasL concentrations increased with diminished lumen diameters (p=0.017), as can be depicted in Fig. 6.

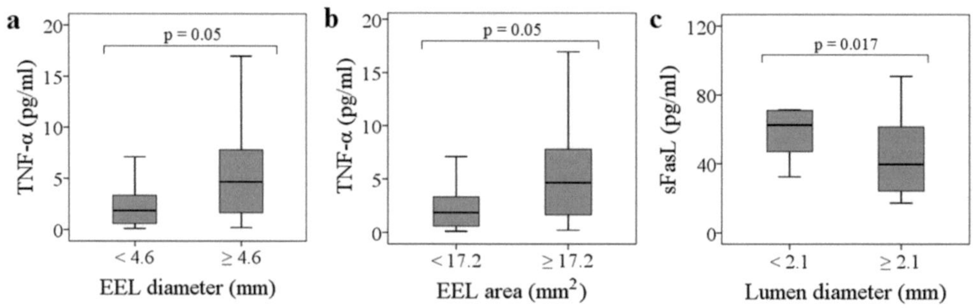

Figure 6. Box-plot representation of the TNF-α and sFasL concentrations relative to indicators of plaque dimensions: a) EEL diameter categories <4.6 mm and ≥4.6 mm; b) EEL area categories <17.2 mm^2 and ≥17.2mm^2; c) Lumen diameter categories <2.1 mm and ≥2.1 mm

The concentrations of ox-LDL in plasma were significantly associated with plaque area as can be depicted in Fig. 7. Large plaque areas, above median value (area ≥13 mm^2), were associated with high ox-LDL concentrations whereas plaque areas below 13 mm^2 were associated with low ox-LDL concentrations, and the differences between median concentration values of ox-LDL in the two groups were significant (p=0.039).

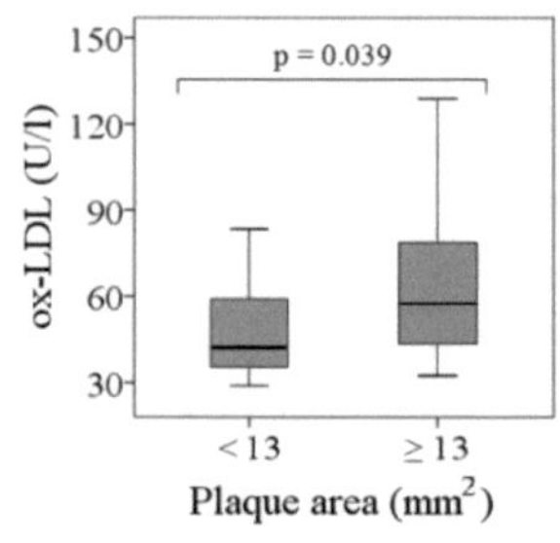

Figure 7. Box-plot representation of ox-LDL concentrations according to plaque area categories <13 mm^2 and ≥13 mm^2.

Concerning the plaque components, only the necrotic content assessed in the plaque region with larger stenosis could be associated with TNF-α concentration in circulation. High concentrations of TNF-α were associated with low necrotic core contents contrasting with the significantly lowered TNF-α concentrations (p=0.016) observed in plaques with large necrotic cores (≥16.5%) (Fig. 8)

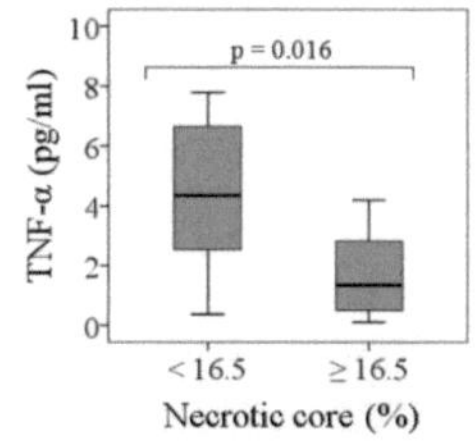

Figure 8. Box-plot representation of TNF-α concentrations according to the necrotic core categories in the larger stenosis region, <16.5 % and ≥16.5 %.

In what concerns T-cell CD3$^+$ populations expressing CD4 and CD8, it was observed that the percentage of T-cells expressing CD3CD8 were associated with the plaque dimensions (T-cell CD3$^+$CD8$^+$ vs EEL diameter r=-0.518, p=0.019; T-cell CD3$^+$CD8$^+$ vs EEL area r=-0.530, p=0.016). T-cells, both CD3$^+$CD4$^+$ and CD3$^+$CD8$^+$, were correlated with the plaque fibrotic and fibro-fatty tissue components along the plaque length, i.e. from distal to proximal regions. Likely, CD3$^+$CD4$^+$ lymphocytes were positively correlated with fibrotic tissue (r=0.579, p=0.009) whereas CD3$^+$CD8$^+$ cells were negatively correlated (r=-0.481, p=0.037) (see Fig. 9 a and c).

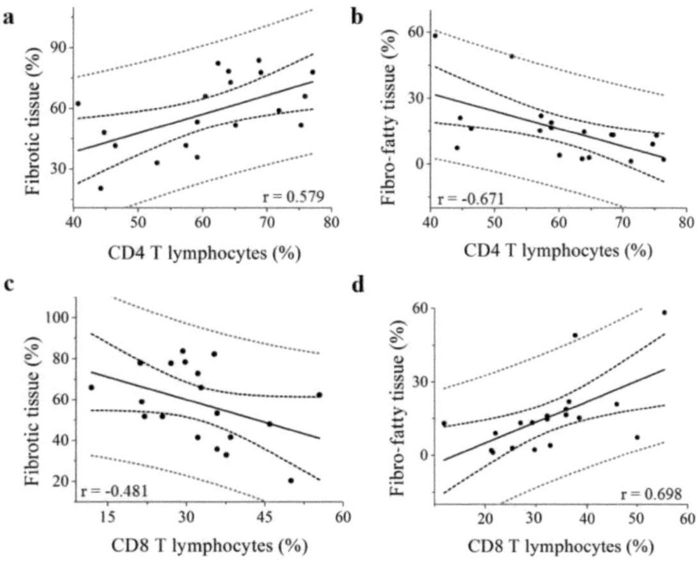

Figure 9. Correlation between plaque fibro-fatty and fibrotic tissue content and CD4$^+$ and CD8$^+$ T lymphocytes. Solid line represents the linear regression, black dashed lines represent 95% confidence bands and grey dashed lines represent prediction bands.

An opposite relationship was found between fibro-fatty tissue component and $CD3^+CD4^+$ lymphocytes (Fig. 9 b and d). The $CD3^+CD4^+$ lymphocytes were negatively correlated with fibro-fatty tissue ($r = -0.671$, $p=0.002$) and $CD3^+CD8^+$ were positively correlated ($r=0.698$, $p=0.001$).

4. Discussion

This prospective study showed that plaque composition is related to plaque morphology and these characteristics were associated with the concentration of biomarkers in blood circulation.

Plaques with higher content in necrotic core showed lower fibrotic and fibro-fatty contents and larger areas of calcified tissue. Increased EEL diameter and area were associated to larger fibrotic and calcium contents, linking these two components to plaques protruding in the vessel wall rather than high-stenosis regions. Together these observations suggest that plaque vulnerability is not strictly linked to high-grade stenosis. Also the angiographic disease severity score was associated with plaque burden. This is in agreement with previous studies demonstrating that plaque ruptures typically occur in large and complex plaques [1,30], and that coronary calcification is associated to acute coronary syndromes [37] and independently predicts all-cause mortality in CAD in addition to traditional risk factors [46]. Prior studies reported that shear stress and circumferential wall stress play an important role in plaque rupture [47]. Sano *et al.* [31] demonstrated that the percentage of fibrous area was the most sensitive parameter for classifying the plaques causing acute coronary syndrome. Also the percentage of lipid area was significant in the classification of vulnerable plaques [31]. Evidences are accumulating by coronary angiography and IVUS and other imaging modalities showing that plaque complexity associates to vulnerable plaques [11,31,37]. Therefore, to differentiate vulnerable plaques from stable plaques, the fragile part of the atheromatous plaque is of major interest and both tissue characteristics of coronary plaques and mechanical stresses on coronary plaques should be taken into account.

Plaque rupture is related to the process in which fibrous caps over lipid core become fragile [3]. Several *in vitro* studies support that continuous inflammatory stimulus in the plaque driven by the infiltration of monocytes, macrophages and T-lymphocytes in the lesion, ultimately lead to disintegration of foam cells, and release of cytokines, such as TNF-α, and matrix metalloproteinases [6,7,18-20]. All this causes the destabilization of plaque lipid rich cores and the thinning of the fibrous cap [3,8].

We have preciously demonstrated [48] that the susceptibility of a plaque to rupture is not strictly linked to significant stenosis. This prospective study supports our previous findings as positive associations between plaque dimensions i.e., EEL diameter and area independent of high-stenosis regions, and the concentrations of TNF-α were found. TNF-α is involved in endothelial cells activation and in the inflammatory response amplification [9,20]. Increasing levels of this pro-inflammatory cytokine promote a continuous systemic inflammatory stimulation that can trigger and/or amplify local inflammatory responses and therefore express the extent of vascular inflammation. Also the relationship found between TNF-α concentration in blood and the percentage of necrotic core area suggests an association between an exacerbation of inflammation and the thinning of the fibrous cap with increases of fibrous and fibro-fatty areas as plaque evolves [30,31].

In addition the process of apoptosis is an important mechanism in the pathophysiology of atherosclerosis. Atherosclerotic plaques include large numbers of apoptotic cells and related receptors, such as FasL, which is a type II membrane protein that induces apoptosis when it binds to its membrane receptor Fas. FasL is expressed by activated T lymphocytes, as well as endothelial cells [49]. It was observed in this study that decreases of lumen diameter as occurring in disease exacerbation, favored the elevation of sFasL in circulation. This supports the view that one of the control mechanisms elicited by FasL in CAD may be the prevention of inflammation by destruction of the activated inflammatory cells invading vascular tissues via FasL/Fas-mediated apoptosis [49,50]. In fact, in this study the percentage of T-cells expressing CD4 and CD8 were associated to the percentage of fibrous and fibro-fatty area reinforcing the notion that Th1 cellular immunity is taking place during the disease process [6]. Also, the opposite relationship between the percentage of $CD4^+$ and $CD8^+$ T-cells and the plaque percentage of fibrous and fibro-fatty areas, as observed in this study call the attention for the balanced action of these immune cells in CAD. However, the role of specific immune responses has remained unclear. Evidence is accumulating that T-cells homing the vessel wall contribute to inflammation [6,9] and that T-cell expressing CD4 promote atherosclerosis particularly when activated by LDL modified by oxidative processes [26,27]. The T-cells expressing CD8, when activated, trigger caspase pathways. However, $CD4^+$ and $CD8^+$ T produce different effectors molecules and then effect different cells and pathways, although redundancy of mechanisms has been described pointing to the importance of lymphocyte homeostasis in disease.

The positive association of plaque area with ox-LDL concentrations in plasma can also be considered a marker of plaque instability and/or plaque rupture [51,52] in addition to disease severity. Extensive experimental data shows that ox-LDL is formed in the arterial wall [14,16] contributing to the plaque progression. It is accepted that ox-LDL in circulation is originated in the vessel wall, being their circulating levels strongly associated to angiographically documented CAD [25]. Increases in plaque area, and therefore in regions where lumen decreases relative to circumferential EEL, may favor plaque outflow. In these regions the vessel wall is exposed to shear stress that may contribute to endothelial denuding and plaque cap erosion [47].

The current forms of imaging enable atherosclerosis assessment at the later stage when the vascular morphology has changed dramatically. However, the evaluation of plaque characteristics by angiography and IVUS-VH was associated to circulating biomarkers levels, and these indicators may reflect plaque vulnerability. The *in vivo* identification of plaque vulnerability whether by characterizing its components or by providing measures of oxidative and inflammation markers may improve diagnostic and eventually allow the detection of vulnerable atheroma before rupture. The relations among the plaque components – fibrotic, fibro-fatty calcified and necrotic core – and plaque dimensions, may be important in the characterization of the plaque and in the assessment of its development. Also, circulating ox-LDL, sFasL, TNF-α and lymphocyte populations may be viable targets to follow as they may reflect the global extend of atherosclerosis and may provide useful information on patient's evolution, together with quantitative angiography-derived plaque parameters. The approach may be incorporated in carefully designed clinical studies for the assessment of coronary atherosclerosis.

5. Study limitations

This prospective study is a single-centre study that has a number of limitations. The small number of patients enrolled did not allow association of parameters with clinical presentation. The measurements of biomarkers that entered into the study do not reflect chronic circulating levels, as more than 50% of patients presented with acute coronary syndromes (STEMI, NSTEMI and UA), which transiently alters levels of inflammatory biomarkers. Some of the measurements may be confounded by concomitant treatments (medication, stenting, etc.), which could not be estimated due to the reduced number of patients. We also wish to emphasize that all angiography and IVUS studies are limited to the analysis of a relatively short segment of coronary arterial tree that does not fully reflect disease characteristics elsewhere. The results obtained of plaque components were not confirmed by histology or other diagnostic modalities, such as optical coherent tomography.

6. Conclusions

The present study using angiography and IVUS-VH revealed that the atherosclerotic plaque components and dimensions were related to the concentration of biomarkers in the blood circulation. We reported on the vascular tissue characteristics that may be associated with vulnerable plaques and the incremental value of biomarkers in addition to invasive imaging modalities.

The association of ox-LDL, sFasL and TNF-α circulating levels with lumen dimension and plaque dimension suggest that these indicators may express not only plaque rupture but plaque vulnerability as well. Also the association of TNF-α and T lymphocytes expressing CD4 and CD8 with plaque percentage of fibrous, fibro-fatty, and necrotic core areas may contribute to an in vivo assessment of vascular inflammation and vulnerable plaques and their detection before rupture.

The results suggest that these biomarkers have clinical implications for identifying vulnerable plaques as well as vulnerable patients. Further studies are needed to evaluate the impact of these biomarkers and angiography and IVUS-VH derived measures on clinical presentation.

Acknowledgements

This work was supported by Fundação para a Ciência e Tecnologia (PIC/IC/82734/2007 and SFRM/BPD/6308/2009); and by Liga dos Amigos do Hospital de Santa Marta.

Author details

Catarina Ramos[1], Patrícia Napoleão[2], Rui Cruz Ferreira[3], Cristina Fondinho[3], Mafalda Selas[3], Miguel Mota Carmo[4], Ana Maria Crespo[4] and Teresa Pinheiro[1*]

*Address all correspondence to: murmur@itn.pt

1 IST/ITN Instituto Superior Técnico, Universidade Técnica de Lisboa, Sacavém, Portugal

2 Unidade de Biologia Microvascular e Inflamação, Instituto de Medicina Molecular, Faculdade de Medicina da Universidade de Lisboa, Lisboa, Portugal

3 Serviço Cardiologia, Hospital Santa Marta, Centro Hospitalar Lisboa Central, Lisboa, Portugal

4 Centro de Estudos de Doenças Crónicas, Faculdade de Ciências Médicas, Universidade Nova de Lisboa & Serviço Cardiologia, Hospital Santa Marta Centro Hospitalar Lisboa Central, Lisboa, Portugal

CESAM & Departamento de Biologia Animal, Faculdade de Ciências da Universidade de Lisboa, Lisboa, Portugal

References

[1] Hoffmann U, Moselewski F, Nieman K, Jang IK, Ferencik M, Rahman AM, Cury RC, Abbara S, Joneidi-Jafari H, Achenbach S, Brady TJ, Noninvasive Assessment of Plaque Morphology and Composition in Culprit and Stable Lesions in Acute Coronary Syndrome and Stable Lesions in Stable Angina by Multidetector Computed Tomography, Am Coll Cardiol 2006; 47: 1655– 62

[2] Red-Horse K, Ueno H, Weissman IL, Krasnow MA, Coronary arteries form by developmental reprogramming of venous cells, Nature 2010; 464: 549-553

[3] Stone GW, Maehara A, Mintz GS, The Reality of Vulnerable Plaque Detection, JACC: Cardiovascular Imaging 2011; 4: 902-904

[4] Roger VL, Go AS, Lloyd-Jones DM, Adams RJ,. Berry JD, Brown TM, Carnethon MR, Dai S, de Simone G,. Ford ES, Fox CS, Fullerton HJ, Gillespie C, Greenlund KJ,. Hail-

pern SM, Heit JA, Ho PM, Howard VJ, Kissela BM, Kittner SJ, Lackland DT, Lichtman JH, Lisabeth LD, Makuc DM, Marcus GM, Mozaffarian D, Mussolino ME, Nichol G, Paynter NP, Rosamond WD, Sorlie PD, Stafford RS, Turan TN, Turner MB, Wong ND, Wylie-Rosett J, Heart Disease and Stroke Statistics—2011 Update, Circulation 2011; 123: e18-e209

[5] Ross R, Atherosclerosis — An Inflammatory Disease, N Engl J Med 1999; 340: 115-126

[6] Libby P, Ridker PM, Hansson GK, Inflammation in Atherosclerosis: From Pathophysiology to Practice, J. Am. Coll. Cardiol. 2009; 54: 2129-2138

[7] Galkina E, Ley K, Vascular Adhesion Molecules in Atherosclerosis, Atherosclero Tromb, Vasc Biol 2007; 27: 2292 - 2301

[8] Vancraeynest D, Pasquet A, Roelants V, Gerber BL, Vanoverschelde JJ, Imaging the Vulnerable Plaque, J Am Coll Cardiol 2011; 57: 1961–79

[9] Hansson GK, Inflammation, Atherosclerosis, and Coronary Artery Disease, N Engl J Med 2005; 352: 1685-95

[10] Goldstein JL, Ross MS, Regulation of low-density lipoprotein receptors: implications for pathogenesis and therapy of hypercholesterolemia and atherosclerosis, Circulation 1987; 76: 504-507

[11] Goldstein JA, Demetriou D, Grines CL, Pica M, Shoukfeh M, O'Neill WW, Multiple complex coronary plaques in patients with acute myocardial infarction, New Engl J Med 2000; 343: 915-22

[12] Fayad ZA, Fuster V, Clinical imaging of the high-risk or vulnerable atherosclerotic plaque, Circ. Res. 2001; 89: 305-316

[13] Choi SH, Chae A, Miller E, Messig M, Ntanios F, DeMaria AN, Nissen SE, Witztum JL, Tsimikas S, Relationship Between Biomarkers of Oxidized Low-Density Lipoprotein, Statin Therapy, Quantitative Coronary Angiography, and Atheroma Volume, J Am Coll Cardiol 2008; 52: 24-32

[14] Greco TP, Conti-Kelly AM, Anthony JR, Greco Jr T, Doyle R, Boisen M, Kojima K, Pharm BA, Matsuura E, Lopez LR, Oxidized-LDL/β_2-Glycoprotein I Complexes Are Associated With Disease Severity and Increased Risk for Adverse Outcomes in Patients With Acute Coronary Syndromes, Am J Clin Pathol 2010;133:737-743

[15] Bronas UG, Dengel DR, Influence of Vascular Oxidative Stress and Inflammation on the Development and Progression of Atherosclerosis, Am J of Lifestyle Med 2010; 4: 521 - 534

[16] Tabas I, The Role of Endoplasmic Reticulum Stress in the Progression of Atherosclerosis, Circ Res 2010; 107: 839-850

[17] van Gils JM, Derby MC, Fernandes LR, Ramkhelawon B, Ray TD, Rayner KJ, Parathath S, Distel E, Feig JL, Alvarez-Leite JI, Rayner AJ, McDonald TO, O'Brien KD,

Stuart LM, Fisher EA, Lacy-Hulbert A, Moore KJ, The neuroimmune guidance cue netrin-1 promotes atherosclerosis by inhibiting the emigration of macrophages from plaques, Nature Immunology 2012; 13: 136–143

[18] Mallat Z, Taleb S, Ait-Oufella H, Tedgui A, The role of adaptive T cell immunity in atherosclerosis, J. Lipid Res. 2009; 50: S364–S369

[19] Keaney Jr JF, Immune Modulation of Atherosclerosis, Circulation 2011; 124: e559 - e560

[20] Zernecke A, Weber C, Chemokines in the vascular inflammatory response of atherosclerosis, Cardiovasc Res 2010; 86: 192 – 201

[21] An G, Wang H, Tang R, Yago T, McDaniel JM, McGee S, Huo Y, Xia L, P-selectin glycoprotein ligand-1 is highly expressed on Ly-6Chi monocytes and a major determinant for Ly-6Chi monocyte recruitment to sites of atherosclerosis in mice, Circulation 2008; 117: 3227–37

[22] Viemann D, Barczyk K, Vogl T, Fischer U, Sunderkötter C, Schulze-Osthoff K, Roth J, MRP8/MRP14 impairs endothelial integrity and induces a caspase-dependent and independent cell death program, Blood 2007; 109: 2453-2460

[23] Ray KK, Morrow DA, Sabatine MS, Shui A, Rifai N, Cannon CP, Braunwald E, Long-Term Prognostic Value of Neopterin: A Novel Marker of Monocyte Activation in Patients With Acute Coronary Syndrome, Circulation 2007; 115: 3071 - 3078

[24] Lopes-Virella MF, Virella G, Clinical Significance of the Humoral Immune Response to Modified LDL, Clin Immunol. 2010; 134(1): 55–65

[25] Tsimikas S, Brilakis ES, Miller ER, McConnell JP, Lennon RJ, Kornman KS, Witztum JL, Berger PB, Oxidized Phospholipids, Lp(a) Lipoprotein, and Coronary Artery Disease, N Engl J Med 2005; 353: 46-57.

[26] Greco TP, Conti-Kelly AM, Greco Jr T, Doyle R, Matsuura E, Anthony JR, Lopez LR, Newer Antiphospholipid Antibodies Predict Adverse Outcomes in Patients With Acute Coronary Syndrome, Am J Clin Pathol 2009; 132: 613-620

[27] Ludewig B, Freigang S, Jäggi M, Kurrer MO, Pei YC, Vlk L, Odermatt B, Zinkernagel RM, Hengartner H, Linking immune-mediated arterial inflammation and cholesterol-induced atherosclerosis in a transgenic mouse model, Proc Natl Acad Sci U S A 2000; 97: 12752–7

[28] Peters RJ, Kok WE, Pasterkamp G, Von Birgelen C, Prins M, Serruys PW, Videodensitometric quantitative angiography after coronary balloon angioplasty, compared to edge-detection quantitative angiography and intracoronary ultrasound imaging, Eur Heart J 2000; 21: 654–661

[29] Leber AW, Knez A, von Ziegler F, Becker A, Nikolaou K, Paul S, Wintersperger B, Reiser M, Becker CR, Steinbeck G, Boekstegers P, Quantification of Obstructive and

Nonobstructive Coronary Lesions by 64-Slice Computed Tomography, J Am Coll Cardiol 2005; 46; 147-154

[30] Böse D, von Birgelen C, Erbel R, Intravascular Ultrasound for the Evaluation of Therapies Targeting Coronary Atherosclerosis, J Am Coll Cardiol 2007; 49:925–32

[31] Sano K, Kawasaki M, Ishihara Y, Okubo M, Tsuchiya K, Nishigaki K, Zhou X, Minatoguchi S, Fujita H, Fujiwara H, Assessment of Vulnerable Plaques Causing Acute Coronary Syndrome Using Integrated Backscatter Intravascular Ultrasound, J Am Coll Cardiol 2006; 47: 734–41

[32] Springer I, Dewey M, Comparison of multislice computed tomography with intravascular ultrasound for detection and characterization of coronary artery plaques: a systematic review, Eur J Radiol 2009; 71: 275-82.

[33] Gao D, Ning N, Guo Y, Ning W, Niu X, Yang J, Computed tomography for detecting coronary artery plaques: a meta-analysis, Atherosclerosis 2011; 219: 603-9.

[34] van der Giessen AG, Toepker MH, Donelly PM, Bamberg F, Schlett CL, Raffle C, Irlbeck T, Lee H, van Walsum T, Maurovich-Horvat P, Gijsen FJ, Wentzel JJ, Hoffmann U, Reproducibility, accuracy, and predictors of accuracy for the detection of coronary atherosclerotic plaque composition by computed tomography: an ex vivo comparison to intravascular ultrasound, Invest Radiol. 2010; 45: 693-701

[35] Rodriguez-Granillo GA, García-García HM, Mc Fadden EP, Valgimigli M, Aoki J, de Feyter P, Serruys PW. In Vivo Intravascular Ultrasound-Derived Thin-Cap Fibroatheroma Detection Using Ultrasound Radiofrequency Data Analysis. J Am Coll Cardiol 2005; 46: 2038–42

[36] Calvert PA, Obaid DR, O'Sullivan M, Shapiro LM, McNab D, Densem CG, Schofield PM, Braganza D, Clarke SC, Ray KK, West NEJ, Bennett MR, Association Between IVUS Findings and Adverse Outcomes in Patients With Coronary Artery Disease, JACC: Cardiovascular Imaging, 2011; 4: 894-901

[37] Nakamura T, Kubo N, Funayama H, Sugawara Y, Ako J, Momomura S, Plaque characteristics of the coronary segment proximal to the culprit lesion in stable and unstable patients, Clin. Cardiol. 2009; 32: e9–e12

[38] Stähr PM, Höfflinghaus T, Voigtländer T, Courtney BK, Victor A, Otto M, Yock PG, Brennecke R, Fitzgerald PJ, Discrimination of Early/Intermediate and Advanced/Complicated Coronary Plaque Types by Radiofrequency Intravascular Ultrasound Analysis, Am J Cardiol. 2002; 9: 19-23

[39] Costa MA, Kozuma K, Gaster AL, van Der Giessen WJ, Sabate M, Foley DP, Kay I, Ligthart J, Thayssen P, van den Brand MJ, de Feyter PJ, Serruys P, Three dimensional intravascular ultrasonic assessment of the local mechanism of restenosis after balloon angioplasty. Heart 2001; 85: 73–79.

[40] Amato M, Montorsi P, Ravani A, Oldani E, Galli S, Ravagnani PM, Tremoli E, Baldassarre D, Carotid intima-media thickness by B-mode ultrasound as surrogate of

coronary atherosclerosis: correlation with quantitative coronary angiography and coronary intravascular ultrasound findings, European Heart Journal, 2007; 28: 2094–2101

[41] Voros S, Rinehart S, Qian Z, Vazquez G, Anderson H, Murrieta L, Wilmer C, Carlson H, Taylor K, Ballard W, Karmpaliotis D, Kalynych A, Brown C, Prospective Validation of Standardized, 3-Dimensional, Quantitative Coronary Computed Tomographic Plaque Measurements Using Radiofrequency Backscatter Intravascular Ultrasound as Reference Standard in Intermediate Coronary Arterial Lesions, J Am Coll Cardiol Intv 2011; 4: 198–208

[42] Peters RJG, Kok WEM, Pasterkamp G, von Birgelen C, Prins M, Serruys PW on behalf of the PICTURE study group. Videodensitometric quantitative angiography after coronary balloon angioplasty, compared to edge-detection quantitative angiography and intracoronary ultrasound imaging. Eur Heart J 2000; 21: 654–661

[43] Leber AW, Knez A, von Ziegler F, Becker A, Nikolaou K, Paul S, Wintersperger B, Reiser M, Becker CR, Steinbeck G, Boekstegers P, Quantification of Obstructive and Nonobstructive Coronary Lesions by 64-Slice Computed Tomography A Comparative Study With Quantitative Coronary Angiography and Intravascular Ultrasound. J Am Coll Cardiol 2005; 46: 147–54.

[44] Naruko T, Furukawa A, Yunoki K, Komatsu R, Nakagawa N, Matsumura Y, Shirai N, Sugioka K, Takagi M, Hozumi T, Itoh A, Haze K, Yoshiyama M, Becker AE, Ueda M. Increased expression and plasma levels of myeloperoxidase are closely related to the presence of angiographically-detected complex lesion morphology in unstable angina. Heart 2010; 96: 1716-1722.

[45] Yun KH, Mintz GS, Farhat N, Marso SP, Taglieri N, Verheye S, Foster MC, Margolis MP, Templin B, Xu K, Dressler O, Mehran R, Stone GW, Maehara A, Relation Between Angiographic Lesion Severity, Vulnerable Plaque Morphology and Future Adverse Cardiac Events (from the Providing Regional Observations to Study Predictors of Events in the Coronary Tree Study), Am J Cardiol. 2012; 110: 471-7.

[46] Budoff MJ, Shaw LJ, Liu ST, Weinstein SR, Mosler TP, Tseng PH, Flores FR, Callister TQ, Raggi P, Berman DS. Long-term prognosis associated with coronary calcification. J Am Coll Cardiol 2007;49:1860-70.

[47] Cheng GC, Loree HM, Kamm RD, Fishbein MC, Lee RT. Distribution of circumferential stress in ruptured and stable atherosclerotic lesions: a structural analysis with histopathological correlation. Circulation 1993;87: 1179 – 87.

[48] P. Napoleão, M. Selas, C. Ramos, A. Turkman, V. Andreozzi, M. Mota Carmo, A. M. Viegas-Crespo, R. Cruz Ferreira, T. Pinheiro. The Role of Inflammatory Biomarkers in the Assessment of Coronary Artery Disease. In: Branislav Baskot (ed.) Coronary Angiography - Advances in Noninvasive Imaging Approach for Evaluation of Coronary Artery Disease: InTech; 2011. p281-314.

[49] Sata M, Walsh K. TNF-alpha regulation of Fas ligand expression on the vascular endothelium modulates leukocyte extravasation. Nat Med 1998; 4 :415-420.

[50] Blanco-Colio LM, Martín-Ventura JL, Tuñón J, García-Camarero T, Berrazueta JR, Egido J. Soluble Fas ligand plasma levels are associated with forearm reactive hyperemia in subjects with coronary artery disease: a novel biomarker of endothelial function? Atherosclerosis. 2008;201:407-12.

[51] P. Napoleão, M. Selas, A. Toste, A. Turkman, V. Andreozzi, A.M. Viegas-Crespo, T. Pinheiro, R. Cruz Ferreira. Serial changes of oxidized low-density lipoprotein associated with culprit vessel in ST-elevation myocardial infarction – a promising marker? Rev Port Cardiol 2009;28:303-308.

[52] M. Mota Carmo, P. Napoleão, S. Andrade, A.M. Selas, C. Freixo, A Turkman, V. Andreozzi, A.M. Viegas-Crespo, T. Pinheiro, R.C. Ferreira, High Oxidized LDL Associate to Low T-Lymphocytes in Acute Myocardial Infarction. Circulation 2010;122: E161.

Section 2

Noninvasive Diagnostic Approach in Coronary Artery Disease

Chapter 3

Radiation Principles and Safety

Jasmin Čaluk

Additional information is available at the end of the chapter

http://dx.doi.org/10.5772/54033

1. Introduction

Interventional cardiology today without the use of x-ray technology cannot even be imagined. This is also true for medicine in general. The radiology era begins with the discovery of the x-rays by Wilhelm Conrad Röntgen, on the November 8th 1895 (following the transliteration conventions for the characters accentuated by 'umlaut', „Röntgen" is in English spelled „Roentgen", and with that spelling is most often found in the literature). On that day he produced and detected for the first time the electromagnetic radiation in the wavelengths today known as the x-rays, for which he received the Nobel prize for physics in 1901 [1]. This was the start of radiology, which has developed tremendously over the years. In time, radiology adopted other forms of human body imaging (magnetic resonance, positron emission tomography etc.), but even today the most radiologic studies in the world are performed using the x-rays, whether in the form of classic x-ray imaging, computer tomography, or various forms of fluoroscopy and/or fluorography, which is used in interventional cardiology. The term 'fluoroscopy' depicts viewing of structures in real time, while 'fluorography' means that different methods of image aquisition and storage for later review are being used.

X-ray radiation is a form of electromagnetic radiation. X-rays are electromagnetic waves with a wavelength in the range of 0.01 to 10 nanometers, which corresponds to frequencies in the range 30 petahertz to 30 exahertz (3×10^{16} Hz to 3×10^{19} Hz) and energies in the range 120 eV to 120 keV. X-rays are shorter in wavelength than ultra-violet rays and longer than gamma rays. In many languages, X-radiation is called Röntgen radiation, after Wilhelm Conrad Röntgen, who is usually credited as its discoverer, and who had actually named it X-radiation to signify the up to then unknown type of radiation [1].

X-ray input doses for fluorography are generally 10-fold higher than those used for fluoroscopy. This is why fluorography is the major source of the radiation dose [2]. Procedures which include the use of x-rays are associated with the exposure of the patients to a certain amount of x-ray radiation, and in some cases, especially in interventional cardiology, the staff is also exposed to this form of radiation. The constant evolution of interventional cardiology, with ever more complex procedures demanding prolonged fluoroscopy and fluorography time, as well as the demands for better imaging of small structures (guidewires, angioplasty balloon- and stent-markers, stents themselves, intravascular ultrasound probes, etc.) associated with higher exposures to larger amounts of x-ray radiation, have all raised the question of radiation protection, both for the patients and the staff inside the catheterization laboratory (cath lab). Occupational doses of radiation in interventional cardiology procedures guided by fluoroscopy are the highest doses registered among medical staff using x-rays. The use of ionizing radiation increases the risk of malignant disease occurrence and can cause skin or eye damage to both the patient and the personnel [3].

2. How the x-ray radiation is produced

2.1. The x-ray tube

The principle of generating the x-rays is basically the same in all x-ray machines. The source of x-rays is the x-ray tube (fig.1, fig. 2). Within it are the cathode and the anode (fig. 1). The electrically positive tungsten anode is bombarded with accelerated electrons originating from the electrically negative cathode. When the high-velocity electrons collide with the anode, they lose most of their energy (~99%) as heat, and a small fraction (~1%) as x-rays. Since the electrons are slowed down within the anode by different segments of atoms and mostly multiple interactions with several atoms within the material itself, they release a variety of x-ray energies. However, when all of the electron's energy is lost in a single interaction, the resultant emitted x-ray has the highest possible energy, equivalent to the voltage applied across the tube. That is reffered to as the kVp, or 'peak kilovoltage' of the emitted x-rays. A typical x-ray tube ranges from 60 kV to 120 kV. The tube current, measured in milliamperes (mA) is defined as the number of electrons that arc from the cathode to the anode per second [4]. Modern x-ray tubes generate the radiation in pulses rather than in a continuous form, and those pulses are synchronized with the other components in the fluoroscopic/fluorographic system. The duration of the time during which the electrons hit the anode is the pulse width, and is measured in milliseconds (ms).

The anode is made of tungsten because this material can withstand very high temperatures without melting. As stated before, some 99% of the energy which the electron beam is losing when hitting the anode is heat. The anode is constructed as a disc, and to reduce the heat strain even more, it is constantly rotated at speeds up to 10,000 rpm (fig. 1). This way, the area bombarded by the small electron beam is not actually a single spot, but a circle track. The small area of the anode which is being bombarded by the electron beam, and from which the x-rays are emitted is called the 'focal spot', and since

http://dx.doi.org/10.5772/54033

the anode is being rotated, the focal spot is actually the already described circular track on the anode disc. The size of the focal spot affects the image quality in different ways. If it is smaller, the images are sharper, but if it is larger, it can produce more x-rays. The cathode is a tungsten wire, and is the source of electrons which are accelerated towards the anode. The cathode is heated to high temperatures by passing the current through it, and is maintained at a large negative voltage relative to the anode. The electrons are 'fired away' from it and accelerate toward the anode, hitting it as they reach their maximum energy, which is 60 kV to 120 kV.

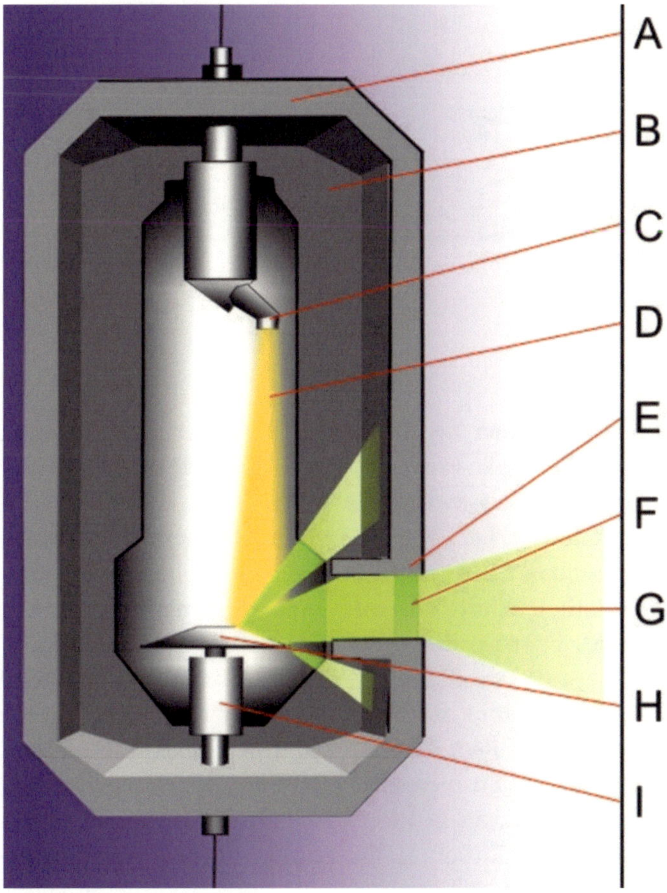

Figure 1. The x-ray tube. Legend: A – housing; B – oil bath for cooling; C – cathode; D – electron beam; E – collimators; F – filters; G – x-rays; H – anode; I – engine for anode rotation (illustration: J. Čaluk).

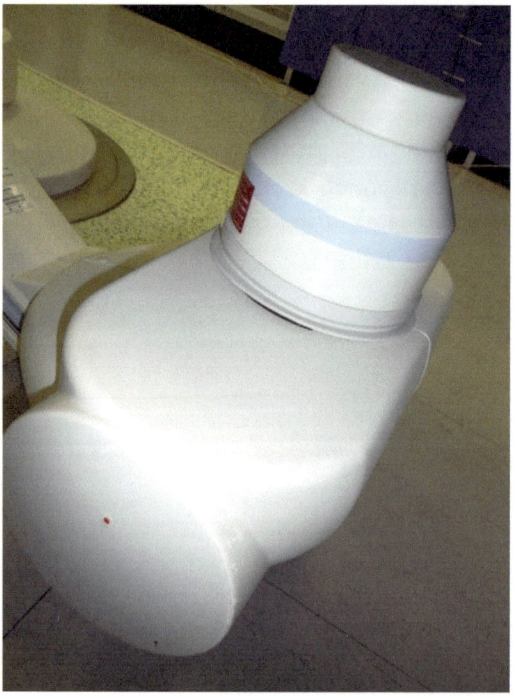

Figure 2. X-ray tube

2.2. Filters

As the electrons are slowed down by the anode, there occurs a spectrum of different wavelength x-rays called the brake-radiation (in German: Bremsstrahlung), with spikes of x-ray energies at characteristic wavelengths when all the energy of an electron is lost at a single collision, as noted earlier. The brake-radiation is mostly of low photon energies (<25-30 keV), and would be mostly absorbed in the patient's superfitial tissues. Therefore, the brake-radiation would not contribute to generating the x-ray image, but would, on the other hand, increase the amount of radiation to which the patient is exposed. This is why these x-rays are filtered in the beam exit port, and the filters applied selectively absorb the x-ray photons from this region of the energy spectrum [4]. Modern systems usually use copper filters 0.2 – 0.9 mm thick. Since these filters attenuate the x-ray beam (fig. 1), this requires an increased tube output, and when this is accomplished, the greater energy output occurs in the energy range of interest. Filters are basically simple, small metal sheets. In addition to the permanent beam filtration that is usually equivalent to 3 mm of aluminium, all cardio-angiographic equipment should have heavily filtered x-ray sources. The number and the mode of filter use differs among manufacturers, but optional filters of 0.1 mm, 0.2 mm, 0.3 mm, etc. should be available to order with the machine. In some products, users can employ different dose-management modes, and these filters might be incorporated into those modes, selectable by the user.

The thickest filters would therefore be used for smaller patients, and the thinnest ones for large patients. Since the filters primarily eliminate the useless part of the x-ray beam, but also do attenuate even a part of the useful beam, the goal of filtration is to produce the best possible compromise between image quality and radiation dose.

2.3. Collimators

In order to adjust the shape and the size of the x-ray field emerging from the tube, lead collimators which completely absorb the x-ray beam are used. They actually limit the exposure of the patient only within the region of interest, and thus reduce the unneccessary exposure to both the patient and the staff. The collimators can be manipulated as to further reduce the port of the x-ray tube (fig. 1) and by that, to reduce the irradiated area. The edges of the collimator blades are then visible in the imaging field as shadows. The amount of absorbed and scattered radiation can be reduced by an adequate collimation –the entrance surface area of the x-ray beam on the patient's skin should be reduced to the smallest possible/needed size [5,6,7].

2.4. X-ray generators

The x-ray generator provides the electric power to heat the cathode, to accelerate the electrons from the cathode to the anode thus generating the x-ray beam, and to turn the x-ray pulses on and off. It automatically adjusts the tube voltage, current, and pulse width to maintain a certain image quality. In interventional cardiology, there is a demand for generators able to provide up to 100 kW of power across all the voltages in the diagnostic range. The modulation of variables of x-ray beams is automated, and it maintains constant brightness at the image receptor as the thickness of patient's tissues varies with different projections and angulations. Very oblique angulations mean that the tissue thickness is bigger, and more powerful radiation is required to generate the image in comparison to less or non-angulated tube positions. Also, the image quality must be maintained regardless of the patient's built, so bigger patients are exposed to higher amounts of radiation, because stronger x-ray beams are required to penetrate their bodies [8,9]. Image brightness at the oputput of the imaging chain is rapidly sampled. The measurements are sent back to the generator to modulate the above mentioned variables and provide the desired image brightness. Beside the pulse width, the voltage, and the current, the parameters which can be altered are camera aperture and electronic amplification gain.

3. X-ray image formation

The x-ray beam directed towards the patient is considered to be uniform. After interacting with different tissues which attenuate it to a variable degree, a non-uniform x-ray beam exits the patient. Its non-uniformity, generated by the process of x-ray absorption in the patient, is the basis for obtaining an x-ray image. The degree of 'darkness' in the x-ray image, which forms the x-ray 'shadow', is determined by the energy of the original x-ray beam generated by the tube, the thickness of the exposed object (patient's tissues), and the elemental makeup of the object (patient's tissues). The removal of the x-ray beam as a function of the object thickness is exponential, but the elemental makeup of the tissue is characteristic for the tissue itself, and as a function is characterized by a linear attenuation coefficient. Half-value layer (HVL) is the parameter defined as the thickness of a tissue sample that absorbes (removes from the beam) one-half of the beam intensity. Regarding the beam energies used in interventional cardiology, HVL for muscle would be 3.2 cm, for bone is 1.5 cm, for iodine is 0.01 cm (100%), and as a comparison, for the lead, the HVL is 0.01 cm [4].

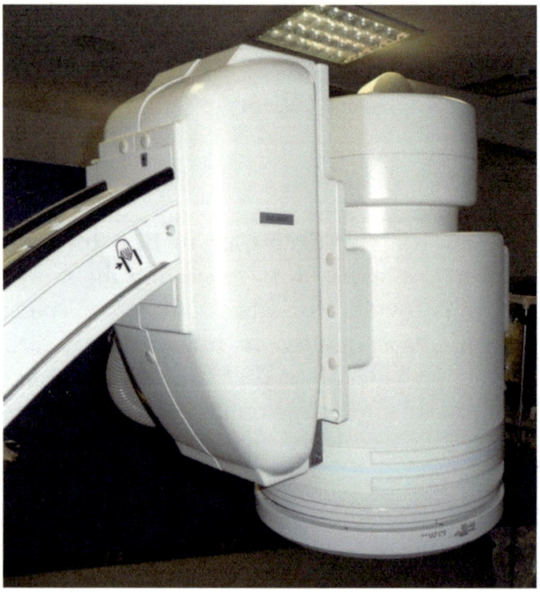

Figure 3. Image intensifier

When a non-uniform x-ray beam leaves the patient's body, its spatial distribution is the basis for forming an x-ray image. It contains the information on the anatomy of the scanned region, and if it is taken within a defined time-frame, it can also be used for the assessment of the patient's physiology. But, since the spectrum of x-rays cannot be detected by the human eyes, it must be 'translated' into visible information. There are several technologies currently in use for that purpose, and the most common being used in interventional cardiology today are image intensifier and digital flat-panel detector technology, both of which are digital. Although our senses use the analogue method to percieve the reality, for the purpose of securely storing the information and being possible to make exact copies, and later review the information without quality loss, that information needs to be digitalized. The digital-flat panel detectors are the state of the art now, but still the vast majority of the systems currently in use employ the image intensifier technology (fig. 3). The main role of

http://dx.doi.org/10.5772/54033

the image intensifier is to convert the x-ray intensity information into the visible light spectrum and expose photographic film or a video camera. The details of the process taking place within the image intensifier are beyond the scope of this chapter and are discussed elsewhere.

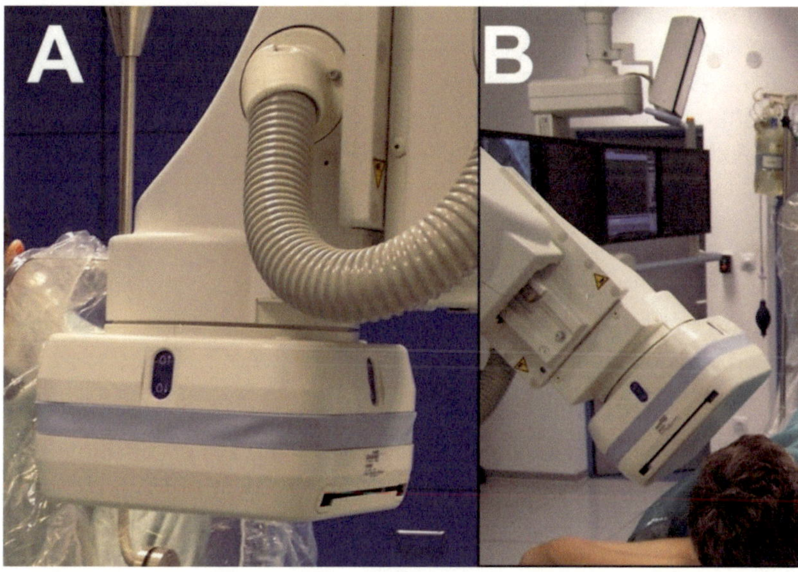

Figure 4. Digital flat-panel detector

However, recently a novel technology has been introduced and its use in cardio-angiography is constantly increasing: the digital flat-panel detector (fig. 4), which consists of (simply speaking) several layers of material. The x-ray photons, upon leaving the patient, hit the input phosphor layer of the detector, and it produces light photons. Behind that layer is the photodiode and the thin-film transistor layer. The generated light photons produce electric signals within this layer, and those signals are captured as voltages in the discrete flat-panel elements [4]. A typical panel consists of 1024 x 1024 elements over a rectangle-shaped field of view. Each flat-panel element's voltage signal is converted from an analogue voltage to a digital representation. The digital image produced like this is represented using a fixed number of values, and those are distributed over a limited set of co-ordinates. This information can then be stored or copied. For viewing, it is fed through conversion system and into the viewing monitor, and we percieve it as an image, with monitor pixels corresponding to flat panel detector's elements which received the beam. In order to standardize the digital communication within the medical community, the DICOM (Digital Imaging Communications in Medicine) system has been introduced. It is used for organizing the image data in such a way that other users of the DICOM system can review those data accurately, and is currently the standard-one in medicine.

4. Radiation management and safety

X-ray radiation is a carcinogen [10]. No dose of radiation may be considered safe or harmless [11]. It can also cause severe injury called radiation burns, but the likelihood of that is extremely low when the fluoroscopy/fluorography is adequately managed. Doctors, nurses, technicians, and other medical staff working in radiation environment, who have accumulated significant doses of radiation through their careers have been shown to develop some form of radiation-induced health-problems, the most important being cancer, cataracts, and skin injury [12,13]. Interventional cardiologists, working at very low distances from x-ray tubes, and the patients who are also the sources of scattered radiation, are at particular health risk.

4.1. Radiation effects

Effects of radiation can be generally divided into two basic groups: the stochastic effects, and the deterministic effects. Both groups are very important for the pathological consequences on the human body.

Stochastic effect occurs within a single cell and makes it adversely functional. This happens because of an alteration of an important macromolecule (such as the DNA) and can result upon a single interaction with radiation. It is therefore logical to assume that this kind of effects may occur with any radiation dose, but in practice, low doses of radiation carry an extremely low risk of stochastic effects on the body. The most important stochastic effects in the clinical sense are the occurrence of radiation-induced tumors and heritable changes in reproductive cells. The risk of these effects occurring rises with the rise of the amount of radiation to which a person is exposed, so the induced cancer becomes measurable in exposed adults at doses over some 100 mSv. In children, and in fetus (if a pregnant woman is exposed to radiation), even lower doses have been defined as carcinogenic. The stochastic risk of inducing malignant disease associated with radiation is small but definite [14].

Deterministic effects are the result of damage to a large number of cells, therefore a certain dose of radiation has to be applied for these effects to take place. This minimal dose for a deterministic effect is called the threshold dose. The higher the dose (above the threshold), the more severe the effects. Some examples of deterministic effects are: skin erythema, epilation, dry or moist desquamation, secondary ulceration, ischemic dermal necrosis, various stages of dermal atrophy, induration, teleangiectasia, late dermal necrosis, vision-impairing cataract [10]. Some authors propose that skin cancer can also be considered to be a deterministic effect of radiation.

For both of these groups of radiation effects there exists a time delay between the exposure to radiation and the clinical manifestation of the effect itself. This delay ranges from days to weeks to months for deterministic effects, and for malignant diseases, from as little as 2 years, to as long as many decades. In many cases, neither the patient, nor the physician (usually a dermatologists or a general practitioner) grasps the connection of a skin disorder (usually an erythema, or a 'radiation burn') and a previous interventional cardiology procedure, because of this time delay – usually several weeks.

4.2. Units of measurement of x-ray radiation

In order to understand and quantify the effects of radiation on humans, different units of measurement have been developed. It is necessary to know these units as to be able to apply the safety measures in radiation environment, as well as to compare the health-risks of different forms of radiation.

Absorbed dose is the amount of radiation energy absorbed by a particular tissue. The x-ray radiation interacts with living tissues upon entering them, and its energy causes molecular changes, and therefore has the potential to have biologic effects. The unit of absorbed dose is gray (Gy), meaning that 1 Gy is the radiation energy of one joule (1 J) concentrated in one kilogram (1 kg) of tissue.

Equivalent dose is an estimate of the biologic potency which a form of radiation might have for an absorbed dose, and is determined by the properties of the radiation itself. Therefore, for different kinds of radiation, the equivalent doses can be different, although the absorbed doses can be the same. This is actually a safety term that can be used to compare the biologic potency of different kinds of radiation. The unit for equivalent dose is sievert (Sv). In interventional cardiology, 1 Sv is considered to be equivalent to 1 Gy [10].

Effective dose is the estimate of a hypothetic dose which would have to be delivered to an interventionist's entire body to have the same risk for the radiation adverse effects as the non-uniform doses which are actually delivered. The need for establishing this unit of measurement occurred because during the procedures in the cath lab (or similar radiation environments), some of the body parts are better protected (e.g. internal organs), while other body parts are less, or not at all protected (e.g. head and limbs), under the assumption that they are less radiosensitive. Therefore, the spatial distribution of radiation exposure is non-uniform. Effective dose eliminates this complexity in radiation risk assessment. The unit to measure the effective dose is sievert (Sv), and in interventional cardiology 1 Sv can be considered to be equal to 1 Gy of x-ray radiation absorbed uniformly in the body.

There are, of course, the proposed limits to which personnel in the radiation environment can be exposed. Regarding the effective dose, the limit for the staff is 100 mSv in a consecutive five year period, subject to a maximum effective dose of 50 mSv in any single year. The equivalent dose for the lenses of the eye should be limited to 150 mSv in a year. The limit on equivalent dose for the skin should be 500 mSv in a year, and the dose for the hands, forearms, feet, and ankles should be limited to 500 mSv in a year [11].

4.3. Limiting the exposure to radiation

The basic rule which can be applied regarding radiation protection is: 'what is good for the patient is also good for the staff'. For this reason, radiation protection measures will be discussed in general, with additional comments regarding the staff or the patient when necessary. The four basic methods of limiting exposure to radiation can be remembered by using the mnemonic TIDS, which stands for: time, intensity, distance, and shielding [10].

The time of fluoroscopy/fluorography should be limited to the necessary minimum. A good measure for orientation regarding this is fluoroscopy time recorded by most machines used for cardio-angiography today. Although, most devices show only fluoroscopy time, and the operator must also think about the fluorography time, knowing that the amount of radiation for the same amount of time is in fluorography 10-fold of that in fluoroscopy. Some devices have the ability to show fluorography time, or a complete beam-on time. In addition, a trend towards less fluoroscopy time is obvious with more experienced operators. However, more experienced operators are more often involved in complex procedures, which actually prolong the fluoroscopy time. Regardless of that, all operators have to be aware that they must reduce the beam-on time to a minimum provided that they can visualize the structures of interest and complete the procedure safely. Complex procedures, such as multivessel interventions, treating chronic total occlusions, or bifurcation lesions demand more procedure time than the simple interventions, and this leads to increased radiation dose when treating more complex coronary disease [16]. Some practical advices: when documenting balloon inflation, just a short single shot should be enough, there is no need to prolong the shot of an inflated balloon; there is no reason to record or observe the gradual balloon deflation, this can be checked with short beam-on shots; the operator's foot should be kept away from the fluoropedal when not actually using fluorography, as to not accidentally step on the pedal and produce unnecessary radiation; a diagnostic fluorography can in most cases (but not always) be limited to a single cardiac cyclus; direct stenting can also be used and is proven to reduce beam-on time [17,18].

Intensity of radiation should also be minimized. This can be done in several ways. As noted earlier, the tube current and voltage can be modulated up to a point. An easier way to reduce the intensity would be by reducing the pulse rate, in some devices marked as 'frame rate'. This can also be done to a point where the radiation is minimal, while the images are adequate for performing the procedure.

Distance from the source of radiation must be maximized. It is advisable for the operator to stand away from the tube as much as possible, while being able to operate the equipment, the catheters, syringes, etc. Regarding the other staff in the cath lab, anyone who is not needed inside the room should leave the room, but be readily available to enter as soon as they are needed. All the members of the staff who must stay inside the cath lab should keep their distance from the radiation source at all times, but be ready to attend the patient, or assist the operator on demand. Even small increase of distance from the source of radiation is important, because for each doubling of distance from the source, the intensity of radiation is reduced 4-fold.

Shielding of personnel from the radiation is also of utmost importance. The radiation shields come in several types. The ones above the patient are connected to an anchor point in the ceiling and should be moveable, so that they can be adjusted to the patient's position and size (fig. 5, fig. 6). These shields protect the operator and the assisting staff from the radiation scattered from the patient's body. Some cardio-angiographic tables have the lower shields attached at the table sides, and the angulation of those shields can be altered to provide the best possible operator and staff protection from the scattered radiation off the posterior aspect of the supine patient, but also from the radiation generated by the tube, which is located beneath the patient (fig. 5, fig. 6). These shielding drapes significantly protect the operator from scattered radiation [19,20]. In some cases these shields are not connected to the tables themselves, but are free-standing. These shields protect the operator's legs and feet, which are among the most exposed body parts of the operator. There is further shielding in the walls, floors, and the ceiling of the cath lab in order to protect the people outside the cath lab.

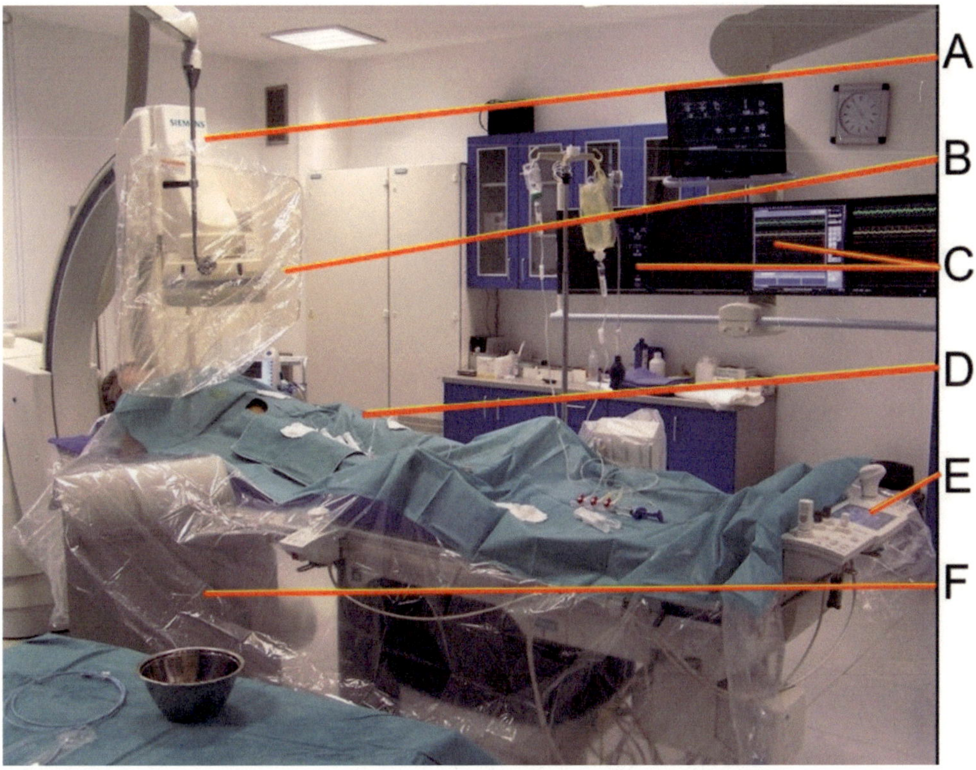

Figure 5. Patient position and shielding in the cath lab. Legend: A – digital flat panel detector mounted on C-arm; B – ceiling-mounted articulated protection screen; C – monitors; D – patient; E – C-arm and image contriol panel; F – table-side protective shielding.

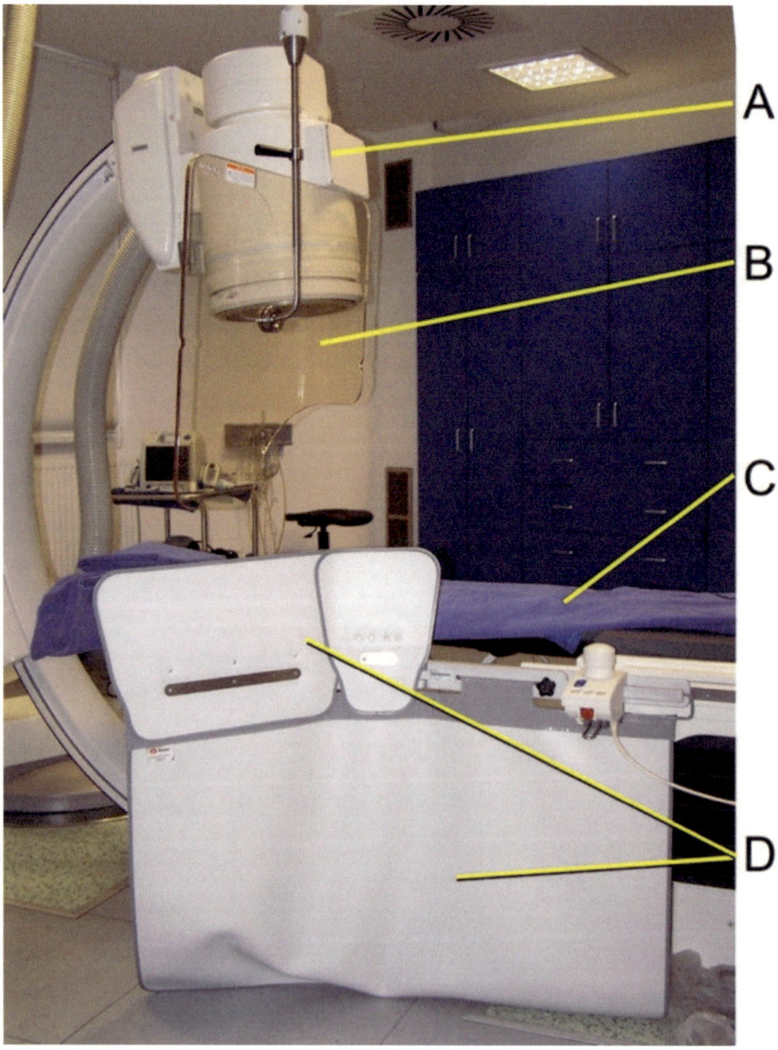

Figure 6. Radiation shields. Legend: A – image intensifier; B – Articulated, ceiling-mounted radiation protection screen; C – patient position; D – table-side shields.

The staff inside the cath lab must also wear the personal protection (fig. 7), which comes in several types and sizes. It is very important that one wears an adequate size protection garments. Firstly, lead apron should be worn. They come in different lead- or lead-equivalent thickness, and can weigh some 15 kg. It is advisable to wear the aprons which cover both the front and the back of the person. Because they may be heavy and put strain to the skeletal system, belts are used to take the weight off the shoulders. The minimum of protection is the equivalent of 0.5 mm of lead at the front. A two piece (blouse-plus-skirt design) is preferred by some operators. Another shield can be worn around the neck to protect the thyroid and neck tissues and organs (fig. 7). An additional small apron can be worn around the waist to increase the protection of the gonads (fig. 7). Since eyes can be affected when exposed to radiation over a prolonged period of time, it is advisable to wear leaded eyeglasses, or face-masks which are secured on the head (fig. 7). Protective eyewear must have at least the equivalent of protection of 0.5 mm of lead. Some recent investigations on the head exposure to radiation have resulted in a recommendation that leaded caps should also be worn.

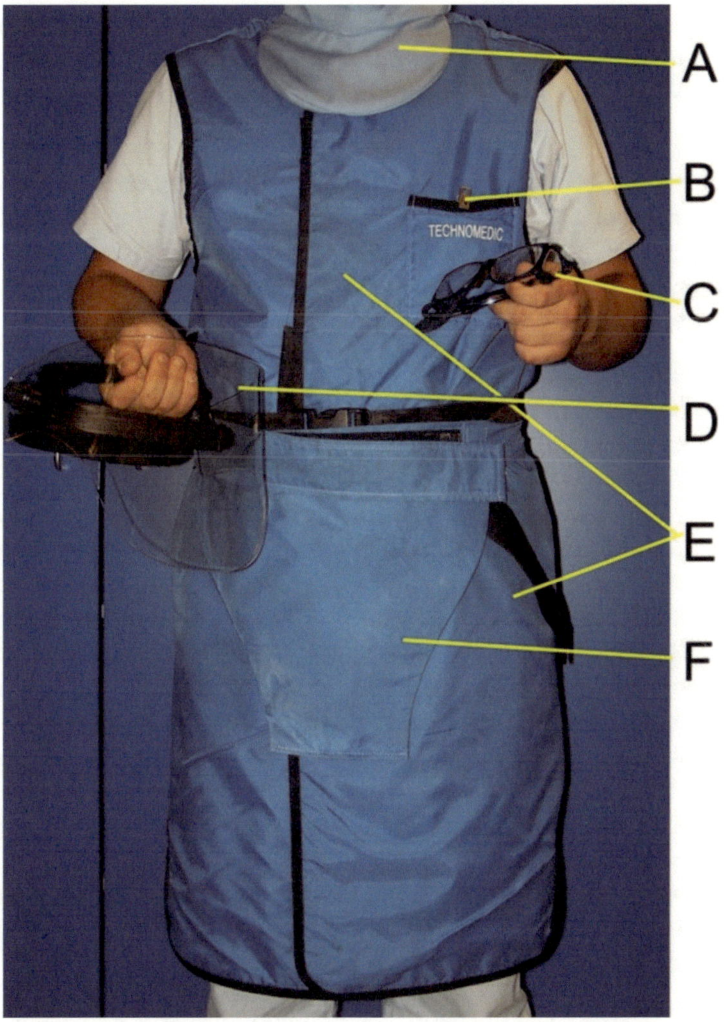

Figure 7. Personal protection for members of the staff in the cath lab. Legend: A –thyroid protection collar; B – outside personal dosimeter (in the pocket); C – protective eyeglasses; D – radiation panoramic full face mask for face shielding (preffered to eyeglasses); E – protective one-piece apron; F – additional protection for the gonads.

A cap with only 0.5 mm lead equivalence was proven to be more protective than a ceiling-mounted shield with 1.0 mm lead equivalence [21] This indicates that a significant amount of secondary scatter radiation, reflected from the walls of the cath lab, may reach the interventionist's head, despite the presence of a ceiling mounted lead glass shield, and this shield is actually designed to protect the operator's head from the primary scatter radiation from the patient. The annual head dose sustained by interventional cardiologists can be quite high, raising the issue of not only the cataract, but also brain tumors. The head dose may reach 60 mSv a year, and may in some cases exceed the occupational limit of 150 mSv a year recommended for the lens of the eye [22]. This information is the cause of the current consideration of the risks of radiation induced cataracts and malignancy, particularly brain cancer [23,24]. Primary scatter to the operator's unprotected head is highest for left anterior oblique (LAO) tube angulations [21]. However, some argue that a careful use of the lead glass shield provides similar protection of the operator's brain [20,25].

The exposure of the operator in general is higher when LAO projections are used, as opposed to RAO projections. The RAO positions are better regarding the operator dose, because the x-ray entrance point into the patient is kept away from the operator [3]. The RAO 90°, for example, exposes the interventionist to some three times less less scattered radiation than the usually used LAO 90° projection [26].

Even the line of interventonist's vision is important in this regard. The monitors in the cath lab are usually placed so that the patient can also follow the procedure, meaning that the monitors are to the interventionist's left front field of vision. For the operator, even leaning the head to the left increases the radiation exposure, and also the whole body posture is affected by this – the interventionist then stands closer to the x-ray tube, and to the source of scattered radiation. Just looking towards the tube exposes the lower parts of the face to levels 4–10 times greater than does looking rightwards [21]. Knowing that the monitor position typically determines the operator's predominant line of vision in interventional cardiology, it is advisable to place the monitors to the operator's right front side. By placing the monitors into the interventionist's right front part of the field of vision (fig. 5), radiation exposure of the interventonist's head can be dramatically reduced. This way, regardless of tube angulation, the lowest scatter towards the operator's head will occur in a line of vision toward the foot of the table. This means that in order to protect the eye lenses and the brain, interventional cardiologists should try to work with monitors positioned to the right [21]. Since the operator's hands might sometimes be directly under an x-ray beam, there are even sets of sterile leaded gloves (for single use, of course) that can be worn, although the material is obviously thicker than that used for normal sterile gloves, and the tactile feeling in the hands and at the operator's fingertips is not very precise.

The cath lab should be in a room of adequate size. Large rooms of some 60 m^2 are preferred not only because they are comfortable to work in, but also because in such rooms it is easy to employ the 'distance' and the 'shielding' principles of radiation protection [10]. A certain amount of space is also required for the ceiling-mounted radiation shields. Since the amount of radiation is reduced by the square distance from the source, in large rooms it is easy to distance and therefore protect oneself from radiation much better than in small rooms with limited space to move or stand. By staying inside the cath lab at the same time, assisting personnel can be readily available to attend the patient when needed.

The equipment used in cardio-angiology is some of the most sophisticated and complex used in medicine today. It must be well-maintained and the users must be well trained in using it. As stated before, in all modern cardiology units, each fluoroscopic image is captured using a short pulse of x-ray beam. The pulse itself lasts for 3-10 ms. Longer pulses would appear blurry since structures observed in cardiology move. The pulse rate is identical to the image capture rate, and between pulses no radiation is being produced. At pulse rate of 30 images per second, the human eye perceives the series of fast changing images as a seemingly continuous motion. However, the amount of radiation at this pulse rate might be excessive. Reducing the pulse rate by half reduces (roughly by half) the amount of radiation to the exposed persons, and slightly affects the sequence quality, but usually not as much as to negatively affect the procedure. For large patients who require larger amounts of radiation to penetrate their bodies, reduction of pulse rate can mean the difference between no skin injury and the occurrence of radiation burns. Dose-rate control can also be achieved through modulating pulse width, tube current, beam energy, and filtration, but not all of these parameters can be controlled by the operator sometimes. The optimal control of these parameters means that the interventionist will choose the dose-rate mode which gives the smallest amount of radiation, while at the same time enabling adequate image quality.

A very important factor in determining the amount of radiation which will be used is the size of the patients. Smaller patients demand less radiation, and the image is brighter, crisper, and with better contrast. Bigger patients, however, demand larger amounts of radiation to obtain the same image quality. That amount is further increased with steeply angulated projections, so the operator must be aware of this while working with larger patients, and choose the projections wisely, to adequately display the region of interest while, at the same time, maintain the lowest radiation dose possible. When the lesions are difficult to treat, that prolongs the beam-on time and doses can be extremely high. Positioning the patient on cardio-angiographic table also plays a role in radiation exposure. To protect the patient against radiation burns, and oneself from scattered radiation, the operator is advised to keep the patient higher, farther away from the radiation source, and at the same time closer to the image receptor [5,6,7].

4.4. Radiation dose monitoring

Today, the modern cardio-angiographic devices are equipped with dose-monitoring systems which record the amount of radiation and calculate the exposure of the patient. There are also simpler methods, such as film-monitoring in which a film layer is positioned beneath the patient, roughly at the site of the beam entrance. The film is sensitive to radiation and becomes darker with higher doses. It is examined after the procedure (or during the procedure if necessary), and a simple device estimates the exposure based on the degree of the film darkening. This method is very good for estimating the skin exposure when the beam enters from posterior, but lacks preciseness if very angulated or lateral projections are used.

Automated devices for exposure measurement usually measure air kerma. The unit of measurement is Gy. It is the sum of initial kinetic energies of all charged particles liberated by the x-rays per mass of air. This measures the amount of radiation at a point in space and can assess the level of hazard at the specified location. Most modern devices used in interventional cardiology have a built-in monitor of total accumulation of air kerma at a reference point, and this point in interventional cardiology approximates the position of the skin where the beam enters the patient. It adds up the radiation from all projections, making it in this sense more convenient than the film monitor, but it approximates, so the true result might be different from the measured value. Some machines have the possibility to measure kerma-area product and dose-area product. The logic of these devices is based on the fact that the beam area increases with the distance from the source, and the air kerma decreases. Theoretically, the product of these values is the same at all positions along the beam. This is primarily a quality control measurement, and if one wants to calculate the dose to the patient, usually a medical physicist must be consulted, because such calculations can be quite complicated.

As for the staff, radiation monitors must be worn at all times during the procedure. This way the exposure of the staff can be measured. It is necessary for interventional cardiologists and other personnel employed in the cath lab to wear personal radiation exposure monitors (dosimeters) on a regular basis, although sometimes this is not the case. Sometimes dosimeters are not worn because of a lack of awareness of risks associated with radiation and/or lack of education in radiation protection [27]. In some institutions or countries, regulatory bodies demand that the monitors are placed outside the protective aprons, while others demand that they must be worn underneath the protection garments. In some hospitals (as is the case in the hospital in which the author works), two monitors must be worn per person: one on the outside, and the other one beneath the protective apron. The one outside records the exposure of the unprotected areas (fig. 7). If only that one is worn, it can be approximated that the dose underneath 0.5 mm of lead equivalent is 0.5% of the dose measured on the outside monitor. Wearing only under-the-apron monitor may give the operator a false sense of security and lead to potentially heavy exposure of the unprotected body parts. Also, the monitoring of the exposure at the hands and legs/feet should be considered, at least periodically. Beside wearing the monitors, the staff working inside the radiation environment must undergo periodical clinical examinations to evaluate the state of their skin, to detect vision impairment, to do blood tests, and to check for chromosomal abnormalities, and possibly other diagnostic measures, as defined by the responsible regulatory bodies. Sometimes, if the doses of radiation exposure found in an employee are larger than recommended, the employee will be ordered to be removed from the radiation environment, temporarily or permanently.

5. Pregnancy and x-ray radiation in the cath lab

There are two ways in which the pregnancy can affect radiologic procedures in a cath lab: either one of the staff is pregnant, or the patient is pregnant. Both situations warrant a careful approach and need to be mentioned.

If a member of the staff is pregnant, different regulatory bodies define different forms of radiologic protection for the woman and the fetus. In some countries, the recommendations are that the fetus must be protected, while not interfering with the future mother's ability to do her job. The employees, both men and women, must be introduced to radiation safety measures in connection with reproductive issues. Usually, there is also a recommendation that all female employees of childbearing potential carry a whole-body dosimeter on the outside of the protective apron, as well as a dosimeter worn under the apron, at the abdominal level. The readings on these dosimeters must not exceed 0.25 mGy per month, thus ensuring that the conceptus receives less than a half of a maximum allowed dose recommended by the professional agencies (which is 0.5 mGy). A pregnant employee must be provided with an option to wear an additional pelvic shield of 0.25 to 0.5 mm of lead equivalent material. The employee should also be provided with duties involving less radiation exposure, if at all possible. In some countries, as is the case in the author's country, the pregnant employee who works in a medical radiation environment has the right to start pregnancy-leave at the very beginning of the pregnancy, and continue with it up to one year postpartum. It is the author's firm belief that all pregnant employees must be given an option to take pregnancy-leave as soon as they learn they are pregnant, so no unnecessary radiation risks, small as they might be, are imposed on the fetus and the pregnant mother-to-be.

When there is a pregnant patient in the cath lab, it is usually a patient with an acute coronary syndrome (ACS). Although pregnant women rarely have ACS, this is possible and the staff must be prepared for such an event. With general population, percutaneous coronary intervention (PCI) is the preferred treatment modality for an acute myocardial infarction. On the other hand, PCI in pregnancy includes the exposure of fetus to ionizing radiation. High doses of radiation carry the risk of a spontaneous abortion, fetal organ deformities, fetal mental retardation and a higher incidence of childhood cancer. However, radiation doses received by fetus during a PCI on a pregnant woman are completely acceptable and PCI can and must be performed in a pregnant woman with an ACS. Before the introduction of the practice of ACS treatment by using PCI, ACS mortality in pregnancy was as high as 20% [28]. Today, by using PCI in the treatment of ACS, the mortality from ACS in pregnancy is reduced to only 5% [29]. During the invasive cardiologic procedures, the x-ray beam is directed to the patient's chest. Some of the radiation does penetrate even to the fetus, and a part of it is scattered radiation from the mother's body. Contemporary cardio-angiography machines, with excellent beam collimation and a precise beam direction, have very little primary beam dissipation. Since that kind of radiation is still theoretically possible, it is mandatory to protect the pregnant patient's abdomen with protective leaded aprons. The mean exposure of a fetus during a PCI procedure is 0.02 mSv, and in very difficult and time-consuming procedures can reach up to 0.1 mSv. These doses are acceptable, and are even relatively small when compared to computer tomography (CT) scan of the abdomen (8 mSv on average, to a maximum of 49 mSv), pelvic CT scan (25 mSv on average, to a maximum of 79 mSv), abdominal radiography (1.4 mSv on average, with a maximum of up to 4.2 mSv), or even a CT-scan of the thorax (0.06 mSv on average, to a maximum of 0.96 mSv). Doses over 50-100 mSv increase the incidence of fetal malformation. The radiation which is scattered from the directly irradiated body part reaches the fetus, but this is only a small fraction of the radiation dose reaching the pregnant patient's thorax [5]. Although it protects from a direct beam, the leaded apron at the patient's abdomen will not protect the fetus from the scattered radiation within the patient's (pregnant woman's) body. Taken into account the spectre of causes of an acute myocardial infarction during pregnancy, PCI will in most cases be the treatment of choice during pregnancy. Not only that it treats the thromboembolic processes, but their causes can be treated also, namely the coronary dissection, which is a disproportionally common cause of ACS in pregnancy, probably because of the alterations in the connective tissue structure (including that within the coronary artery walls) mediated by pregnancy hormones. Once again, PCI is considered to be relatively safe during pregnancy, both for the pregnant patient and for the fetus and it must be employed as the first line of treatment for ACS in pregnancy because it dramatically reduces ACS mortality for pregnant women.

6. Conclusion

In conclusion, although the discovery of the x-ray radiation is more than 100 years old, the x-ray technology is developing as fast as ever. As much as we need to learn about its usefulness and the different forms of its application, we must always be aware of its dangers, risks, and limitations, and use it with care and adequately protect ourselves and our patients.

Author details

Jasmin Čaluk

BH Heart Center, Department of interventional cardiology, Tuzla, Bosnia and Herzegovina

References

[1] Novelline R. Squire's Fundamentals of Radiology. Harvard University Press. 5th edition. 1997.

[2] Tsapaki V, Maniatis PN, Magginas A et al.: What are the clinical and technical factors that influence the kerma-area product in percutaneous coronary intervention? Br. J. Radiol 2008;81:949–945.

[3] Saunamaki KI. Radiation Protection in the Cardiac Catheterization Laboratory. Interv Cardiol 2010;2(5):667-672.

[4] Cusma JT. X-Ray Cinefluorographic Systems. In: King SB & Yeung AC (eds.) Interventional Cardiology. The McGraw-Hill Companies, Inc, 2007.p109-119.

[5] Hirshfeld JW, Balter S, Brinker et al.: ACCF/AHA/SCAI Clinical competence statement on physician knowledge to optimize patient safety and image quality in fluoroscopically guided invasive cardiovascular procedures. Circulation 2005;111:511–532.

[6] Kuon E, Dahm JB, Robinson DM, et al: Radiation-reducing planning of cardiac catherization. Z. Kardiol 2005; 94: 663–673.

[7] Bashore TM: Radiation safety in the catherization laboratory. Am. Heart J 2004;147:375–378.

[8] Vano E, Gonzales L, Fernandez JM, et al: Influence of patient thickness and operation modes on occupational and patient radiation doses in interventional cardiology. Radiat. Prot. Dosimetry 2006;118:325–330.

[9] Reay J, Chapple CL, Kotre CJ: Is patient size important in dose determination and optimization in cardiology? Phys. Med. Biol 2003;48:3843–3850.

[10] Wagner LK. Operational Radiation Management for Patients and Staff. In: King SB & Yeung AC (eds.) Interventional Cardiology. The McGraw-Hill Companies, Inc, 2007.p121-135.

[11] Miller SW, Castronovo FP. Radiation exposure and protection in cardiac catheterisation laboratories.Am J Cardiol 1985;55:171–6.

[12] Yoshinaga S, Mabuchi K, Sigurdson AJ, et al. Cancer risks among radiologists and radiologic technologists: review of epidemiologic studies. Radiology 2004;233(2): 313-21.

[13] Wagner LK. Overconfidence, overexposure, and overprotection. Radiology. 2004;233(2):307-8.

[14] Venneri L, Rossi F, Botto N et al.: Cancer risk from professional exposure in staff working in cardiac catheterization laboratory: insights from the National Research Council's Biological Effects of Ionizising Radiation VII Report. Am. Heart J 2009;157:118–124.

[15] International Commission on Radiological Protection. ICRP Publication 85. Avoidance of radiation injuries from medical interventional procedures. Annals ICRP 2000;30(2). Oxford: Pergamon, Elsevier Science Ltd.

[16] Mercuri M, Xie C, Levy M, et al: Predictors of increased radiation dose during percutaneous coronary intervention. Am. J. Cardiol 2009;104:1241–1244.

[17] Caluk J, Osmanovic E, Barakovic F, et al. Direct coronary stenting in reducing radiation and radiocontrast consumption. Radiol Oncol 2010; 44(3): 153-157.

[18] Larrazet F, Dibie A, Philippe F, et al: Factors influencing fluoroscopy time and dose–area product values during ad hoc one-vessel percutaneous coronary angioplasty. Br. J. Radiol 2003;76:473–477.

[19] Miller DL, Vano E, Bartal G et al.: Occupational radiation protection in interventional radiology: a Joint Guideline of the Cardiovascular and and Interventional Radiology Society of Europe and the Society of Interventional Radiology. J Vasc Interv Radiol 2010;21(5):607-15.

[20] Shortt CP, Al-Hashimi H, Malone L, Lee MJ: Staff radiation doses to the lower extremities in interventional radiology. Cardiovasc. Interv. Radiol 2007;30:1206–1209.

[21] Kuon E, Birkel J, Schmitt M, Dahm JB. Radiation exposure benefit of a lead cap in invasive cardiology. Heart 2003;89:1205–1210.

[22] Renaud L. A 5-year follow up of the radiation exposure to in-room personnel during cardiac catheterization. Health Phys 1992;62:10–15.

[23] Folkerts KH, Münz A, Jung S. Estimation of radiation exposure and radiation risk to staff of cardiac catheterization laboratories. Z Kardiol 1997;86:258–63.

[24] Finkelstein MM. Is brain cancer an occupational disease of cardiologists? Can J Cardiol 1998;14:1385–8.

[25] Maeder M, Brunner-La Rocca HP, Wolber T et al.: Impact of lead glass screen on scatter radiation to eyes and hands in interventional cardiologists. Catheter. Cardiovasc. Interv 2006;67:18–23.

[26] Kuon E, Dahm JB, Empen K, et al: Identification of less-irradiating tube angulations in invasive cardiology. J. Am. Coll. Cardiol 2004;44:1420–1428.

[27] Niklason LT, Marx MV, Chan HP. Interventional radiologists: occupational radiation doses and risks. Radiology 1993;187:729–33.

[28] Roth A, Elkayam U. Acute myocardial infarction associated with pregnancy. Ann Intern Med. 1996;125(9):751-62.

[29] James AH, Jamison MG, Biswas MS et al.: Acute myocardial infarction in pregnancy: a United States population-based study. Circulation 2006;113(12):1564-1571.

Chapter 4

Noninvasive Modalities for Coronary Angiography

Karthikeyan Ananthasubramaniam,
Sabha Bhatti and Abdul Hakeem

Additional information is available at the end of the chapter

http://dx.doi.org/10.5772/54082

1. Introduction

Optimal diagnostic quality non-invasive alternatives for visualization of the coronary arteries has been a major goal with the advent of newer cardiovascular imaging modalities such as coronary computed tomography angiography (CCTA) and magnetic resonance coronary angiography (MRCA). The challenges in imaging coronaries are obvious. The technology must be capable of visualizing arteries as small as 1.5 mm to delineate luminal and wall pathology which becomes challenging as many of the arteries are engulfed in tissue of similar composition. Coronary arteries exhibit rapid motion which poses major issues with blurring of images due to substantial limitations of temporal resolution. Invasive coronary angiography current enjoys the best temporal resolution (less than 20 msec) for real time visualization of coronaries and its branches but comes with its obvious limitations. CCTA has rapidly risen to this challenge and is already widely employed using 64 slice detector technology and is outstanding for exclusion of CAD with substantial advances in radiation reduction and speed of acquisition. MRCA has made significant improvements in technology which has made coronary imaging less challenging using navigator gating, whole heart imaging and using 3Tesla magnets, with the big advantage of no radiation and capability of non-contrast coronary imaging and most of all the promise of a true " one stop " comprehensive assessment. However, it is still suboptimal compared to CCTA as discussed subsequently in detail. This chapters aims to discuss MRCA and CCTA with regards to coronary imaging and compare and contrast both these imaging modalities with one another and also highlight some emerging comparisons of CCTA to invasive coronary luminal assessment technologies.

2. Magnetic Resonance Coronary Angiography (MRCA)

Introduction: MRCA has been performed for close to 20 years with numerous advances in technical and imaging aspects during this period although slower than CCTA explaining its slower adoption [1]. Initially 2 dimensional k space segmented imaging was done, but most centers now use whole heart free breathing navigator coronary MRI or targeted 3D imaging to enable better reconstruction capabilities. Published studies from experienced centers have shown excellent accuracy and superiority to conventional coronary angiography (CA) using 2 and 3 dimensional k space gradient echo MRCA (Table 1)[2]..

Although whole heart MRCA was initially performed with 4 channel cardiac coils and a parallel imaging factor of 2 [3, 4] it has been limited due longer acquisition times and image deterioration from diaphragmatic drift. Thirty two channel cardiac coils and higher parallel imaging factor of 4 [5] has potential for enhanced coronary imaging with whole heart MRCA. 3T MRCA gives higher signal to noise ratio (approximately 30%) but has its own limitations such as constructive/destructive interference in images causing dark and bright areas due to inherent in-homogeneities which worsen with strong magnetic fields [6]. Also specific absorption rates can increase upto 4 fold with 3T systems limiting use of certain imaging sequences. There are multiple components of MRCA namely cardiac triggering to suppress cardiac motion, respiratory motion suppression (navigator, breath hold) pre-pulses to enhance contrast noise ratio and image acquisition to enhance coronary arterial image quality. Overall image sequences for coronaries include black blood (fast spin echo and dual inversion) bright blood (segmented k space gradient echo and SSFP) all of which can be used either with 2D or 3D imaging.

Investigator	Technique	Respiratory Compensation	Number of Subjects	RCA	LM	LAD	LCX
Manning, 1993	2D GRE	BH	25	100%	96%	100%	76%
Pennell, 1993	2D GRE	BH	26	95%	95%	91%	76%
Duerinckx, 1994	2D GRE	BH	20	100%	95%	86%	77%
Sakuma, 1994	2D GRE cine	BH	18	100%	100%	100%	67%
Masui, 1995	2D GRE	BH	13	85%	92%	100%	92%
Davis, 1996	2D GRE	BH	33*	100%	100%	100%	100%
Li, 1993	3D GRE	Multiple Averages	14	100%	100%	86%	93%
Post, 1996	3D GRE	Retro Nav G	20	100%	100%	100%	100%
Wielopoiski, 1998	3D Seg EPI	BH	32	100%	100%	100%	100%
Botnar, 1999	3D GRE	Pro Nav G/C	13	97%	100%	100%	97%
Weber, 2003	3D SSFP	Pro Nav G/C	12	100%	100%	100%	100%

Abbreviations: BH, breath hold; GRE, gradient echo; LAD, left anterior descending coronary artery; LCX, left circumflex coronary artery; LM, left main coronary artery; PRO Nav GAC, prospective navigator gating with correction; RCA, right coronary artery; Retro Nav, retrospective navigator gating; Seg EPL, segmented EPI; SSFP, steady state free precession, 3D

Table 1. Successful visualization of native coronary arteries using 2 and 3 dimensional k space gradient echo MRCA [2].Obtained with permission

http://dx.doi.org/10.5772/54082

3. Challenges for MRCA

Achieving optimal spatial and temporal resolution, accurate motion compensation, wide anatomical coverage, and high signal and contrast to noise ratios are inherent challenges in MRCA. Improvement in one parameter occurs at the expense of another. Other factors that limit its widespread application in the acute setting include longer exam time, limited clinical monitoring in the scanner, device implants and other metallic objects that may need clearance prior to scanning.

Cardiac motion compensation deserves special mention. Since the heart moves due to both inherent motion and due to diaphragmatic movement and as the magnitude of this motion is greater than the diameter of the coronary vessels substantial blurring occurs if motion suppression techniques are not utilized [7]. A regular cardiac rhythm and reliable ECG gating is crucial for cardiac motion suppression techniques to work. Also time intervals of acquisition has to be determined in advance to plan the preparatory pulses which is a limitation. Acquisition is usually in mid-diastole due to least coronary motion and lasts for 50-150 milliseconds per cardiac cycle [8, 9].

As breath holds may be long during coronary imaging and impossible for some patients free breathing MRCA is an alternative and numerous correction techniques such as multiple averaging, chest wall bellows and navigator techniques have been attempted of which the latter is the most widely used [10].

MRCA Acquisition Methods:

1. Pulse sequences:

Pulse sequence design has evolved from black blood spin echo sequences to bright blood sequences such as gradient echo and steady state free precession (SSFP) imaging. Currently GRE is the chosen acquisition scheme in the majority of MRCA studies.

2. Acquisition strategies:

This includes k-space acquisition, contrast –enhanced (intrinsic and extrinsic) MRCA, 2D and 3D acquisitions. Despite many advances, the speed of acquisition and signal to noise ratio (SNR) remain limited. New strategies such as real time, parallel, time resolved and whole heart imaging have been developed.

1. CONVENTIONAL SPIN ECHO MRI: A spin echo signal results from a 90^0 RF pulse followed by a 180^0 pulse which refocuses the dephased spins up to a decay curve determined by the T2 relaxation time.

2. 2D SEGMENTED k SPACE GRADIENT ECHO MRI: The most widely available MRCA sequence is a 2D segmented k-space gradient echo acquisition usually performed in a single breath hold of fewer than 12 heartbeats. Thick slices and breath hold variability can limit registration of images from slice to slice however this sequence is adequate for applications such as evaluation for anomalous coronaries.

3. 3D MRI: The use of navigator respiratory gating has given access to three-dimensional (3D) coronary magnetic resonance imaging techniques, allowing a 3D dataset to be obtained in a single acquisition. It provides higher spatial resolution and is less operator dependent. However, it relies on a reproducible respiratory pattern, which is not always present. Furthermore, 3D techniques are hampered by the saturation of blood signal, which decreases the signal to-noise ratio and the contrast of blood to myocardium.

4. CONTRAST ENHANCED CORONARY MRI: The use of interstitial paramagnetic contrast agents allows an improvement of signal and contrast. The disadvantage is the rapid leakage out of the intravascular space, amounting to 50% during the first pass. Multiple injections are necessary to cover the whole coronary artery tree. With the introduction of intravascular paramagnetic contrast agents [11, 12], the signal from blood no longer relies on inflow of blood but rather on the presence of the contrast agent itself. The imaging time can be prolonged with potential increased signal and in contrast, allowing a larger volume coverage and higher resolution.

5. 3T MRI: Imaging at higher field strength can enhance signal-to-noise ratio (SNR) and enable higher spatial resolution. However, image quality may be hampered by increased susceptibility artifacts and RF inhomogeneity which may be addressed by shortening the TE and acquisition time. High-field imaging at 3 Tenhances spiral MRCA. A number of research groups already have demonstrated the feasibility of cardiac imaging at 7 T and beyond and have shown improved contrast between blood and epicardial fat, better coronary vessel sharpness, and increased blood signal intensity of the coronaries are obtained at 7 T than at 3 T [13].

Clinical Applications:

1. Anomalous coronary arteries:

C-MRA provides a 3D spatial relationship to great vessels, allowing evaluation of the origin and course of anomalous coronary arteries. Accurate delineation of proximal course has been shown with a sensitivity of 88-100% and specificity of 100% [14-19] MRI can often provide a definitive diagnosis in patients in whose X ray angiography is inconclusive. See Table 2

Investigator	Number of patients	Correctly Classified Anomalous Vessels
McConnell, 1995	15	14 (93%)
Post, 1995	19	19 (100%)
Vilegen, 1997	12	11 (92%)
Taylor, 2000	25	24 (96%)
Bunce, 2003	26	26 (100%)
Razmi, 2001	12	12 (100%)

Table 2. Anomalous coronary assessment by MRCA.[2] (reproduced with permission)

2. Coronary Artery Disease:

Clinical studies have produced variable results. Kim et al [20] performed the first multicenter trial in 109 patients with suspected CAD. Overall sensitivity and specificity was 93 and 42%, respectively. 84% of coronary segments were of diagnostic quality. Table 1 shows the comparative sensitivities of MRCA to CA. An example of MRCA coronary artery delineation is shown in Figures 1A and 1B

Sakuma et al [21] evaluated over 130 patients with significant CAD and found an overall accuracy of 87%, per patient sensitivity of 82% and specificity of 90%

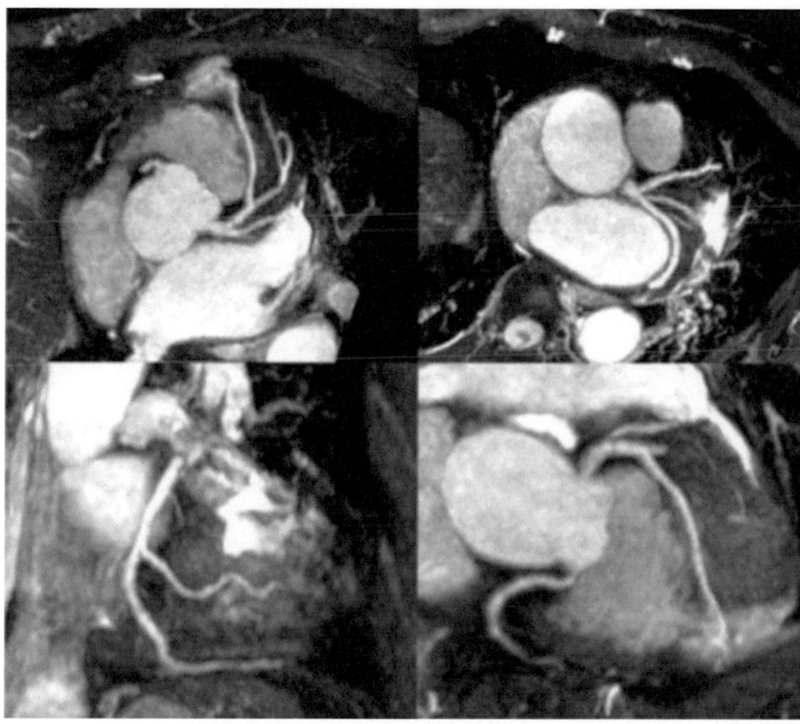

Figure 1. Sliding partial MIP images of 3 T whole heart coronary MRA acquired with a patient-specific narrow acquisition window (50 ms) in the cardiac cycle Journal of Cardiovascular Magnetic Resonance **Vol.** 11 **Issue** Suppl 1 2009-01-2

4. Coronary Computed Tomoraphy Angiography (CCTA)

Introduction: CCTA has been rapidly adopted in a short time span by institutions across the world as the most widely used anatomic noninvasive imaging modality for coronary artery assessment. A major reason for this is the existing wide use of CT for non-cardiac applications and most institutions have access to a CT scanner. Thus, investing in a state of the art

CT scanner serves multiple purposes and makes financial sense with opportunity for cardiac and non-cardiac use. Although initially limited to electron beam scanners in the 1980's where imaging of the heart arteries took several seconds and processing several hours, with the advent of multi-detector coronary computed CT technology (MDCT or multi slice (MSCT)) in the late 1990's, rapid advancement in scanner technology has enabled rapid whole heart acquisitions in a few seconds. With such scanners post processing capabilities on a 3D dataset is usually achievable in about 15-20 minutes.

CCTA requires high temporal resolution to minimize motion artifacts caused by cardiac motion and breathing. This requires a fast gantry rotation with multiple detectors. Because the coronaries are seen best when there is least motion, the diastolic phase is most optimal for imaging and thus the temporal resolution must be less than the length of the diastolic phase. High spatial resolution is also necessary to allow imaging of the coronary arteries which are small and tortuous. At present, 64-detector row CT systems are the most widely employed platform for performing CCTA. The 64 detectors allow an x-,y- axis (in-plane) spatial resolution of near 0.4mm and the z-axis spatial resolution or slice thickness is almost 0.6mm. Fast contiguous coverage of the heart is required to allow imaging of the entire heart in one breath hold. This requires the multi-slice helical CT technique, each slice of the heart is collected in one or more heartbeats. There is a 30%-50% overlap between each slice. The scan must be triggered to the heartbeat to allow gating so that imaging in multiple slices occurs across multiple heartbeats. Table 3 below, is a summary of the state of art 64 slice CT scanners with their various technical specifications [22].

Scanner	X-ray sources, n	Detector rows, n	Detector-row x-axis dimension, mm*	Total nominal beam width, mm	Fastest gantry rotation time, second	Temporal resolution for each cross-sectional image, second†
GE Discovery CT750 HD	1	64	0.625	40	0.35	0.175
Hitachi SCENARIA	1	64	0.625	40	0.35	0.175
Philips Brilliance iCT	1	128‡	0.625	80	0.27	0.135
Siemens SOMATOM Definition FLASH	2 (95° apart)	64‡	0.6	40	0.28	0.075
Toshiba Aquilion ONE	1	320	0.5	160	0.35	0.175

*Values measured at scanner isocenter.
†Values do not reflect the use of multisegment reconstruction.
‡Uses z-axis flying focal spot to sample each detector twice per rotation.

Table 3. Reproduced under permission from [22]

Patient preparation:

On the day of the test, patients should take medications as scheduled especially betablockers. Metformin should be avoided because of the potential adverse effects when used concomitantly with iodinated contrast agents. Phosphodiesterase inhibitors should be avoided 48 hours before a CCTA because nitrates are needed to dilate the coronary arteries. Premedication with mucomyst and hydration are recommended if the creatinine is elevated. If a contrast allergy is present, premedication with steroids and antihistamines is required. A right antecubital IV that is at least 18-gauge is preferred. If heart rate is not low enough with oral beta-blockers, IV beta-blockers may be useful.

Data Acquisition:

Two types of ECG gating are possible, prospective and retrospective. Prospective is where the scanner emits radiation only at a predefined point after the R wave. Mid-diastole occurs at 70-75% of the R-R interval and during this time in the cardiac cycle, there is minimum amount of motion enabling better coronary imaging. The CT beam is off during all other points in the cycle. This requires a regular heart rate and is the preferred method of imaging because of the low radiation dose. In retrospective triggering a continuous heart scan is utilized. Imaging is performed throughout systole and diastole. Left ventricular function data is hence available. This method of gating is used if the patient's heart rate is irregular or not low enough for 64 slice CT scanners. Figure 2 below shows the different modes of CCCT acquisition [22].

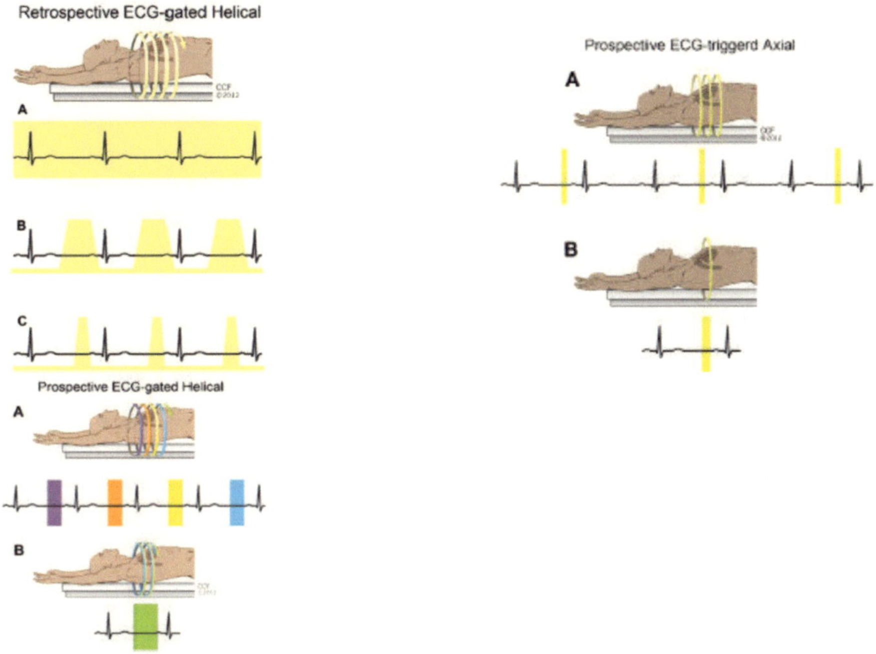

Figure 2. Reproduced under permission from [22]

Radiation Exposure: Reported CTA effective radiation dose is higher than many other cardiac diagnostic procedures as described by the International Commission on Radiological Protection (ICRP) 60 [23]. The rapid expansion of CCTA magnifies the importance of dose reduction within the population. The clinical acceptance of CCTA will partially depend on the radiation exposure and its consequences, particularly if it is going to be used at an earlier stage of CAD detection. Some commonly used dose reduction strategies include:

1. Restricting scan field to anatomy of interest (~1 cm above left main to ~1 cm below heart)
2. Reducing peak mAs based on body size (non-contrast scout films may be used to estimate image noise)
3. Using ECG dependant current modulation with lowest mAs during systole. Narrowing the width of the peak mAs phase
4. Reducing kV to 100 if body Wt is <85 kg
5. Use prospective gating if available.

With regards to radiation exposure numerous algorithms and acquisition techniques have been developed as discussed previously to reduce exposure specifically prospective triggered acquisition [24] and high pitch acquisition with dual source CCTA [25].

5. Limitations

There are several limitations with CCTA. Patients unable to cooperate with scanning instructions should be considered for other imaging modalities. Uncontrollable arrhythmias can result in significant motion artifacts and multiple uninterpretable coronary segments. Contraindications to iodinated contrast use include pregnancy, prior severe/anaphylactic contrast reaction and renal insufficiency (but end-stage renal disease is not a contraindication) for contrast-induced nephropathy. Certain conditions should raise concerns for the use of pre-scan beta-blocker (chronic obstructive pulmonary disease/asthma, decompensated heart failure, and advanced atrioventricular block) and nitroglycerin (severe aortic stenosis, hypertrophic cardiomyopathy, recent phosphodiesterase-5 inhibitor use). Metallic objects such as pacemakers, intra-cardiac defibrillator leads, prosthetic valves cause beam-hardening and streaking artifact over adjacent coronary arteries. Dense concentric coronary calcification causes a blooming artifact, which often leads to overestimation of degree of stenosis.

Clinical Applications:

Most Important Appropriate indications for CCTA

Chest pain evaluation after an uninterpretable or equivocal stress test
Chest pain evaluation in patients with an intermediate probability, an uninterpretable EKG and unable to exercise
Acute chest pain evaluation, an intermediate pretest probability, no EKG changes, and serial enzymes negative
Suspected coronary anomalies in symptomatic patients
Coronary evaluation in new onset heart failure

Table 4.

1. **Anomalous coronary arteries:** CTA provides a 3D spatial relationship to great vessels, allowing evaluation of the origin and course of anomalous coronary arteries in a non–invasive manner. It is the "gold standard" test for evaluating anomalous coronary arteries and has the highest level of appropriateness use for this indication.

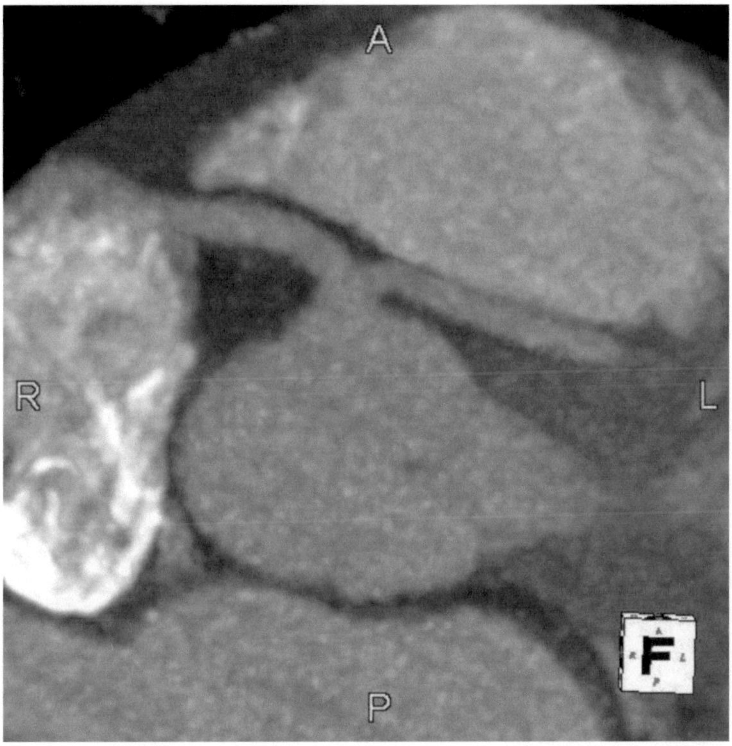

Figure 3. 40 year old male with syncope during exercise. CCTA shows anomalous left main coronary artery take off from right coronary cusp between aorta and RVOT

2. **Coronary artery disease**

i. **Detection of Coronary Stenosis:** With ongoing technical development, the diagnostic performance of CT with respect to detection and quantification of obstructive CAD is steadily improving. The confidence and accuracy to assess stenosis is better in larger branches and in the absence of extensive coronary calcification. For the assessment of individual coronary segments, the sensitivity to detect significant coronary artery stenosis ranges between 64-99%, the specificity between 84- 98%, with pooled average sensitivity of 87% and specificity of 96%. The positive predictive value is approximately 80% whereas the negative predictive value has been consistently high in all the studies with a pooled average of 98%. Calcified coronary disease causes blooming artifacts, which increases apparent stenosis severity of a lesion. The ability to quantify coronary stenosis severity has been modest compared to invasive angiography given the limited spatial resolution of CT and blooming artifacts of calcified lesions. There are numerous single-center [26-34] and three multicenter studies [35-37] using different scanner technologies (Table 4) [35-37] in symptomatic patients with suspected CAD.

				Per-patient base analysis			
Author	Year	Patients	CAD prevalence (%)	Sensitivity	Specificity	Positive predictive value	Negative predictive value
Budoff *et al.*	2008	230	25	95	83	64	99
Miller *et al.*	2008	291	56	85	90	91	83
Meijboom *et al.*	2008	360	68	99	64	86	97

CAD, coronary artery disease.

Table 5. Adapted with permission from Chang et al [38].

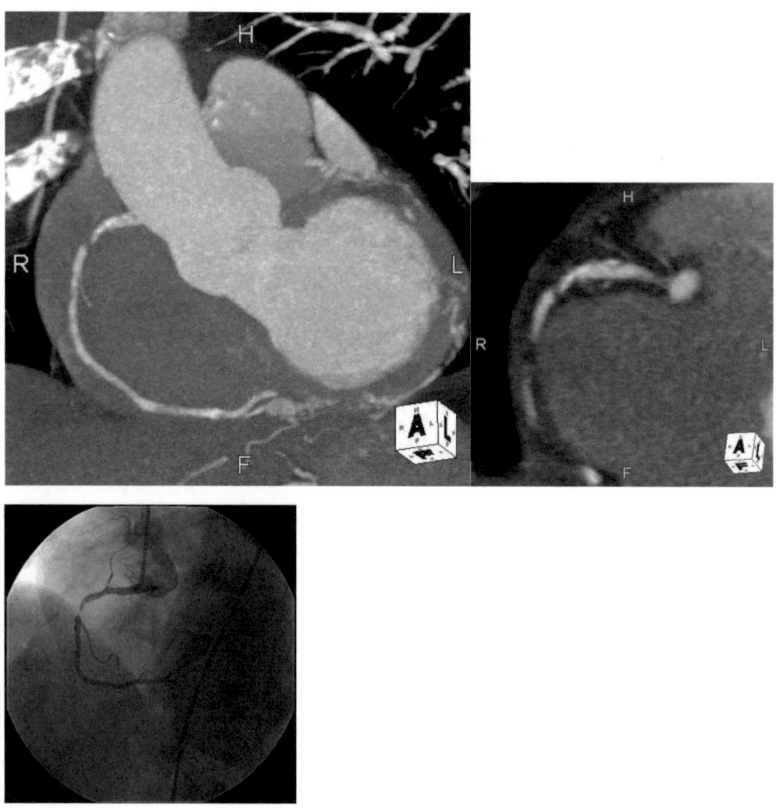

Figure 4. CCTA of a 60 year old smoker with atypical chest pain and sub-maximal negative stress echo. Thick maximum intensity projection (MIP) images and multiplanar reconstruction images (MPR) are shown showing focal high grade stenosis in proximal-mid RCA accompanied by scattered calcified plaques throughout RCA, Coronary angiogram was performed confirming CCTA findings.

http://dx.doi.org/10.5772/54082

ii. **Stents:** CCTA is not optimal for the evaluation of coronary stents because the spatial resolution is not quite good enough to visualize the intrastent lumen, thus should not be routinely used for the evaluation of coronary stents. Small stents tend to cause blooming and beam hardening issues leading to poor delineation of lumen. Lack of contrast in lumen is a sign of in-stent restenosis. Currently, larger stents >3.5-4.0 mm may be adequately assessed [39].

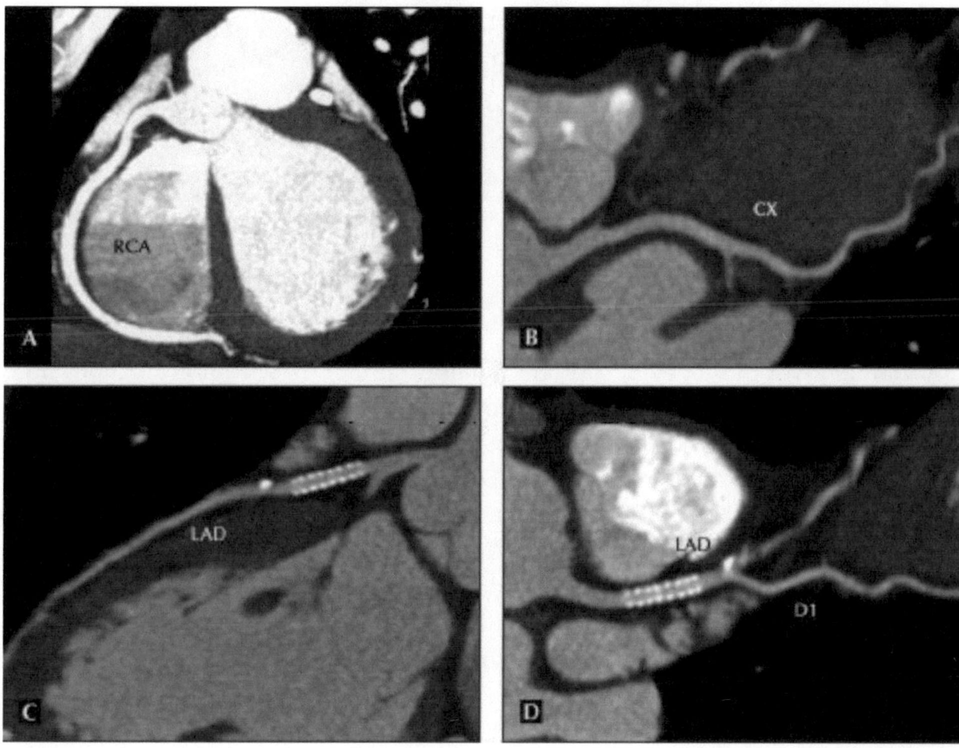

Figure 5. Shows multiplanar reformats of the left anterior descending coronary artery with clear visualization of patent stents and normal right and left circumflex coronary arteries. Reproduced from Cademartiri et al [39].

iii. **Bypass Graft Analysis:** CCTA may be used to assess bypass graft patency as well as to evaluate the patient undergoing repeat bypass surgery. In repeat bypass surgery CCTA is utilized to identify the location of a previously utilized graft. Clips may often create challenges in assessing bypass grafts because of beam hardening artifact and their potential to obscure the graft lumen or anastomosis point. Below is an example of a 3d surface rendering of patient with prior coronary artery bypass surgery (Figure 6) [40]. The saphenous vein graft (SVG) to the right coronary artery is seen taking off from the aorta and inserting into the RCA. The origins of 2 other SVG are also noted adjacent to the SVG to RCA going to the left coronary system. The maximum intensity projection reveals a significant stenosis in the insertion site of the SVG to RCA [40].

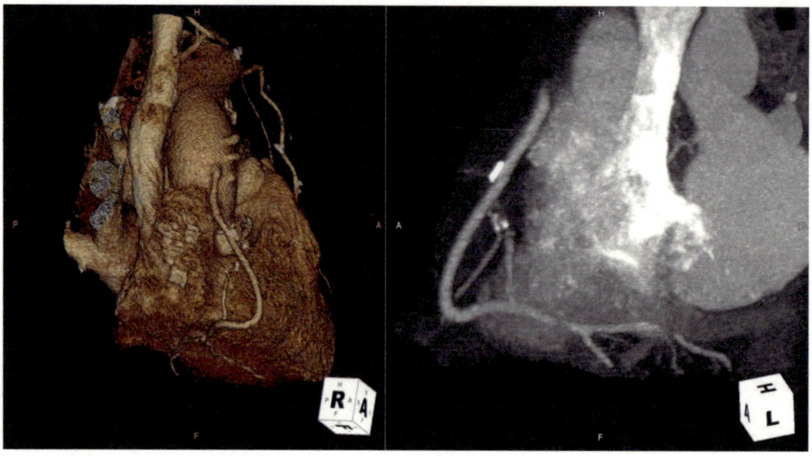

Figure 6.

3. Role of CCTA in Emergency Department:

A significant amount of money is wasted on inappropriate chest pain evaluations and admissions. Given CTA's high NPV, the test would most benefit the intermediate-probability patients in the ED. By using CTA, hospitalization could be avoided in patients presenting to ED with chest pain. Logistic issues such as ED scanner availability and 24 hour expertise in CTA interpretation limit use of CTA in most institutions. Triple rule out protocols have been developed and studied to rule out coronary disease, pulmonary embolism and aortic dissection [27, 41, 42]. These are however not used widely due to logistic issues and since often one or more of these 3 etiologies can be ruled out clinically. A recent meta analysis by Samad et al [43] synthesized data from 9 studies involving 1349 patients presenting to the emergency room with suspected acute coronary syndrome (ACS). Endpoint was the diagnostic performance of CTA for ACS. The bivariate summary estimate of sensitivity of CTA for ACS diagnosis was 95% (95% CI 88-100) and specificity was 87% (95% CI 83-92), yielding a negative likelihood ratio of 0.06 (95% CI 0-0.14) and positive likelihood ratio of 7.4 (95% CI 4.8-10). Based on this meta analysis of all the clinical studies, coronary CTA with its high sensitivity and a low negative likelihood ratio of 0.06, is effective in ruling out the presence of ACS in low to intermediate risk patients presenting to the ED with acute chest pain. More recently the role of CCTA in ER has been studied in 2 important randomized trials the ACRIN-PA [44] and the ROMICAT-2. Both studies showed that CCTA has an outstanding negative predictive value with low subsequent event rates although conventional management including stress testing also achieved comparable results. There was shorter length of stay and quicker discharge directly from ED in CCTA arm although costs were the same between CCTA and conventional testing in ROMICAT-2. Also radiation doses and downstream testing were higher in CCTA arm in ROMICAT-2 [45]. An important point with regards to use of CCTA in ED is that although a zero calcium score makes obstructive CAD highly unlikely as a cause of chest pain it is now clear that young patients (age < 50, smokers) may present

http://dx.doi.org/10.5772/54082

with non-calcified obstructive disease and thus should not be triaged based on a negative calcium score alone (see Figure 7 below)

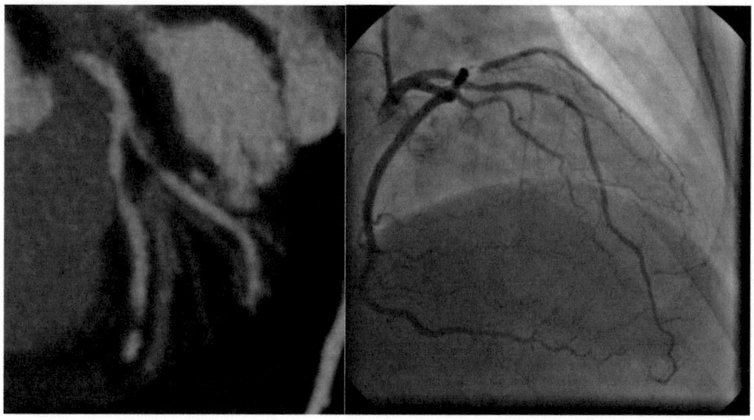

Figure 7. 30 year old male with history of 15 pack history of smoking, cocaine abuse presents with intermittent substernal pressure of 3 days duration. Coronary CT was done. Non-contrast scan showed zero calcium score but CCTA showed high grade stenosis in the LAD and diagonal. The image on left is a view of the mid LAD showing mainly non-calcified obstructive plaque. Coronary angiography confirms high grade LAD.

4. Role of CCTA in Assessing Etiology of Cardiomyopathy

It is extremely important to define the etiology of cardiomyopathies to enable appropriate management and therapies. CCTA can be of critical importance to rule out ischemic cardiomyopathy in a non-invasive manner. CCTA has immensely robust accuracy at evaluating the proximal vascular bed with accuracy approaching almost 97-100%. This attribute becomes most relevant in the context of ischemic cardiomyopathy which per the standardized definition proposed by Felker et al [46][Patients with 75% stenosis of left main or proximal LAD, patients with 75% stenosis of two or more epicardial vessels] yields a very high diagnostic odds ratio for ischemic cardiomyopathy. Several studies have evaluated the diagnostic accuracy of CCTA in comparison with invasive angiography. We performed a meta analysis of all 6 studies involving 452 patients with cardiomyopathy of undetermined cause who underwent CTA. All patients also underwent diagnostic invasive angiography. The pooled summary estimate of sensitivity was 98% and specificity 97% yielding a negative likelihood ratio of 0.06 for ischemic cardiomyopathy. The receiver operator curve analysis showed a robust discriminate diagnostic accuracy of ischemic etiology with an AUC of 0.99(Figure 8). With a pooled sensitivity of 98%, an ischemic etiology of left ventricular systolic dysfunction can be accurately "ruled out" with CTA (>16 slices). A negative study hence essentially excludes the presence of ischemic cardiomyopathy. A positive CTA effectively "rules in" the probability that an underlying cardiomyopathy could be related to significant epicardial coronary stenosis. Hence, CTA can be considered as an invaluable imaging modality for evaluating patients with left ventricular dysfunction of a suspected ischemic etiology [47].

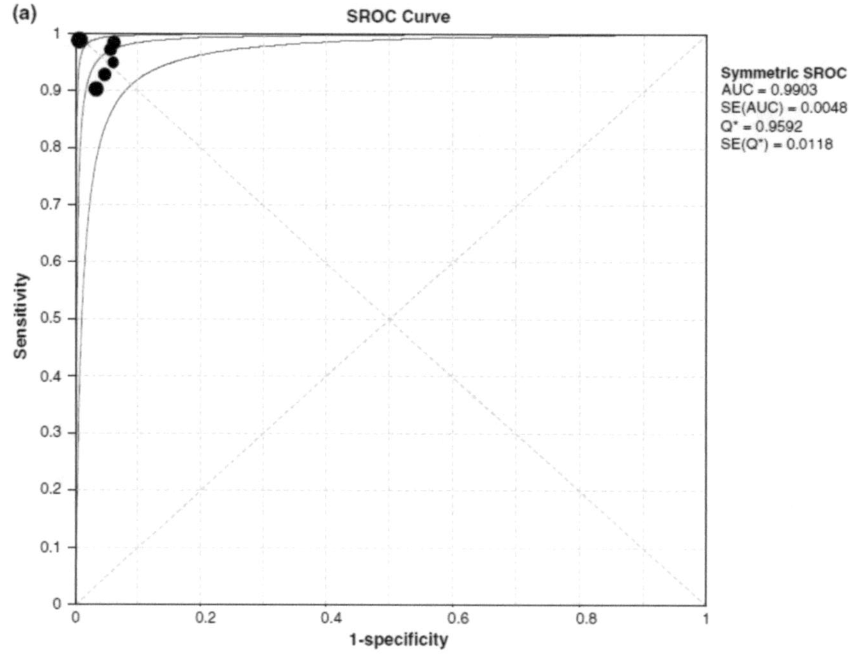

Figure 8. Diagnostic accuracy of CCTA for ischemic cardiomyopathy. Adapted with permission from Bhatti et al [47].

6. Comparison of MSCT angiography and Invasive angiography

Since the first report of Moshage et al over 17 years ago [48], numerous studies and meta analyses have been published confirming the superior diagnostic performance of MSCT in comparison with invasive angiography as the reference standard.. The largest meta analysis to date collated data from 89 studies with 7516 patients [49]. Bivariate analysis yielded a mean sensitivity and specificity were 97.2% (95% CI, 96.2% to 98.0%) and 87.4% (CI, 84.5% to 89.8%) for CT. Negative likelihood ratio was 0.03 (0.02-0.04) whereas the positive likelihood ratio was modest at 7.7(6.2-9.5) area under the curve was 0.98 (CI, 0.96 to 0.99) for CT. The resulting sensitivity of 98.1% for scanners with more than 16 detector rows was significantly higher ($P < 0.050$) than that for scanners with a maximum of 16 rows (95.6%). The high negative predictive value of CTA best suites it as an effective rule-out test for significant CAD.

Despite the use of newer generation scanners (>64 slice), coronary calcification remains the Achilles heel of CTA. A recent analysis from the CORE 64 study demonstrated that the robust AUC of CTA (0.93) significantly decreased to (0.81) in patients with calcium score >600 [50]. Furthermore, the negative predictive value of CTA decreased from 0.93 in patients with Calcium score <100 to 0.75 in patients with calcium score >100. High pretest probability of CAD and high calcium score negatively impacts the diagnostic performance of CTA and must be carefully considered in test selection.

7. Prognostic value

Whereas the diagnostic accuracy of CCTA has been rigorously established, increasing number of studies have also evaluated the prognostic value of CCTA. A recent meta analysis included eighteen studies involving 9,592 patients with a median follow-up of 20 months for adverse cardiac events [51]. The authors computed a pooled annualized event MACE rate of 8.8% for obstructive (any vessel with >50% luminal stenosis) disease versus 0.17% per year for normal CCTA ($p < 0.05$) and 3.2% versus 0.15% for death or MI ($p < 0.05$) Figure 9. Furthermore, the pooled negative likelihood ratio for MACE after normal CCTA findings was 0.008 (95% CI: 0.0004 to 0.17, $p < 0.001$). Patients with a normal CTA can hence be confidently reassured given a very low risk of death, MI or revascularization fairly comparable to an otherwise healthy population(<1%). Furthermore, the low event rate for normal CTA (0.16%) is comparable to other well established non invasive risk stratification modalities including stress echocardiography (0.45%) and myocardial perfusion stress imaging (0.54%). CTA has hence emerged as a well established clinical tool that carries not only robust diagnostic accuracy but also has powerful predictive accuracy as well [51].

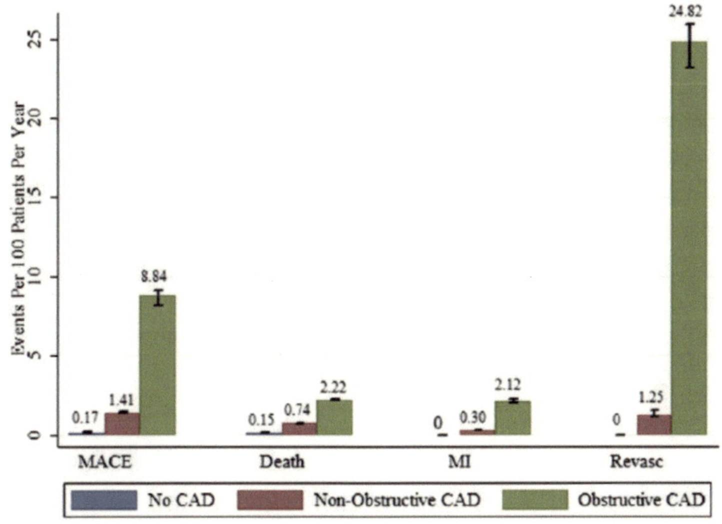

Figure 9. Adapted with permission from Hulten et al [51]

8. Physiological significance of stenoses identified by CTA

That, coronary angiography is merely a "luminogram" and does not provide much insight into the hemodynamic significance of a stenotic lesion, is a fact that has been rigorously established for the past two decades. This well-recognized limitation has been documented repeatedly by intravascular ultrasound imaging and stress testing. It has been known that coronary angiography often leads to overestimation of the functional significance of epicardial coronary stenoses. In this regard, fractional flow reserve (FFR) has emerged as a powerful catheter based tool that provides robust information about the functional severity of the lesion. FFR calculated from coronary pressure measurement, is a reliable, invasive index to indicate if a stenosis is ischemia-related and can be determined in the catheterization laboratory in a simple and rapid way. By taking the ratio of the coronary pressure measured distal to the stenosis to aortic pressure as the normal perfusion pressure (distal coronary pressure/ aortic pressure) and obtaining these measurements when the microvascular resistance was minimal and assumed to be constant (that is, at maximal hyperemia), the percentage of normal coronary flow, or a fraction of normal flow (i.e., FFR), can be calculated. FFR has a uniform normal value of 1.0 for every patient and every coronary artery; it is not dependent on changes in heart rate, blood pressure, or contractility; it accounts for collateral flow; and it has a sharp threshold value to indicate inducible ischemia: FFR < 0.75 always indicates inducible ischemia; FFR > 0.80 excludes ischemia in 90% of the cases [15, 17-20, 23, 46, 52-54]. The grey zone is very limited, which is important for clinical decision making in an individual patient. Coronary pressure measurements can be easily performed by a pressure wire, with almost identical mechanical properties as normal guide wires, and barely prolong the procedure, even when multiple vessels are interrogated. The ischemic threshold of FFR has been replicated independently with different noninvasive functional tests in numerous studies (including exercise electrocardiography, dobutamine stress echocardiography, and MPI) as well as alongside one another in the same population. An FFR >0.75 identified coronary stenoses in patients with inducible myocardial ischemia with high sensitivity (88%), specificity (100%), positive predictive value (100%), and overall accuracy (93%). FFR has a high reproducibility and low intra-individual variability. Several randomized clinical trials including DEFER, FAME and now FAME II have established the prognostic utility of FFR.Consequently, now, measurement of FFR during invasive coronary angiography is the gold standard for identifying coronary artery lesions that cause ischemia and improves clinical decision-making for revascularization.

Similar limitations of stenoses especially in the intermediate range (50-70%) are widely seen in CT angiograms. This poses both diagnostic and therapeutic challenges. Meijboom et al [55] evaluated 89 lesions in 79 patients with stable angina. Lesion correlation with invasive angiography was performed and FFR of stenoses was measured. The authors demonstrated very poor correlation between CTA and invasive coronary angiography with hemodynamically significant stenosis (FFR<0.75); diagnostic accuracy 64% for FFR <0.8 and 49% for FFR< 0.75. CTA overestimated the functional significance of coronary stenoses (poor specificity/ high false positive rate) even after excluding segments with high calcification and coronary motion. Hence patients with intermediate stenoses on CTA require further evaluation by either FFR evaluation of stress testing.

Recently, evaluation of FFR from CCTA data (FFRCT) has been proposed as a noninvasive method for identifying ischemic lesions. This employs the concept of computational fluid dynamics (CFD) Koo et al [56] correlated FFR from CT data with invasive FFR in 103 patients (159 vessels) in a prospective multicenter DISCOVER-FLOW (Diagnosis of Ischemia-Causing Stenoses Obtained via Noninvasive Fractional Flow Reserve) study. On a per-vessel basis, the accuracy, sensitivity, specificity, positive predictive value, and negative predictive value were 84.3%, 87.9%, 82.2%, 73.9%, 92.2%, respectively, for FFRCT and were 58.5%, 91.4%, 39.6%, 46.5%, 88.9%, respectively, for CCTA stenosis yielding an AUC of 0.9 for FFR CT and 0.75 for CTA. There was fair correlation between invasive FFR and FFRCT ($r = 0.717$, $p < 0.001$) although FFR Ct had slight underestimation (0.022 ± 0.116, $p = 0.016$). The results of the larger 285 patient DEFACTO trial comparing CT FFR and invasive FFR are awaited later this year and would further consolidate the role of non invasive FFR in the evaluation of intermediate coronary lesions see on CTA.

9. Complimentary role of CTA in guiding complex PCI like Chronic total occlusion (CTOs)

The unprecedented spatial resolution and 3D reconstruction of the epicardial coronary vessels has led to its role as an indispensable tool in guiding complex coronary interventions including recanalizing chronic total occlusions (CTO); the most challenging subset of complex coronary lesions. The display of CTA images as a 3D roadmap, side-by-side with live angiography images is instrumental in providing the interventional team access to the occluded channel. Furthermore, synchronization of the CTA image orientation with the C-arm, allows for selection of the ideal treatment projection angle without additional contrast medium or radiation exposure. Several studies have validated the use of CTA in guiding CTO intervention [57].

10. Diagnostic accuracy of CTA for in-stent restenosis

Despite the introduction of drug eluting stents, instent restenosis (ISR) from neointimal hyperplasia remains a real issue. For patients with recurrent chest pain following stent implantation, invasive coronary angiography is often performed to evaluate the presence of ISR. However, the need for a noninvasive alternative approach for ISR detection is more desirable. The experience with older generation CTA systems (4 and 16 slice) in evaluation of ISR was very disappointing largely related to motion and blooming artifacts. The improved spatial and temporal resolution with 64,128 and 256 slice scanners seems to have ameliorated those limitations. Carrabba et al [58] performed a meta analysis of nine studies involving 598 participants with 978 stents evaluated for ISR with CTA (64 slice) using invasive coronary angiography as the reference standard. More than 60% of the studied stents were >3 mm in diameter. Approximately 10% of the stents were unassessable. The pooled sensitivity and specificity of CTA was 86% (95% CI 80-91%) and 93%(95% CI 91-95%) respectively yielding an AUC of 0.94 for per stent analysis. The calculated positive and negative predictive values were 70.4% and 97.2%, respectively. CTA can hence 64-MDCT can hence reliably rule out ISR and further evaluation by means of invasive coronary angiography can be avoided.

Caution is still advised for smaller stents and the fact that almost 10% of the studies were still uninterpretable despite the use of 64 detector scanners.

11. Comparison of coronary computed tomography angiography and magnetic resonance coronary angiography

This section aims to compare the techniques of coronary computed tomography angiography (CCTA) with magnetic resonance coronary angiography (MRCA) from the standpoint of coronary and cardiac imaging.

12. Comparison of technical aspects CCTA to MRCA

Currently the majority of the institutions utilize 64 slice technology (in-plane spatial resolution of 0.4 x 0.4 mm with a slice thickness of 0.6 mm and a 360° gantry rotation in about 330 milliseconds). More recently dual source CCTA technology has pushed the envelope further and has delivered a temporal resolution of 70-83 msec with an in plane resolution of 0.4 mm [59]. Furthermore, 256 and 320 slice CT- scanners are available in limited institutions across the world which can image the entire heart in 1 beat thus obviating many limitations with current 64 slice scanners such as irregular heart rhythm, breath hold issues and opening options for perfusion CCCTA imaging.

The tremendous advantages that CCTA holds over MRCA with such high spatial resolution relates to: 1. ability to visualize small diameter vessels including distal coronary branches, 2. increased ability to quantify calcium and reduce blooming artifacts, 3. better visualization of stents, and 4. better plaque morphology assessment. The temporal resolution advances in CCTA has enabled: 1. enhanced ability to freeze cardiac motion, 2. additional reconstruction capabilities within cardiac cycle, and 3. reduced scan time.

The obvious disadvantages of CCTA compared to MRCA are: 1. radiation exposure which depending on the scanner, mode of acquisition and protocol modifications can range from 1 milliseivert to > 15 milliseiverts[60, 61], 2. use of iodinated contrast which could pose issues for patients with underlying renal dysfunction, and 3. need for slow heart rates which require use of beta-blockers.

13. One stop shop imaging : MRCA versus CCTA

A very attractive advantage with MRCA is that it can combined with detailed cardiac MRI exam to provide a "one stop shop" assessment is easily achievable where coronary disease, valves, stress/rest perfusion for ischemia and viability and overall cardiac and adjacent thoracic and extra-thoracic anatomy can be all studied without concern for nephrotoxic contrast or repetitive exposure to radiation. Furthermore, imaging sequences or views can easily be repeated. Thus, a hybrid anatomic and functional assessment is clinically feasible at present in centers with experience with MRCA. With CCTA, valves and ventricular function assessment comes at the cost of higher radiation exposure as retrospective triggered acquisition is needed. CT perfusion imaging for ischemia and viability is still not well validated compared to cardiac MRI but has been performed for both viability [62, 63] and perfusion [64, 65] and is being tested against SPECT in ongoing clinical trials. Promising new studies with CCTA with lower radiation doses encompassing a complete anatomical-functional assessment compared to traditional SPECT imaging has been published recently [66] but this aspect of CCTA is not ready for clinical use. Although MRCA does offer high temporal resolution, good spatial resolution, high soft tissue contrast and the ability to generate any three dimensional image without need for ionizing radiation it is much more challenging to perform as it requires selection of the correct pulse sequences and each pulse sequence needs many parallel slices or slab volumes to cover the entire heart. Free breathing MRCA acquisitions can take 5-15 minutes compared to a few seconds with current 64-320 slice CCTA. Spatial resolution of CCTA is superior to MRCA (0.4 to -0.6 mm with CCTA compared to 1.5 mm with MRCA). The disadvantage for MRCA compared to CCTA in terms of speed of acquisition is difficult to overcome although breath hold MRCA may offer some improvement in time required for acquisition compared to free breathing techniques [67]. The temporal resolution of CCTA is limited by the gantry rotation speed and hence cannot be altered. On the contrary free breathing MRCA temporal resolution can be flexibly determined using imaging parameters. The acquisition window position and the length within the RR interval can be individually set [68]. This is an important advantage with MRCA.

14. Diagnostic accuracy of CCTA versus MRCA for CAD

The diagnostic accuracy of CCTA is well established with it outstanding negative predictive value (97.2%) and moderate-to good positive predictive value (87.4%) based on cumulative data from 89 studies of 7519 patients(69). This compares much more favorably to MRCA which has a sensitivity of 87.1% and specificity of 70.3 % based on 20 studies of 989 patients [69]. Furthermore, in patients suspected of CAD or with acute disease at presentation, CCTA has an outstanding negative likelihood ratio of 0.03(0.02-0.04) and 0.06(0.02-0.19) respectively [69]. A meta-analysis of CCTA versus MRCA [49] and a recent study comparing state of art 64 slice CCTA to 32 channel 3T MRCA [70] both concluded that although both modalities performed well for CAD detection CCTA outperformed MRCA. Furthermore CCTA was completed in 13.9+/= 1.1 sec compared to 17 +/- 4.7 minutes for MRCA [70]. The expert consensus document on "appropriate" use of CT and MRI imaging published in 2006 gave an appropriate indication for CCTA to rule out significant CAD in patients with chest pain and intermediate likelihood of CAD. On the contrary the document gave a recommendation of "inappropriate" for MRCA for the same indication [71]. This reflects the lack of adequate data demonstrating the feasibility and accuracy for MRCA on a practical level across many institutions.

15. Assessment of coronary anomalies and aneurysms: CCTA versus MRCA

One important indication where MRCA could be very helpful is imaging for anomalous coronaries in children and young adults where exposure to radiation from CCTA is undesirable [72]. Coronary arteries in MRCA can be imaged without nephrotoxic contrast administration. The high T2/T1 signal in steady state free precession imaging (SSFP) acts as a natural contrast agent providing coronary lumen definition [73]. However, SSFP imaging has greater susceptibility to artifacts and newer sequences such as fast low angle shots (FLASH) show better imaging characteristics at 3.0T compared to SSFP [74] also showing a 50% reduction in scan time [75]. CCTA offers outstanding spatial resolution and is the widely preferred technique at least in adults to evaluate anomalous coronaries as long as there are no inherent contraindications to its use. ACC/AHA appropriate use guidelines for CCTA /MRI [71] gives CCTA and MRCA an " appropriate" indication score with CCTA receiving a higher score of 9 compared to MRCA which also receives a high score of 8. MRCA may also be used for serial follow-up of coronary aneurysms which can be a sequelae of Kawasaki disease particularly in adolescents and young adults who otherwise may need repeated angiography.[76, 77] CCTA again is excellent to delineate these aneurysms but suffers from limitations of repetitive radiation exposure.

16. Comparison of Technical Challenges in Imaging for CCTA and MRCA

16.1. Motion artifact issues : CCTA versus MRCA

Motion artifacts pose a significant problem with both MRCA and CCTA. In MRCA this can be intrinsic related to cardiac contraction /relaxation or extrinsic attributable to diaphragm and chest wall movement during respiration [35]. Furthermore, MRCA requires expertise to perform and interpret and is currently limited largely to academic centers with a dedicated 1.5 or a 3T cardiac magnet at least in North America. In CCTA motion artifacts are related to patient motion and respiratory based artifact (as CCTA imaging is during breath hold). In contrast 64 slice CCTA is available in most large institutions and practices and the training and interpretation process is much more feasible for physicians desiring to practice this technology.

16.2. Calcification issues: CCTA versus MRCA

Calcification of coronary arteries is seen in at least 50-70% of patients with atherosclerotic plaques [78]. Calcium poses a significant limitation for accuracy of CCTA due to blooming/beam hardening artifacts compromising lumen assessment [79]. However it is not a limitation for MRCA for assessing the lumen of the coronary arteries as MRI does not have issues with beam hardening or blooming. Thus lumen visualization is not compromised [80]. The flip side of this is the added advantage of detection of coronary calcium during the non-contrast portion of CCTA which serves both to diagnose atherosclerosis [81] and in its absence make obstructive CAD highly unlikely both in asymptomatic patients and in patient with suspected cardiac etiology of chest pain [82, 83]. Coronary calcium also provides powerful prognostic information and is incremental in risk assessment beyond traditional risk scores like Framingham risk scores [84]. Furthermore, identifying substantial calcium may also help in decision making for the physician as the CCTA portion of the test could be cancelled and more definitive testing towards significance of underlying lesion could be pursued wither with stress testing or angiography. MRCA lack this important " heads up" diagnostic advantage that CCTA possess as part of its armamentarium due to its inability to image calcium. More recently some investigators have tried to exploit the different capabilities of CCTA and MRCA by combining both technologies in patients with significant calcification. In a small study of 18 patients who underwent 64 slice CCTA, 3D free breathing MRCA and coronary angiography, MRCA had better diagnostic image quality and performed better in detection of obstructive CAD in coronary segments with focal rather than diffuse calcification and overall performed better than CCTA in detecting significant CAD in patients with high calcium scores [80].

17. Imaging bypass grafts and stents: CCTA versus MRCA

CCTA is an outstanding modality for imaging bypass grafts. In a study by Liu and colleagues [85] 228 patients underwent 64 slice CCTA to evaluate diagnostic accuracy of CCTA for bypass graft disease. The sensitivity, specificity, positive negative predictive value and overall accuracy were reported at an impressive 93.3%, 98.1%, 93.3%, 98.1%, and 97.7 % respectively. Major disadvantages include higher contrast dose, increased radiation from longer scanning to cover the anatomy of origin and course of grafts and artifacts related to clips from surgery. The anastamotic sites in particular can sometimes be challenging to evaluate. In comparison, in a study by Langerak et al,[86] MRCA showed a sensitivity and specificity of 83 and 100% for graft occlusion,82%, and 88% for graft stenosis >/= 50% and 73% and 80% for graft stenosis >/= 70%. MRCA also suffers from signal void artifacts from metallic implants, clips, etc. In addition it seems to perform inferior to CCTA in consistently identifying severely diseased yet patent vessels [86] making its widespread applicability for bypass graft evaluation less feasible. Furthermore even though CCTA has limitations with radiation the population with CABG are older and hence the lifetime risk of cancer is less of a concern. Newer generation 64 slice CCTA has also shown promise in imaging stent lumen although stents less than 3 mm tend to cause unacceptable degree of lumen visualization and blooming artifacts (highest with tantalum stents and lowest with titanium and nitinol based alloys) and CCTA is not recommended below this size. A recent study on coronary stent patency with CCTA showed a promising 89% sensitivity and 95% specificity [87]. MRCA data with stents is limited but the stainless steel composition of stents make imaging challenging as in-stent integrity and persistent assessment can be compromised. The attractive force and local heart generated with stent imaging at 1.5 T and 3T is not a major issue the local susceptibility artifacts can be a big problem [88, 89]. This is less of problem with tantalum compared to stainless steel stents. In the USA both Cypher and Taxus Liberte stents are approved for imaging with MRI immediately after implantation.

18. Contrast issues: CCTA versus MRCA

CCTA has to utilize iodinated contrast agents between 80-120 ml for opacification of coronary vessels. This is an obvious limitation for those with underlying chronic kidney disease particularly Stage 3 and above as it is potentially nephrotoxic. MRCA on the other hand utilizes the natural signal differences seen in SSFP imaging to visualize coronaries and does not require gadolinium contrast although it can be utilized. Currently used gadolinium compounds remain intravascular only for a short period of time thus limiting the benefit of contrast enhancement for MRCA for a short period of time. However some advances in MRI contrast agents have been made with newer agents with more prolonged intravascular time now being available. These agents increase contrast to noise ratio with MRCA and hold promise to improve diagnostic accuracy although no large scale studies have been performed as yet. It is important o note that gadolinium chelates can cause nephrogenic systemic fibrosis and are usually contraindicated in patients with glomerular filtration rates of < 30 ml/min.

19. Plaque imaging: CCTA versus MRCA

Plaque imaging is an exciting area of intense research and potential application of CCTA given its capacity to image the vessel wall and provide information beyond luminal narrowing. It can detect and characterize atherosclerotic plaques as calcified, non-calcified and mixed composition (Figure 10).[90] It is now known that regardless of degree of luminal stenosis even non-obstructive plaques as detected by CCTA carries adverse prognosis [91]. However, inter-observer variability of measurement of plaque dimensions is substantial and routine plaque measurements is not feasible at this time. However CCTA shows promise in identifying certain high risk characteristics such as bulky plaques, spotty calcification and positive remodeling all of which have been shown to be related to acute coronary syndromes [92]. With MRI, although once felt to be not possible, several investigators have imaged the coronary vessel wall and plaque successfully including subclinical wall thickening [93, 94], although from point of practical applicability this has yet to find a place in the clinical arena. Because of the lack of radiation exposure in MRCA it is ideally suited for follow-up imaging for assessing plaque progression [95] or to follow-up intermediate range stenosis where anatomy can be combined with a functional assessment of significance of lesion with stress –rest perfusion sequences [96].

http://dx.doi.org/10.5772/54082

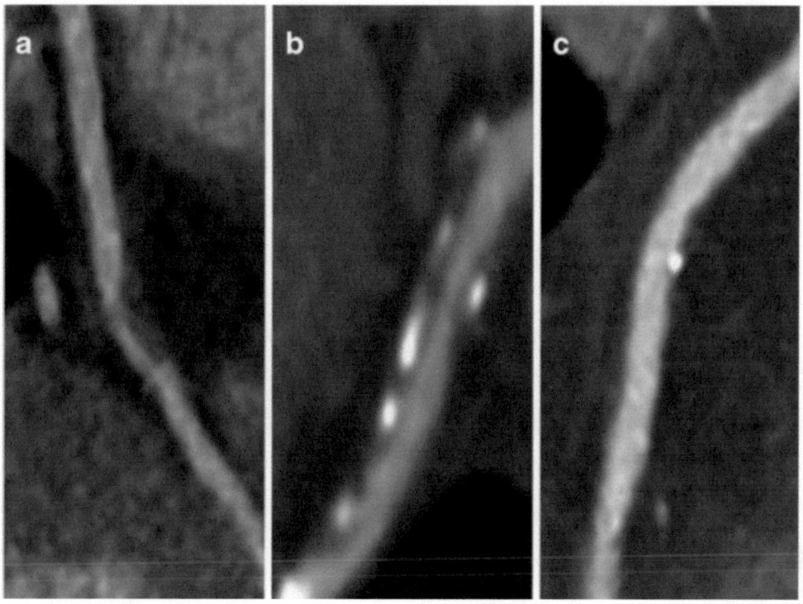

Figure 10.

20. Patient acceptance of CCTA versus MRCA

CCTA enjoys a much shorter time to completion of study compared to MRCA (20 versus 60 minutes respectively) which is a major attraction from the patient perspective [97]. For a modality to be overall successful in clinical practice it should not only be accurate, demonstrate clinical benefit and cost effective but also preferred by patients [98]. Studies have shown that patients prefer CCTA to MRCA [99]. This is mainly driven by longer imaging times, confinement in closed space and noise associated with MR imaging.

21. Training issues CCTA versus MRCA

Guidelines exist both from American College of Radiology [100] and the American College of Cardiology [101] for specific training requirements for gaining expertise in CCTA. Unfortunately no such guidelines exist for MRCA and given the complexity involved in image acquisition the degree of expertise needed to independently perform and interpret MRCA is likely to substantially greater with regards to training requirements. CCTA program clearly is easier to establish and execute than a MRCA program.

Table 5 summarizes various advantages and disadvantages from the authors perspective of CCTA and MRCA.

Properties	CTA	MRI
Time and patient preference	short duration and preffered	long duration, many breath holds, more claustrophobic
Comprehensive assessment	YES with higher radiation exposure, viability still not widely validated	one stop shop complete function, perfusion, viability and ischemic, myopathic assessment
Resolution	Higher spatial resolution	better temporal resolution
Diagnostic issues	superb negative predictive value and moderate positive predictive value	very good prognostic value in limited studies. Diagnostic values close to CT with 32C/3T
Radiation	yes	no
Calcification	interferes with interpretation	cannot be assessed. not limitation to assess coronaries
Radiocontrast	yes	no
Mettalic interference	yes but not contraindicated	currently contraindicated in pacemakers, defibrillators, metallic implants, shrapnel intracranial clips
Bypass Grafts	Excellent	Limited by artifacts
Stents	Large stents good	not good ?
Experience	Widespread	Limited
Availability	Widespread	Limited
Scanner	16Slice and Higher	1.5 T reasonable 3T better
Claustrophobia	Not a big issue	It is an issue
Irregular rhythm	Problem	Problem
Need premedication	Yes (mostly)	Not needed

Table 6.

22. Future perspectives

Noninvasive coronary angiography involving CCTA and MRCA has revolutionized delineation of coronary anatomy in a safe and fast way. CCTA has advanced much more in this aspect with fast imaging with single breath holds and 1 beat acquisition lasting a few seconds. The radiation and iodine based contrast are the major disadvantages although currently radiation doses below 1 millisievert are achievable with CCTA. MRCA with whole heart 3D imaging and 32 channel coils and 3T magnets have improved coronary imaging significantly but still lags behind and is not available widely. We foresee that CCTA will become mainstream for coronary imaging in low to intermediate risk populations with chest pains syndromes in the near future with exciting prospects of comprehensive cardiac imaging of perfusion and viability and plaque imaging.

http://dx.doi.org/10.5772/54082

Acknowledgements

We are indebted for the expert manuscript preparation assistance of Mrs Nandita S. Mani, MLIS, Sladen Library, Henry Ford Hospital, Detroit MI, USA

Author details

Karthikeyan Ananthasubramaniam[1*], Sabha Bhatti[1] and Abdul Hakeem[2]

*Address all correspondence to: kananth1@hfhs.org

1 Henry Ford Hospital, Heart and Vascular Institute, Detroit MI, USA

2 William Beaumont Hospital Royal Oak MI, USA

References

[1] Stuber M, Weiss RG. Coronary magnetic resonance angiography. Journal of magnetic resonance imaging: JMRI. 2007;26(2):219-34. Epub 2007/07/05.

[2] Manning WJ, Nezafat R, Appelbaum E, Danias PG, Hauser TH, Yeon SB. Coronary magnetic resonance imaging. Magnetic resonance imaging clinics of North America. 2007;15(4):609-37, vii. Epub 2007/11/03.

[3] Jahnke C, Paetsch I, Nehrke K, Schnackenburg B, Gebker R, Fleck E, et al. Rapid and complete coronary arterial tree visualization with magnetic resonance imaging: feasibility and diagnostic performance. European heart journal. 2005;26(21):2313-9. Epub 2005/07/01.

[4] Sakuma H, Ichikawa Y, Suzawa N, Hirano T, Makino K, Koyama N, et al. Assessment of coronary arteries with total study time of less than 30 minutes by using whole-heart coronary MR angiography. Radiology. 2005;237(1):316-21. Epub 2005/08/30.

[5] Nehrke K, Bornert P, Mazurkewitz P, Winkelmann R, Grasslin I. Free-breathing whole-heart coronary MR angiography on a clinical scanner in four minutes. Journal of magnetic resonance imaging : JMRI. 2006;23(5):752-6. Epub 2006/03/25.

[6] Wansapura J, Fleck R, Crotty E, Gottliebson W. Frequency scouting for cardiac imaging with SSFP at 3 Tesla. Pediatric radiology. 2006;36(10):1082-5. Epub 2006/07/11.

[7] Wang Y, Riederer SJ, Ehman RL. Respiratory motion of the heart: kinematics and the implications for the spatial resolution in coronary imaging. Magnetic resonance in

medicine : official journal of the Society of Magnetic Resonance in Medicine / Society of Magnetic Resonance in Medicine. 1995;33(5):713-9. Epub 1995/05/01.

[8] Botnar RM, Stuber M, Danias PG, Kissinger KV, Manning WJ. Improved coronary artery definition with T2-weighted, free-breathing, three-dimensional coronary MRA. Circulation. 1999;99(24):3139-48. Epub 1999/06/22.

[9] Jahnke C, Paetsch I, Achenbach S, Schnackenburg B, Gebker R, Fleck E, et al. Coronary MR imaging: breath-hold capability and patterns, coronary artery rest periods, and beta-blocker use. Radiology. 2006;239(1):71-8. Epub 2006/02/24.

[10] Ehman RL, Felmlee JP. Adaptive technique for high-definition MR imaging of moving structures. Radiology. 1989;173(1):255-63. Epub 1989/10/01.

[11] Johansson LO, Nolan MM, Taniuchi M, Fischer SE, Wickline SA, Lorenz CH. High-resolution magnetic resonance coronary angiography of the entire heart using a new blood-pool agent, NC100150 injection: comparison with invasive x-ray angiography in pigs. Journal of cardiovascular magnetic resonance : official journal of the Society for Cardiovascular Magnetic Resonance. 1999;1(2):139-43. Epub 2001/09/12.

[12] Li D, Dolan RP, Walovitch RC, Lauffer RB. Three-dimensional MRI of coronary arteries using an intravascular contrast agent. Magnetic resonance in medicine : official journal of the Society of Magnetic Resonance in Medicine / Society of Magnetic Resonance in Medicine. 1998;39(6):1014-8. Epub 1998/06/11.

[13] Snyder CJ, DelaBarre L, Metzger GJ, van de Moortele PF, Akgun C, Ugurbil K, et al. Initial results of cardiac imaging at 7 Tesla. Magnetic resonance in medicine : official journal of the Society of Magnetic Resonance in Medicine / Society of Magnetic Resonance in Medicine. 2009;61(3):517-24. Epub 2008/12/20.

[14] Bunce NH, Lorenz CH, Keegan J, Lesser J, Reyes EM, Firmin DN, et al. Coronary artery anomalies: assessment with free-breathing three-dimensional coronary MR angiography. Radiology. 2003;227(1):201-8. Epub 2003/02/26.

[15] Gharib AM, Ho VB, Rosing DR, Herzka DA, Stuber M, Arai AE, et al. Coronary artery anomalies and variants: technical feasibility of assessment with coronary MR angiography at 3 T. Radiology. 2008;247(1):220-7. Epub 2008/03/29.

[16] McConnell MV, Ganz P, Selwyn AP, Li W, Edelman RR, Manning WJ. Identification of anomalous coronary arteries and their anatomic course by magnetic resonance coronary angiography. Circulation. 1995;92(11):3158-62. Epub 1995/12/01.

[17] Post JC, van Rossum AC, Bronzwaer JG, de Cock CC, Hofman MB, Valk J, et al. Magnetic resonance angiography of anomalous coronary arteries. A new gold standard for delineating the proximal course? Circulation. 1995;92(11):3163-71. Epub 1995/12/01.

[18] Taylor AM, Thorne SA, Rubens MB, Jhooti P, Keegan J, Gatehouse PD, et al. Coronary artery imaging in grown up congenital heart disease: complementary role of

magnetic resonance and x-ray coronary angiography. Circulation. 2000;101(14): 1670-8. Epub 2000/04/12.

[19] Vliegen HW, Doornbos J, de Roos A, Jukema JW, Bekedam MA, van der Wall EE. Value of fast gradient echo magnetic resonance angiography as an adjunct to coronary arteriography in detecting and confirming the course of clinically significant coronary artery anomalies. The American journal of cardiology. 1997;79(6):773-6. Epub 1997/03/15.

[20] Kim WY, Danias PG, Stuber M, Flamm SD, Plein S, Nagel E, et al. Coronary magnetic resonance angiography for the detection of coronary stenoses. The New England journal of medicine. 2001;345(26):1863-9. Epub 2002/01/05.

[21] Sakuma H, Ichikawa Y, Chino S, Hirano T, Makino K, Takeda K. Detection of coronary artery stenosis with whole-heart coronary magnetic resonance angiography. Journal of the American College of Cardiology. 2006;48(10):1946-50. Epub 2006/11/23.

[22] Halliburton S, Arbab-Zadeh A, Dey D, Einstein AJ, Gentry R, George RT, et al. State-of-the-art in CT hardware and scan modes for cardiovascular CT. Journal of cardiovascular computed tomography. 2012;6(3):154-63. Epub 2012/05/04.

[23] 1990 Recommendations of the International Commission on Radiological Protection. Annals of the ICRP. 1991;21(1-3):1-201. Epub 1991/01/01.

[24] Alkadhi H, Stolzmann P, Scheffel H, Desbiolles L, Baumuller S, Plass A, et al. Radiation dose of cardiac dual-source CT: the effect of tailoring the protocol to patient-specific parameters. European journal of radiology. 2008;68(3):385-91. Epub 2008/11/04.

[25] Lell M, Marwan M, Schepis T, Pflederer T, Anders K, Flohr T, et al. Prospectively ECG-triggered high-pitch spiral acquisition for coronary CT angiography using dual source CT: technique and initial experience. European radiology. 2009;19(11):2576-83. Epub 2009/09/18.

[26] Gallagher MJ, Ross MA, Raff GL, Goldstein JA, O'Neill WW, O'Neil B. The diagnostic accuracy of 64-slice computed tomography coronary angiography compared with stress nuclear imaging in emergency department low-risk chest pain patients. Annals of emergency medicine. 2007;49(2):125-36. Epub 2006/09/19.

[27] Goldstein JA, Gallagher MJ, O'Neill WW, Ross MA, O'Neil BJ, Raff GL. A randomized controlled trial of multi-slice coronary computed tomography for evaluation of acute chest pain. Journal of the American College of Cardiology. 2007;49(8):863-71. Epub 2007/02/27.

[28] Hoffmann U, Bamberg F, Chae CU, Nichols JH, Rogers IS, Seneviratne SK, et al. Coronary computed tomography angiography for early triage of patients with acute chest pain: the ROMICAT (Rule Out Myocardial Infarction using Computer Assisted Tomography) trial. Journal of the American College of Cardiology. 2009;53(18): 1642-50. Epub 2009/05/02.

[29] Hollander JE, Chang AM, Shofer FS, McCusker CM, Baxt WG, Litt HI. Coronary computed tomographic angiography for rapid discharge of low-risk patients with potential acute coronary syndromes. Annals of emergency medicine. 2009;53(3): 295-304. Epub 2008/11/11.

[30] Leber AW, Knez A, von Ziegler F, Becker A, Nikolaou K, Paul S, et al. Quantification of obstructive and nonobstructive coronary lesions by 64-slice computed tomography: a comparative study with quantitative coronary angiography and intravascular ultrasound. Journal of the American College of Cardiology. 2005;46(1):147-54. Epub 2005/07/05.

[31] Leschka S, Alkadhi H, Plass A, Desbiolles L, Grunenfelder J, Marincek B, et al. Accuracy of MSCT coronary angiography with 64-slice technology: first experience. European heart journal. 2005;26(15):1482-7. Epub 2005/04/21.

[32] Pugliese F, Mollet NR, Hunink MG, Cademartiri F, Nieman K, van Domburg RT, et al. Diagnostic performance of coronary CT angiography by using different generations of multisection scanners: single-center experience. Radiology. 2008;246(2): 384-93. Epub 2008/01/09.

[33] Raff GL, Gallagher MJ, O'Neill WW, Goldstein JA. Diagnostic accuracy of noninvasive coronary angiography using 64-slice spiral computed tomography. Journal of the American College of Cardiology. 2005;46(3):552-7. Epub 2005/08/02.

[34] Rubinshtein R, Halon DA, Gaspar T, Jaffe R, Karkabi B, Flugelman MY, et al. Usefulness of 64-slice cardiac computed tomographic angiography for diagnosing acute coronary syndromes and predicting clinical outcome in emergency department patients with chest pain of uncertain origin. Circulation. 2007;115(13):1762-8. Epub 2007/03/21.

[35] Bluemke DA, Achenbach S, Budoff M, Gerber TC, Gersh B, Hillis LD, et al. Noninvasive coronary artery imaging: magnetic resonance angiography and multidetector computed tomography angiography: a scientific statement from the american heart association committee on cardiovascular imaging and intervention of the council on cardiovascular radiology and intervention, and the councils on clinical cardiology and cardiovascular disease in the young. Circulation. 2008;118(5):586-606. Epub 2008/07/01.

[36] Meijboom WB, Meijs MF, Schuijf JD, Cramer MJ, Mollet NR, van Mieghem CA, et al. Diagnostic accuracy of 64-slice computed tomography coronary angiography: a prospective, multicenter, multivendor study. Journal of the American College of Cardiology. 2008;52(25):2135-44. Epub 2008/12/20.

[37] Miller JM, Rochitte CE, Dewey M, Arbab-Zadeh A, Niinuma H, Gottlieb I, et al. Diagnostic performance of coronary angiography by 64-row CT. The New England journal of medicine. 2008;359(22):2324-36. Epub 2008/11/29.

[38] Chang SM, Bhatti S, Nabi F. Coronary computed tomography angiography. Current opinion in cardiology. 2011;26(5):392-402. Epub 2011/07/12.

[39] Cademartiri F, Maffei E, Palumbo A, Carrabba N, Ardissino D, Mollet N, et al. Multislice CT coronary angiography for the detection of in-stent restenosis. Current Cardiovascular Imaging Reports. 2008;1(2):119-24.

[40] Lu M, Jen-Sho Chen J, Awan O, White CS. Evaluation of Bypass Grafts and Stents. Radiologic clinics of North America. 2010;48(4):757-70.

[41] Gallagher MJ, Raff GL. Use of multislice CT for the evaluation of emergency room patients with chest pain: the so-called "triple rule-out". Catheterization and cardiovascular interventions : official journal of the Society for Cardiac Angiography & Interventions. 2008;71(1):92-9. Epub 2007/12/22.

[42] Gruettner J, Fink C, Walter T, Meyer M, Apfaltrer P, Schoepf UJ, et al. Coronary computed tomography and triple rule out CT in patients with acute chest pain and an intermediate cardiac risk profile. Part 1: Impact on patient management. European journal of radiology. 2012. Epub 2012/07/04.

[43] Samad Z, Hakeem A, Mahmood SS, Pieper K, Patel MR, Simel DL, et al. A meta-analysis and systematic review of computed tomography angiography as a diagnostic triage tool for patients with chest pain presenting to the emergency department. Journal of nuclear cardiology : official publication of the American Society of Nuclear Cardiology. 2012;19(2):364-76. Epub 2012/02/11.

[44] Litt HI, Gatsonis C, Snyder B, Singh H, Miller CD, Entrikin DW, et al. CT angiography for safe discharge of patients with possible acute coronary syndromes. The New England journal of medicine. 2012;366(15):1393-403. Epub 2012/03/28.

[45] Hoffmann U, Truong QA, Schoenfeld DA, Chou ET, Woodard PK, Nagurney JT, et al. Coronary CT angiography versus standard evaluation in acute chest pain. The New England journal of medicine. 2012;367(4):299-308. Epub 2012/07/27.

[46] Felker GM, Shaw LK, O'Connor CM. A standardized definition of ischemic cardiomyopathy for use in clinical research. Journal of the American College of Cardiology. 2002;39(2):210-8. Epub 2002/01/15.

[47] Bhatti S, Hakeem A, Yousuf MA, Al-Khalidi HR, Mazur W, Shizukuda Y. Diagnostic performance of computed tomography angiography for differentiating ischemic vs nonischemic cardiomyopathy. Journal of nuclear cardiology : official publication of the American Society of Nuclear Cardiology. 2011;18(3):407-20. Epub 2011/02/18.

[48] Moshage WE, Achenbach S, Seese B, Bachmann K, Kirchgeorg M. Coronary artery stenoses: three-dimensional imaging with electrocardiographically triggered, contrast agent-enhanced, electron-beam CT. Radiology. 1995;196(3):707-14. Epub 1995/09/01.

[49] Schuetz GM, Zacharopoulou NM, Schlattmann P, Dewey M. Meta-analysis: noninvasive coronary angiography using computed tomography versus magnetic resonance imaging. Annals of internal medicine. 2010;152(3):167-77. Epub 2010/02/04.

[50] Arbab-Zadeh A, Miller JM, Rochitte CE, Dewey M, Niinuma H, Gottlieb I, et al. Diagnostic accuracy of computed tomography coronary angiography according to pretest probability of coronary artery disease and severity of coronary arterial calcification. The CORE-64 (Coronary Artery Evaluation Using 64-Row Multidetector Computed Tomography Angiography) International Multicenter Study. Journal of the American College of Cardiology. 2012;59(4):379-87. Epub 2012/01/21.

[51] Hulten EA, Carbonaro S, Petrillo SP, Mitchell JD, Villines TC. Prognostic value of cardiac computed tomography angiography: a systematic review and meta-analysis. Journal of the American College of Cardiology. 2011;57(10):1237-47. Epub 2010/12/15.

[52] Bax JJ, Poldermans D, Schuijf JD, Scholte AJ, Elhendy A, van der Wall EE. Imaging to differentiate between ischemic and nonischemic cardiomyopathy. Heart failure clinics. 2006;2(2):205-14. Epub 2007/03/28.

[53] Dilsizian V, Pohost GM. Cardiac CT, PET, and MR. 2nd ed. Chichester, West Sussex, UK ; Hoboken, NJ: Wiley-Blackwell; 2010. ix, 374 p. p.

[54] Mark DB, Berman DS, Budoff MJ, Carr JJ, Gerber TC, Hecht HS, et al. ACCF/ACR/AHA/NASCI/SAIP/SCAI/SCCT 2010 expert consensus document on coronary computed tomographic angiography: a report of the American College of Cardiology Foundation Task Force on Expert Consensus Documents. Catheterization and cardiovascular interventions : official journal of the Society for Cardiac Angiography & Interventions. 2010;76(2):E1-42. Epub 2010/08/06.

[55] Meijboom WB, Van Mieghem CA, van Pelt N, Weustink A, Pugliese F, Mollet NR, et al. Comprehensive assessment of coronary artery stenoses: computed tomography coronary angiography versus conventional coronary angiography and correlation with fractional flow reserve in patients with stable angina. Journal of the American College of Cardiology. 2008;52(8):636-43. Epub 2008/08/16.

[56] Koo BK, Erglis A, Doh JH, Daniels DV, Jegere S, Kim HS, et al. Diagnosis of ischemia-causing coronary stenoses by noninvasive fractional flow reserve computed from coronary computed tomographic angiograms. Results from the prospective multicenter DISCOVER-FLOW (Diagnosis of Ischemia-Causing Stenoses Obtained Via Noninvasive Fractional Flow Reserve) study. Journal of the American College of Cardiology. 2011;58(19):1989-97. Epub 2011/10/29.

[57] Hoe J. CT coronary angiography of chronic total occlusions of the coronary arteries: how to recognize and evaluate and usefulness for planning percutaneous coronary interventions. The international journal of cardiovascular imaging. 2009;25 Suppl 1:43-54. Epub 2009/01/24.

[58] Carrabba N, Schuijf JD, de Graaf FR, Parodi G, Maffei E, Valenti R, et al. Diagnostic accuracy of 64-slice computed tomography coronary angiography for the detection of in-stent restenosis: a meta-analysis. Journal of nuclear cardiology : official publication of the American Society of Nuclear Cardiology. 2010;17(3):470-8. Epub 2010/04/10.

[59] Flohr TG, Raupach R, Bruder H. Cardiac CT: how much can temporal resolution, spatial resolution, and volume coverage be improved? Journal of cardiovascular computed tomography. 2009;3(3):143-52. Epub 2009/06/17.

[60] Einstein AJ, Moser KW, Thompson RC, Cerqueira MD, Henzlova MJ. Radiation dose to patients from cardiac diagnostic imaging. Circulation. 2007;116(11):1290-305. Epub 2007/09/12.

[61] Gerber TC, Carr JJ, Arai AE, Dixon RL, Ferrari VA, Gomes AS, et al. Ionizing radiation in cardiac imaging: a science advisory from the American Heart Association Committee on Cardiac Imaging of the Council on Clinical Cardiology and Committee on Cardiovascular Imaging and Intervention of the Council on Cardiovascular Radiology and Intervention. Circulation. 2009;119(7):1056-65. Epub 2009/02/04.

[62] Higgins CB, Siemers PT, Newell JD, Schmidt W. Role of iodinated contrast material in the evaluation of myocardial infarction by computerized transmission tomography. Investigative radiology. 1980;15(6 Suppl):S176-82. Epub 1980/11/01.

[63] Mahnken AH, Koos R, Katoh M, Wildberger JE, Spuentrup E, Buecker A, et al. Assessment of myocardial viability in reperfused acute myocardial infarction using 16-slice computed tomography in comparison to magnetic resonance imaging. Journal of the American College of Cardiology. 2005;45(12):2042-7. Epub 2005/06/21.

[64] George RT, Arbab-Zadeh A, Miller JM, Kitagawa K, Chang HJ, Bluemke DA, et al. Adenosine stress 64- and 256-row detector computed tomography angiography and perfusion imaging: a pilot study evaluating the transmural extent of perfusion abnormalities to predict atherosclerosis causing myocardial ischemia. Circulation Cardiovascular imaging. 2009;2(3):174-82. Epub 2009/10/08.

[65] Rumberger JA, Feiring AJ, Lipton MJ, Higgins CB, Ell SR, Marcus ML. Use of ultrafast computed tomography to quantitate regional myocardial perfusion: a preliminary report. Journal of the American College of Cardiology. 1987;9(1):59-69. Epub 1987/01/01.

[66] Williams MC, Reid JH, McKillop G, Weir NW, van Beek EJ, Uren NG, et al. Cardiac and coronary CT comprehensive imaging approach in the assessment of coronary heart disease. Heart. 2011;97(15):1198-205. Epub 2011/07/12.

[67] Foo TK, Ho VB, Saranathan M, Cheng LQ, Sakuma H, Kraitchman DL, et al. Feasibility of integrating high-spatial-resolution 3D breath-hold coronary MR angiography with myocardial perfusion and viability examinations. Radiology. 2005;235(3): 1025-30. Epub 2005/05/26.

[68] Plein S, Jones TR, Ridgway JP, Sivananthan MU. Three-dimensional coronary MR angiography performed with subject-specific cardiac acquisition windows and motion-adapted respiratory gating. AJR American journal of roentgenology. 2003;180(2): 505-12. Epub 2003/01/24.

[69] Dewey M. Coronary CT versus MR angiography: pro CT--the role of CT angiography. Radiology. 2011;258(2):329-39. Epub 2011/01/29.

[70] Hamdan A, Asbach P, Wellnhofer E, Klein C, Gebker R, Kelle S, et al. A prospective study for comparison of MR and CT imaging for detection of coronary artery stenosis. JACC Cardiovascular imaging. 2011;4(1):50-61. Epub 2011/01/15.

[71] Hendel RC, Patel MR, Kramer CM, Poon M, Hendel RC, Carr JC, et al. ACCF/ACR/SCCT/SCMR/ASNC/NASCI/SCAI/SIR 2006 appropriateness criteria for cardiac computed tomography and cardiac magnetic resonance imaging: a report of the American College of Cardiology Foundation Quality Strategic Directions Committee Appropriateness Criteria Working Group, American College of Radiology, Society of Cardiovascular Computed Tomography, Society for Cardiovascular Magnetic Resonance, American Society of Nuclear Cardiology, North American Society for Cardiac Imaging, Society for Cardiovascular Angiography and Interventions, and Society of Interventional Radiology. Journal of the American College of Cardiology. 2006;48(7):1475-97. Epub 2006/10/03.

[72] Kleinerman RA. Cancer risks following diagnostic and therapeutic radiation exposure in children. Pediatric radiology. 2006;36 Suppl 2:121-5. Epub 2006/07/25.

[73] McCarthy RM, Shea SM, Deshpande VS, Green JD, Pereles FS, Carr JC, et al. Coronary MR angiography: true FISP imaging improved by prolonging breath holds with preoxygenation in healthy volunteers. Radiology. 2003;227(1):283-8. Epub 2003/03/05.

[74] Liu X, Bi X, Huang J, Jerecic R, Carr J, Li D. Contrast-enhanced whole-heart coronary magnetic resonance angiography at 3.0 T: comparison with steady-state free precession technique at 1.5 T. Investigative radiology. 2008;43(9):663-8. Epub 2008/08/19.

[75] Yang Q, Li K, Liu X, Bi X, Liu Z, An J, et al. Contrast-enhanced whole-heart coronary magnetic resonance angiography at 3.0-T: a comparative study with X-ray angiography in a single center. Journal of the American College of Cardiology. 2009;54(1):69-76. Epub 2009/06/27.

[76] Greil GF, Stuber M, Botnar RM, Kissinger KV, Geva T, Newburger JW, et al. Coronary magnetic resonance angiography in adolescents and young adults with kawasaki disease. Circulation. 2002;105(8):908-11. Epub 2002/02/28.

[77] Mavrogeni S, Papadopoulos G, Douskou M, Kaklis S, Seimenis I, Baras P, et al. Magnetic resonance angiography is equivalent to X-ray coronary angiography for the evaluation of coronary arteries in Kawasaki disease. Journal of the American College of Cardiology. 2004;43(4):649-52. Epub 2004/02/21.

[78] Wang L, Jerosch-Herold M, Jacobs DR, Jr., Shahar E, Detrano R, Folsom AR, et al. Coronary artery calcification and myocardial perfusion in asymptomatic adults: the MESA (Multi-Ethnic Study of Atherosclerosis). Journal of the American College of Cardiology. 2006;48(5):1018-26. Epub 2006/09/05.

[79] Brodoefel H, Burgstahler C, Tsiflikas I, Reimann A, Schroeder S, Claussen CD, et al. Dual-source CT: effect of heart rate, heart rate variability, and calcification on image quality and diagnostic accuracy. Radiology. 2008;247(2):346-55. Epub 2008/03/29.

[80] Liu X, Zhao X, Huang J, Francois CJ, Tuite D, Bi X, et al. Comparison of 3D free-breathing coronary MR angiography and 64-MDCT angiography for detection of coronary stenosis in patients with high calcium scores. AJR American journal of roentgenology. 2007;189(6):1326-32. Epub 2007/11/22.

[81] McCarthy JH, Palmer FJ. Incidence and significance of coronary artery calcification. British heart journal. 1974;36(5):499-506. Epub 1974/05/01.

[82] Hecht HS, Budoff MJ, Berman DS, Ehrlich J, Rumberger JA. Coronary artery calcium scanning: Clinical paradigms for cardiac risk assessment and treatment. American heart journal. 2006;151(6):1139-46. Epub 2006/06/20.

[83] McLaughlin VV, Balogh T, Rich S. Utility of electron beam computed tomography to stratify patients presenting to the emergency room with chest pain. The American journal of cardiology. 1999;84(3):327-8, A8. Epub 1999/09/25.

[84] Greenland P, LaBree L, Azen SP, Doherty TM, Detrano RC. Coronary artery calcium score combined with Framingham score for risk prediction in asymptomatic individuals. JAMA : the journal of the American Medical Association. 2004;291(2):210-5. Epub 2004/01/15.

[85] Liu ZY, Gao CQ, Li BJ, Wu Y, Xiao CS, Ye WH, et al. [Diagnostic study on the coronary artery bypass grafts lesions using 64 multi-slice computed tomography angiography]. Zhonghua wai ke za zhi [Chinese journal of surgery]. 2008;46(4):245-7. Epub 2008/08/08.

[86] Langerak SE, Vliegen HW, de Roos A, Zwinderman AH, Jukema JW, Kunz P, et al. Detection of vein graft disease using high-resolution magnetic resonance angiography. Circulation. 2002;105(3):328-33. Epub 2002/01/24.

[87] Antoniucci D, Valenti R, Santoro GM, Bolognese L, Trapani M, Cerisano G, et al. Restenosis after coronary stenting in current clinical practice. American heart journal. 1998;135(3):510-8. Epub 1998/03/20.

[88] Hug J, Nagel E, Bornstedt A, Schnackenburg B, Oswald H, Fleck E. Coronary arterial stents: safety and artifacts during MR imaging. Radiology. 2000;216(3):781-7. Epub 2000/08/31.

[89] Maintz D, Botnar RM, Fischbach R, Heindel W, Manning WJ, Stuber M. Coronary magnetic resonance angiography for assessment of the stent lumen: a phantom study. Journal of cardiovascular magnetic resonance : official journal of the Society for Cardiovascular Magnetic Resonance. 2002;4(3):359-67. Epub 2002/09/18.

[90] Maurovich-Horvat P, Ferencik M, Bamberg F, Hoffmann U. Methods of plaque quantification and characterization by cardiac computed tomography. Journal of cardiovascular computed tomography. 2009;3 Suppl 2:S91-8. Epub 2010/02/05.

[91] Pundziute G, Schuijf JD, Jukema JW, Boersma E, de Roos A, van der Wall EE, et al. Prognostic value of multislice computed tomography coronary angiography in pa-

tients with known or suspected coronary artery disease. Journal of the American College of Cardiology. 2007;49(1):62-70. Epub 2007/01/09.

[92] Motoyama S, Sarai M, Harigaya H, Anno H, Inoue K, Hara T, et al. Computed tomographic angiography characteristics of atherosclerotic plaques subsequently resulting in acute coronary syndrome. Journal of the American College of Cardiology. 2009;54(1):49-57. Epub 2009/06/27.

[93] Botnar RM, Stuber M, Lamerichs R, Smink J, Fischer SE, Harvey P, et al. Initial experiences with in vivo right coronary artery human MR vessel wall imaging at 3 tesla. Journal of cardiovascular magnetic resonance : official journal of the Society for Cardiovascular Magnetic Resonance. 2003;5(4):589-94. Epub 2003/12/11.

[94] Fayad ZA, Fuster V, Fallon JT, Jayasundera T, Worthley SG, Helft G, et al. Noninvasive in vivo human coronary artery lumen and wall imaging using black-blood magnetic resonance imaging. Circulation. 2000;102(5):506-10. Epub 2000/08/02.

[95] Botnar RM, Stuber M, Kissinger KV, Kim WY, Spuentrup E, Manning WJ. Noninvasive coronary vessel wall and plaque imaging with magnetic resonance imaging. Circulation. 2000;102(21):2582-7. Epub 2000/11/22.

[96] Nikolaou K, Alkadhi H, Bamberg F, Leschka S, Wintersperger BJ. MRI and CT in the diagnosis of coronary artery disease: indications and applications. Insights into imaging. 2011;2(1):9-24. Epub 2012/02/22.

[97] Dewey M, Teige F, Schnapauff D, Laule M, Borges AC, Wernecke KD, et al. Noninvasive detection of coronary artery stenoses with multislice computed tomography or magnetic resonance imaging. Annals of internal medicine. 2006;145(6):407-15. Epub 2006/09/20.

[98] Genders TS, Meijboom WB, Meijs MF, Schuijf JD, Mollet NR, Weustink AC, et al. CT coronary angiography in patients suspected of having coronary artery disease: decision making from various perspectives in the face of uncertainty. Radiology. 2009;253(3):734-44. Epub 2009/10/30.

[99] Schonenberger E, Schnapauff D, Teige F, Laule M, Hamm B, Dewey M. Patient acceptance of noninvasive and invasive coronary angiography. PloS one. 2007;2(2):e246. Epub 2007/03/01.

[100] Jacobs JE, Boxt LM, Desjardins B, Fishman EK, Larson PA, Schoepf J, et al. ACR practice guideline for the performance and interpretation of cardiac computed tomography (CT). Journal of the American College of Radiology : JACR. 2006;3(9):677-85. Epub 2007/04/07.

[101] Budoff MJ, Cohen MC, Garcia MJ, Hodgson JM, Hundley WG, Lima JA, et al. ACCF/AHA clinical competence statement on cardiac imaging with computed tomography and magnetic resonance: a report of the American College of Cardiology Foundation/American Heart Association/American College of Physicians Task Force on Clinical Competence and Training. Journal of the American College of Cardiology. 2005;46(2):383-402. Epub 2005/07/19.

Chapter 5

Non-Invasive Study of Coronary Circulation by Means of a Transthoracic Dipyridamole Stress Echocardiography with Coronary Flow Reserve Evaluation

Maurizio Turiel, Luigi Gianturco,
Vincenzo Gianturco and Bruno Dino Bodini

Additional information is available at the end of the chapter

http://dx.doi.org/10.5772/54042

1. Introduction

Ultrasound techniques represent easy and useful diagnostic tools able to detect cardiac morphological and functional damage.

Transthoracic echocardiography is a reliable, cheap and non-invasive technique that allows an accurate evaluation of valvular abnormalities, pericardial diseases and ventricular wall motion defects, while Doppler analysis is useful to study left ventricular diastolic filling, valvularfuctioning and pulmonary pressures. Rexhepaj et al [1] found significant differences in early diastolic flow velocity (E), atrial flow velocity (A) and E/A ratio in rheumatoid arthritis (RA) patients compared to the control group, suggesting that a subclinical impairment of left and right ventricular function is present in RA patients, when left ventricular thickness, dimensions and myocardial performance indexes were still normal.

A new clinical application of ultrasound imaging is represented by the transthoracic dipyridamole stress echocardiography with coronary flow reserve (CFR) evaluation. CFR is assessed in the distal left anterior descending coronary artery (LAD) defined by the ratio between peak diastolic velocity during stress and at baseline(Fig. 1-2). It is a highly sensitive (>90%) diagnostic marker for coronary artery disease (CAD)[2, 3] and, when associated with the evaluation of the regional wall motion analysis, it becomes also highly specific [4]. In literature reports, a value of CFR < 2 has been shown to accurately predict the presence of coronary stenosis. In absence of epicardial coronary stenosis, an abnormal CFR may reflect an impaired coronary microcirculation in patients with reperfused myocardial infarct, arterial hypertension with or without left ventricular hypertrophy, diabetes mellitus, hypercholesterolemia, syndrome X, hypertrophic cardiomyopathy and other diseases [5].The assessment of CFR has also a prognostic value, so that a reduced CFR correlates with a negative prognosis [6]. Recently, new evidence underlined that not only the binary (normal-abnormal) response in CFR but the continuous spectrum of CFR value is a strong independent prognostic predictor in patients with known or suspected CAD [7].

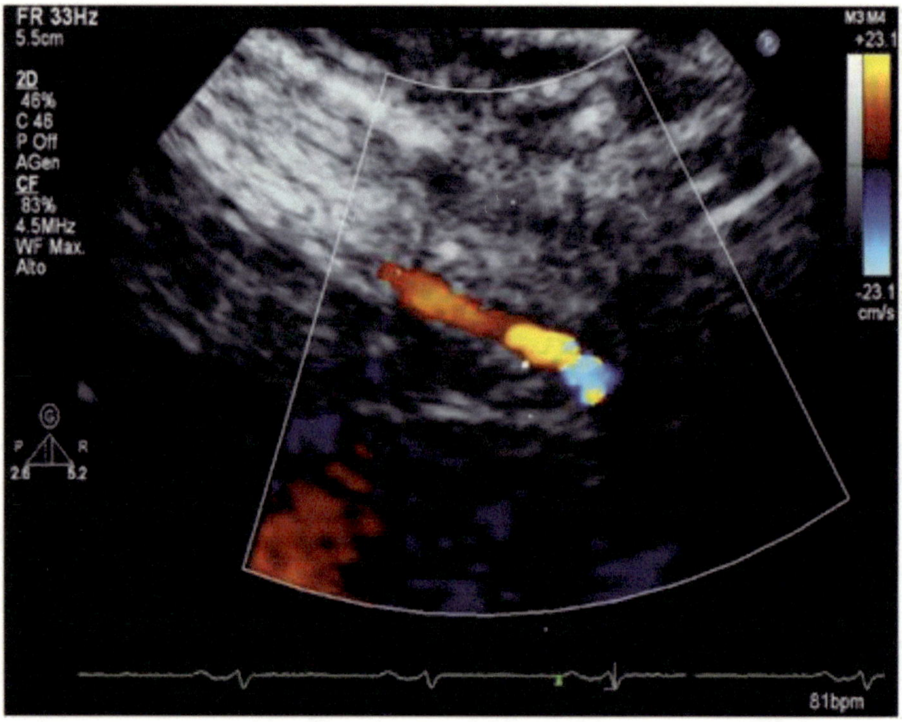

Figure 1. Distal left anterior descending (LAD) flow at color-Doppler.

Hirata et al [8] found a significant reduction of CFR in premenopausal women with SLE compared with age- and sex-matched controls. They concluded that microvascular impairment in SLE could be explained by functional alteration of endothelium which is responsible for the decrease vasodilation in response to pharmacological stress.

Turiel et al. 9 detected a significant impairment of CFR in 25 early RA patients, with disease duration less than 1 year and without any anti-rheumatic therapy. The reduced CFR in absence of wall motion abnormalities at rest and during pharmacological stress showed a coronary microcirculation involvement present in early RA and was associated with endothelial dysfunction.

Tissue Doppler Imaging (TDI) representsa new imaging modality which allows the measurement of myocardial velocities. Till now, TDI has been considered a reliable tool for the assessment of myocardial deformation, but this method is limited by angle-dependency and only deformation along the ultrasound beam can be derived from velocities, while myocardium deforms simultaneously in 3 dimensions [10]. Recently, Birdane et al [11] demonstrated that RA patients had a significant impairment of TDI biventricular diastolic functional parameters compared to healthy controls depending on age and use of steroids. To overcome TDI limitations, speckle tracking analysis has been introduced to evaluate myocardial strain along the longitudinal, circumferential and radial axis [12].

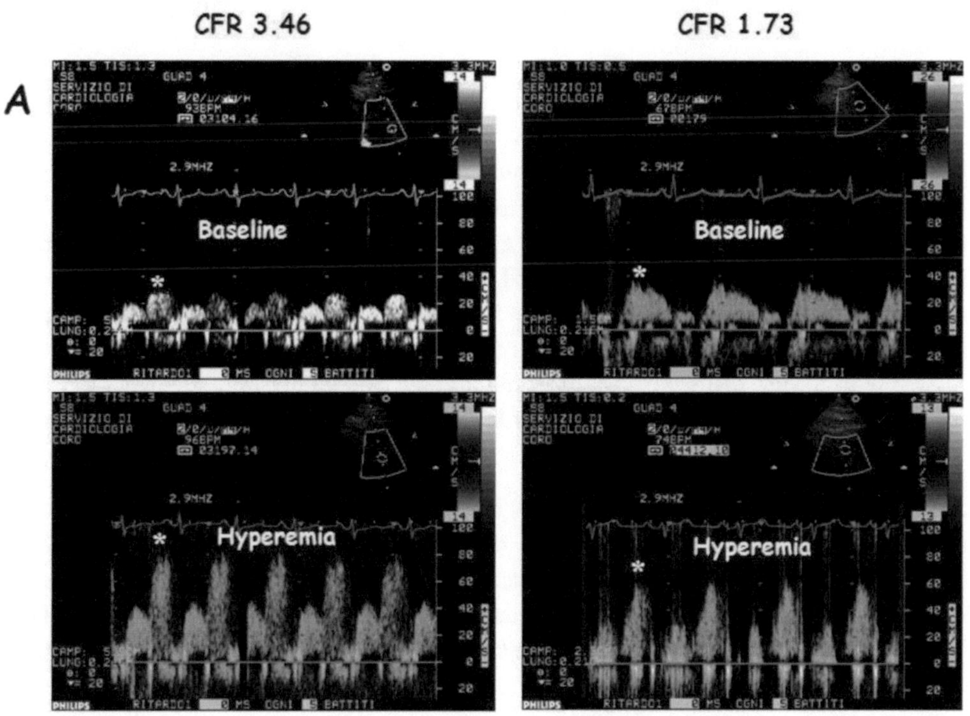

Figure 2. Doppler sampling of LAD: ratio between peak diastolic velocity during stress and at baseline.

Another very useful application of echocardiography in systemic autoimmune diseases is the echo transesophageal approach which is widely recognized as more sensitive than the transthoracic evaluation for the detection of valvular lesions [13] and identification of intracardiac masses.

In particular, Turiel et al [14] observed a large prevalence (61%) of valvular thickening or vegetations and/or potential embolic sources by transesophageal echocardiographic approach in 56 patients with primary antiphospholipid syndrome followed up for 5 years.

2. Utility of coronary flow reserve assessment in systemic autoimmune diseases

Patients suffering from systemic autoimmune diseases (SADs), especially RA, present higher risk of acute myocardial infarction and stroke [15], correlated with disease duration [16] with higher frequency of silent myocardial infarction and sudden death compared to general population [17]. This increase in cardiovascular (CV) risk seems not depending on traditional risk factors, thus suggesting a dominating role of RA-related risk factors [18, 19]. During these last years, attempts of explaining the accelerated atherosclerosis pathogenic pathways in RA were made; Attention particularly focused importance of chronic systemic inflammatory processwith high pro-inflammatory cytokines plasmatic levels. Presence of pro-atherogenic alterations such as dislipidemy, insulin-resistance, trombofilia and oxidative stress look favoring development of endothelial dysfunction that may be the initial stage of the atherosclerotic process [20, 21]. Arosio et al. [22], showed a reduced vasodilatation endothelium-dependant, changes in micro circle reactivity and an increased arterial stiffness in RA female patients.

Today non invasive evaluation of carotid median intimal thickness (IMT) is considered an early atherosclerosis clinical marker [23]. Kumeda et al. [24] observed in RA patients an increased IMT of common carotid and femoral artery, related to disease severity and duration. According to these evidences, Ciftci et al. [25] confirmed increased IMT and presence of reduced coronary flow reserve (CFR) in RA patients, correlating CV risk to disease duration. Moreover, Chung et al. [26], studied extension of coronary calcifications with CT, showing that patient with a long history of RA presents greater prevalence and severity of coronary calcifications compared to patients with early RA, also correlated with smoking and increase eritrosedimentation rate (ESR).

Nowadays, trans-thoracic echocardiographic evaluation of CFR by pharmacological stress (adenosine or dipyridamole)is considered a very useful exam as diagnose marker highly sensible (>90%) for coronary disease [27]. If associated with LV regional kinesis evaluation, acquires high specificity too. CFR value< 2 measured about at middle-distal tract of left anterior descending artery can accurately predict the presence of coronary significative stenosis. If epicardial vessels are free from significant stenosis a reduced CFR can be evidence of an alteration in coronary microcirculation in patients with reperfused myocardial infarction, high blood pressure with or without LV hypertrophy, diabetes mellitus, hypercholesterolemia, X syndrome, hypertrophic cardiomyopathy and collagen diseases. CFR measure has prognostic value in different pathologic conditions too[28].

Turiel et al. [29] showed a statistically significative variation of CFR among RA patients related with disease duration.

Endothelium function can be also studied through measure of asymmetric dymethilarginine(ADMA) plasmatic levels. Many clinical evidences support a close association between ADMA level and CV involvement in patients autoimmune diseases [30].

http://dx.doi.org/10.5772/54042

Higher ADMA plasmatic levels are reported in many conditions associated with high CV risk such as hypercholesterolemia, hypertriglyceridemia [31], peripheral artery disease [32], diabetes mellitus type II [33], acute coronary syndrome [34], chronic renal failure [35]. Moreover, Surdacki et al [36] evidenced in RA patient an association between high ADMA plasmatic levels and increased IMT at common carotid artery. Turiel et al. [37]observed an inverse correlation between ADMA and CFR in early stages of RA thus indicating a subclinical heart involvement already present at the beginning of the development of the disease.

Many clinical trials evidenced potential effects against atherosclerosis of therapies lead with disease modifying anti-rheumatic drugs (DMARDs), going beyond the simple control of inflammatory process and of disease activity (Tab. 1). In particular Hurlimann et al. [38] showed that anti-TNFα can not only reduce disease activity indexes, but also increase endothelial function in RA. Moreover, Sitia et al. [39] observed that long time treatment with DMARDs can reverse endothelial dysfunction, in early stages of disease.

Farmaco	Posologia	Tempo approssimativo per l' azione	Documentazione attività ref.	Costo per terapia annuale ($)
Idrossiclorochina	200 mg 2 volte al giorno	2 – 6 mesi	11,12	1.056
Oro intramuscolo	25-.50 mg i.m. ogni 2-4 sett	3 – 6 mesi	13	198
Azatioprina	50-150 mg al giorno	2 - 3 mesi	14	579 - 1.737
D-penicillamina	250-750 mg/die	3 – 6 mesi	15	865 - 2.595
Ciclosporina	25-4 mg/Kg/die	2 – 4 mesi	16	4.432 – 8.859
Methotrexate	7,5-20 mg/sett i.m o per os	1 – 2 mesi	17,18	orale 697 –1.859 i.m. 419 - 806
Sulfasalazina	100 mg 2-3 volte die	1 - 3 mesi	19 - 21	509 - 763
Leflunomide	20 mg al giorno	4 - 12 sett.	22,23	2.938
Infliximab (+ Methotrexate)	3-10 mg/Kg i.v. ogni 8 sett	da pochi giorni a 4 mesi	24 - 26	13.940 - 36.694
Etanercept	25 mg sc 2 volte/sett.	da pochi giorni a 4 sett.	27 - 29	15.436
Anakinra	100 mg sc quotidie	-	30,31	-

Table 1. Disease modifying anti-rheumatic drugs (DMARDs) in common use. (From American College of Rheumatology Subcommittee on Rheumatoid Arthritis Guidelines. Guidelines for the management of rheumatoid arthritis. Arthritis Rheum 2002; 46: 328-46, modified).

In addition, Mäki-Petäjä et al. [40] in a recent study confirmed the efficacy of associating ezetimibe and simvastatin in reducing the inflammatory process, but also in improving aortic stiffness in RA. Anyway, the possible validation of efficacy of the therapy with statin and/or biological drugs in modifying the evolution of atherosclerosis needs further perspective clinical trials.

3. Conclusions

Subclinical CV involvement related to specific and non-specific risk factors is frequent in systemic autoimmunity diseases. It begins rapidly after the onset of the disease and progresses with disease duration. All cardiac structures may be affected, and the cardiac complications include a variety of clinical manifestations. As CV involvement is associated with an unfavorable prognosis, the early detection of subclinical cardiac involvement in asymptomatic SADs patients is essential and then modern techniques nowhere existing and in this chapter illustrated are very very important to reach such goal.

Conflict of interest

None

Author details

Maurizio Turiel[1], Luigi Gianturco[1], Vincenzo Gianturco[2] and Bruno Dino Bodini[3]

*Address all correspondence to: maurizio.turiel@unimi.it

1 Cardiology Unit, IRCCS Galeazzi Orthopedic Institute, Department of Biomedical Sciences for Health, University of Milan, Milan, Italy

2 Department of Cardiovascular, Respiratory, Nephrological, Anesthesiological and Geriatrics Sciences, Sapienza University of Rome, Italy

3 Rehabilitation Unit, IRCCSGaleazzi Orthopedic Institute, Italy

References

[1] NoneRexhepaj N, Bajraktari G, Berisha I, Beqiri A, Shatri F, Hima F, Elezi S, Ndrepepa G. Left and right ventricular diastolic functions in patients with rheumatoid ar-

thritis without clinically evident cardiovascular disease. Int J Clin Pract 2006; 60: 683-688.

[2] Caiati C, Zedda N, Montaldo C, Montisci R, Ruscazio M, Lai G, Cadeddu M, Meloni L, Iliceto S. Contrast-enhanced transthoracic second harmonic echo Doppler with adenosine: a noninvasive, rapid and effective method for coronary flow reserve assessment. J Am Coll Cardiol 1999; 34:122-130.

[3] Hozumi T, Yoshida K, Ogata Y, Akasaka T, Asami Y, Takagi T, Morioka S. Non invasive assessment of significant left anterior descending coronary artery stenosis by coronary flow velocity reserve with transthoracic color Doppler echocardiography. Circulation 1998; 97: 1557-1562.

[4] Rigo F, Richieri M, Pasanisi E, Cutaia V, Zanella C, Della Valentina P, Di Pede F, Raviele A, Picano E. Usefulness of coronary flow reserve over regional wall motion when added to dual-imaging dipyridamole echocardiography. Am J Cardiol 2003; 91: 269-273.

[5] Dimitrow PP. Coronary flow reserve-measurement and application: focus on transthoracic Doppler echocardiography. Boston/Dordrecht/London: Kluwer Academic Publishers. 2002.

[6] Rigo F, Gherardi S, Galderisi M, Pratali L, Cortigiani L, Sicari R, Picano E. The prognostic impact of coronary flow-reserve assessed by Doppler echocardiography in non-ischemic dilated cardiomyopathy. Eur Heart J 2006;27:1319-1323.

[7] Cortigiani L, Rigo F, Gherardi S, Bovenzi F, Picano E, Sicari R. Implication of the continuous prognostic spectrum of Doppler echocardiographic derived coronary flow reserve on left anterior descending artery. Am J Cardiol 2010; 105:158-162.

[8] Hirata K, Kadirvelu A, Kinjo M, Sciacca R, Sugioka K, Otsuka R, Choy A, Chow SK, Yoshiyama M, Yoshikawa J, Homma S, Lang CC. Altered coronary vasomotor function in young patients with Systemic Lupus Erythematosus. Arthritis and Rheum 2007; 56: 1904-1909.

[9] Turiel M, Tomasoni L, Sitia S, Cicala S, Gianturco L, Ricci C, Atzeni F, De Gennaro Colonna V, Longhi M, Sarzi-Puttini P. Effects of long-term disease-modifying antirheumatic drugs on endothelial function in patients with early rheumatoid arthritis. Cardiovasc Ther. 2010 Oct;28(5):e53-64.

[10] Dandel M, Hetzer R. Echocardiographic strain and strain rate imaging – Clinical applications. Int J Cardiol 2009; 132: 11-24.

[11] Birdane A, Korkmaz C, Ata N, Cavusoglu Y, Kasifoglu T, Dogan SM, Gorenek B, Goktekin O, Unalir A, Timuralp B. Tissue Doppler imaging in the evaluation of the left and right ventricular diastolic functions in Rheumatoid Arthritis. Echocardiography 2007; 24: 485-493.

[12] Sitia S, Tomasoni L, Turiel M. Speckle tracking echocardiography: a new approach to myocardial function. World J Cardiol 2010; 2: 1-5.

[13] Turiel M, Muzzupappa S, Gottardi B, Crema C, Sarzi-Puttini P, Rossi E. Evaluation of cardiac abnormalities and embolic sources in primary antiphospholipid syndrome by transesophageal echocardiography. Lupus 2000;9: 406-412.

[14] Turiel M, Sarzi-Puttini P, Peretti R, Bonizzato S, Muzzupappa S, Atzeni F, Rossi E, Doria A. Five-year follow-up by transesophageal echocardiographic studies in primary antiphospholipid syndrome. Am J Cardiol 2005; 96: 574-579.

[15] Solomon DH, Goodson NJ, Katz JN, Weinblatt ME, Avorn J, Setoguchi S, Canning C, Schneeweiss S. Patterns of cardiovascular risk in rheumatoid arthritis. Ann Rheum Dis. 2006;65:1608-12.

[16] Solomon DH, Karlson EW, Rimm EB, Cannuscio CC, Mandl LA, Manson JE, Stampfer MJ, Curhan GC. Cardiovascular morbidity and mortality in women diagnosed with rheumatoid arthritis. Circulation. 2003;107:1303-7.

[17] Maradit-Kremers H, Crowson CS, Nicola PJ, Ballman KV, Roger VL, Jacobsen SJ, Gabriel SE. Increased unrecognized coronary heart disease and sudden deaths in rheumatoid arthritis: a population-based cohort study. Arthritis Rheum. 2005;52:402-11.

[18] Del Rincón ID, Williams K, Stern MP, Freeman GL, Escalante A. High incidence of cardiovascular events in a rheumatoid arthritis cohort not explained by traditional cardiac risk factors. Arthritis Rheum. 2001;44:2737-45.

[19] Del Rincón I, O'Leary DH, Freeman GL, Escalante A. Acceleration of atherosclerosis during the course of rheumatoid arthritis. Atherosclerosis. 2007;195:354-60.

[20] Voskuyl AE. The heart and the cardiovascular manifestations in rheumatoid arthritis. Rheumatology 2006;45:iv4-7.

[21] Dhawan SS, Quyyumi AA. Rheumatoid arthritis and cardiovascular disease. Curr Atheroscler Rep. 2008 Apr;10(2):128-33.

[22] Arosio E, De Marchi S, Rigoni A, Prior M, Delva P, Lech A. Forearm haemodynamics, arterial stiffness and microcirculatory reactivity in rheumatoid arthritis. J Hypertens. 2007;25:1273-8.

[23] Sidhu PS, Allen PL. Ultrasound assessment of internal carotid artery stenosis. Clin Radiol 1997;52: 654-8.

[24] Kumeda Y, Inaba M, Goto H, Nagata M, Henmi Y, Furumitsu Y, Ishimura E, Inui K, Yutani Y, Miki T, Shoji T, Nishizawa Y. Increased thickness of arterial intima-media detected by ultrasonography in patients with rheumatoid arthritis. Arthritis Rheum 2002; 46:1489-97.

[25] Ciftci O, Yilmaz S, Topcu S, Caliskan M, Gullu H, Erdogan D, Pamuk BO, Yildirir A, Muderrisoglu H. Imapired coronary microvascular function and increased intima-media thickness in rheumatoid arthritis. Atherosclerosis 2008; 198: 332-7.

[26] Chung CP, Oeser A, Raggi P, Gebretsadik T, Shintani AK, Sokka T, Pincus T, Avalos I, Stein CM. Increased coronary-artery atherosclerosis in rheumatoid arthritis. Arthritis Rheum 2005;52: 3045-53.

[27] Kerekes G, Soltész P, Nurmohamed MT, Gonzalez-Gay MA, Turiel M, Végh E, Shoenfeld Y, McInnes I, Szekanecz Z. Validated methods for assessment of subclinical atherosclerosis in rheumatology. Nat Rev Rheumatol 2012; 8(4): 224-34.

[28] Sitia S, Atzeni F, Sarzi-Puttini P, Di Bello V, Tomasoni L, Delfino L, Antonini-Canterin F, Di Salvo G, De Gennaro Colonna V, La Carrubba S, Carerj S, Turiel M. Cardiovascular involvement in systemic autoimmune diseases. Autoimmunity Rev 2009; 8: 281-286.

[29] Atzeni F, Sarzi-Puttini P, Delfino L, et al. Decreased coronary flow reserve in patients with rheumatoid arthritis. Ann Rheum Dis 2004;63:S196.

[30] De Gennaro Colonna V, Pascale V, Bianchi M, Ferrario P, Morelli F, Pascale W, Tomasoni L, Turiel M. Asymmetric dimethylarginine (ADMA): an endogenous inhibitor of nitric oxide sinthase and a novel cardiovascular risk molecole. Medical Science Monitor 2008; 15(4): 91-101.

[31] Lundman P, Eriksson MJ, Stuhlinger M, Cooke JP, Hamsten A, Tornvall P. Mild-to-moderate hypertriglyceridemia in young men is associated with endothelial dysfunction and increased plasma concentrations of asymmetric dimethylarginine. J Am Coll Cardiol 2001; 38: 111-6.

[32] Boger RH, Bode-Boger SM, Thiele W, Junker W, Alexander K, Frölich JC. Biochemical evidence for impaired nitric oxide synthesis in patients with peripheral arterial occlusive disease. Circulation 1997; 95:2068-74.

[33] Stuhlinger MC, Abbasi F, Chu JW, Lamendola C, McLaughlin TL, Cooke JP, Reaven GM, Tsao PS. Relationship between insulin resistance and an endogenous nitric oxide synthase inhibitor. JAMA 2002; 287: 1420-6.

[34] Bae SW, Stuhlinger MC, Yoo HS, Yu KH, Park HK, Choi BY, Lee YS, Pachinger O, Choi YH, Lee SH, Park JE. Plasma asymmetric dimethylarginine concentrations in newly diagnosed patients with acute myocardial infarction or unstable angina pectoris during two weeks of medical treatment. Am J Cardiol 2005;95: 729-33.

[35] MacAllister RJ, Rambausek MH, Vallance P, Williams D, Hoffmann KH, Ritz E. Concentration of dimethyl-l-arginine in the plasma of patients with end-stage renal failure. Nephrol Dial Transplant 1996; 11: 2449-52.

[36] Surdacki A, Martens-Lobenhoffer J, Wloch A, Marewicz E, Rakowski T, Wieczorek-Surdacka E, Dubiel JS, Pryjma J, Bode-Böger SM. Elevated plasma asymmetric dimethyl- L-arginine levels are linked to endothelial progenitor cell depletion and carotid atherosclerosis in rheumatoid arthritis. Arthritis Rheum 2007; 56: 809-19.

[37] Turiel M, Tomasoni L, Delfino L, Bodini B, Bacchiani G, Atzeni F, Sarzi-Puttini P, De Gennaro Colonna V. Clinical implications of assessing coronary flow reserve and

plasma asymmetric dimethylarginine in early rheumatoid arthritis. Eur J Echocardiogr 2007; 8: S35.

[38] Hurlimann D, Forster A, Noll G, Enseleit F, Chenevard R, Distler O, Béchir M, Spieker LE, Neidhart M, Michel BA, Gay RE, Lüscher TF, Gay S, Ruschitzka F. Anti-tumor necrosis factor-alpha treatment improves endothelial function in patients with rheumatoid arthritis. Circulation 2002; 106: 2184-7.

[39] Sitia S, Tomasoni L, Cicala S, Delfino L, Atzeni F, Sarzi-Puttini P, De Gennaro Colonna V, Turiel M. Effects of long-term disease-modifying antirheumatic drugs on endothelial function in patients with early rheumatoid arthritis. Eur J Echocardiogr 2008; 9:166.

[40] Mäki-Petäjä KM, Booth AD, Hall FC, Wallace SM, Brown J, McEniery CM, Wilkinson IB. Ezetimibe and simvastatin reduce inflammation, disease activity, and aortic stiffness and improve endothelial function in rheumatoid arthritis. J Am Coll Cardiol 2007; 50: 852-8.

Chapter 6

Computed Tomography Imaging of the Coronary Arteries

G.J. Pelgrim, M. Oudkerk and R. Vliegenthart

Additional information is available at the end of the chapter

http://dx.doi.org/10.5772/54044

1. Introduction

In this chapter the possibilities of computed tomography (CT) for imaging of the coronary arteries are examined. Only in the last decades CT has entered the field of cardiac imaging, due to technical developments. First the history of CT in cardiac imaging is described. When did this technique enter clinical practice and what level of temporal and spatial resolution does it reach nowadays?

The goal of the CT technique described in this chapter is to image the coronary arteries. It is important to know how a CT scan for coronary imaging is made. This is discussed in the second part of the chapter. Contraindications to coronary CT angiography (CCTA) are put forward followed by the explanation of scan acquisition techniques. A detailed overview is provided regarding different CCTA scan protocols and types of acquisitions.

One of the main disadvantages of CCTA is the patient exposure to radiation to acquire the imaging data. Therefore, an important goal in CCTA imaging is to reduce the radiation dose while maintaining diagnostic image quality. There are multiple developments in the area of CT radiation reduction, which are discussed in the next section.

The diagnostic accuracy of CCTA has been investigated extensively in recent years. In this section the diagnostic accuracy of different CT scanner generations for calcium scoring and CCTA are expanded upon. This includes results for different parameters used in diagnostic accuracy studies, such as sensitivity and specificity.

What are the indications for CCTA examinations? This is the question which is answered in the fifth section. While this is a dynamic field, the main indications, supported by different consensus statements, are discussed. Approximately ten indications are described and ordered by relevance. Examples of different indications are shown by patient CCTA images.

The future of cardiac CT is the last topic discussed. There are ample opportunities for future cardiac CT research such as CT perfusion imaging. These options are briefly mentioned.

2. Computed tomography

Computed tomography (CT) has been utilized in numerous fields in clinical practice since its invention in the 1970s. The first CT scanner was developed in 1971 by Geoffrey Hounsfield and installed at the Atkinson-Morley hospital in England. CT uses X-ray radiation to acquire 2D cross-sectional images of the body. X-ray imaging uses the different properties of different tissues to distinguish them in the image data. These images are acquired by a rapid 360 degree circular motion of the X-ray tube. The images are registered by the circular ray of X-ray detectors located in the gantry surrounding the patient. Then, a 2 dimensional reconstruction is made using the principle that an internal structure of the body can be made using multiple X-ray projections. To reconstruct a CT image, data from approximately 180^0 of gantry rotation are required. From the start in 1972, CT has had an important role in diagnostics as non-invasive imaging technique.

In cardiac imaging, however, CT did not gain ground until developments in recent years. Early CT modalities were limited in their ability to display cardiac morphological information due to the interference of cardiac motion and spatial resolution. The diameter of coronary arteries varies from large, 3 mm, to small, 1.5 mm. Therefore, the spatial resolution of the angiography technique should be at least 1 mm. [1] Temporal resolution was not sufficient to display the heart due to cardiac motion. Therefore, until recently, invasive coronary angiography (ICA) was the only accurate method for coronary imaging. [2, 3]

CT for cardiac imaging first entered the field with the development of electron beam computed tomography (EBCT) in the 1980s. EBCT was specifically developed for cardiac imaging, combining very high temporal resolution (50-100ms) with prospective electrocardiographic (ECG) triggering. The high temporal resolution combined with ECG triggering greatly reduced cardiac motion artifacts. The main clinical application of EBCT was the quantification of coronary calcium deposits in a so-called calcium score. The calcium score is correlated with degree and severity of coronary artery disease (CAD) and is a strong predictor of coronary events. [4, 5]The application of calcium scoring is explained in more detail further in this chapter. Main limitation of EBCT is the spatial resolution of between 1.5 mm and 3 mm in the z-axis. This prevents EBCT to accurately determine the severity of CAD, especially in CCTA setting. After the introduction of multidetector CT (MDCT) scanners in 1990s (see below) and due to limited availability of EBCT scanners, EBCT was used less frequently and eventually replaced by MDCT systems from 2003 onwards.

The developments in CT were rapid, compared to other imaging fields in the last decades. These developments have led to considerably improved temporal and spatial resolution. MDCT scanners use multiple detectors to acquire the data, scanning multiple detector rows in one rotation. Already 4- and 16-row MDCT scanners caused a revolution in cardiac imaging, however diagnostic accuracy in terms of specificity was generally low. [6-10] Sensitivity and negative predictive value were already good. MDCT proved useful in evaluation of coronary anomalies and bypass graft patency. Although the 16-row MDCT scanners had improved spatial resolution, making detection and characterization of coronary plaques and coronary wall changes possible, high heart rates, stents and severely calcified arteries, however, affected the image quality negatively. [11, 12]

In 2004, the next generation of MDCT scanners was introduced, with 32, 40 and 64 slices, another step forward in speed of volume coverage. Compared to 16-row MDCT scanners, the gantry rotation time of 64-row MDCT scanners improved from 500 ms to 330 ms. This translates in an improvement in temporal resolution from 250 ms to 165 ms, as only half a rotation is needed to acquire the data required for the image reconstruction. The visualization of the coronary arteries was again markedly improved, with a high sensitivity and specificity achieved for evaluation of coronary stenosis. [13-15] Examinations in patients with high heart rates were reported to still yield diagnostic images, with the use of multisegment reconstruction algorithms, reducing influence of motion artifacts. [16, 17]

Dual source computed tomography (DSCT) is one of the latest improvements in CT imaging modalities. The DSCT scanners consist of 2 tube-detector systems mounted in the same gantry, off-set by 90 degrees (perpendicular). Compared with conventional single-source CT scanners, the temporal resolution of this CT scanner is twice as high. This is because the temporal resolution is equal to a quarter of the gantry rotation. The other parameters, such as gantry rotation time, are equal to single-source CT scanners. In DSCT, the temporal resolution is further improved to 83 ms, further reducing the influence of motion artifacts on the image quality. Studies have shown an improvement in the assessment of the moving heart at a high heart rate without the need to use medication to control the heart rate during the examination. [18-22] Multiple studies have assessed the difference in image quality and accuracy of DSCT compared to 64-row scanners. [23-25] The higher temporal resolution resulted in better image quality and diagnostic accuracy.

Recent expansion of the detector width in MDCT has resulted in CT scanners with 256 and 320 detector rows. These systems allow for coverage of up to 320 slices during one rotation and in one heartbeat. This allows coverage of the whole heart in one gantry rotation. The principle of these CT scanners is the use of a cone beam. The X-ray tube can reach the detectors at the edges of the gantry readout, possibly displaying the whole heart in one scan. However, the 320-slice coverage comes at a cost as the temporal resolution is lowered to 350 ms and the edge of the scan range is prone to artifacts. [26-28]

The introduction of CT and different generations of CT scanners over time is described in Table 1. Continuously, new technologies are developed to improve the diagnostic performance of the CT technique for imaging the coronary arteries, including the spatial and temporal resolution.

Computed tomography development	
Year	**Technique**
1971	**First computed tomography scanner**
1980s	**Electron beam computed tomography (EBCT)**
1990s	**Multidetector CT scanner**
2004	**32-, 40-, 60-row multidetector CT**
2006	**Dual source computed tomography (DSCT)**
2007	**256- and 320-slice CT**

Table 1. Development in computed tomography with highlights through the years

3. Imaging the coronary arteries by CCTA

The goal of coronary CT angiography (CCTA) is to image the coronary arteries, detect coronary artery calcification, and evaluate coronary stenosis or occlusion. Final aim is to aid the cardiologist in determining the best patient treatment and management.

High quality images are the most important prerequisite in the diagnostic assessment of the coronary arteries. Certain factors need to be taken into account to ensure a high-quality CCTA examination in the correct patient. These factors include selecting the right patients for the examination, proper patient preparation, an adequate CT scanner, optimal CT scan protocol, including synchronization of the CT data with the ECG information and proper reconstruction of image data, and dedicated software for evaluation of the coronary CT images. Furthermore, a prerequisite for CCTA is the injection of iodinated contrast material to delineate the lumen of the coronary arteries. Therefore, an absolute contraindication for CCTA is an allergy for iodine. An overview of contraindications for CCTA are listed in table 2. [29] Apart from general contraindications for CT, there are some specific contraindications for CCTA, such as high or irregular heart rates.

CCTA Contraindications
Atrial fibrillation (permanent or at time of the study)
Heart rate "/> 65 beats/minute refractory to heart-rate lowering agents
Bigeminy, Trigeminy, high degree heart block
Severe asthma
Creatinine "/> 1.8 (estimated Glomerular Filtration < 60), measurement of kidney function
Failed steroid preparation for contrast allergy
Morbid obesity (body mass index "/> 40)
Calcium score "/> 1000
Pregnancy
Inability to cooperate with scan acquisition and/or breath hold instructions

Table 2. Contraindications for coronary CTA

As stated before, motion artifacts on CCTA are observed more frequently in patients with higher and irregular heart rates. This negatively affects the image quality and reliability of detecting or excluding coronary stenoses. For earlier generation 16- to 64-row MDCT scanners it has been proven that the highest image quality is achieved in patients with a low heart rate (< 65 beats per minute). [30-32] It was shown that breath hold at end-inspiration reduces the heart rate by (on average) 6 beats per minute, which can be tested prior to performing the CCTA acquisition. In case of a patient's heart rate higher than 70 per minute it is advised to reduce the heart rate by medication. This can be done by administration of intravenous injection of 5-25 mg metoprolol.

Patients are positioned on the CT table in supine position. The three ECG leads are attached to the patient body to acquire an adequate ECG tracing, which is synchronized with the raw image data. Furthermore, an 18-gauge intravenous-line is inserted to ensure a correct injection of the contrast agent. The actual acquisition protocol consists of three steps: a topogram, a determination of the contrast arrival time using a test contrast bolus or acquisition of repetitive images during contrast injection for bolus tracking and the actual CCTA scan.

First, a low-energy topogram is acquired to enable accurate positioning of the scan volume. Afterwards, a non-contrast scan can be performed to obtain a coronary artery calcification (CAC) score. The coronary calcium score is a calculation of the amount of coronary artery calcium. The most commonly used method for coronary calcium quantification is the calcium score according to Agatston. [33] A negative CT scan for coronary calcium shows no calcification in the coronaries. A positive test means CAD is present, also when a patient is asymptomatic. The amount of calcification, expressed in the calcium score, can help to predict the risk of coronary events. The extent of CAD is graded according to the calcium, shown in table 3. The height of the calcium score is also strongly related to the risk of coronary heart disease. [34-37] At this moment, the strongest indication for coronary calcium scoring is in asymptomatic individuals at intermediate risk based on risk factors, to improve risk stratification. [38] For 64-row MDCT and earlier CT generations, a calcium score above 1000 is generally considered a contraindication for performing CCTA. The reason is twofold: patients with a very high calcium score have a considerable probability of having one or more significant stenosis, and severe calcifications cause blooming artifacts that limit the assessment of luminal narrowing.

Two techniques are available to correctly start the CCTA acquisition, based on arrival of contrast in the coronary arteries: the bolus tracking and the bolus timing technique. Bolus tracking involves a series of axial low-dose images to track the bolus of contrast material (every 2 seconds), monitoring the contrast enhancement in a region of interest (ROI) in the ascending aorta. The CCTA imaging sequence is initiated when the Hounsfield Unit (HU) in the ROI reaches a certain predefined level, usually 100 HU. The bolus timing technique involves an extra low-dose scan acquisition of a single slice. Here, a small contrast bolus followed by a saline flush is injected to determine the contrast arrival time. An axial low-dose image is generated every 2 seconds at a predefined ROI in the ascending aorta. The time between the start of the contrast injection and the arrival of contrast bolus in ROI is used as the scan delay for the actual CCTA. Both methods have similar results and have proven its usefulness in multiple research studies.

Cardiac calcium score	Extent of CAD, risk of coronary events in the next 5 year
0	No evidence of CAD, very low risk of coronary events
1-10	Minimal evidence of CAD, low risk of coronary events
11-100	Mild evidence of CAD, low-moderate risk of coronary events
101-400	Moderate evidence of CAD, moderate risk of coronary events
"/>400	Severe evidence of CAD, high risk of coronary events

Table 3. Cardiac calcium score related to the extent of CAD

When the correct volume and scan delay have been selected, the actual CCTA scan can be performed. A volume dataset of the coronary arteries is required, covering the entire heart. The scan is acquired during breath hold. A contrast agent with a high concentration of iodine is used (300mg/ml) to ensure adequate opacification of the coronary arteries. A total amount of 60-80 ml of contrast agent is injected with an injection speed of approximately 4-6 ml/s, which is flushed by a saline bolus of 40-70 ml (4-6 ml/s).

The scanning parameters are different from vendor to vendor and per scanner generation. These parameters are beyond the scope of this chapter and can be obtained from the vendor of the CT scanner.

CCTA scans are usually acquired in spiral mode, with continuous acquisition of data throughout the whole cardiac cycle (see Figure 1). The quality of the reconstructed axial images is determined by multiple parameters.

The use of retrospective ECG-triggering enables the reconstruction of CCTA images at different time points in the R-R interval. The R-R interval is the time between two R-tops in a normal cardiac cycle. In previous studies it has been shown that the optimal visualization window for coronary imaging, nearly free of motion artifacts is mid-diastole, at 60% to 70% of the R-R interval. In patients with higher or irregular heart rates however, better image quality is usually obtained at 25% to 35% of the R-R interval.

Slice thickness is dependent on the parameters of the specific CT scanner. Thinner slices improve the quality of the 3-dimensional dataset and the quality of the reconstructed images; on the downside it also increases the image noise which could potentially limit the diagnostic accuracy of the CCTA examination.

The CCTA images are usually reconstructed with a medium smooth reconstruction kernel. The reconstruction kernel, also referred to as 'filter' or 'algorithm' by some CT vendors, is one of the most important parameters affecting the image quality. In general, there is a tradeoff between the spatial resolution and noise for each kernel. Smooth kernels generate images with low noise, resulting in lower spatial resolution. A sharp kernel however, generates images with high spatial resolution but also have increased noise levels. [39] Recently, iterative reconstruction techniques have been introduced. These techniques reduce image noise by iteratively comparing the acquired image to a modeled projection. This algorithm is developed to reduce the radiation dose and enhance tube current modulation. These reconstruction techniques have shown to reduce image noise and improve image quality. [40, 41]

Prospective ECG-triggering is a technique used in cardiac CT that uses forward-looking prediction of R wave timing (see Figure 1). This is step-and-shoot non-spiral acquisition without table motion during imaging. Main advantage of prospective ECG-triggering is the lower radiation dose compared to retrospective ECG-triggering, see below. A disadvantage is the possibility of non-diagnostic coronary artery segments in case of unexpected changes or irregularity in the heart rate, as retrospective manipulation of the CT image data is generally not possible. [42-44]

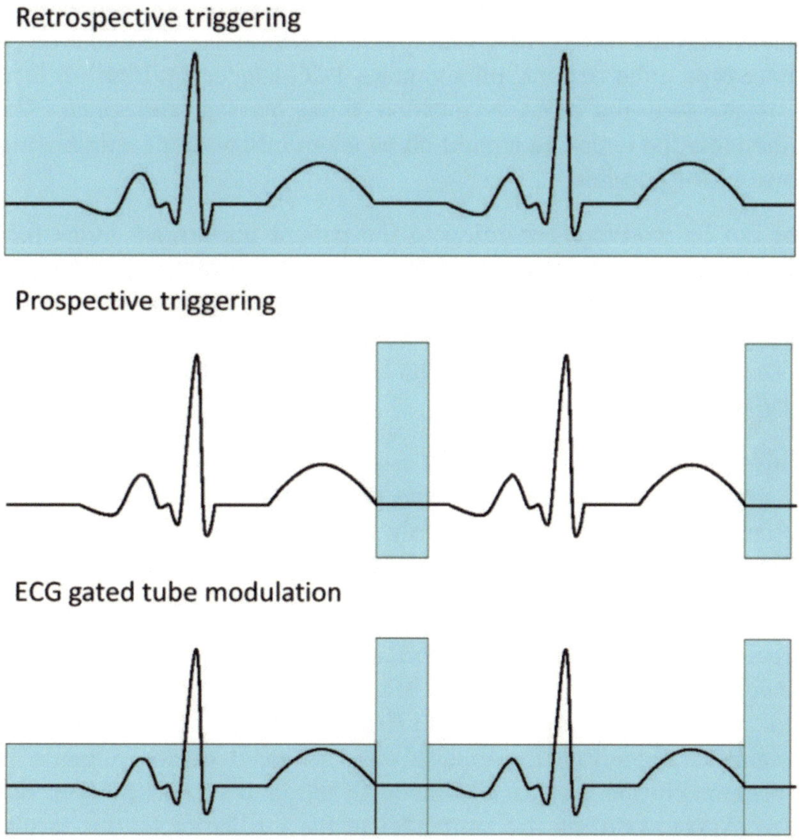

Figure 1. Different triggering techniques used to lower radiation dose. In retrospective triggering, the acquisition is constant and afterwards, the best cardiac phase is reconstructed for analysis. In prospective triggering, the acquisition is only performed during small parts of the cardiac phase, reducing radiation dose. In ECG-gated tube current modulation, the tube current is lowered during phases more likely to have motion artifacts and normal in the area of interest.

4. CCTA radiation exposure

The retrospectively ECG-gated CT is associated with relatively high radiation dose because of low pitch and overlapping data. Effective doses that have been published vary between 2 and 30 mSv, a prospective triggering mode has an effective radiation dose of between 1-3 mSv in adults. [42-45]

Radiation is a potential threat, which can cause harm to the human body. Therefore, minimizing radiation exposure to patients is of critical importance for physicians. The International Commission on Radiological Protection (ICRP) estimated that chance of acquiring fatal radiogenic cancer in the adult population is approximately 0.005%/mSv. Furthermore, it is assumed that there is no safe amount of radiation; any radiation amount is potentially harmful. Thus, effort should be taken to keep radiation doses as low as possible while maintaining diagnostic scan relevance. This radiological principle is also expressed as 'As Low As Reasonably Achievable' or ALARA. Multiple factors influence the radiation exposure, including scanner type, tube current, tube voltage, ECG triggering, high pitch helical scanning, scan range, slice thickness, acquisition time, overlap and pitch. Those factors influencing the radiation exposure should all be taken into account, minimizing the radiation to the lowest level possible.

Tube current can be modified according to the patient body mass index (BMI). Higher tube current increases the amount of photons per exposure time, reducing the image noise, but at the same time increasing the radiation dose. Patients with higher BMI need higher tube current to reduce the noise level, generated by the higher amount of tissue penetrated. The tube current should only be increased to a level necessary for acquiring adequate diagnostic images.

Increasing tube voltage will lead to higher energy X-ray beams with higher tissue penetration, and substantially increased radiation dose. Generally, 100 to 120 KeV tube voltages are sufficient for cardiac imaging. Only in really large patients, 140 KeV could be used. Reducing tube voltage will reduce radiation dose in proportion to the square of changes in tube voltage. [46, 47]

ECG synchronization is of particular importance for the amount of radiation exposure. As aforementioned, in retrospective ECG triggering data are acquired throughout the whole cardiac cycle and only the data with the least motion are used for reconstruction. In prospective ECG triggering, the tube is only activated during a predefined cardiac phase with presumably the greatest likelihood of minimal cardiac motion. Because there is no radiation exposure during the remainder of the cardiac cycle, this results in a dose reduction potential of 31%-86%. [25] In case of retrospective ECG triggering, ECG-based tube current modulation is an effective form of dose reduction (see Figure 1). This modulation utilizes the concept that coronary motion is least during end-systole and end-diastole. Therefore, the tube current is reduced by up to 96% during periods with presumably more cardiac motion and ramped up during diastole, when motion is at its lowest (for heart rates up to 65 bpm). [46] The image quality of phases with lower tube

http://dx.doi.org/10.5772/54044

current is reduced, which is a downside of this technique. The potential dose reduction of ECG-gated tube current modulation is 13%-46%. [25].

The introduction of the second generation DSCT scanners made high-pitch helical scanning possible. This prospectively ECG triggered technique involves a high speed of the patient table. Due to this high pitch, the heart can be scanned in a fraction of one heartbeat. This eliminates overlapping volume coverage of sequential sections. Early results show dose reductions of up to 80% and CCTA examinations with <1 mSv radiation dose. [25]

Scan range is a term that indicates the z range (length) of the body which is scanned. Therefore, the larger the scan range is set, the higher the radiation exposure will be. The scan range should be limited to the range that is ultimately necessary to clarify the diagnostic questionnaire. A scan of the coronaries should not include the aortic root unless this is specifically asked by the referring physician. This will limit unnecessary radiation exposure.

Some factors of minor importance are slice thickness, acquisition time, overlap and pitch. Thinner slices will increase radiation dose because of the larger overlap and lower pitch, which increases acquisition time. The thinner slices need equal amounts of data to have same contrast-to-noise ratio compared to thicker slices. Because of this effect, the table speed needs to be slower with more overlap. This results in higher radiation exposure. With wider detector ranges and dynamic scanning, these factors become less important. A summary of important dose reduction parameters in CCTA is given in table 4.

The options to reduce radiation dose are numerous and radiation dose is gradually declining. As stated before, radiation dose of CTA acquisition over time ranges from 2 to 30 mSv. [45] In more recent scanners with optimal, up-to-date scanning protocols, the radiation dose will generally be around 3 to 4 mSv with a maximum of up to 7 mSv. [24, 25]

Radiation dose reduction
Scanner type (Multidetector, DSCT, etc.)
Tube current
Tube voltage
Triggering (Retrospective, prospective or ECG-gated tube current modulation)
High pitch helical scanning
Image reconstruction
Scan range
Slice thickness
Pitch
Overlap
Acquisition time

Table 4. Factors in radiation dose reduction

5. Diagnostic and prognostic accuracy

Scientific consensus documents have been published that address the appropriate use, diagnostic performance, prognostic value and interpretation of CCTA. [29, 48] Coronary artery calcium (CAC) is one of the parameters that can be assessed as part of a coronary CT acquisition protocol. As indicated, this involves a separate, non-contrast-enhanced CT scan prior to CCTA. The diagnostic and prognostic value of CAC was assessed in a systematic review by Sarwar et al. in 2009. [49] Only 146 of 25.903 asymptomatic individuals without CAC (0.56%) experienced a cardiovascular event during mean follow-up of 51 months. In 7 studies assessing the prognostic value of CAC in a symptomatic population, 1.8% of the patients without CAC had a cardiovascular event during mean follow-up of 42 months. Furthermore, the combined 18 studies indicated that the presence of CAC had a sensitivity and negative predictive value of 98% and 93%, respectively, for the detection of significant CAD on invasive coronary angiography. Prospective, population-based studies have shown that the calcium score is a very strong predictor of coronary events in asymptomatic individuals, with relative risks up to 10.

A systematic review and meta-analysis by Den Dekker et al. assessed the sensitivity and specificity of CCTA with 16-MDCT and newer CT scanner generations for significant stenosis at different degrees of coronary calcification. [50] 51 studies reported on the impact of calcium scoring on diagnostic performance of CCTA and were included the review. 27 out of 51 were suitable for the meta-analysis. Calcium scores were categorized as 0-100, 101-400, 401-1000, and >1000. On a patient-basis, sensitivity of CCTA for significant stenosis was 95.8%, 95.6%, 97.6% and 99.0%, respectively. Specificity of CCTA was 91.2%, 88.2%, 50.6% and 84.0%, respectively, for 64-row MDCT and newer scanners. The 16-row MDCT generation performed significantly worse than the more recently introduced scanners. Specificity was lower in the group with a calcium score of 401-1000, mainly because of low numbers of patients. These results suggest that even in severely calcified coronary arteries, the sensitivity and specificity of CCTA for significant stenosis is high, in case of 64-row MDCT or newer scanners. A cut-off for calcium scoring for CCTA in newer CT systems no longer seems necessary.

A systematic review and meta-analysis from 2007 by Abdulla et al. evaluated the diagnostic accuracy of 64-multidetector CT compared with conventional invasive coronary angiography (ICA) for coronary stenosis. [51] Mean sensitivity and specificity of CCTA to detect and exclude significant stenosis on a patient basis were 98% and 91% respectively. Single center studies have shown that the negative predictive value (NPV) of CCTA for 64-row MDCT scanners is high (>95%) and are clinically useful to rule out significant CAD. [15, 52, 53]

The diagnostic accuracy of ECG-gated 64-row MDCT in individuals without known CAD was assessed in a prospective multicenter trial named ACCURACY. [54] A total of 230 subjects underwent both CCTA and ICA. On a patient-based level the sensitivity, specificity, PPV and NPV to detect >50% stenosis were 95%, 83%, 64% and 99% respectively. The test characteristics for >70% stenosis were 94%, 83%, 48% and 99%, respectively. 64-row MDCT was shown to have a high diagnostic accuracy in detecting coronary stenosis, both at >50% and >70%. Even more importantly, the 99% NPV establishes CCTA as an alternative for ICA to rule out significant CAD.

Miller et al. (2008) also examined the accuracy of 64-row multidetector CT compared to conventional ICA. [55] In 291 patients with calcium score below 600, coronary segments with a diameter of >1.5 mm were analyzed by CCTA and ICA. 56% of the patients had obstructive CAD. Patient-based diagnostic accuracy of CCTA for ruling out stenosis >50% according to ICA revealed an area under the curve (AUC) of 0.93, with sensitivity, specificity, PPV, NPV of 85%, 90%, 91% and 83% respectively. The PPV and NPV in this study indicated that CCTA cannot replace ICA at that time.

Baumuller et al. compared CCTA with DSCT and 64-row MDCT in the diagnosis of significant coronary stenosis in 200 patients. [24] Of these patients, 100 underwent DSCT and 100 underwent MDCT. On a segment basis, sensitivity and specificity for DSCT were 96.4% and 97.4% respectively. For 64-row MDCT the sensitivity and specificity were 92.4% and 95.3% respectively. The NPV for DSCT and 64-row MDCT was 99.5% and 98.8% respectively. DSCT showed significantly improved accuracy and specificity for the diagnosis of significant stenosis on a segment basis, but shows comparable diagnostic accuracy compared to 64-row MDCT on a per patient-analysis.

In a study by Leber et al., DSCT was performed in 88 patients. [20] Results showed an overall sensitivity and specificity on a segment base of 95% and 90% respectively. DSCT accurately ruled out coronary stenosis in patients with intermediate pretest likelihood for CAD, independent of the heart rate. Higher heart rates did not show significant decrease in diagnostic accuracy.

A non-comprehensive overview of studies regarding the diagnostic accuracy of CT (64-row and DSCT) for significant stenosis versus ICA is shown in table 5. It can be concluded from most studies that CCTA has a good sensitivity, specificity and excellent NPV. Thus, CCTA can be used to rule out or detect the presence of CAD in selected symptomatic populations suspected of CAD.

Another important aspect of CCTA is the possibility to predict coronary events in symptomatic patients. This may have consequences for clinical management. Hulten et al. performed a systematic review and meta-analysis on the prognostic value of CCTA. In 18 studies 9.592 patients were evaluated with a median follow-up time of 20 months. [63] Major adverse cardiac events (MACE) occurred at an absolute rate of 0.6% (myocardial infarction (MI) or death) in patients with negative scan results. Occurrence of MACE in the positive scan group was 8.2%, with MI or death in 3.7%. Adverse cardiovascular events among patients with a normal CCTA are very rare and comparable to the baseline risks among healthy patients. The negative likelihood ratio of CCTA with normal findings is comparable to reported values for stress myocardial perfusion scans and stress echocardiography.

Author	Sensitivity (%)	Specificity (%)	PPV (%)	NPV (%)	Number of patients
Meijboom et al.[56]	99	64	86	97	360
Miller et al.[55]	85	90	91	83	291
Budoff et al.[54]	95	83	64	99	230
Baumuller et al.[24]	96.4	97.4	83.2	99.5	200
Tsiflikas et al.[57]	94	79	88	90	170
Sun et al.[58]	84.3	98.6	92.2	96.9	103
Ropers et al.[59]	98	81	79	99	100
Brodoefel et al.[19]	100	81.5	93.6	100	100
Weustink et al.[60]	99	87	96	95	100
Leber et al.[20]	95	90	74	99	88
Oncel et al.[53]	100	100	100	99	80
Raff et al.[15]	95	90	93	98	70
Ehara et al.[61]	98	86	98	86	69
Mollet et al.[52]	99	95	76	99	51
Achenbach et al.[62]	100	82	72	100	50
Johnson et al.[22]	100	89	89	100	35

Table 5. Accuracy of DSCT and 64-row CT in the detection of coronary stenosis on a segment level in comparison to ICA.

6. Indications

Even though CCTA has only become a viable potential alternative for ICA for selected patients since the development of 64-MDCT, already a number of indications are supported by scientific societies, and the number of indications is rapidly increasing. In 2008, a report of a writing group deployed by the Working Group Nuclear Cardiology and Cardiac CT of the European Society of Cardiology (ESC) and the European Council of Nuclear Cardiology (ECNC) was written with the indications, applications, limitations and training requirements for CCTA analysis. [64] In 2010, the American College of Cardiology Foundation (ACCF) along with key- and subspecialty societies conducted an appropriate use review of common clinical scenarios where CCTA is frequently considered and applied. [48] For potential clinical applications, the advantages and disadvantages of CCTA must be weighed against ICA. The following section lists the potential clinical indications for the use of CTA. This list starts with the strongest indication and reports to less frequent and less strong indications, taking different opinions of aforementioned societies into account.

The strongest indication for CCTA is to rule out significant luminal stenosis in stable patients with suspected CAD, at low-intermediate pretest likelihood of disease. As stated above, literature convincingly demonstrates that CCTA has a high negative predictive value and allows to reliably rule out CAD. [48, 64-66] Here, the aim is to avoid ICA when CT shows the absence of clinically relevant CAD. Based on clinical and statistical considerations, CCTA will be most useful in patients with an intermediate likelihood of CAD. The false-positive rate may be too high, for patients with a very low pretest likelihood. In patients with high pretest likelihood, it is not likely that a negative CT result excludes significant CAD.

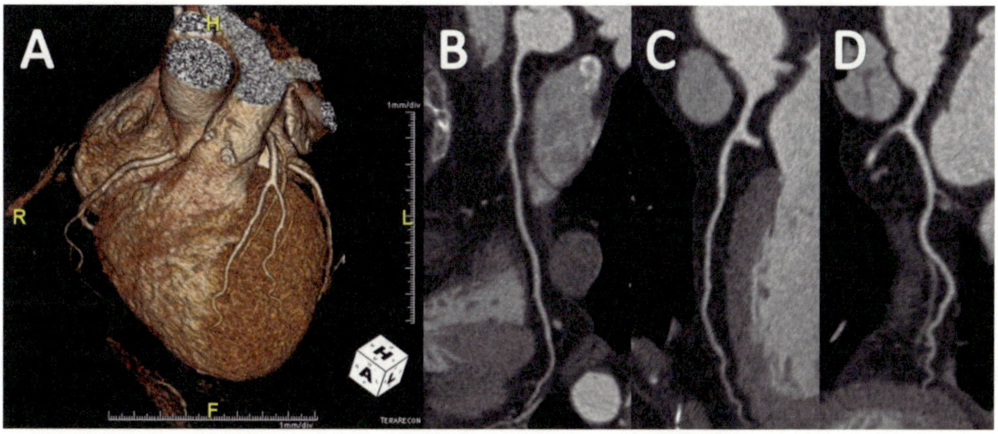

Figure 2. CCTA of a 61 year old women. A) 3D volume rendered reconstruction of the heart and the coronaries. The coronary arteries can be seen in the 3D reconstruction. B) Reconstruction of the right coronary artery (RCA) without CAD. C) Reconstruction of the left anterior descending artery of the same patient, also without stenosis. D) Circumflex (CX) reconstruction, not showing any disease.

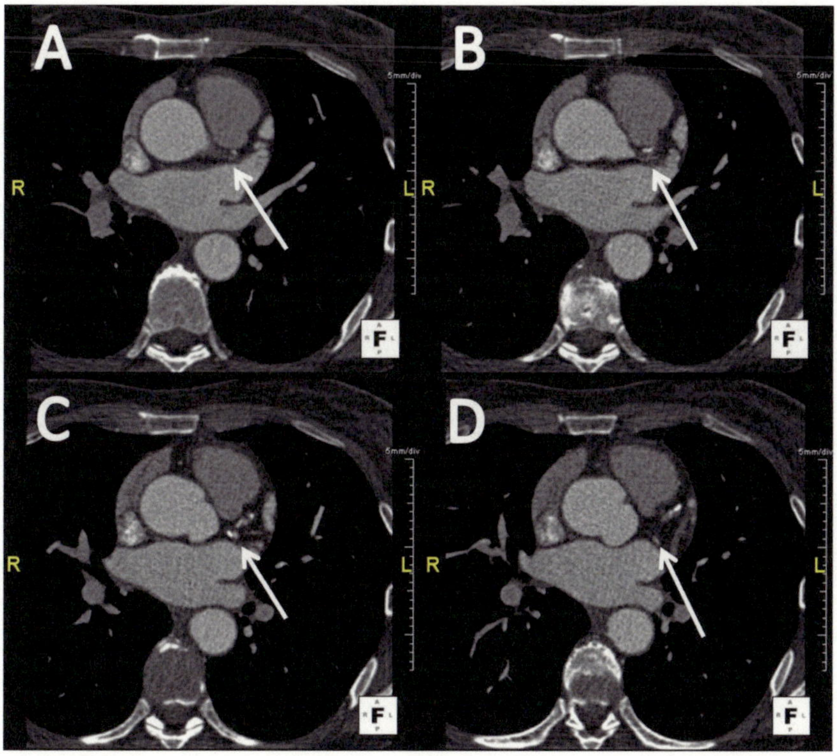

Figure 3. Overview of transverse CCTA images of a patient with an occlusion of the left main artery. In figs. A to C the arrow indicates the origin of the total occlusion. In image D the CX artery (retrograde filled) is pointed out.

Another application of CCTA is to rule out CAD in acute chest pain. This concerns patients presenting to the emergency room with acute chest pain, without direct evidence of myocardial infarction based on e.g. electrocardiogram or myocardial enzymes. In these patients, further testing is often necessary in order to rule out significant CAD, or prolonged observation in the emergency room. Coronary CTA has been found useful in these patients to rapidly assess the coronary arteries for the presence of luminal stenosis. Recent studies have shown the efficiency of applying CCTA in the emergency room. [67, 68]

CCTA can determine the complex course of anomalous coronary arteries. CCTA is the technique of choice for patient workup in known anomalous coronary vessels or vessels suspected to be anomalous because of the ease of data acquisition and the high resolution of the data set. CT has been qualified as an appropriate technique for evaluation of coronary anomalies. [48, 69-71] An example of CCTA analysis of coronary anomalies is shown in figure 4.

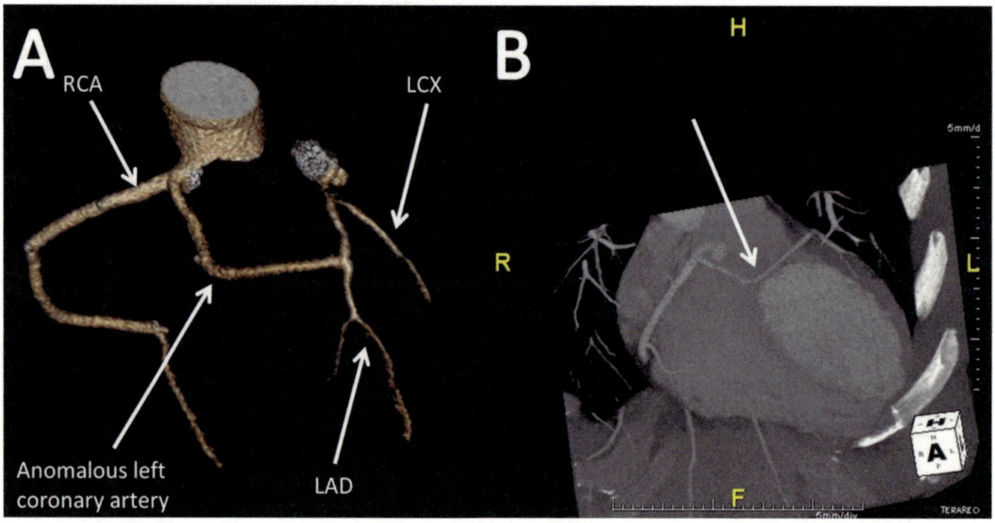

Figure 4. Patient with a coronary anomaly. A) The anomalous left coronary artery arises from the proximal RCA, through the septum into the LAD. B) Maximum intensity projection of the anomalous left coronary artery.

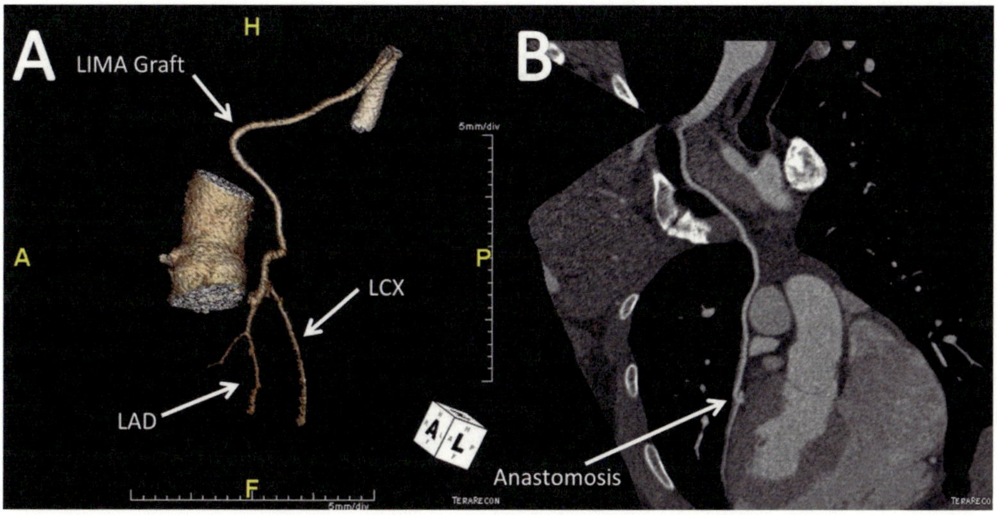

Figure 5. Evaluation after bypass-surgery, same patient as in figure 4. A) The distal left internal mammary artery (LIMA) is anastomosed with the proximal LAD at the location of the former anomalous left coronary artery. B) The graft and distal LAD show good contrast filling.

Significant coronary artery disease, mainly left main disease, needs to be ruled out before non-coronary cardiac surgery. Cardiothoracic surgeons often request coronary angiography to rule out CAD in patients scheduled for cardiac surgery, for instance valve replacement. For this purpose, stress testing is not reliable enough, as ischemia could possibly be masked by the underlying pathology. CCTA may be a useful technique to analyze the coronary arteries, without having to perform an ICA. Meijboom et al. addressed the use of CCTA in the detection of CAD prior to aortic valve replacement. [72] The overall sensitivity and specificity of CCTA for detecting CAD was, respectively 100% and 82%. So, it can be assumed that patients scheduled for cardiac surgery can be evaluated by CCTA for the detection of CAD, without subgroups such as arrhythmias and unstable patients.

It has been determined that CCTA has a high accuracy for the detection of bypass graft stenosis and occlusion. [73-77] Bypass grafts are arteries or veins from elsewhere in the patient's body, grafted to the coronary arteries to bypass coronary stenosis and improve blood supply to the myocardium, shown in figure 5. Especially venous grafts have a larger diameter and are less prone to motion, which is an advantage for image quality. Coronary artery calcifications and dimensions of native coronary arteries complicate assessment of native coronary arteries in patients with bypass grafts. Recent studies showed that the sensitivity and specificity is lower in bypass graft patients. [75] Therefore, in clinical cases in which only bypass graft evaluation is required, CCTA use may be beneficial. If the coronary arteries also require assessment, value of CCTA will be limited.

Recent statements agree on the value of coronary calcium scoring in asymptomatic individuals at intermediate risk of cardiovascular disease. In these patients, the calcium score has shown to improve risk stratification compared to cardiovascular risk factors. [36, 37]

Multiple less frequent and less strongly supported applications for CCTA imaging are known. For instance, CTA can be used as an alternative when cardiac catheterization is impossible or carries too much risk. Percutaneous coronary intervention (PCI) planning could also be an indication for CCTA. CT can more reliably identify parameters influencing PCI outcome such as length and extent of the stenosis than ICA. [78] Assessment of coronary stent lumen is also a possibility with CCTA. The ability to assess the stents depends on many factors including stent type and diameter.

CCTA Indications
Detection of CAD in symptomatic patients with suspected CAD
Detection of CAD in asymptomatic individuals without known CAD
Detection of CAD in a newly diagnosed heart failure without known CAD
Rule out CAD before non-coronary cardiac surgery
Clarify unclear findings in other noninvasive imaging techniques
Assessment post CABG (Graft evaluation)
Assessment post PCI (Stent evaluation)
Evaluation of anomalies of coronary arterial and thoracic arteriovenous vessels
Evaluation of complex adult congenital heart disease
Evaluation of ventricular morphology and systolic function

Table 6. Table Indications for CCTA analysis

7. Potential new application

It is important to realize that the presence of a significant stenosis on CCTA does not equate with hemodynamically significant CAD. Not all stenoses result in reduced myocardial perfusion in stress, and not all patients with a positive ischemia test have coronary stenosis. Thus, whereas angiographic evaluation of coronary artery pathology (morphological information) is needed on the one hand, assessment of inducible ischemia (functional information) due to coronary narrowing is necessary on the other hand. The number of different examinations that a patient has to undergo may be considerably reduced by combining morphological and functional data acquisition in one technique. CT, PET/CT and SPECT/CT have the potential of providing both functional and morphological information. [79] CT perfusion imaging is still early in development. It has different imaging options such as dynamic perfusion CT and (static) dual energy CT. Dynamic perfusion CT acquires multiple images of the contrast buildup in the myocardium, which can be monitored. Myocardial segments perfused by a stenotic artery will have a slower and lower contrast upslope resulting in a hypodense area in the myocardium. In dual-energy imaging, the amount of iodine contrast in the myocardium can be derived based on images at different KeV energy levels, an indication of blood distribution in the myocardium.

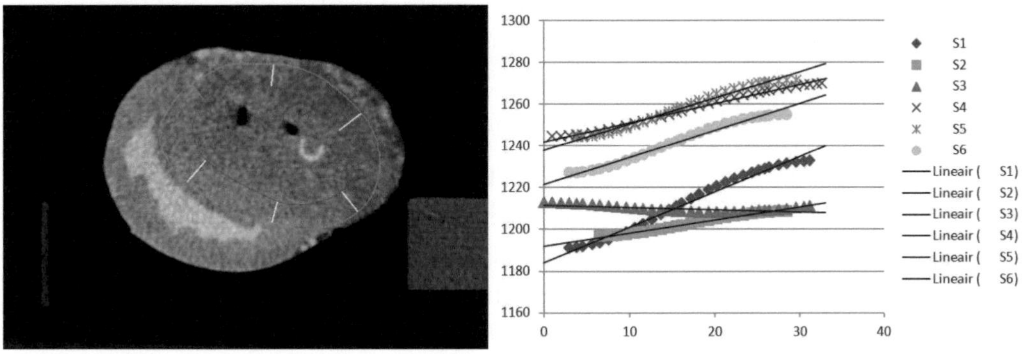

Figure 6. Dynamic CT perfusion analysis in a pig heart. The heart is divided into 6 segments (5 white lines and 1 blue line). Mean attenuation over time is monitored. B) Upslope of contrast enhancement in the 6 different segments in HU (not corrected for baseline -1024). Segments S2 and S3 have significantly lower upslope, corresponding with an applied stenosis in the CX artery.

8. Conclusion

Recent advances in modern CT technique have established CCTA as an accepted modality for coronary angiography in specific patients groups. One of the most important uses of CCTA is to exclude significant CAD in symptomatic patients at low-intermediate probability of significant stenosis. To yield most benefit from CCTA, patient selection remains important. Appropriate use will largely depend on patient characteristics, for instance pre-test likelihood of CAD. The advances in CT scanner technology have reduced the concerns about radiation dose, an important prior disadvantage. Exciting new imaging techniques in cardiac CTA could evolve in a comprehensive test for the assessment of CAD, making analysis of both anatomy and function possible in one modality.

Author details

G.J. Pelgrim[1,2*], M. Oudkerk[2] and R. Vliegenthart[1,2]

*Address all correspondence to: g.j.pelgrim@umcg.nl

1 Department of Radiology, University of Groningen, University Medical Center Groningen, Groningen, Netherlands

2 Center for Medical Imaging – North East Netherlands, University of Groningen, University Medical Center Groningen, Groningen, Netherlands

References

[1] Dodge JT, Jr., Brown BG, Bolson EL, Dodge HT. (1992) Lumen diameter of normal human coronary arteries. Influence of age, sex, anatomic variation, and left ventricular hypertrophy or dilation. Circulation; 86: 232-46.

[2] Harell GS, Guthaner DF, Breiman RS et al. (1977) Stop-action cardiac computed tomography. Radiology; 123: 515-7.

[3] Ritman EL, Kinsey JH, Robb RA et al. (1980) Three-dimensional imaging of heart, lungs, and circulation. Science; 210: 273-80.

[4] Keelan PC, Bielak LF, Ashai K et al. (2001) Long-term prognostic value of coronary calcification detected by electron-beam computed tomography in patients undergoing coronary angiography. Circulation; 104: 412-7.

[5] Guerci AD, Spadaro LA, Goodman KJ et al. (1998) Comparison of electron beam computed tomography scanning and conventional risk factor assessment for the prediction of angiographic coronary artery disease. Journal of the American College of Cardiology; 32: 673-9.

[6] Achenbach S, Giesler T, Ropers D et al. (2001) Detection of coronary artery stenoses by contrast-enhanced, retrospectively electrocardiographically-gated, multislice spiral computed tomography. Circulation; 103: 2535-8.

[7] Nieman K, Oudkerk M, Rensing BJ et al. (2001) Coronary angiography with multislice computed tomography. Lancet; 357: 599-603.

[8] Achenbach S. (2004) Detection of coronary stenoses by multidetector computed tomography: it's all about resolution. Journal of the American College of Cardiology; 43: 840-1.

[9] Flohr TG, Schoepf UJ, Kuettner A et al. (2003) Advances in cardiac imaging with 16-section CT systems. Academic radiology; 10: 386-401.

[10] Kuettner A, Trabold T, Schroeder S et al. (2004) Noninvasive detection of coronary lesions using 16-detector multislice spiral computed tomography technology: initial clinical results. Journal of the American College of Cardiology; 44: 1230-7.

[11] Stein PD, Beemath A, Kayali F et al. (2006) Multidetector computed tomography for the diagnosis of coronary artery disease: a systematic review. The American journal of medicine; 119: 203-16.

[12] Herzog C, Britten M, Balzer JO et al. (2004) Multidetector-row cardiac CT: diagnostic value of calcium scoring and CT coronary angiography in patients with symptomatic, but atypical, chest pain. European radiology; 14: 169-77.

[13] Pugliese F, Mollet NR, Runza G et al. (2006) Diagnostic accuracy of non-invasive 64-slice CT coronary angiography in patients with stable angina pectoris. European radiology; 16: 575-82.

[14] Ong TK, Chin SP, Liew CK et al. (2006) Accuracy of 64-row multidetector computed tomography in detecting coronary artery disease in 134 symptomatic patients: influence of calcification. American heart journal; 151: 1323 e1-6.

[15] Raff GL, Gallagher MJ, O'Neill WW, Goldstein JA. (2005) Diagnostic accuracy of noninvasive coronary angiography using 64-slice spiral computed tomography. Journal of the American College of Cardiology; 46: 552-7.

[16] Herzog C, Nguyen SA, Savino G et al. (2007) Does two-segment image reconstruction at 64-section CT coronary angiography improve image quality and diagnostic accuracy? Radiology; 244: 121-9.

[17] Wintersperger BJ, Nikolaou K, von Ziegler F et al. (2006) Image quality, motion artifacts, and reconstruction timing of 64-slice coronary computed tomography angiography with 0.33-second rotation speed. Investigative radiology; 41: 436-42.

[18] Flohr TG, McCollough CH, Bruder H et al. (2006) First performance evaluation of a dual-source CT (DSCT) system. European radiology; 16: 256-68.

[19] Brodoefel H, Burgstahler C, Tsiflikas I et al. (2008) Dual-source CT: effect of heart rate, heart rate variability, and calcification on image quality and diagnostic accuracy. Radiology; 247: 346-55.

[20] Leber AW, Johnson T, Becker A et al. (2007) Diagnostic accuracy of dual-source multi-slice CT-coronary angiography in patients with an intermediate pretest likelihood for coronary artery disease. European heart journal; 28: 2354-60.

[21] Klepzig H. (2008) Diagnostic accuracy of dual-source multi-slice CT-coronary angiography in patients with an intermediate pretest likelihood for coronary artery disease. European heart journal; 29: 680.

[22] Johnson TR, Nikolaou K, Busch S et al. (2007) Diagnostic accuracy of dual-source computed tomography in the diagnosis of coronary artery disease. Investigative radiology; 42: 684-91.

[23] Nakashima Y, Okada M, Washida Y et al. (2011) Evaluation of image quality on a per-patient, per-vessel, and per-segment basis by noninvasive coronary angiography with 64-section computed tomography: dual-source versus single-source computed tomography. Japanese journal of radiology; 29: 316-23.

[24] Baumuller S, Leschka S, Desbiolles L et al. (2009) Dual-source versus 64-section CT coronary angiography at lower heart rates: comparison of accuracy and radiation dose. Radiology; 253: 56-64.

[25] Fink C, Krissak R, Henzler T et al. (2011) Radiation dose at coronary CT angiography: second-generation dual-source CT versus single-source 64-MDCT and first-generation dual-source CT. AJR American journal of roentgenology; 196: W550-7.

[26] Mizuno N, Funabashi N, Imada M et al. (2007) Utility of 256-slice cone beam tomography for real four-dimensional volumetric analysis without electrocardiogram gated acquisition. International journal of cardiology; 120: 262-7.

[27] Dewey M, Zimmermann E, Deissenrieder F et al. (2009) Noninvasive coronary angiography by 320-row computed tomography with lower radiation exposure and maintained diagnostic accuracy: comparison of results with cardiac catheterization in a head-to-head pilot investigation. Circulation; 120: 867-75.

[28] Rybicki FJ, Otero HJ, Steigner ML et al. (2008) Initial evaluation of coronary images from 320-detector row computed tomography. The international journal of cardiovascular imaging; 24: 535-46.

[29] Abbara S, Arbab-Zadeh A, Callister TQ et al. (2009) SCCT guidelines for performance of coronary computed tomographic angiography: a report of the Society of Cardiovascular Computed Tomography Guidelines Committee. Journal of cardiovascular computed tomography; 3: 190-204.

[30] Pugliese F, Mollet NR, Hunink MG et al. (2008) Diagnostic performance of coronary CT angiography by using different generations of multisection scanners: single-center experience. Radiology; 246: 384-93.

[31] Hoffmann MH, Shi H, Manzke R et al. (2005) Noninvasive coronary angiography with 16-detector row CT: effect of heart rate. Radiology; 234: 86-97.

[32] Sun Z, Choo GH, Ng KH. (2012) Coronary CT angiography: current status and continuing challenges. The British journal of radiology; 85: 495-510.

[33] Agatston AS, Janowitz WR, Hildner FJ et al. (1990) Quantification of coronary artery calcium using ultrafast computed tomography. Journal of the American College of Cardiology; 15: 827-32.

[34] Budoff MJ, Shaw LJ, Liu ST et al. (2007) Long-term prognosis associated with coronary calcification: observations from a registry of 25,253 patients. Journal of the American College of Cardiology; 49: 1860-70.

[35] Greenland P, Bonow RO, Brundage BH et al. (2007) ACCF/AHA 2007 clinical expert consensus document on coronary artery calcium scoring by computed tomography in global cardiovascular risk assessment and in evaluation of patients with chest pain: a report of the American College of Cardiology Foundation Clinical Expert Consensus Task Force (ACCF/AHA Writing Committee to Update the 2000 Expert Consensus Document on Electron Beam Computed Tomography). Circulation; 115: 402-26.

[36] McClelland RL, Chung H, Detrano R et al. (2006) Distribution of coronary artery calcium by race, gender, and age: results from the Multi-Ethnic Study of Atherosclerosis (MESA). Circulation; 113: 30-7.

[37] Elias-Smale SE, Proenca RV, Koller MT et al. (2010) Coronary calcium score improves classification of coronary heart disease risk in the elderly: the Rotterdam study. Journal of the American College of Cardiology; 56: 1407-14.

[38] Piers LH, Salachova F, Slart RH et al. (2008) The role of coronary artery calcification score in clinical practice. BMC cardiovascular disorders; 8: 38.

[39] Achenbach S, Boehmer K, Pflederer T et al. (2010) Influence of slice thickness and reconstruction kernel on the computed tomographic attenuation of coronary atherosclerotic plaque. Journal of cardiovascular computed tomography; 4: 110-5.

[40] Leipsic J, Labounty TM, Heilbron B et al. (2010) Adaptive statistical iterative reconstruction: assessment of image noise and image quality in coronary CT angiography. AJR American journal of roentgenology; 195: 649-54.

[41] Scheffel H, Stolzmann P, Schlett CL et al. (2012) Coronary artery plaques: cardiac CT with model-based and adaptive-statistical iterative reconstruction technique. European journal of radiology; 81: e363-9.

[42] Gutstein A, Wolak A, Lee C et al. (2008) Predicting success of prospective and retrospective gating with dual-source coronary computed tomography angiography: development of selection criteria and initial experience. Journal of cardiovascular computed tomography; 2: 81-90.

[43] Huang B, Li J, Law MW et al. (2010) Radiation dose and cancer risk in retrospectively and prospectively ECG-gated coronary angiography using 64-slice multidetector CT. The British journal of radiology; 83: 152-8.

[44] Hirai N, Horiguchi J, Fujioka C et al. (2008) Prospective versus retrospective ECG-gated 64-detector coronary CT angiography: assessment of image quality, stenosis, and radiation dose. Radiology; 248: 424-30.

[45] Hausleiter J, Meyer T, Hermann F et al. (2009) Estimated radiation dose associated with cardiac CT angiography. JAMA : the journal of the American Medical Association; 301: 500-7.

[46] Hausleiter J, Meyer T, Hadamitzky M et al. (2006) Radiation dose estimates from cardiac multislice computed tomography in daily practice: impact of different scanning protocols on effective dose estimates. Circulation; 113: 1305-10.

[47] Siegel MJ, Schmidt B, Bradley D et al. (2004) Radiation dose and image quality in pediatric CT: effect of technical factors and phantom size and shape. Radiology; 233: 515-22.

[48] Taylor AJ, Cerqueira M, Hodgson JM et al. (2010) ACCF/SCCT/ACR/AHA/ASE/ASNC/NASCI/SCAI/SCMR 2010 appropriate use criteria for cardiac computed tomography. A report of the American College of Cardiology Foundation Appropriate Use Criteria Task Force, the Society of Cardiovascular Computed Tomography, the American College of Radiology, the American Heart Association, the American Soci-

ety of Echocardiography, the American Society of Nuclear Cardiology, the North American Society for Cardiovascular Imaging, the Society for Cardiovascular Angiography and Interventions, and the Society for Cardiovascular Magnetic Resonance. Journal of the American College of Cardiology; 56: 1864-94.

[49] Sarwar A, Shaw LJ, Shapiro MD et al. (2009) Diagnostic and prognostic value of absence of coronary artery calcification. JACC Cardiovascular imaging; 2: 675-88.

[50] den Dekker MA, de Smet K, de Bock GH et al. (2012) Diagnostic performance of coronary CT angiography for stenosis detection according to calcium score: systematic review and meta-analysis. European radiology.

[51] Abdulla J, Abildstrom SZ, Gotzsche O et al. (2007) 64-multislice detector computed tomography coronary angiography as potential alternative to conventional coronary angiography: a systematic review and meta-analysis. European heart journal; 28: 3042-50.

[52] Mollet NR, Cademartiri F, van Mieghem CA et al. (2005) High-resolution spiral computed tomography coronary angiography in patients referred for diagnostic conventional coronary angiography. Circulation; 112: 2318-23.

[53] Oncel D, Oncel G, Tastan A, Tamci B. (2007) Detection of significant coronary artery stenosis with 64-section MDCT angiography. European journal of radiology; 62: 394-405.

[54] Budoff MJ, Dowe D, Jollis JG et al. (2008) Diagnostic performance of 64-multidetector row coronary computed tomographic angiography for evaluation of coronary artery stenosis in individuals without known coronary artery disease: results from the prospective multicenter ACCURACY (Assessment by Coronary Computed Tomographic Angiography of Individuals Undergoing Invasive Coronary Angiography) trial. Journal of the American College of Cardiology; 52: 1724-32.

[55] Miller JM, Rochitte CE, Dewey M et al. (2008) Diagnostic performance of coronary angiography by 64-row CT. The New England journal of medicine; 359: 2324-36.

[56] Meijboom WB, Meijs MF, Schuijf JD et al. (2008) Diagnostic accuracy of 64-slice computed tomography coronary angiography: a prospective, multicenter, multivendor study. Journal of the American College of Cardiology; 52: 2135-44.

[57] Tsiflikas I, Brodoefel H, Reimann AJ et al. (2010) Coronary CT angiography with dual source computed tomography in 170 patients. European journal of radiology; 74: 161-5.

[58] Sun ML, Lu B, Wu RZ et al. (2011) Diagnostic accuracy of dual-source CT coronary angiography with prospective ECG-triggering on different heart rate patients. European radiology; 21: 1635-42.

[59] Ropers U, Ropers D, Pflederer T et al. (2007) Influence of heart rate on the diagnostic accuracy of dual-source computed tomography coronary angiography. Journal of the American College of Cardiology; 50: 2393-8.

[60] Weustink AC, Meijboom WB, Mollet NR et al. (2007) Reliable high-speed coronary computed tomography in symptomatic patients. Journal of the American College of Cardiology; 50: 786-94.

[61] Ehara M, Surmely JF, Kawai M et al. (2006) Diagnostic accuracy of 64-slice computed tomography for detecting angiographically significant coronary artery stenosis in an unselected consecutive patient population: comparison with conventional invasive angiography. Circulation journal : official journal of the Japanese Circulation Society; 70: 564-71.

[62] Achenbach S, Goroll T, Seltmann M et al. (2011) Detection of coronary artery stenoses by low-dose, prospectively ECG-triggered, high-pitch spiral coronary CT angiography. JACC Cardiovascular imaging; 4: 328-37.

[63] Hulten EA, Carbonaro S, Petrillo SP et al. (2011) Prognostic value of cardiac computed tomography angiography: a systematic review and meta-analysis. Journal of the American College of Cardiology; 57: 1237-47.

[64] Schroeder S, Achenbach S, Bengel F et al. (2008) Cardiac computed tomography: indications, applications, limitations, and training requirements: report of a Writing Group deployed by the Working Group Nuclear Cardiology and Cardiac CT of the European Society of Cardiology and the European Council of Nuclear Cardiology. European heart journal; 29: 531-56.

[65] Hamon M, Biondi-Zoccai GG, Malagutti P et al. (2006) Diagnostic performance of multislice spiral computed tomography of coronary arteries as compared with conventional invasive coronary angiography: a meta-analysis. Journal of the American College of Cardiology; 48: 1896-910.

[66] Vanhoenacker PK, Heijenbrok-Kal MH, Van Heste R et al. (2007) Diagnostic performance of multidetector CT angiography for assessment of coronary artery disease: meta-analysis. Radiology; 244: 419-28.

[67] Meijboom WB, van Mieghem CA, Mollet NR et al. (2007) 64-slice computed tomography coronary angiography in patients with high, intermediate, or low pretest probability of significant coronary artery disease. Journal of the American College of Cardiology; 50: 1469-75.

[68] Hoffmann U, Truong QA, Schoenfeld DA et al. (2012) Coronary CT angiography versus standard evaluation in acute chest pain. The New England journal of medicine; 367: 299-308.

[69] Hollander JE, Litt HI, Chase M et al. (2007) Computed tomography coronary angiography for rapid disposition of low-risk emergency department patients with chest pain syndromes. Academic emergency medicine : official journal of the Society for Academic Emergency Medicine; 14: 112-6.

[70] Deibler AR, Kuzo RS, Vohringer M et al. (2004) Imaging of congenital coronary anomalies with multislice computed tomography. Mayo Clinic proceedings Mayo Clinic; 79: 1017-23.

[71] Datta J, White CS, Gilkeson RC et al. (2005) Anomalous coronary arteries in adults: depiction at multi-detector row CT angiography. Radiology; 235: 812-8.

[72] Meijboom WB, Mollet NR, Van Mieghem CA et al. (2006) Pre-operative computed tomography coronary angiography to detect significant coronary artery disease in patients referred for cardiac valve surgery. Journal of the American College of Cardiology; 48: 1658-65.

[73] Nieman K, Pattynama PM, Rensing BJ et al. (2003) Evaluation of patients after coronary artery bypass surgery: CT angiographic assessment of grafts and coronary arteries. Radiology; 229: 749-56.

[74] Meyer TS, Martinoff S, Hadamitzky M et al. (2007) Improved noninvasive assessment of coronary artery bypass grafts with 64-slice computed tomographic angiography in an unselected patient population. Journal of the American College of Cardiology; 49: 946-50.

[75] Ropers D, Pohle FK, Kuettner A et al. (2006) Diagnostic accuracy of noninvasive coronary angiography in patients after bypass surgery using 64-slice spiral computed tomography with 330-ms gantry rotation. Circulation; 114: 2334-41; quiz

[76] Salm LP, Bax JJ, Jukema JW et al. (2005) Comprehensive assessment of patients after coronary artery bypass grafting by 16-detector-row computed tomography. American heart journal; 150: 775-81.

[77] Feuchtner GM, Schachner T, Bonatti J et al. (2007) Diagnostic performance of 64-slice computed tomography in evaluation of coronary artery bypass grafts. AJR American journal of roentgenology; 189: 574-80.

[78] Mollet NR, Hoye A, Lemos PA et al. (2005) Value of preprocedure multislice computed tomographic coronary angiography to predict the outcome of percutaneous recanalization of chronic total occlusions. The American journal of cardiology; 95: 240-3.

[79] Flohr TG, Klotz E, Allmendinger T et al. (2010) Pushing the envelope: new computed tomography techniques for cardiothoracic imaging. Journal of thoracic imaging; 25: 100-11.

Chapter 7

Clinical and Research Applications of Optical Coherence Tomography Imaging in Coronary Artery Disease

Takao Hasegawa and Kenei Shimada

Additional information is available at the end of the chapter

http://dx.doi.org/10.5772/54078

1. Introduction

Optical coherence tomography (OCT) is an optical analog of intravascular ultrasound (IVUS) that allows microscopic visualization of coronary plaque types and intracoronary tissue. The high-resolution images of OCT produce an intense interest in adopting this imaging technique for both clinical and research purposes.

In clinical aspects, OCT imaging for undergoing percutaneous coronary intervention (PCI) is feasible and provides superior resolution of arterial pathology than IVUS. During PCI, OCT can assess pre-procedural coronary plaque morphology and acute effects of coronary intervention (dissection, tissue prolapse, thrombi, and incomplete stent apposition (ISA)). Moreover, OCT provides more useful information to consider PCI strategy, such as distal protection, optimal stent landing zone.

In research aspects, OCT provides characterization of coronary plaque to assess factors associated with acute coronary syndrome (ACS) and vessel healing process after stent implantation. Recent studies have shown that OCT is useful for the assessment of coronary atherosclerotic plaques (plaque rupture, erosion, thin-cap fibroatheroma (TCFA), and intracoronary thrombi) in patients with ACS. In addition, OCT can detect the proliferation of vasa vasorum and the distribution of macrophages surrounding vulnerable plaques. OCT provides cardiologists with the tool they need to better understand the pathological condition of ACS.

According to vessel healing after stent implantation, OCT can provide stent strut coverage, ISA, and restenotic tissue characteristics at follow up. Previous OCT studies have shown that delayed neointimal coverage after drug-eluting stent (DES) implantation vs. bare metal stent (BMS) implantation. Pathological studies have indicated that the proportion of delayed neointimal coverage represents the best morphometric predictor of late stent thrombosis. Recent OCT studies demonstrate that restenotic tissue characteristics is completely different between BMS and DES. Therefore, OCT can play an important role to assess the safety profile of novel DES systems.

Finally, we introduce usefulness of 3-dimensional reconstruction of the OCT images and 1-μm resolution OCT.

2. Differences between IVUS and OCT

OCT is an optical analog of IVUS, used to examine the coronary arteries. There is a pressing need for improved characterization of coronary pathology to better recognize the factors associated with coronary vessel disease and to guide the selection of better interventional strategies. The resolution and contrast of OCT is attractive for these applications and suitable catheters to access the coronary arteries in detail. There are several differences between IVUS and OCT, as shown in Table 1 [1]. The resolution of OCT (10-20 μm) is 10-fold higher than that of IVUS (100-150 μm), but the penetration depth is lower with OCT (1-2 mm) than with IVUS (4-8 mm) [2]. According to other important difference between IVUS and OCT, the removal of blood is not need for IVUS examination but OCT examination. To examine coronary arteries, blood must first be removed during an OCT examination because of the strong attenuation of light by blood [3].

OCT imaging uses an interferometry technique based on time-delay measurements of the light reflected or backscattered from the tissues [4]. We can use two processing modes used for intracoronary OCT imaging, the first generation time-domain OCT (TD-OCT) imaging systems and the more recently available second generation frequency-domain OCT (FD-OCT) imaging systems [5, 6].

The first-generation OCT (ImageWire and M2/3 OCT system; LightLab Imaging, Inc., Westford, Massachusetts) incorporated both an OCT imaging wire and an over-the-wire occlusion balloon. To deliver the image wire and remove blood from the target lesion, an over-the-wire occlusion balloon catheter was used. The OCT imaging procedure started with advancing a 0.014-inch coronary guide wire distal to the target lesion. The occlusion catheter is passed along the guide wire through the lesion. After the guide wire and OCT image wire were exchanged, the occlusion balloon is pulled back proximal to the lesion. Then, ringer's solution was continuously flushed at 0.5–0.6 ml/s through the occlusion catheter lumen using a power injector, and the balloon was inflated to 0.3–0.5 atm by an inflation device to block blood flow. When an OCT image well appeared, a motorized pullback was initiated from the imaging system console. The first-generation OCT was not user-friendly and had several disadvantages of complex procedure, such as balloon occlusion and relatively short length of image acquisition due to the limited frame rate. To improve these disadvantage, a new generation of OCT systems, termed FD-OCT imaging methods, has been developed.

FD-OCT imaging methods, utilize a light source with variable wavelength that is tuned to continuously oscillate between 1250 and 1350 nm, a so-called wavelength swept laser, instead of the broadband light source used in TD-OCT. As a result, FD-OCT system can enable faster image acquisition and greater scan depths compared with TD-OCT system. Intravascular OCT examination has been frustrated by requiring blood removal. However, FD-OCT system can enable faster image acquisition and greater scan depths compared with TD-OCT system. As a result, only intermittent injection of transparent fluid through guiding catheter for a few seconds enables to obtain entire coronary images [6, 7]. FD-OCT system has been developed (Dragonfly imaging catheter and C7- XR OCT system; LightLab Imaging, Inc., St Jude Medical,St Paul, Minnesota, USA). Differences between TD- (M3) and FD-OCT (C7-XR) systems are shown in Table 1 [8]. This advance may provide dramatic improvements in understanding coronary atherosclerosis and response to intravascular interventions such as angioplasty and stenting.

3. Clinical applications of OCT imaging

In clinical aspects, OCT imaging for undergoing PCI is feasible and provides superior resolution of arterial pathology than intravascular ultrasound. During PCI, OCT can assess pre-procedural coronary plaque morphology.

Regarding to plaque characterization, OCT can differentiate three types of coronary plaques, such as fibrous, calcified, and lipid-rich. Fibrous plaque is characterized by a homogenous high signal region with low attenuation, calcified plaque by a well-delineated, low-signal region with sharp borders, and lipid-rich plaques as a low-signal region with diffuse borders [9]. Importantly, a histology-controlled OCT study showed >90% sensitivity and specificity for detecting lipid-rich plaque in comparisons with pathological specimens. [9, 10]. Moreover, OCT can recognize vulnerable plaques, such as plaque rupture, erosion, intracoronary thrombus, TCFA.

Assessment of plaque characteristics before PCI is useful to choose optimal interventional strategy. Tanaka et al. showed that TCFA was often observed at target lesions of the patients with no reflow after PCI compared with good reflow (50% versus 16%, $P = 0.005$). The frequency of the no reflow phenomenon increased according to the lipid arc assessed by OCT [11]. When OCT detects lipid-rich plaque and TCFA especially in patients with ACS, we should consider to use distal protection devices to prevent no-reflow phenomenon.

Another aspect, plaque type at the stent edges has an impact on the occurrence of edge dissections. Gonzalo et al. showed that presence of edge dissection was significantly more frequent when the plaque type at the edge was fibrocalcific (43.8%) or lipid rich (37.5%) than when the plaque was fibrous (10%) [12]. This study demonstrated that complex plaque type at the stent edge might influence on the presence of edge dissections from OCT observation. The OCT guide stenting might be a useful assistance to achieve optimal landing zone.

After PCI, OCT can assess acute effects of coronary intervention (dissection, tissue prolapse, and ISA). Dissection, tissue prolapse, and ISA were observed more often with OCT than with IVUS [13, 14]. Coronary dissection is frequently observed at the distal stent edge because of the oversized stent diameter or complex types of plaque at the stent edge by OCT. When there is no limited coronary flow by angiography and adequate area of the true lumen by OCT, no additional procedure might be necessary for the treatment of coronary dissection [15].

There are 2 types of tissue prolapse, plaque prolapse or thrombus prolapse. OCT can distinguish between plaque prolapse and thrombus prolapse. Plaque prolapse is characterized by smooth surface with no signal attenuation, and thrombus protrusion by irregular surface with significant signal attenuation. Minor tissue prolapse identified by IVUS was not found to be associated with angiographic in-stent restenosis [16]. However, the relationship tissue prolapse identified by OCT and angiographic in-stent restenosis has not been elucidated.

ISA by OCT was identified as clear separation between at least one stent strut and the vessel wall. To check the stent apposition to the vessel wall, the distance between surface of stent strut and adjacent inatima border should be measured because of differences of stent and polymer thickness [8]. Small ISA, which is detected by only OCT but not by IVUS, could disappear by neointimal growth during follow-up period [15].

4. Research applications of OCT imaging

In research aspects, OCT can provide characterization of coronary plaque to assess factors associated with ACS and vessel healing process after stent implantation.

The first OCT study to assess in vivo culprit lesion morphology in patients with ACS showed that higher frequency of TCFA in ACS compared with stable angina pectoris (72% in acute myocardial infarction (AMI), 50% in unstable angina pectoris, and 20% in stable angina pectoris; $P = 0.012$) [2]. Kubo et al. showed superiorities of TD-OCT for the detection of plaque rupture (73% vs. 40% vs. 43%, $P = 0.021$), erosion (23% vs. 0% vs. 3%, $P = 0.003$), and thrombus (100% vs. 33% vs. 100%, $P < 0.001$) compared with IVUS and coronary angioscopy in patients with AMI [17]. The frequency of vulnerable plaque (plaque rupture, erosion, and thrombus) by detected OCT was similar to that of the pathological reports. As described above, OCT is more useful to assess atherosclerotic plaque instability compared to other intracoronary imaging devices.

OCT has been proposed as a high resolution imaging modality that can identify vasa vasorum as microchannels with tiny black holes (50-100 μm). The proliferation of vasa vasorum has been identified recently as a common feature of vulnerable plaque [18]. Kitabata et al. demonstrated increase of microvessels counts in TCFA [19]. An observational study of OCT revealed that the presence of microvessels in the plaques was also associated with positive remodeling and elevated high-sensitive C-reactive protein levels [19]. The OCT evaluation of microvessels counts might be helpful for assessing plaque vulnerability.

Moreover, the other unique aspect of OCT is the detection of macrophages. Degradation of the fibrous cap matrix by macrophages is associated with atherosclerotic plaque instability

[20]. Macrophages detected by OCT were observed as a 'bright spot', with a high signal variance from the surrounding tissue. Tearney et al. [21] and MacNeill et al. [16] descried OCT is capable to evaluate cap macrophage content accurately. High degree of positive correlation was observed between OCT and histological measurements of macrophage density in fibrous cap ($r < 0.84$, $P < 0.0001$). OCT provided to detect a cap macrophage density > 10% with 100% sensitivity and specificity [19].

According to vessel healing after stent implantation, OCT can provide stent strut coverage, ISA, and restenotic tissue characteristics at follow up. Previous OCT studies have shown that delayed neointimal coverage after DES implantation vs. BMS implantation [22]. Pathological studies have indicated that the proportion of delayed neointimal coverage represents the best morphometric predictor of late stent thrombosis [23, 24]. Recent OCT studies demonstrate that restenotic tissue characteristics is completely different between BMS and DES [21, 25]. Therefore, OCT can play an important role to assess the safety profile of novel DES systems.

5. Future directions of OCT imaging

Recently, a second-generation OCT technology, termed FD-OCT, has been developed that solves the TD-OCT limitations by imaging at much higher frame rates with slightly deeper penetration depth and greater scan area. In combination with a short, non-occlusive flush and rapid spiral pullback, the higher frame rates generated by FD-OCT enable imaging of the 3-dimensional reconstruction of longer segments of coronary arteries. The 3-dimensional OCT can express all of the coronary microanatomy and pathology previously visualized by OCT, including lipid pools, calcium, macrophages, thin fibrous caps, cholesterol crystals, thrombus, stent, and stents with neointimal hyperplasia [26]. The 3-dimensional OCT may be useful as a research tool for assessing human coronary pathophysiology and as a clinical tool for guiding the management of coronary artery disease.

Progress in understanding, diagnosis, and treatment of coronary artery disease has been hindered because of inability to observe cells and extracellular components associated with human coronary atherosclerosis *in situ*. A μOCT system with a very broad bandwidth light source and common-path spectral-domain OCT technology provides 1-μm axial resolution ranging in tissue [27]. The μOCT is possible to visualize many key cellular and subcellular features relevant to atherogenesis, plaque rupture, thrombosis, and neointimal healing after stenting *in situ*. The μOCT technology has the potential to make a significant impact in cardiovascular pathology.

6. Conclusion

The high resolution of OCT provides histology-grade definition of the microstructures of coronary atherosclerosis in vivo. Introduction of this attractive imaging method contributes significant progression in both clinical and research aspects. Clinically, OCT can provide more useful information to consider PCI strategy for getting the optimal interventional results. On the other hand, OCT is a useful imaging device for understanding, diagnosis, and treatment of coronary artery disease. In the future direction of OCT systems, 3-dimensional OCT and μOCT may be upcoming in the field of coronary artery disease. These novel OCT technologies will play an important role for investigation of coronary artery disease.

	IVUS	TD-OCT (M3)	FD-OCT (C7)
Axial resolution, μm	100-150	15-20	12-15
Lateral resolution, μm	150-300	39	19
Frame rate, fps	30	20	100
Pullback speed, mm/s	0.5-2.0	0.5-2.0	10-25
Scan diameter, mm	8-10	6.8	10
Penetration depth, mm	4-8	1-2	1-2
Balloon occlusion	Unnecessary	Necessary	Unnecessary

IVUS, intravascular ultrasound; OCT, optical coherence tomography; TD, time-domain; FD, frequency-domain; fps, frames per second.

Modified from Terashima M et al, korean j intern med 2012;27:1-12.

Table 1. Differences among IVUS, TD-OCT, and FD-OCT

	IVUS	OCT
Dissection	○	◎
Tissue prolapse	△	◎
ISA	○	◎
Stent expansion	◎	○
Lesion coverage	○	○

IVUS, intravascular ultrasound; OCT, optical coherence tomography; ISA, incomplete stent apposition.

Table 2. Acute effects of coronary intervention between IVUS and OCT

Author details

Takao Hasegawa and Kenei Shimada

*Address all correspondence to: shimadak@med.osaka-cu.ac.jp

Department of Internal Medicine and Cardiology, Osaka City University Graduate School of Medicine, Abeno-ku, Osaka, Japan

References

[1] Yamaguchi T, Terashima M, Akasaka T, Hayashi T, Mizuno K, Muramatsu T, et al. Safety and feasibility of an intravascular optical coherence tomography image wire system in the clinical setting. The American journal of cardiology. 2008;101(5):562-7.

[2] Jang IK, Tearney GJ, MacNeill B, Takano M, Moselewski F, Iftima N, et al. In vivo characterization of coronary atherosclerotic plaque by use of optical coherence tomography. Circulation. 2005;111(12):1551-5. Epub 2005/03/23.

[3] Kataiwa H, Tanaka A, Kitabata H, Imanishi T, Akasaka T. Safety and usefulness of non-occlusion image acquisition technique for optical coherence tomography. Circulation journal : official journal of the Japanese Circulation Society. 2008;72(9):1536-7.

[4] Huang D, Swanson EA, Lin CP, Schuman JS, Stinson WG, Chang W, et al. Optical coherence tomography. Science. 1991;254(5035):1178-81.

[5] Suter MJ, Nadkarni SK, Weisz G, Tanaka A, Jaffer FA, Bouma BE, et al. Intravascular optical imaging technology for investigating the coronary artery. JACC Cardiovascular imaging. 2011;4(9):1022-39.

[6] Yun SH, Tearney GJ, Vakoc BJ, Shishkov M, Oh WY, Desjardins AE, et al. Comprehensive volumetric optical microscopy in vivo. Nature medicine. 2006;12(12):1429-33.

[7] Imola F, Mallus MT, Ramazzotti V, Manzoli A, Pappalardo A, Di Giorgio A, et al. Safety and feasibility of frequency domain optical coherence tomography to guide decision making in percutaneous coronary intervention. EuroIntervention : journal of EuroPCR in collaboration with the Working Group on Interventional Cardiology of the European Society of Cardiology. 2010;6(5):575-81.

[8] Terashima M, Kaneda H, Suzuki T. The role of optical coherence tomography in coronary intervention. The Korean journal of internal medicine. 2012;27(1):1-12.

[9] Yabushita H, Bouma BE, Houser SL, Aretz HT, Jang IK, Schlendorf KH, et al. Characterization of human atherosclerosis by optical coherence tomography. Circulation. 2002;106(13):1640-5.

[10] Kume T, Akasaka T, Kawamoto T, Watanabe N, Toyota E, Neishi Y, et al. Assessment of coronary arterial plaque by optical coherence tomography. The American journal of cardiology. 2006;97(8):1172-5.

[11] Tanaka A, Imanishi T, Kitabata H, Kubo T, Takarada S, Tanimoto T, et al. Lipid-rich plaque and myocardial perfusion after successful stenting in patients with non-ST-segment elevation acute coronary syndrome: an optical coherence tomography study. European heart journal. 2009;30(11):1348-55.

[12] Gonzalo N SP, Okamura T, Shen ZJ, Garcia-Garcia HM, Onuma Y, van Geuns RJ, Ligthart J, Regar E. Relation between plaque type and dissections at the edges after

stent implantation: an optical coherence tomography study. Int J Cardiol 2011;150(2): 151-5.

[13] Bouma BE, Tearney GJ, Yabushita H, Shishkov M, Kauffman CR, DeJoseph Gauthier D, et al. Evaluation of intracoronary stenting by intravascular optical coherence tomography. Heart. 2003;89(3):317-20.

[14] Diaz-Sandoval LJ, Bouma BE, Tearney GJ, Jang IK. Optical coherence tomography as a tool for percutaneous coronary interventions. Catheterization and cardiovascular interventions : official journal of the Society for Cardiac Angiography & Interventions. 2005;65(4):492-6.

[15] Kume T, Okura H, Miyamoto Y, Yamada R, Saito K, Tamada T, et al. Natural history of stent edge dissection, tissue protrusion and incomplete stent apposition detectable only on optical coherence tomography after stent implantation - preliminary observation. Circulation journal : official journal of the Japanese Circulation Society. 2012;76(3):698-703.

[16] Hoffmann R, Mintz GS, Dussaillant GR, Popma JJ, Pichard AD, Satler LF, et al. Patterns and mechanisms of in-stent restenosis. A serial intravascular ultrasound study. Circulation. 1996;94(6):1247-54.

[17] Kubo T, Imanishi T, Takarada S, Kuroi A, Ueno S, Yamano T, et al. Assessment of culprit lesion morphology in acute myocardial infarction: ability of optical coherence tomography compared with intravascular ultrasound and coronary angioscopy. Journal of the American College of Cardiology. 2007;50(10):933-9.

[18] Kolodgie FD, Gold HK, Burke AP, Fowler DR, Kruth HS, Weber DK, et al. Intraplaque hemorrhage and progression of coronary atheroma. The New England journal of medicine. 2003;349(24):2316-25.

[19] Kitabata H, Tanaka A, Kubo T, Takarada S, Kashiwagi M, Tsujioka H, et al. Relation of microchannel structure identified by optical coherence tomography to plaque vulnerability in patients with coronary artery disease. The American journal of cardiology. 2010;105(12):1673-8. Epub 2010/06/12.

[20] Moreno PR, Falk E, Palacios IF, Newell JB, Fuster V, Fallon JT. Macrophage infiltration in acute coronary syndromes. Implications for plaque rupture. Circulation. 1994;90(2):775-8.

[21] Tearney GJ, Yabushita H, Houser SL, Aretz HT, Jang IK, Schlendorf KH, et al. Quantification of macrophage content in atherosclerotic plaques by optical coherence tomography. Circulation. 2003;107(1):113-9.

[22] Chen BX, Ma FY, Luo W, Ruan JH, Xie WL, Zhao XZ, et al. Neointimal coverage of bare-metal and sirolimus-eluting stents evaluated with optical coherence tomography. Heart. 2008;94(5):566-70.

[23] Finn AV, Joner M, Nakazawa G, Kolodgie F, Newell J, John MC, et al. Pathological correlates of late drug-eluting stent thrombosis: strut coverage as a marker of endothelialization. Circulation. 2007;115(18):2435-41.

[24] Joner M, Finn AV, Farb A, Mont EK, Kolodgie FD, Ladich E, et al. Pathology of drug-eluting stents in humans: delayed healing and late thrombotic risk. Journal of the American College of Cardiology. 2006;48(1):193-202.

[25] Gonzalo N, Serruys PW, Okamura T, van Beusekom HM, Garcia-Garcia HM, van Soest G, et al. Optical coherence tomography patterns of stent restenosis. American heart journal. 2009;158(2):284-93.

[26] Tearney GJ, Waxman S, Shishkov M, Vakoc BJ, Suter MJ, Freilich MI, et al. Three-dimensional coronary artery microscopy by intracoronary optical frequency domain imaging. JACC Cardiovascular imaging. 2008;1(6):752-61.

[27] Liu L, Gardecki JA, Nadkarni SK, Toussaint JD, Yagi Y, Bouma BE, et al. Imaging the subcellular structure of human coronary atherosclerosis using micro-optical coherence tomography. Nature medicine. 2011;17(8):1010-4.

Chapter 8

Multidector CT Imaging of Coronary Artery Stent and Coronary Artery Bypass Graft

Bong Gun Song

Additional information is available at the end of the chapter

http://dx.doi.org/10.5772/54085

1. Introduction

Coronary artery stenting has become the most important nonsurgical treatment for coronary artery disease. However, in-stent restenosis occurs at a relatively high rate and this problem has led to the routine use of invasive angiography for assessing stent patency. Although coronary angiography is the clinical gold standard and it is a very effective diagnostic tool for detecting such in-stent restenosis, it's clearly an invasive procedure with its associated morbidity and mortality risks. Therefore, a noninvasive technique for detecting in-stent restenosis would be of great interest and use for following up patients after coronary angioplasty. Multidetector-row CT (MDCT) is being increasingly used for noninvasive coronary artery imaging as it has high diagnostic accuracy for detecting coronary artery stenosis in native, non-stented, coronary arteries. The recently introduced 64-slice CT offers more improved spatial and temporal resolution than does 4 and 16-slice CT and this results in superior visualization of the stent lumen and in-stent restenosis. However, although 64-slice MDCT allows for improved stent visualization, a relevant part (up to 47%) of the stent lumen is still not assessable (Mahnken et al., 2006). The metal of the stents can cause blooming artifacts that prevent the accurate interpretation of a lumen's patency. To improve a stent's visualization, numerous methods have been attempted such as dedicated post-processing or the use of dual-source CT. However, because of its presently limited sensitivity and high radiation exposure, MDCT should not be used as the first-line test to screen for in-stent restenosis in asymptomatic patients. Given its high specificity and negative predictive value, MDCT might be valuable for confirming stent occlusion in symptomatic patients.

Coronary artery bypass graft (CABG) surgery is the standard care in the treatment of advanced coronary artery disease. Notwithstanding the clear benefits of bypass grafting, recurrent chest pain after myocardial revascularization surgery is a common postoperative presentation and the long-term clinical outcome after myocardial revascularization surgery is largely dependent on graft patency and the progression of coronary artery disease. Therefore, assessment of the status of the grafts and graft disease after CABG surgery is an important issue in cardiology. Although conventional coronary angiography is still standard method for assessment of the status of naïve and recipient vessels after CABG surgery, it is an invasive and costly procedure that is not risk-free. Recently, MDCT with retrospective electrocardiographic (ECG) gating has gained rapid acceptance as a diagnostic cardiac imaging modality, allowing assessment of coronary bypass graft patency with high spatial resolution. Initial assessment of bypass grafts was done with single-slice scanners and electron-beam CT. Subsequently, the addition of electrocardiographic (ECG) gating and the improved capabilities available with 4- or 16-slice MDCT scanners for rapid scanning of the area of interest led to promising results in the imaging of bypass grafts (Marano et al., 2005; Ueyama et al., 1999). Recently, the introduction of 64-slice MDCT permitted improved temporal resolution (94 to 200 msec) and spatial resolution (upto submillimeter) and reduction of both cardiac and respiratory motion, leading to improved assessment of graft stenosis and occlusion (Frazier et al., 2005; Lee et al., 2010). Moreover, 3-dimensional (3D) image processing and advanced volumetric visualization techniques now allow radiologists and cardiologists to evaluate coronary grafts in multiple planes using various projections. With the capability of acquiring 3D data volumes along with its tomographic nature, it shares many of the advantages of intravascular ultrasound and thus has the potential to enhance the practice of percutaneous coronary intervention (PCI) in the catheterization laboratory by providing data which was difficult to obtain by invasive coronary angiography (Song et al., 2010; Dikkers et al., 2007; Vembar et al., 2003). MDCT scanners characterized by submillimeter spatial resolution and a temporal resolution of 94 to 200 ms are now available and are increasingly used for cardiac imaging with promising results.

2. Imaging acquisition

2.1. Image protocol

Cardiac CTA technique requires rapid injection of nonionic, iodinated, low-osmolar intravenous contrast. A bolus of 100 to 120 mL nonionic contrast material (high iodine concentration is recommended) is administered intravenously using an automatic injector at a flow rate of 3 to 4 mL/s. A region of interest was placed in the descending aorta by using a preset threshold of 150 HU; a 10-second delay followed before scanning was begun to ensure filling of the distal vessels with contrast material. Axial images are reconstructed in the mid-to-late diastolic phase, using a fraction (percentage; relative delay) of the R-R interval of the cardiac cycle. Images are acquired with a heart rate < 70 beats per minute, if possible, and with breath-holding during mid-inspiration to prevent substantial inflow of unopacified blood into the right atrium, which may result in heterogeneity of contrast. Low heart rates (< 65 beats/min for 16-slice MDCT or < 70 beats/min for 64-slice MDCT) are recommended to obtain high-quality CT scans, and in the absence of contraindications (heart failure, systolic BP < 100 mm Hg, atrioventricular blockade greater than grade I, and referred adverse reaction), beta-blockers can be administered before CT acquisition (Frazier et al., 2005; Marano et al., 2005). Oral or intravenous beta-adrenergic blocking medications, specifically metoprolol (Lopressor; Novartis Pharmaceuticals Corp., East Hanover, NJ), are administered prior to scanning to prevent heart rate variabilityand tachycardia. Retrospective ECG-gated CTA is essential for optimal image acquisition and reconstruction of evenly spaced phases of the cardiac cycle. The images are acquired in a limited field of view with axial images centered on the heart. Using 60% to 80% of the R-R interval, with 0.6-0.75 mm thick images reconstructed in 0.4-0.5 mm increments, axial source images, three-dimensional (3D) volume-rendered images, and multiplanar reformatted (MPR) images are generated.

There are a variety of protocols for image acquisition in the evaluation of patients after CABG surgery. In many respects, the protocol is similar to that for coronary CT angiography (CTA). One important difference is that the scan should be extended superiorly to include the origins of the internal mammary arteries. Scanning is performed with the patient in the supine position, during breath-hold. After placement of the leads for ECG recording on the chest wall and a check of the heart rate, a noncontrast CT scan image is acquired through the entire thorax in order to define the volume of the subsequent CT angiography and to detect associated or unsuspected findings. Hence, MDCT angiography is performed during ECG recording, from the subclavian arteries to the cardiac base; in patients with venous grafts, a smaller scanning volume starting from the lower third of the ascending aorta is usually sufficient. On the contrary, when a right gastroepiploic artery (RGEA) has been used, the scanning volume should include the upper abdomen. Since the left internal mammary artery (LIMA) is the most frequently used graft to the anterior cardiac wall, a right arm venous access is preferable in order to avoid streak artifacts from the left subclavian vein that may hamper a complete evaluation of LIMA course and takeoff. Both 3D volume-rendering and MPR images are used to assess the bypass grafts, proximal and/or distal graft anastomoses, and the cardiac anatomy. In particular, curved multiplanar images with centerlines through the bypass grafts and native coronary arteries are obtained. To correctly assess graft patency and/or the presence of significant stenosis and occlusion, a thorough knowledge of CABG anatomy and its configuration on CTA is important for radiologists and cardiologists. There are 2 types of bypass grafts, arterial and venous. Venous grafts are generally larger in caliber than arterial grafts, and for this reason, jointly to the absence of surgical clips along their course, venous grafts are usually better assessable by noninvasive imaging techniques. In order of frequency of use, graft arteries include the internal mammary arteries (IMAs), radial arteries (RAs), right gastroepiploic artery (RGEA), and inferior epigastric artery. Although arterial grafts have better long-term outcomes, venous grafts, specifically saphenous vein grafts (SVGs), are more readily available. CTA following CABG surgery is done by first assessing the morphology and size of the ascending aorta and the origin of the in situ vessel such as the IMA. Then, graft patency is assessed for homogeneous, contrast-enhanced graft lumen and for regular shape and border of the graft wall. The graft is usually divided into 3 different segments: the origin or proximal anastomosis of the graft, the body of the graft, and the single (or sequential) distal anastomosis. During the CTA evaluation of bypass grafts, the proximal anastomosis is usually better visualized than the distal anastomosis. In cases in which the distal anastomosis is not well evaluated, the bypass graft is usually considered patent as long as contrast is evident within the graft lumen.

2.2. Image noise

The advantages of MDCT are the relatively rapid imaging time and high spatial resolution attributable to the multi-row detector system. Numerous studies dealing with MDCT coronary bypass angiography have reported cardiac and respiratory motion artifacts as the most significant limitations in the reliable assessment of graft patency and stenosis of recipient vessels. It is well known that heart rate greatly influences image quality and stenosis detection. The introduction of 64-slice MDCT scanners, with faster gantry rotation times and shorter breath-hold times, improved diagnostic image quality by reducing cardiac and respiratory motion artifacts. However, optimum performance was observed primarily in patients with heart rates below 70 beats per minute. Even with improved spatial and temporal resolution with 64-slice technology, routine administration of β-blockers is still required. If graft segment image quality is suboptimal due to motion artifacts, a potential remedy is to obtain additional image reconstructions in smaller increments throughout the cardiac cycle. The other limitations of MDCT are the presence of calcification and metal clip artifacts, which make assessment of graft patency difficult, and accurate evaluation of the degree of stenosis impossible. Nevertheless, the thinner slices of 64-slice MDCT give increased temporal resolution, and 3-dimentional reconstructions show consistent detail in every plane. Moreover, bypass grafts are characterized by minor calcification compared to naive vessels, allowing more accurate analysis in most cases. Coronary calcifications and metal clip artifacts still remain a challenging issue with 64-slice cardiac CT despite improvements with the use of sharper image filters, e.g. the B46 Kernel (Siemens Medical Solutions) (Seifarth et al., 2005). The another important limitation is the high radiation dose required for 64-slice MDCT, although electrocardiogram-dependent dose modulation can reduce this by 30%–50%. The minimization of radiation exposure as well as optimization of the diagnostic accuracy in calcified vessels remain the chief goals for future MDCT advances.

2.3. Strategies for reduction of radiation dose and image noise

Current limitations of coronary CTA include image noise and radiation dose. As a result, a number of techniques and strategies have become available on newer CT platforms to enable dose reduction in coronary CT. These include sequential or prospective ECG triggering, reduced tube voltage scanning, and high-pitch helical scanning. Recently, iterative reconstruction (Adaptive Statistical Iterative Reconstruction [ASIR], GE Healthcare) has been introduced as a new reconstruction algorithm (Rajiah et al., 2012; Leipsic et al., 2007; Min et al., 2009). In comparison with filtered back projection (FBP), ASIR reduces image noise (increase contrast-to-noise ratio [CNR]) by iteratively comparing the acquired image to a modeled projection. This reconstruction algorithm is used to help deal with one of the primary issues of dose and tube current reduction for coronary CTA with FBP: increased image noise with decreased tube current. Recently, a high-definition CT (HDCT) scanner, with improved in-plane spatial resolution of 230 μm and the ability to reconstruct images with the use of a novel applied ASIR algorithm, has been developed (Min et al., 2009).

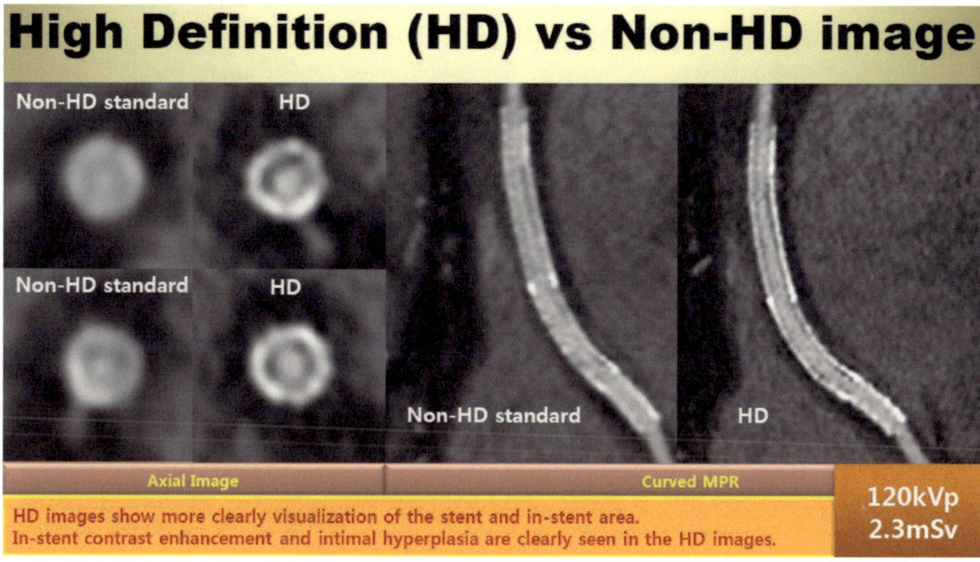

Scheme 1. High definition (HD) versus non-HD CT imagings. HD images show more clearly visualization of the stent and in-stent area.

3. Coronary artery stent imaging with MDCT

Coronary artery stenting is currently the standard practice in nonsurgical myocardial revascularization. However, coronary in-stent restenosis attributable to intimal hyperplasia remains problematic, with an incidence rate of 20% to 30%. The evaluation of stent patency is a major issue in the follow-up after stent placement. It would be desirable to obviate the use of invasive and costly angiography in the evaluation of stent patency. Initial studies using 4-detector coronary CTA for the evaluation of stent patency showed difficulties in imaging small and high-attenuating structures such as coronary stents (Table 1). With 16-detector coronary CTA, coronary artery stent patency has been assessed on the basis of contrast enhancement measurements or pixel count methods. However, stent diameter (≤ 3 mm), strut thickness, and stent material are still a cause of poor lumen visualization. In a study by Gilard et al, 232 stents were evaluated in vivo with 16-detector CT. Lumen interpretability depended on stent diameter: for stents with diameter > 3mm, 81% of lumens were interpretable, compared with 51% for stents with diameter ≤ 3 mm (Gilard et al., 2006). Restenosis detection depended on stent diameter: for stents with diameter > 3 mm, sensitivity and specificity of MDCT were 86% and 100%, respectively. For small stents with diameter ≤ 3 mm, corresponding values were 54% and 100% (Lefebvre et al., 2007; Pugliese et al., 2006). As stated by Kitagawa et al, the importance of metal artifacts and partial volume effect of stents is related to the stent material, the stent diameter and thickness, and the strut design (Kitagawa et al., 2006). In vitro studies comparing 16-slice CT with 4-slice CT showed improvement in lumen visibility, with the same medium smooth body kernel (B30f) for reconstruction (Maintz et al., 2003). The use of a dedicated high spatial resolution reconstruction kernel (sharp kernel or "B46f"), compared with a standard reconstruction kernel (medium-smooth kernel or "B30f"), resulted in a further improvement of the visible stent lumen diameter because, with the B46f-kernel, the stent boundary was depicted more sharply than on the B30f-kernel images. Further, a larger window width to suppress the high attenuation of the stent strut seemed to contribute better delineation and more accurate measurement of the in-stent lumen. In a phantom study, Seifarth et al. showed that the use of 64-slice CT results in superior visualization of the stent lumen and in-stent stenosis, compared with 16-slice CT (Seifarth et al., 2006). In addition to evaluating the in vitro and in vivo performance of 64-slice CT for stent analysis, further developments could focus on the design of stents to reduce artifacts.

Authors	CT technique	Number of Patients	Number of Stents	Stent Caliber (mm)	Criteria for patency	Sensitivity (%)	Specificity (%)
Pump, et al., 2000	Electron beam	202	321	-	Distal runoff	78	98
Knollman, et al., 2004	Electron beam	117	152	2.5- 3.0	Distal runoff	72	60
Maintz, et al., 2003	4-MDCT	29	47	3.0-5.0	Distal runoff	100	100
Ligabue, et al., 2004	4-MDCT	48	72	2.5-4.5	Distal runoff	100	100
Schuijf, et al., 2004	16-MDCT	22	68	2.25-5.0	Distal runoff	78	100
Gilard, et al., 2006	16-MDCT	143	232	2.5-4.5	visualize lumen	100	92

Table 1. Results of studies of the use of MDCT to evaluate coronary stent patency.

3.1. Beam hardening and blooming effect

Metallic struts cause a severe CT artifact known as blooming effect. Blooming effect results from beam hardening and causes the stent struts to appear thicker than they are and, often, to overlap the vessel lumen. As a result the in-stent luminal diameter is underestimated. The energy spectrum of the x-ray beam increases as it passes through a hyperattenuating structure because lower-energy photons are absorbed more rapidly than are higher-energy photons, resulting in the beam being more intense when it reaches the detectors. Calcified spots of vessel wall near or at the outer surface of an implanted stent also contribute to beam hardening, which further erodes the assessability of the stent lumen. Depending on the metal type and the design of the stent, the magnitude of this artifact varies. As a rule, the depiction of stents with the slimmest profile is least affected by blooming artifacts (Lefebvre et al., 2007; Pugliese et al., 2006).

3.2. Partial volume averaging and interpolation

Another obstacle to coronary stent imaging is related to partial volume averaging and interpolation. Inherent in all digital tomographic imaging techniques, partial volume averaging yields a CT number that represents average attenuation of the materials within a voxel. At stent imaging in vessels with a large diameter, such as the aorta or iliac arteries, partial volume averaging effects are present but are limited to the proximity of the vessel wall. In coronary arteries with smaller diameters, the artifacts are of the same magnitude, but a reliable assessment of the lumen is much more problematic. The smaller the stent, the more detrimental the effect of partial volume averaging on the assessability of the in-stent lumen. The thinner detector width on 64-section CT scanners partly solves this problem by reducing the voxel size and thereby the general assessability of the stent lumen (Lefebvre et al., 2007; Pugliese et al., 2006).

3.3. Stent type

The visibility of lumens of different stents varies and this largely depends upon the stent type and the diameter. The blooming effect is more disturbing for smaller coronary stents with thicker struts. Uninterpretable images tend to be obtained for stents with thicker struts and/or a smaller diameter. When the lumen diameter is less than 3mm, the lumen visibility is worse. Regarding the type of stent, the most severe artifacts are found with tantalum, gold or gold-coated stents, or with covered stent grafts as compared with stainless steel stents. Maintz et al. recently evaluated 68 different stents in vitro with using 64-slice MDCT and they created a catalogue of the CT appearance of most of the currently available coronary stents (Maintz et al., 2009). They confirmed that the high variability for stent lumen visibility depended on the stent type, and this was previously reported on with using 4-slice and 16-slice CT. They also concluded that while in vivo studies will be required to verify their results, it can be assumed that a reliable evaluation of lumens of stents in the more advantageous stent types, such as the Radius, Teneo, Symbiot or Flex standard stents, will be possible with using 64-slice MDCT. First-generation drug-eluting stents, which released sirolimus or paclitaxel, were shown to be superior to bare-metal stents and to balloon angioplasty in reducing the magnitude of neointimal proliferation, the incidence of clinical restenosis, and the need for reintervention. Unfortunately, late stent thrombosis (thrombosis that occurs 30 days or more after implantation of the stent) is more likely to occur with drug-eluting stents than with bare-metal stents. The gradual release of the antiproliferative agent effectively inhibits endothelialization of the stent struts, thereby allowing them to continue to serve as a nidus for platelet aggregation and thrombus formation. Second or third-generation drug-eluting stents are designed to provide better stent deployment, safety, and efficacy. They differ from the first-generation stents with respect to the antiproliferative agent, the polymer layer (which acts as a reservoir for controlled drug delivery), and the stent frame. Improvements in stent structure may result in better stent apposition to the vessel wall, improved endothelialization (a thin stent strut elicits less neointimal proliferation and requires less endothelialization to cover the struts completely), and reduced platelet aggregation and thrombus formation, thereby reducing the incidence of stent thrombosis.

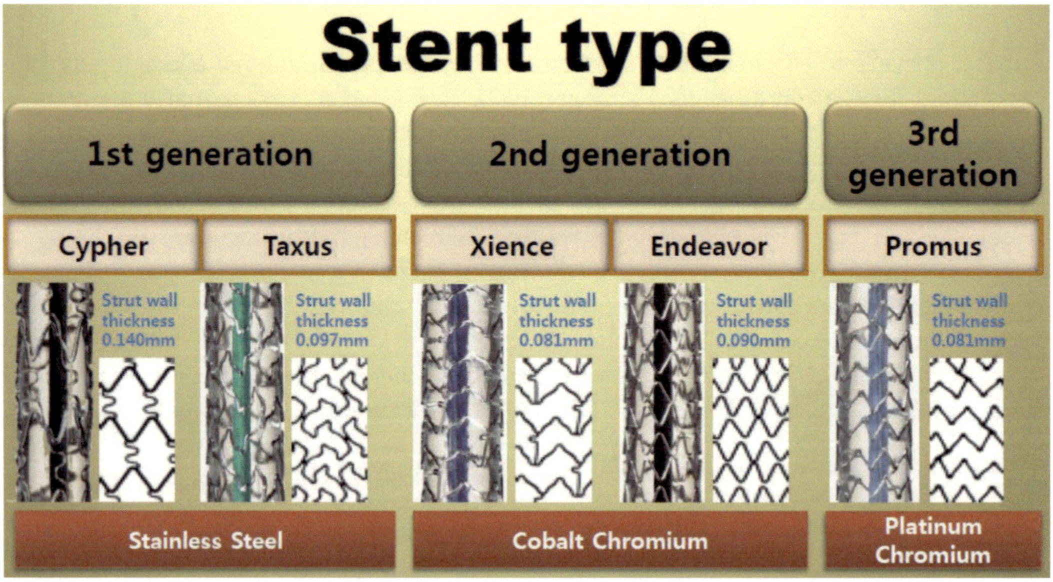

Scheme 2. Detail render of drug-eluting stents. Diverse drug-eluting stents are currently available, differing in the type of metal used, stent design, and drug coating.

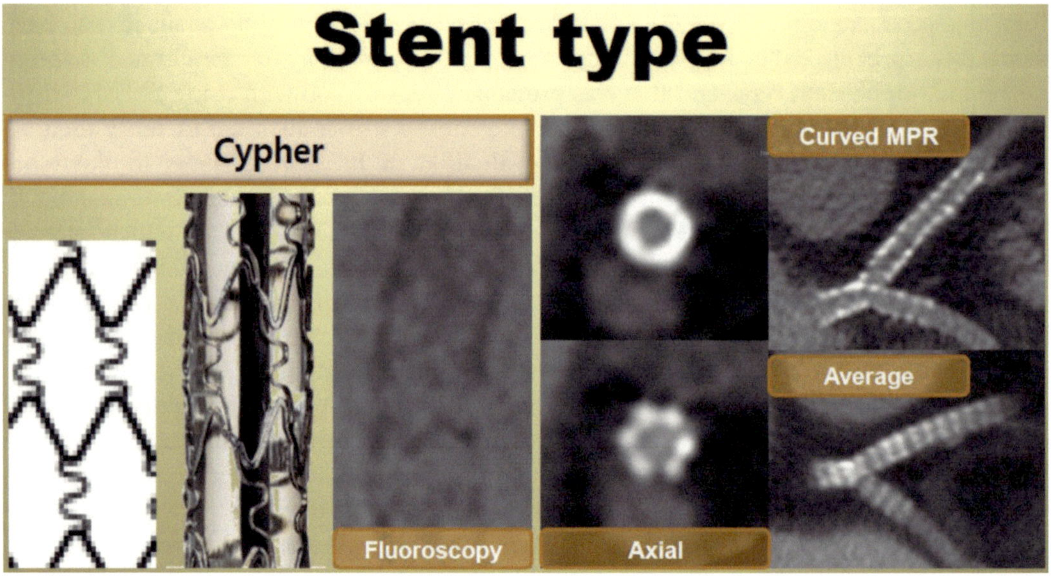

Scheme 3. Type of metal used, stent design, and images of fluoroscopy and 64-slice MDCT of Cypher, first-generation Sirolimus-eluting stent.

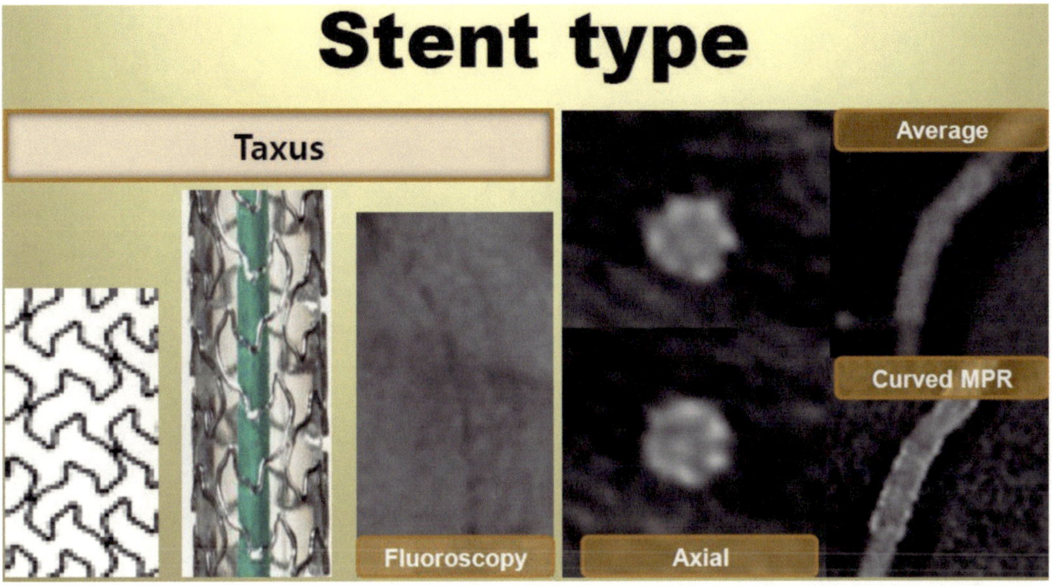

Scheme 4. Type of metal used, stent design, and images of fluoroscopy and 64-slice MDCT of Taxus, first-generation Paclitaxel-eluting stent.

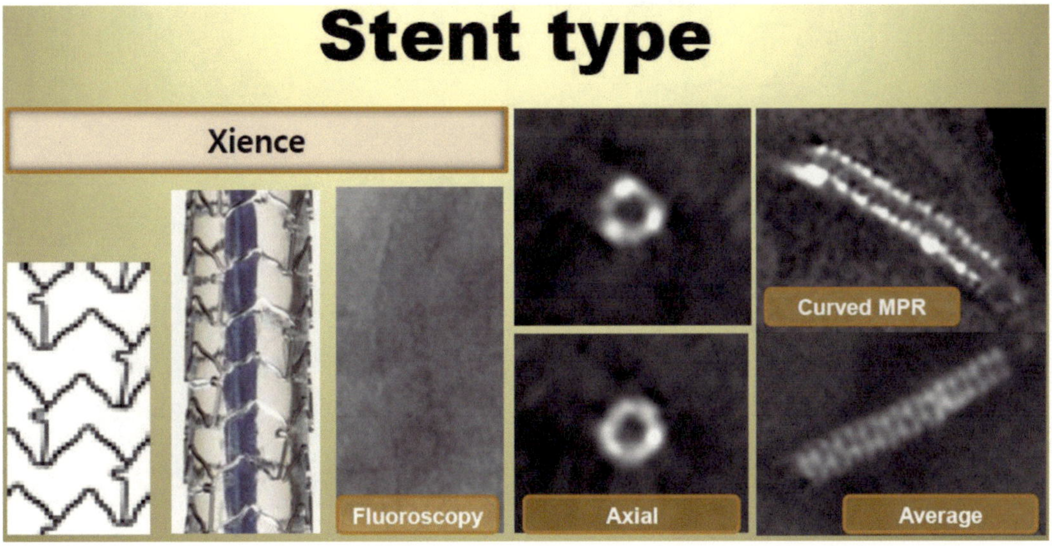

Scheme 5. Type of metal used, stent design, and images of fluoroscopy and 64-slice MDCT of Xience, second-generation Everolimus-eluting stent.

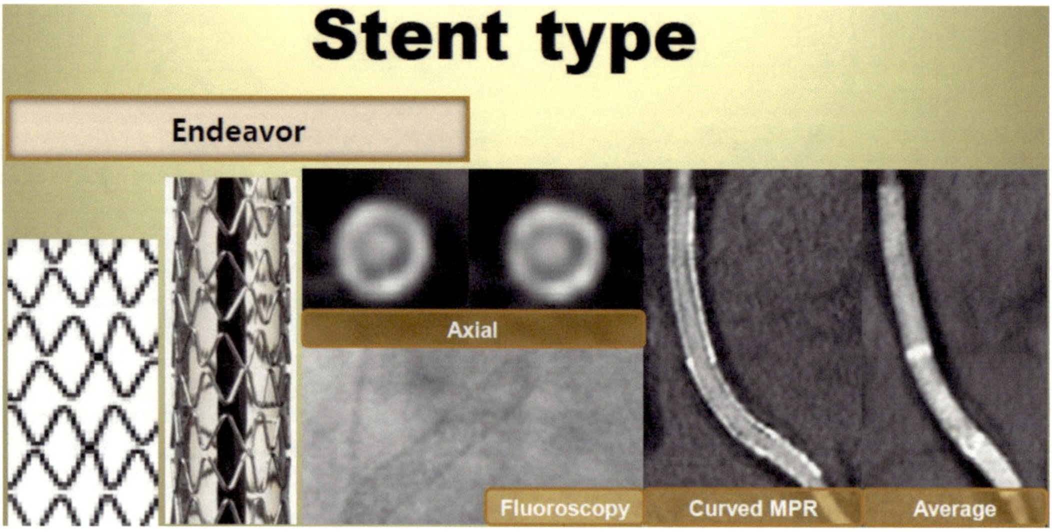

Scheme 6. Type of metal used, stent design, and images of fluoroscopy and 64-slice MDCT of Endeavor, second-generation Zotarolimus-eluting stent.

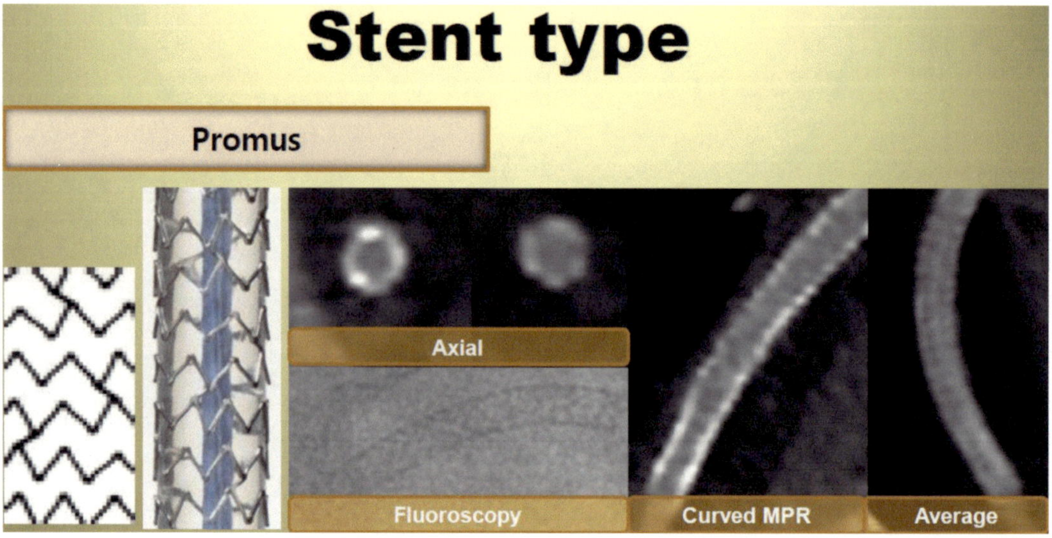

Scheme 7. Type of metal used, stent design, and images of fluoroscopy and 64-slice MDCT of Promus, third-generation Everolimus-eluting stent.

http://dx.doi.org/10.5772/54085

Stent trade name	Metal platform	Coating drug used
Cypher	Stainless steel	Sirolimus (Rapamune)
Endeavor	Cobalt-chromium	Zotarolimus
Taxus	Stainless steel	Paclitaxel (Taxol)
Xience, Promus	Cobalt-chromium	Everolimus (Afinitor)

Table 2. Types of Drug-Eluting Stents Available for Clinical Use

3.4. Optimization of contrast enhancement

Prominent contrast enhancement in the lumen is a prerequisite for robust coronary CT angiography. It is achieved not only by optimizing the contrast material injection parameters (example, using a high-concentration contrast agent and a fast injection rate) but also by accurately synchronizing CT data acquisition with the passage of the contrast agent by means of bolus tracking or a test bolus. Edge-enhancing convolution filters, which may be used for better delineation of stents, have the drawback of producing noisier data sets. If such convolution filter is used, the assessability of in-stent lumen particularly benefits from the presence of high degree of intraluminal contrast enhancement, which somewhat compensates for the kernel-related noise. A high degree of intraluminal enhancement is recommended especially for the investigation of stent patency in vessels that have a small diameter and thus contain less blood (Lefebvre et al., 2007; Pugliese et al., 2006).

3.5. Residual cardiac motion

Residual cardiac motion is of the utmost importance as a cause of vessel non-assessability at MDCT. Residual cardiac motion also plays a role in exacerbating metal-related artifacts such as beam hardening or partial volume averaging effects. The use of high gantry rotation speeds, multisegmental reconstruction techniques, and beta-blockers to lower the heart rate consistently improves the interpretability of MDCT. ECG-based editing techniques allow improvement of image quality for patients with mild irregularities in sinus rhythm, such as premature beats, and for those with bundle-branch block (Lefebvre et al., 2007; Pugliese et al., 2006).

3.6. In-stent lumen evaluation

As mentioned earlier, the direct visualization of the in-stent lumen is important for assessing patency, because collateral vessels may be feeding vessel segment distal to the occluded stent in a retrograde direction. An accurate intraluminal evaluation can best be performed by means of multiplanar reformation of the CT data volume. The stent may be considered to be occluded if the lumen inside the device appears darker than the contrast-enhanced vessel lumen proximal to the stent. Unless severe artifacts affect the CT data set, stent evaluation may proceed beyond a judgment of patency or occlusion. Nonocclusive in-stent neointimal hyperplasia is characterized by the presence of a darker rim between the stent and the contrast-enhanced vessel lumen and is secondary to the healing response to procedurerelated vessel injury. If neointimal hyperplasia exceeds a luminal diameter reduction of 50%, the process is consistent with hemodynamically significant in-stent restenosis. Instent restenosis typically occurs as a localized nonenhancing lesion, often (but not invariably) associated with complex lesion anatomy and discontinuity in lesion coverage. Restenosis may occur either within or adjacent to the stent (within 5 mm of the stent extremities). Edge restenosis might occur because of a decrease in local drug availability, incomplete lesion coverage due to a gap between two stents, procedure-related trauma, or damage to the polymer coating of a stent from calcifications or an overlapping stent.

3.7. Coronary stent fracture

Stent fracture (SF) is an important and potentially serious complication of drug-eluting stents (DES), resulting in thrombosis and in-stent restenosis. Recent reports suggest that the prevalence of fracture ranges between 1.9% and 2.6% (Dimitrios et al., 2011; Lim et al., 2008). SF is probably related to mechanical fatigue of the metallic stent strut, which may be aggravated by highly pulsatile structures such as myocardial bridge, use of long stents or DES unsupported by neointimal tissue. SF may also result from a manufacturing defect. Various factors that have been implicated for a stent fracture include vessel tortuosity, the presence of a right coronary artery lesion, overlapping stents, and the use of a DES such as a sirolimus-eluting stent. In general stent fractures have been reported to be more common when placed in the right coronary artery (RCA) probably due to its curved course, than in the left anterior descending (LAD) or circumflex (LCX) coronary arteries. The type of stent also influences its risk for fracture. The Cypher stent is more prone to fracture as compared to Taxus and Endeavor stents. Overlapping stents are more likely to fracture rather than isolated stents. The presence of stent fracture was classified as grade I to V: I = involving a single-strut fracture; II = 2 or more strut fractures without deformation; III = 2 or more strut fractures with deformation; IV = multiple strut fractures with acquired transection but without gap; and V = multiple strut fractures with acquired transection with gap in the stent body (Nakazawa et al., 2009).

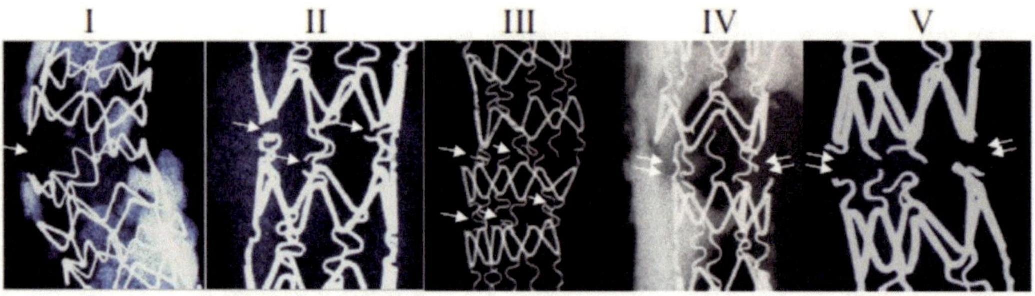

Scheme 8. Classification of stent fracture.

http://dx.doi.org/10.5772/54085

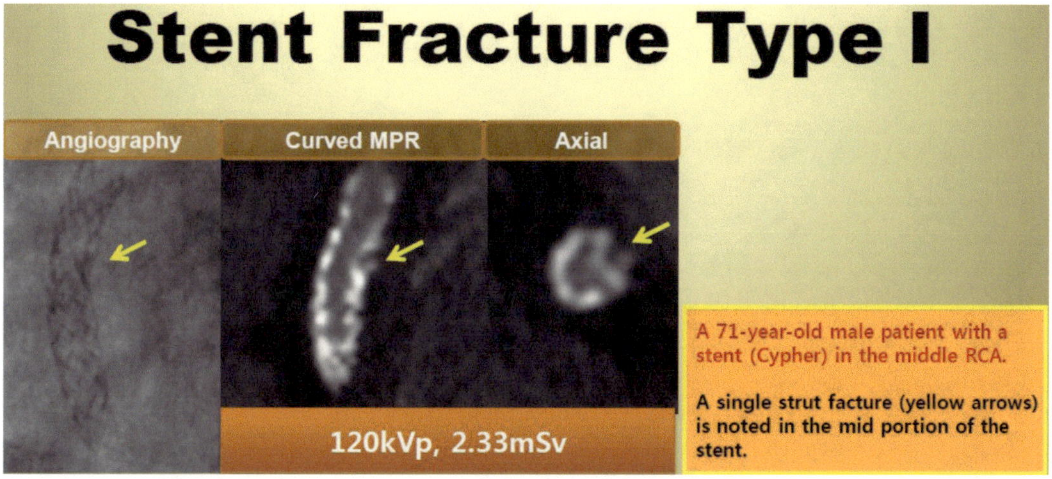

Scheme 9. Images of fluoroscopy and 64-slice MDCT of stent fracture type I. A single strut fracture is seen in the mid portion of the stent in RCA.

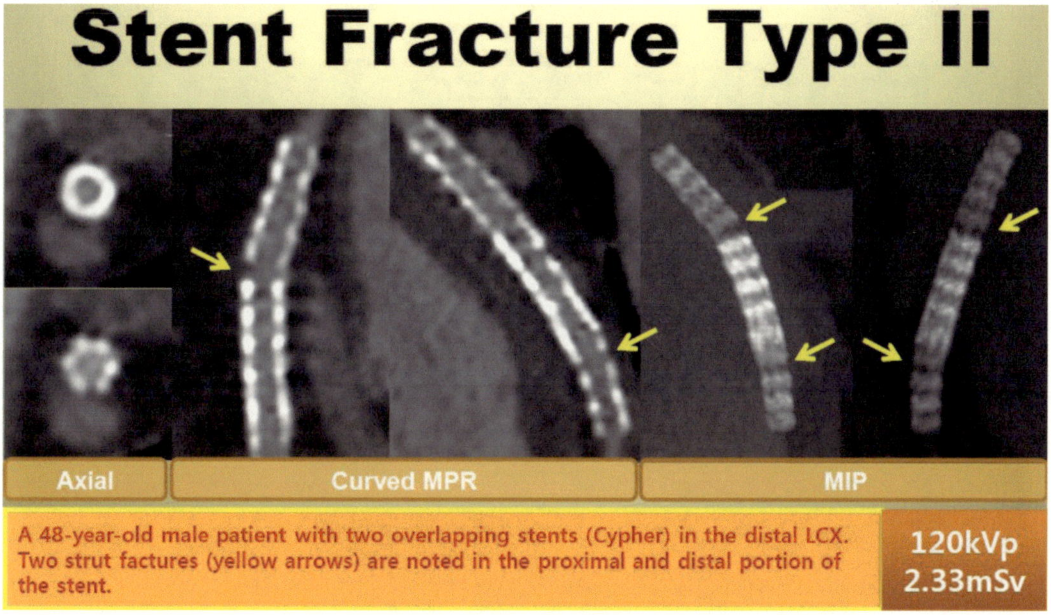

Scheme 10. Images of fluoroscopy and 64-slice MDCT of stent fracture type II. Two strut fractures are seen in the proximal and distal portion of the stent in LCX.

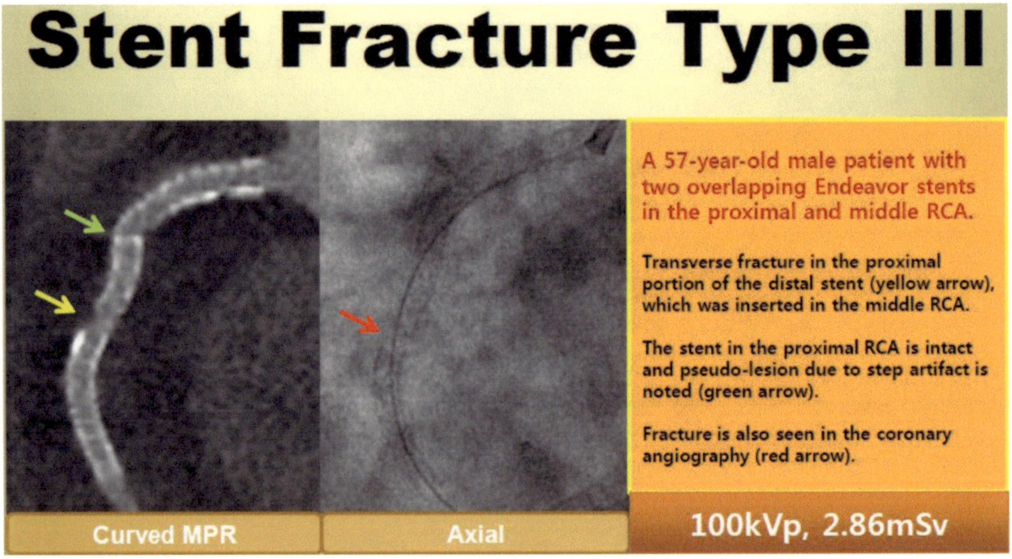

Scheme 11. Images of fluoroscopy and 64-slice MDCT of stent fracture type III. Transverse fracture with deformation is seen in the proximal portion of the stent in middle RCA. The stent in proximal RCA is intact in coronary angiography suggesting pseudo-lesion due to step artifact in MDCT.

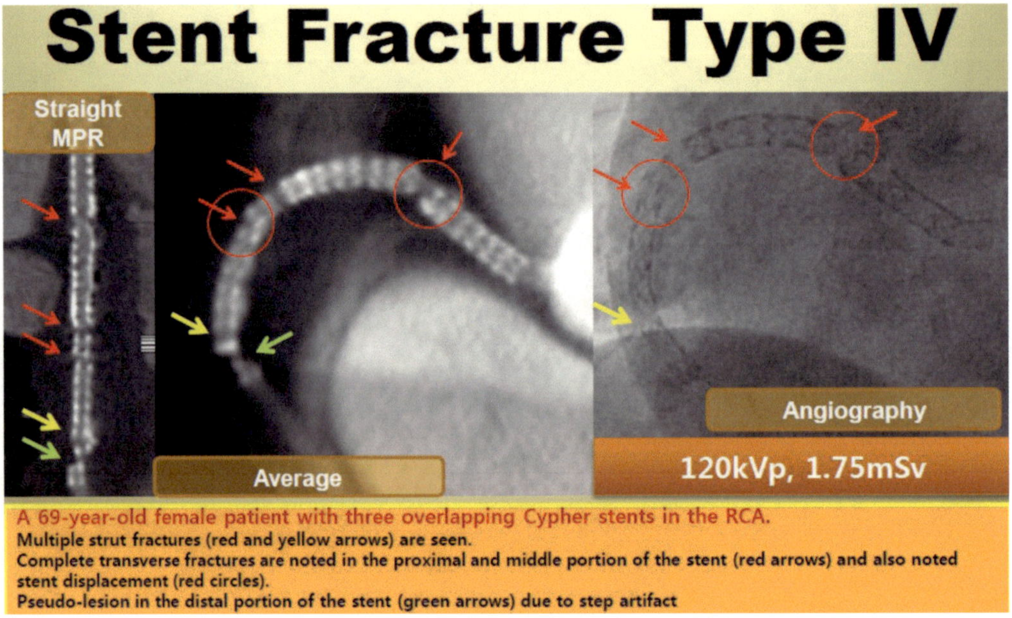

Scheme 12. Images of fluoroscopy and 64-slice MDCT of stent fracture type IV. Multiple strut fractures with acquired transection without gap are seen in the proximal and mid portion of the stent in RCA. The distal portion of the stent is intact in coronary angiography suggesting pseudo-lesion due to step artifact in MDCT.

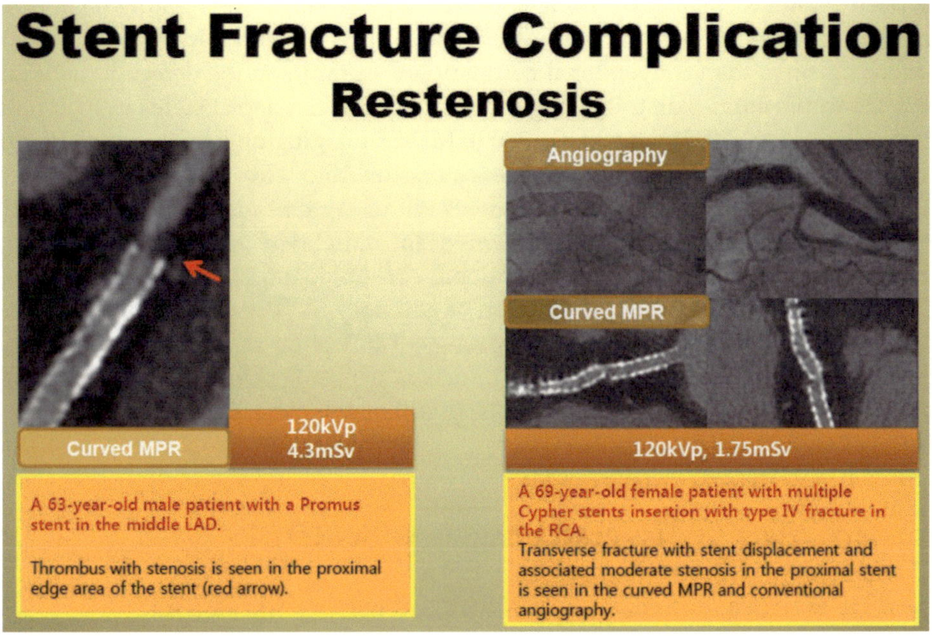

Scheme 13. Images of fluoroscopy and 64-slice MDCT of restenosis due to stent fracture. (Left) Thrombus with stenosis is seen in the proximal edge of the LAD stent. (Right) Transverse fracture with stent displacement and moderate stenosis is seen in the RCA stent.

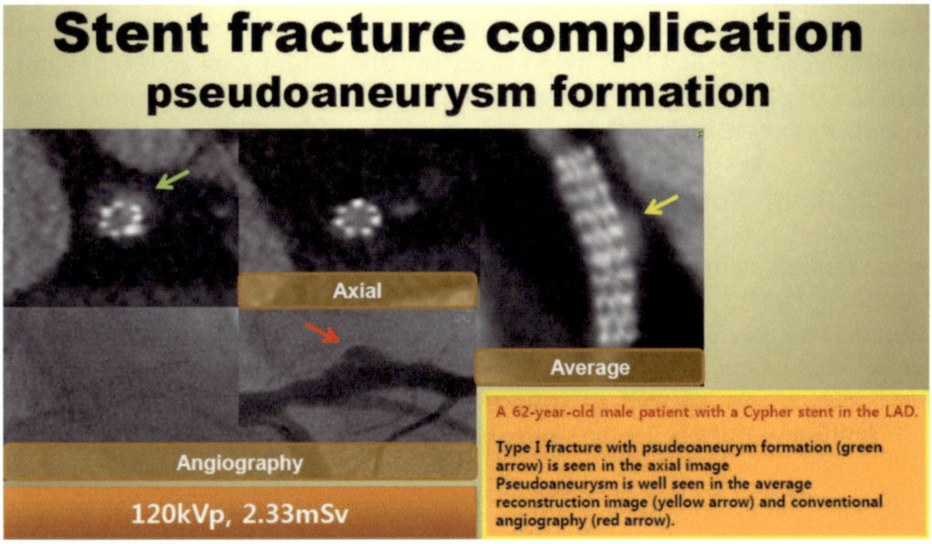

Scheme 14. Images of fluoroscopy and 64-slice MDCT of pseudoaneurysm due to stent fracture. Type I fracture with pseudoaneurysm formation is seen in the LAD stent.

SF has been evaluated mainly by using conventional coronary angiography or fluoroscopy and in selected cases by intravascular ultrasound (IVUS). Recently, MDCT has been found to be more sensitive than conventional coronary angiography in the detection of SF, due to its nearly isotropic multi-planar imaging capabilities, that can depict stents in their long and short axes (Lim et al., 2008; Pang et al., 2009). MDCT imaging on 64-slice scanners provide most of the relevant details required to assess stents on follow-up. In a retrospective evaluation, 64-slice MDCT angiography of 371 patients with 545 stents identified 24 SFs, of which 6 were not detected on conventional angiograms at the initial readings (Lim et al., 2008). An *in vitro* comparison of 64-slice MDCT, conventional cine-angiography, and IVUS revealed that MDCT had high accuracy for the evaluation of coronary SF (Pang et al., 2009). The important features that must be evaluated in all post-stent follow-up include not only the evaluation of in-stent thrombosis, but also features such as stent migration, fracture, buckling, and rarely coronary perforation and aneurysms or pseudoaneurysms (Dimitrios et al., 2011).

4. Coronary artery bypass graft imaging with MDCT

4.1. Coronary bypass graft lumen assessment: Graft patency and stenoses

Coronary bypass graft CT can be performed with 2 different objectives, each with a separate clinical context and goal: the evaluation of graft patency, and the evaluation of graft and anastomotic stenoses. Within the first postoperative month, the main cause of graft failure is thrombosis.75 Graft closure from thrombosis at 1 month is a known complication in 10% to 15% of cases. Coronary bypass graft patency assessment has been shown to be excellent with ECG-gated 4-detector CT, with mean sensibility and specificity for occlusion of 97% and 98%, respectively, in comparison with catheter angiography (Nieman K et al., 2003; Marano R et al., 2004). With 16-detector CT, accuracy is also excellent, with mean sensitivity of 100 % and mean specificity of 99% for detecting bypass graft occlusion, in comparison with catheter angiography (Chiurlia E et al., 2005; Anderson K et al., 2006). Recent studies using 64-slice MDCT have reported sensitivity and specificity values of 95% to 100% and 93% to 100%, respectively, for graft occlusion and high-grade stenosis with > 50% luminal narrowing. Since naïve coronary arteries and coronary grafts are small vessels, 2 to 4 mm in diameter, and are characterized by both complex anatomy and continuous movements, high spatial and temporal resolutions are mandatory to visualize these vessels at MDCT. Vascular clips in the proximity of grafts and their anastomoses, as well as artifacts owing to residual cardiac motion, can be a cause of significant artifacts for the evaluation of graft stenoses.

4.2. Type of arterial or vein graft

4.2.1. Saphenous vein Graft (SVG)

The SVG was first successfully used in a CABG operation by Sabiston in 1962. Both the benefits and limitations of SVG have been well documented in the literature (Bourassa et al., 1985; Campeau et al., 1983). Saphenousveins are fairly simple to access and harvest from the lower extremities, and they are more versatile and widely available than arterial grafts. In addition, during the intra- and perioperative period, saphenous veins are resistant to spasm versus their arterial counterparts. However, the use of SVG is limited by distortion from varicose and sclerotic disease as well as a higher occurrence of intimal hyperplasia and atherosclerotic changes after exposure to systemic blood pressure, resulting in lower patency rates. Graft occlusion can also occur due to vascular damage during harvesting of the saphenous vein. In a large study, the SVG patency was 88% perioperatively, 81% at 1 year, 75% at 5 years, and 50% at greater than or equal to 15 years (Fitzgibbon et al., 1996). The graft attrition rate between 1 and 6 years after CABG surgery is 1% to 2% per year, and between 6 and 10 years is 4% per year. The great saphenous vein is the vein routinely used for CABG surgery. The proximal anastomosis of the venous graft with the ascending aorta is usually performed cranial to the origin of coronary arteries and as distal as the proximal portion of the aortic arch. The SVG can be sutured directly to the anterior portion of the ascending aorta or attached with an anastomotic device, allowing faster, sutureless attachment. The device, called the Symmetry Bypass System aortic connector (St Jude Medical, St Paul, Minn), alters the common appearance of the bypass graft by requiring the aortic connector to be anastomosed perpendicularly to the aorta (Mack et al., 2003; Poston et al., 2004). Recent reports have documented the development of significant stenosis and occlusion in 13.7%-15.5% of vein grafts attached with the aortic connector (Carrel et al., 2003; Wiklund et al., 2002). In order to support the course of the aortovenous anastomosis, the left-sided SVG is connected to the left side of the aorta, stabilizing the graft on top of the main pulmonary artery. A right-sided SVG is attached either to the lower aspect or right side of the ascending aorta, allowing the graft to traverse the right arterio-ventricular groove. SVGs tend to appear as large contrast-filled vessels (Fig.1).

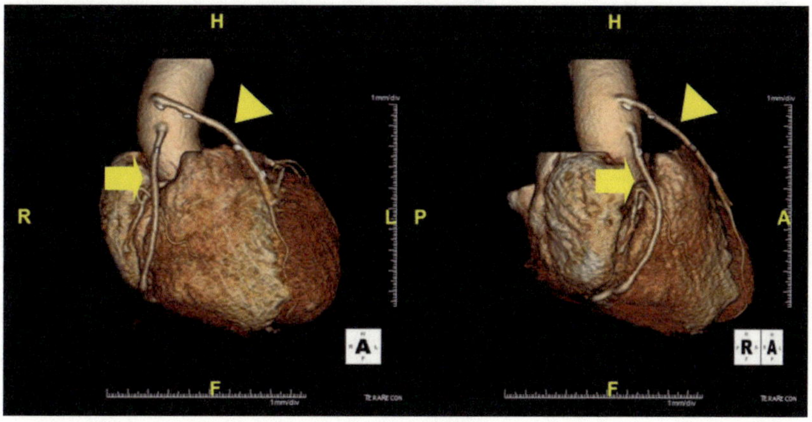

Figure 1. Saphenous vein grafts. Three-dimensional volume-rendered images show the typical appearance of right (arrow) and left (arrowhead) saphenous vein grafts (SVGs) sutured to the anterior aorta. The left SVG is attached to

the mid-portion of left anterior descending (LAD) artery and the right SVG is attached to the distal-portion of right coronary artery (RCA).

An SVG to the right side is attached to the distal right coronary artery (RCA), posterior descending artery (PDA), or distal LAD artery. The distal anastomosis may lie on the phrenic wall of the heart. An SVG to the left side is attached distally to the LAD artery, diagonal artery, left circumflex (LCx) artery, or the obtuse marginal (OM) arteries, by traversing anteriorly and superiorly to the right ventricular outflow tractor main pulmonary artery (Fig. 2, 3, 4).

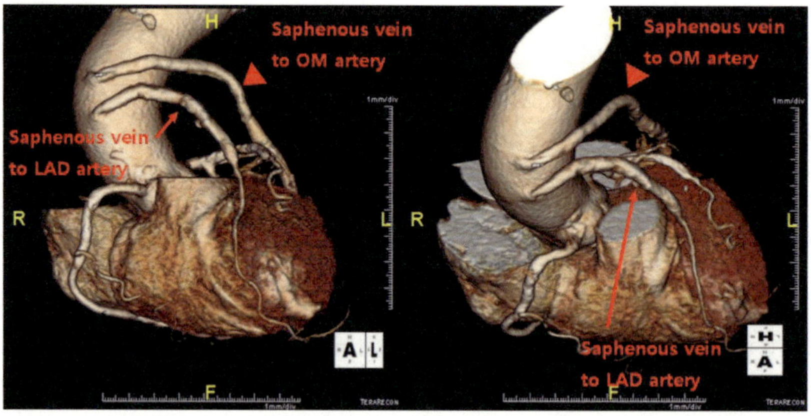

Figure 2. Saphenous vein grafts. Three-dimensional volume-rendered images show the typical appearance of right (arrow) and left (arrowhead) saphenous vein grafts (SVGs) sutured to the anterior aorta. The right SVG is attached to the mid-portion of left anterior descending (LAD) artery and the left SVG is attached to the obtuse marginal (OM) artery.

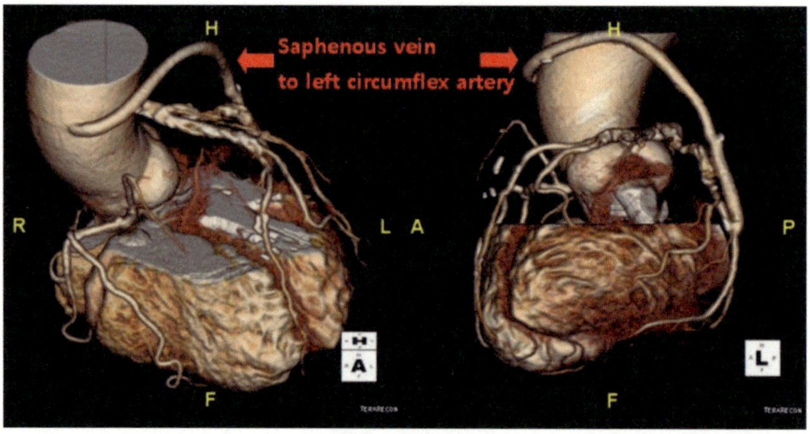

Figure 3. Saphenous vein graft. Three-dimensional volume-rendered images show the left saphenous vein graft (SVG) with its anastomosis with the left circumflex (LCx) artery.

SVG may present a horizontal or slightly oblique course on axial images, especially when the distal anastomosis is placed on the LCx or a diagonal branch to supply the left cardiac wall. In these cases, the graft can be recognized in the fatty tissue of mediastinum, posterior to the sternum and anterior to the RVOT. On occasion, the distal SVG is anastomosed sequentially to greater than or equal to 2 coronary vessels or in the same vessel, using side-to-side and end-to-side anastomoses. The naive vessel distal to the anastamotic site should be assessed and is recognized by its position and smaller caliber compared with the SVG (Fig. 3, 4). Typically, venous grafts are larger than arterial grafts and are not accompanied by surgical clips along their course. Sometimes a circumferential clip can be identified at the site of proximal anastomosis with the ascending aorta (Fig.1).

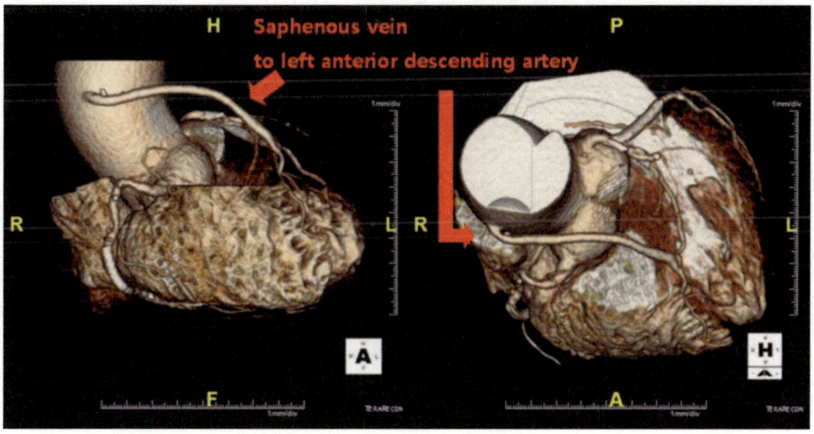

Figure 4. Saphenous vein graft. Three-dimensional volume-rendered images show the left saphenous vein graft (SVG), which is attached to the mid-portion of left anterior descending (LAD) artery.

4.2.2. Internal Mammary Artery (IMA)

The internal mammary artery (IMA) is characterized by unique resistance to atherosclerosis and extremely high long-term patency rates compared with the saphenous vein. The IMA has a nonfenestrated internal elastic laminawithout vaso vasorum inside the vessel wall, which tends to protect against cellular migration and intimal hyperplasia. Moreover, the medial layer of IMA is thin and poor of muscle cells with poor vasoreactivity. In addition, the endothelium produces vasodilator(nitric oxide) and platelet inhibitor (prostacyclin). Glycosaminoglycan and lipid compositions of IMA result in being less atherogenetic in comparison with venous grafts. Therefore, use of the IMA decreases all postoperative cardiac events and mortality, and is associated with a long-term patency rate well >90% at 10 years (Loop et al., 1986; Motwani & Topol, 1998).

4.2.3. Left IMA

The Left IMA (LIMA) is the vessel of choice for the surgical revascularization of the left anterior descending (LAD) artery for its biological and anatomical characteristiscs, being the conduit more proximal to the LAD artery and the easiest to harvest both in median sternotomy and mini-thoracotomy. Due to anatomical proximity to the LAD artery and favorable patency rates, the left IMA (LIMA) is most commonly used as an in situ graft to revascularize the LAD or diagonal artery, supplying the anterior or anterolateral cardiac wall. The LIMA extends from its origin at the subclavian artery and courses through the anterior mediastinum along the right ventricular outflow tract after being separated surgically from its original position in the left parasternalRegion (Fig. 5).

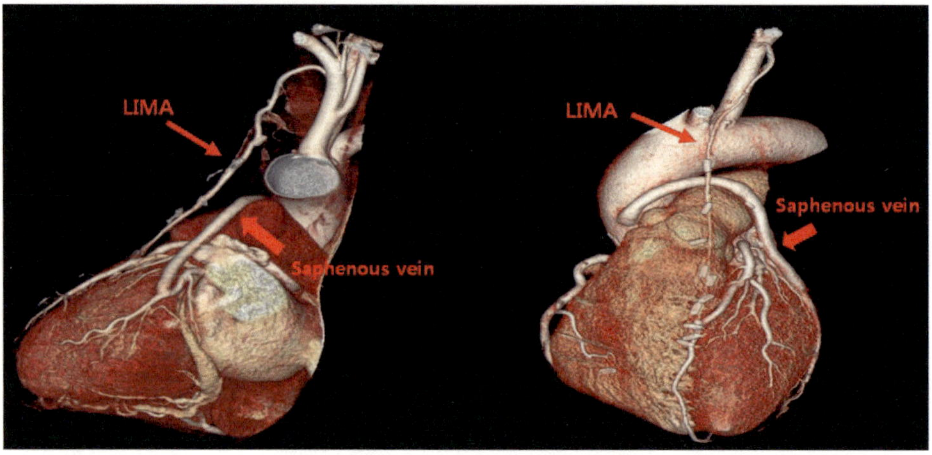

Figure 5. Left internal mammary artery (IMA) graft. Three-dimensional volume-rendered images show the left IMA graft from its origin at the left subclavian artery to its anastomosis with the left anterior descending (LAD) artery. There is also a left saphenous vein graft (SVG), which is attached to the obtuse marginal (OM) artery. Note the smaller diameter of the arterial graft compared with that of the venous graft.

Infrequently, sequential distal anastomoses, with side-to-side and end-to-side anastomoses to the diagonal and LAD arteries, respectively, or involving separate sections of the LAD artery, are performed. On axial images, the LIMA is no longer visible in its usual site, on the left side of the sternum, but courses as a small vessel in the anterior mediastinum along the right ventricle outflow tract (RVOT). Although in most cases LIMA grafts show a single distal anastomosis to the left anterior descending artery (LAD) or a diagonal branch, multiple sequential anastomoses to both the LAD and diagonal branches are sometimes performed. Surgical clips are routinely used to occlude collaterals and to avoid arterial bleeding and can be seen either adjacent to the graft or at the original site of the LIMA. As with other grafts, on CTA, the distal anastamosis is typically most difficult to visualize. Surgical clips are used routinely to occlude branch vessels of the IMA, and metallic artifact may limit assessment in some instances (Fig. 6).

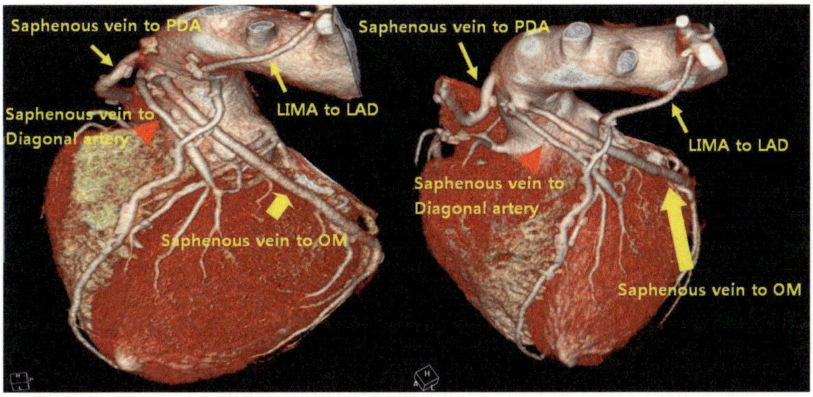

Figure 6. Left internal mammary artery (IMA) graft. Three-dimensional volume-rendered images show the left IMA graft from its origin at the left subclavian artery to its anastomosis with the left anterior descending (LAD) artery. There is also a right saphenous vein graft (SVG) sutured to the anterior aorta with its anastomosis with the posterior descending artery (PDA). The left saphenous vein grafts (SVG) are attached to diagonal artery and the obtuse marginal (OM) artery.

4.2.4. Right IMA

The right IMA (RIMA) is used less frequently than the LIMA. The RIMA may be used in a variety of ways. As an in situ graft, The RIMA remains attached to the right subclavian artery proximally and anastomoses with the target coronary artery distally. However, it is more commonly used as "free" graft from the ascending aorta to the RCA or from the LIMA to the left circumflex artery (LCx) or obtuse marginal (OM) branches. In cases in which both in situ IMAs are necessary for revascularization of the left heart, either the RIMA is connected to the LCx artery or OM branches by extension through the transverse sinus of the pericardium and the LIMA is attached to the LAD artery or the RIMA is attached to the LAD artery and the LIMA is anastomosed to the LCx artery or other side branches (OM or diagnonal branches). Otherwise, the RIMA can be removed from the right subclavian artery and used as a composite or free graft. As a segment of a composite graft to perform an arterial "T" or "Y" graft, the RIMA is anastomosed proximally to LIMA, allowing total arterial revascularization instead of using a venous graft with LIMA. As a free graft, a RIMA is anastomosed to the anterior ascending aorta and used in the same way as an SVG. The CTA appearance of the RIMA is similar to that of the LIMA. As already described for LIMA grafts, surgical clips are used to occlude collaterals. Studies have shown that total arterial myocardial revascularzation has the advantages of decreased recurrent angina and superior patency rates at 1 year when compared with those of conventional coronary artery bypass surgery in which a LIMA graft is coupled with an SVG (Muneretto et al., 2003).

4.2.5. Radial Artery (RA)

The first use of the radial artery (RA) as arterial conduit for coronary revascularization has been de-scribed by Carpentier et al in 1971 (Carpentier et al., 1973). As a muscular artery from the forearm, the RA has a prominent medial layer and elevated vasoreactivity, which results in a lower patency rate than that of IMA grafts (Possati et al., 2003). The RA is usually harvested from the nondominant arm and is used as a third arterial graft, either as a free or composite graft or to avoid using a venous graft in case of unavailability of IMA grafts. The RA is often grafted to supply the left cardiac wall (LCx, OM). On CTA, the caliber of the RA is similar to the IMA, but it typically is visualized coursing from the ascending aorta to the naïve coronary artery (Fig. 7). In the early postoperative period, the RA may be reduced in caliber and may be difficult to identify because of vasospasm. In addition, because the RA is a muscular artery, the number of surgical clips used to close collaterals along the graft is usually higher than with IMA. This may represent a limit for noninvasive assessment of RA grafts with MDCT because of artifacts from surgical clips limiting a full CTA evaluation of an RA graft.

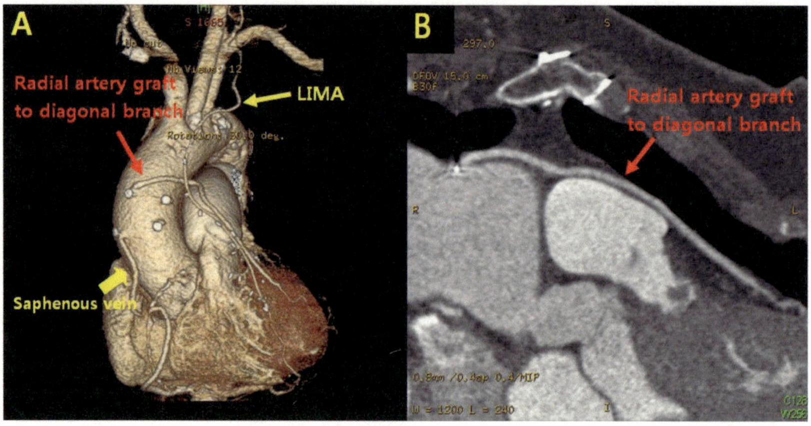

Figure 7. Radial artery (RA) graft. (A) Three-dimensional volume-rendered image shows radial artery graft sutured to the anterior aorta with its anastomosis with diagonal artery. There are also left internal mammary artery (LIMA) graft from its origin at the left subclavian artery to its anastomosis with the left anterior descending (LAD) artery and right saphenous vein graft (SVG), which is attached to the distal right coronary artery (RCA). Note the diameter of the RA is similar to the IMA, but it typically is visualized coursing from the ascending aorta to the diagonal artery. (B) Curved multiplanar reformation image shows patent RA graft within the anterior mediastinum. The full extent of the graft is seen from the ascending aorta to diagonal artery.

4.2.6. Right gastroepiploic artery (RGEA) and inferior epigastric artery (IEA)

The use of right gastroepiploic and inferior epigastric arteries in CABG procedures has been limited because of the need to extend the median sternotomy to expose the abdominal cavity (Buche et al., 1992; Manapat et al., 1994; Pym et al., 1987). Although the use of these arteries increases surgical time and technical difficulty of the surgery, these arteries can be used as a free graft to perform total arterial revascularization. The use of the RGEA was first described by Pym et al in June 1984 (Pym et al., 1987). Although it has been originally used in reoperation, in the absence of other suitable conduits, RGEA is now used as secondary, tertiary, or quaternary arterial conduit to provide all-arterial revascularization. The biological characteristics of RGEA are similar to IMA, but unclear benefits for third or fourth arterial grafts, the increment of surgery time, and the involvement of an additional body cavity are the main drawbacks limiting the widespread use of this conduit. Occasionally, the RGEA is used to supply the inferior cardiac wall and is anastomosed as an in situ graft to the posterior descending artery (PDA). In these cases, the mobilized artery is seen coursing anterior to the liver and through the diaphragm to reach the site of anastomosis. Small clips can be identified at the original site of the RGEA, near the small curvature of stomach. These instances require that the surgical history be conveyed to the radiologist so the CTA protocol can be modified to include the upper abdomen, because the gastroepiploic artery is freed to course anteriorly to the liver and through the diaphragm to reach the target vessel. The inferior epigastric artery (IEA) is an arterial branch of the abdominal wall, arising from the external iliac artery and coursing inside the abdominal rectus muscle. Similar to the radial artery (RA), the IEA has a predominant muscular structure, while the limited length of the vessel with an adequate caliber is a constraint to using this vessel only as a lateral branch of a multiple arterial graft.

4.3. Complication

4.3.1. Graft failure

Bypass graft failures are classified either as early or late following CABG surgery. During the early phase, usually within 1 month after CABG surgery, the most common cause of graft failure is thrombosis from platelet dysfunction at the site of focal endothelial damage during surgical harvesting and anastomosis. Graft closure from thrombosis at 1 month is a recognized complication in 10-15% of cases (Fitzgibbon et al., 1996). Perioperative venous graft failure after off-pump CABG procedures is chiefly determined by the two factors of graft endothelial damage and patient hypercoagulability. Early bypass graft failure can also be due to a malpositioned graft (Ricci et al., 2000). If the graft is too long, it may twist or kink. Technical factors associated with use of an aortic connector may predispose venous grafts to kinking (Traverse et al., 2003). Late-phase venous graft failure is due primarily to progressive changes related to systemic blood pressure exposure. One month after surgery, the venous graft starts to undergo neointimal hyperplasia. Although this process does not produce significant stenosis, it is the foundation for later development of graft atheroma. Beyond 1 year, atherosclerosis is the dominant process, resulting in graft stenosis and occlusion. On the other hand, arterial grafts, specifically IMA graft, are resistant to atheroma development. Late IMA graft failure is more commonly due to progression of atherosclerotic disease in the native coronary artery distal to the graft anastomosis. CTA can delineate multiple findings associated with graft stenosis and occlusion. Calcifiedand noncalcified atherosclerotic plaque is readily identified, and the calculation of the extent of graft narrowing is straightforward. Occlusion can be determined by non-visualization of a vessel which is known to have been used for surgical grafting. In many instances, the most proximal part of an occluded aortocoronary graft fills with contrast, creating a small out-pouching from the ascending aorta, allowing a diagnosis. Acute or chronic graft occlusion can sometimes be differentiated by the diameter of the bypass graft. In chronic occlusion, the diameter is usually reduced from scarring, as compared with acute occlusion in which the diameter is usually enlarged.

4.3.2. Graft vasospasm

Radial artery (RA) grafts are susceptible to vasospasm because the RA is a muscular artery with elevated vasoreactivity. The appearance is similar to fixed graft stenosis, although the luminal narrowing is more extensive in length. Nevertheless, the administration of intraoperative alpha-adrenergic antagonist solution or posteroperative calcium channel blockers can overcome many cases of graft vasospasm postoperatively (Locker et al., 2002; Myers & Fremes, 2003).

4.3.3. Graft aneurysm

There are 2 types of bypass graft aneurysms: true aneurysms and pseudoaneurysms (Dubois & Vandervoort, 2001; Mohara et al., 1998). True aneuryms are usually found 5 to 7 years after CABG surgery and are related to atherosclerotic disease. On the other hand, pseudoaneuryms more commonly occur within 6 months after surgery, although they may also arise several years later. Pseudoaneurysms arise at either proximal or distal anastomotic sites. Pseudoaneurysm cases that are found earlier may be related to infection or tension at the anastomotic site, resulting in suture rupture. In late-onset pseudoaneurysms, similar to true aneurysms, atherosclerotic changes likely played a role. Currently, there is no clear guideline for surgery. Nevertheless, size >2 cm has been a cause for concern (Memon et al., 2003). Graft aneurysms may lead to various complications, including compression and mass effect on adjacent structures, thrombosis and embolization of the bypass graft leading to an acute coronary event, formation of fistula to the right atrium and ventricle, sudden rupture leading to hemothorax, hemopericardium, or death.

4.3.4. Pericardialand pleuraleffusions

Approximately 22%-85% of patients have postoperative pericardial effusions after CABG surgery (Meurin et al., 2004; Pepi et al., 1994). Although pericardial effusions are common, only 0.8%-6% of patients progress to cardiac temponade (Katara et al., 2003). Risk factors include postoperative coagulation abnormality or use of anticoagulation agents that are often related to the use of cardiopulmonary bypass. Nearly all significant pericardial effusions are diagnosed within 5 days postoperatively, peak in 10 days, and resolve within a month (Kuvin et al., 2002). Postoperative pleural effusions are even more numerous after surgery, a prevalence of 89% within 7 days after surgery (Hurlbut et al., 1990; Vargas et al., 1994). These pleural effusions are usually unilateral, small, left-sided, and without clinical significance. Only 1%-4% of CABG surgery patients proceed to develop clinically significant effusions that require thoracentesis (Peng et al., 1992).

http://dx.doi.org/10.5772/54085

4.3.5. Sternal infection

The sternal infection is an important complication of the CABG surgery, with a prevalence of 1% to 20% (Roy, 1998). Three different compartments may be affected: the presternal (cellulitis, sinus tracts, and abscess), sternal (osteomyelitis, and dehiscence), or retrosternal (mediastinitis, hematoma, and abscess) compartments (Li & Fishman, 2003). Risk factors include diabetes mellitus, obesity, current cigarette smoking, and steroid therapy. Surgical risk factors include complexity of surgery, type of bone saw used, type of sternal closure, length of surgical time, blood transfusions, and early reexploration to control hemorrhage. The CTA is important in revealing the extent and depth of infection, which, in turn, will help guide treatment planning. Usually, the preservation of mediastinalfat planes in CTA excludes surgical intervention. On the other hand, obliteration of mediastinalfat planes and diffuse soft tissue infiltration without or with gas collection, or low-density fluid collections within the mediastinum, are concerning for sternal infection. Recently published studies reported a 1-year mortality rate of approximately 22% (Loop et al., 1986; Sarr et al., 1984).

4.3.6. Pulmonary embolism

Clinical diagnosis of deep vein thrombosis and pulmonary embolism may be especially challenging because postoperative atelectasis, pleural effusion, or fluid overload may all contribute to the development of chest pain and dyspnea after CABG surgery. A recent report regarding pulmonary embolism in the post-CABG surgery population showed an overall prevalence of 23% for deep vein thrombosis by 1 week after surgery, with less than 2% of these cases identified clinically (Shammas, 2000).

4.3.7. Incidental findings

Although the intent of CTA after CABG surgery is to assess bypass graft patency and surgical complications, incidental findings are also frequently detected. In a recent study, 13.1% of patients in the immediate postoperative period had unsuspected noncardiac findings, including pulmonary embolism, pulmonary nodules, pneumonia, mucous plugging, and pneumothorax. (Mueller et al., 2007) Therefore, radiologists need to be aware of clinically significant findings with possible life-threatening consequences. 5. Conclusions

Despite image-degrading effects caused by the metallic scaffold of the stent, recent experience with the current generation of 64-section scanners suggests improved assessability of the in-stent lumen with the capability to appreciate more subtle degrees of in-stent neointimal hyperplasia. Knowledge of the different types of artifacts and how they can be compensated for with dedicated postprocessing and appropriate image views and window settings is a prerequisite for reliable depiction of the in-stent lumen and leads to a more robust application of CT findings. In future, the development of biodegradable stents may create optimal conditions for noninvasive post-implantation follow-up with MDCT. In recent years, MDCT with retrospective ECG gating has gained rapid acceptance as a diagnostic cardiac imaging modality, allowing assessment of coronary bypass graft patency with high spatial resolution. This tool could play an important role in patients with recurrence of chest pain or with unclear stress test results after myocardial revascularization surgery. Therefore, it is crucial that cardiologists and radiologists understand CABG anatomy with knowledge of the type and number of bypass grafts used during myocardial revascularization surgery.

Author details

Bong Gun Song

Cardiovascular Imaging Center, Cardiac and Vascular Center, Konkuk University Medical Center, Republic of Korea

References

[1] Achenbach, S.; Moshage, W.; Ropers, D.; Nossen, J. & Bachmann, K. (1997). Noninvasive, three-dimensional visualization of coronary artery bypass grafts by electron beam tomography. *American Journal of Cardiology,* Vol.79, No.7, (Apr 1 1997), pp. 856-861, ISSN 0002-9149

[2] Alexopoulos D.; Xanthopoulou I. (2011). Coronary stent fracture: how frequent it is? Does it matter? *Hellenic J Cardiol*, Vol.52, No.1, pp. 1-5, ISSN 1109-9666

[3] Anders, K.; Baum, U.; Schmid, M.; Ropers, D.; Schmid, A.; Pohle, K.; Daniel, W. G.; Bautz, W. & Achenbach, S. (2006). Coronary artery bypass graft (CABG) patency: assessment with high-resolution submillimeter 16-slice multidetector-row computed tomography (MDCT) versus coronary angiography. *European Journal of Radiology*, Vol.57, No.3, (Mar 2006), pp. 336-344, ISSN 0720-048X

[4] Bourassa, M. G.; Fisher, L. D.; Campeau, L.; Gillespie, M. J.; McConney, M. & Lesperance, J. (1985). Long-term fate of bypass grafts: the Coronary Artery Surgery Study (CASS) and Montreal Heart Institute experiences. *Circulation*, Vol.72, No.6 Pt 2, (Dec 1985), pp. V71-78, ISSN 0009-7322

[5] Buche, M.; Schoevaerdts, J. C.; Louagie, Y.; Schroeder, E.; Marchandise, B.; Chenu, P.; Dion, R.; Verhelst, R.; Deloos, M.; Gonzales, E. & et al. (1992). Use of the inferior epigastric artery for coronary bypass. *Journal of Thoracic and Cardiovascular Surgery,* Vol. 103, No.4, (Apr 1992), pp. 665-670, ISSN 0022-5223

[6] Campeau, L.; Enjalbert, M.; Lesperance, J.; Vaislic, C.; Grondin, C. M. & Bourassa, M. G. (1983). Atherosclerosis and late closure of aortocoronary saphenous vein grafts: sequential angiographic studies at 2 weeks, 1 year, 5 to 7 years, and 10 to 12 years after surgery. *Circulation,* Vol.68, No.3 Pt 2, (Sep 1983), pp. II1-7, ISSN 0009-7322

[7] Carpentier, A.; Guermonprez, J. L.; Deloche, A.; Frechette, C. & DuBost, C. (1973). The aorta-to-coronary radial artery bypass graft. A technique avoiding pathological

changes in grafts. *Annals of Thoracic Surgery*, Vol.16, No.2, (Aug 1973), pp. 111-121, ISSN 0003-4975

[8] Carrel, T. P.; Eckstein, F. S.; Englberger, L.; Windecker, S. & Meier, B. (2003). Pitfalls and key lessons with the symmetry proximal anastomotic device in coronary artery bypass surgery. *Annals of Thoracic Surgery*, Vol.75, No.5, (May 2003), pp. 1434-1436, ISSN 0003-4975

[9] Chiurlia E.; Menozzi M.; Ratti C.; Romagnoli R.; Modena MG. (2005). Follow-up of coronary artery bypass graft patency by multislice computed tomography. *Am J Cardiol*, Vol.95, No.9, pp 1094-1097, ISSN 0002-9149

[10] Dikkers, R.; Willems, T. P.; Tio, R. A.; Anthonio, R. L.; Zijlstra, F. & Oudkerk, M. (2007). The benefit of 64-MDCT prior to invasive coronary angiography in symptomatic post-CABG patients. *International Journal of Cardiovascular Imaging*, Vol.23, No. 3, (Jun 2007), pp. 369-377, ISSN 1569-5794

[11] Dubois, C. L. & Vandervoort, P. M. (2001). Aneurysms and pseudoaneurysms of coronary arteries and saphenous vein coronary artery bypass grafts: a case report and literature review. Acta Cardiologica, Vol.56, No.4, (Aug 2001), pp. 263-267, ISSN 0001-5385

[12] Engelmann, M. G.; von Smekal, A.; Knez, A.; Kurzinger, E.; Huehns, T. Y.; Hofling, B. & Reiser, M. (1997). Accuracy of spiral computed tomography for identifying arterial and venous coronary graft patency. *American Journal of Cardiology*, Vol.80, No.5, (Sep 1 1997), pp. 569-574, ISSN 0002-9149

[13] Fitzgibbon, G. M.; Kafka, H. P.; Leach, A. J.; Keon, W. J.; Hooper, G. D. & Burton, J. R. (1996). Coronary bypass graft fate and patient outcome: angiographic follow-up of 5,065 grafts related to survival and reoperation in 1,388 patients during 25 years. *Journal of the American College of Cardiology*, Vol.28, No.3, (Sep 1996), pp. 616-626, ISSN 0735-1097

[14] Frazier, A. A.; Qureshi, F.; Read, K. M.; Gilkeson, R. C.; Poston, R. S. & White, C. S. (2005). Coronary artery bypass grafts: assessment with multidetector CT in the early and late postoperative settings. *Radiographics*, Vol.25, No.4, (Jul-Aug 2005), pp. 881-896, ISSN 1527-1323

[15] Fullerton, D. A.; St Cyr, J. A.; Fall, S. M. & Whitman, G. J. (1994). Protection of the patent internal mammary artery by-pass graft from subsequent sternotomy. *Journal of Cardiovascular Surgery*, Vol.35, No.6, (Dec), pp. 499-501, ISSN 0021-9509

[16] Gilkeson, R. C.; Markowitz, A. H. & Ciancibello, L. (2003). Multisection CT evaluation of the reoperative cardiac surgery patient. *Radiographics*, Vol.23 Spec No, (Oct 2003), pp. S3-17, ISSN 1527-1323

[17] Gillinov, A. M.; Casselman, F. P.; Lytle, B. W.; Blackstone, E. H.; Parsons, E. M.; Loop, F. D. & Cosgrove, D. M., 3rd (1999). Injury to a patent left internal thoracic artery

graft at coronary reoperation. *Annals of Thoracic Surgery*, Vol.67, No.2, (Feb 1999), pp. 382-386, ISSN 0003-4975

[18] Gilard M, Cornily JC, Pennec PY, Le Gal G, Nonent M, Mansourati J, Blanc JJ, Boschat J. (2006). Assessment of coronary artery stents by 16 slice computed tomography. *Heart*, Vol.92, No.1, (Jan 2006), pp.58-61, ISSN 1468-201X

[19] Hecht, H. S. & Roubin, G. (2007). Usefulness of computed tomographic angiography guided percutaneous coronary intervention. *American Journal of Cardiology*, Vol.99, No.6, (Mar 15 2007), pp. 871-875, ISSN 0002-9149

[20] Hurlbut, D.; Myers, M. L.; Lefcoe, M. & Goldbach, M. (1990). Pleuropulmonary morbidity: internal thoracic artery versus saphenous vein graft. *Annals of Thoracic Surgery*, Vol.50, No.6, (Dec 1990), pp. 959-964, ISSN 0003-4975

[21] Katara, A. N.; Samra, S. S. & Bhandarkar, D. S. (2003). Thoracoscopic window for a post-coronary artery bypass grafting pericardial effusion. *Indian Heart Journal*, Vol.55, No.2, (Mar-Apr 2003), pp. 180-181, ISSN 0019-4832

[22] Kitagawa T.; Fujii T.; Tomohiro Y.; Maeda K.; Kobayashi M.; Kunita E.; Sekiguchi Y. (2006). Noninvasive assessment of coronary stents in patients by 16-slice computed tomography. *Int J Cardiol*, Vol.109, No.2, (Jul 2005), pp. 188-194, ISSN 0167-5273

[23] Kuvin, J. T.; Harati, N. A.; Pandian, N. G.; Bojar, R. M. & Khabbaz, K. R. (2002). Postoperative cardiac tamponade in the modern surgical era. *Annals of Thoracic Surgery*, Vol.74, No.4, (Oct 2002), pp. 1148-1153, ISSN 0003-4975

[24] Lee, R.; Lim, J.; Kaw, G.; Wan, G.; Ng, K. & Ho, K. T. (2010). Comprehensive noninvasive evaluation of bypass grafts and native coronary arteries in patients after coronary bypass surgery: accuracy of 64-slice multidetector computed tomography compared to invasive coronary angiography. *Journal of Cardiovascular Medicine (Hagerstown)*, Vol.11, No.2, (Feb 2010), pp. 81-90, ISSN 1558-2035

[25] Leipsic J.; Labounty TM.; Heilbron B.; Min JK.; Mancini GB.; Lin FY.; Taylor C.; Dunning A.; Earls JP. (2010). Adaptive statistical iterative reconstruction: assessment of image noise and image quality in coronary CT angiography. *AJR Am J Roentgenol*, Vol.195, No.3, pp. 649-54, ISSN 1546-3141

[26] Li, A. E. & Fishman, E. K. (2003). Evaluation of complications after sternotomy using single- and multidetector CT with three-dimensional volume rendering. *AJR. American Journal of Roentgenology*, Vol.181, No.4, (Oct 2003), pp. 1065-1070, ISSN 0361-803X

[27] Lim HB.; Hur G.; Kim SY.; Kim YH.; Kwon SU.; Lee WR.; Cha SJ. (2008). Coronary stent fracture: detection with 64-section multidetector CT angiography in patients and in vitro. Radiology, Vol.249, No.3, pp. 810-819, ISSN 1527-1323

[28] Locker, C.; Mohr, R.; Paz, Y.; Lev-Ran, O.; Herz, I.; Uretzky, G. & Shapira, I. (2002). Pretreatment with alpha-adrenergic blockers for prevention of radial artery spasm. *Annals of Thoracic Surgery*, Vol.74, No.4, (Oct 2002), pp. S1368-1370, ISSN 0003-4975

[29] Loop, F. D.; Lytle, B. W.; Cosgrove, D. M.; Stewart, R. W.; Goormastic, M.; Williams, G. W.; Golding, L. A.; Gill, C. C.; Taylor, P. C.; Sheldon, W. C. & et al. (1986). Influence of the internal-mammary-artery graft on 10-year survival and other cardiac events. *New England Journal of Medicine*, Vol.314, No.1, (Jan 1986), pp. 1-6, ISSN 0028-4793

[30] Mack, M. J.; Emery, R. W.; Ley, L. R.; Cole, P. A.; Leonard, A.; Edgerton, J. R.; Dewey, T. M.; Magee, M. J. & Flavin, T. S. (2003). Initial experience with proximal anastomoses performed with a mechanical connector. *Annals of Thoracic Surgery*, Vol.75, No.6, (Jun 2003), pp. 1866-1870; discussion 1870-1871, ISSN 0003-4975

[31] Mahnken AH.; Mühlenbruch G.; Seyfarth T.; Flohr T.; Stanzel S.; Wildberger JE.; Günther RW.; Kuettner A. (2006). 64-slice computed tomography assessment of coronary artery stents: a phantom study. *Acta Radiol*, Vol. 47, No.1, pp. 36-42, ISSN 0284-1851

[32] Maintz D.; Burg MC.; Seifarth H.; Bunck AC.; Ozgün M.; Fischbach R.; Jürgens KU.; Heindel W. (2009). Update on multidetector coronary CT angiography of coronary stents: in vitro evaluation of 29 different stent types with dual-source CT. *Eur Radiol*, Vol.19, No.1, pp. 42-49, ISSN 1432-1084

[33] Maintz D.; Seifarth H.; Flohr T.; Krämer S.; Wichter T.; Heindel W.; Fischbach R. (2003). Improved coronary artery stent visualization and in-stent stenosis detection using 16-slice computed-tomography and dedicated image reconstruction technique. *Invest Radiol*, Vol.38, No.12, pp.790-795, ISSN 0020-9996

[34] Manapat, A. E.; McCarthy, P. M.; Lytle, B. W.; Taylor, P. C.; Loop, F. D.; Stewart, R. W.; Rosenkranz, E. R.; Sapp, S. K.; Miller, D. & Cosgrove, D. M. (1994). Gastroepiploic and inferior epigastric arteries for coronary artery bypass. Early results and evolving applications. *Circulation*, Vol.90, No.5 Pt 2, (Nov 1994), pp. II144-147, ISSN 0009-7322

[35] Marano, R.; Storto, M. L.; Maddestra, N. & Bonomo, L. (2004). Non-invasive assessment of coronary artery bypass graft with retrospectively ECG-gated four-row multidetector spiral computed tomography. *European Radiology*, Vol.14, No.8, (Aug 2004), pp. 1353-1362, ISSN 0938-7994

[36] Marano, R.; Storto, M. L.; Merlino, B.; Maddestra, N.; Di Giammarco, G. & Bonomo, L. (2005). A pictorial review of coronary artery bypass grafts at multidetector row CT. *Chest*, Vol.127, No.4, (Apr 2005), pp. 1371-1377, ISSN 0012-3692

[37] Memon, A. Q.; Huang, R. I.; Marcus, F.; Xavier, L. & Alpert, J. (2003). Saphenous vein graft aneurysm: case report and review. *Cardiology in Review*, Vol.11, No.1, (Jan-Feb 2003), pp. 26-34, ISSN 1061-5377

[38] Meurin, P.; Weber, H.; Renaud, N.; Larrazet, F.; Tabet, J. Y.; Demolis, P. & Ben Driss, A. (2004). Evolution of the postoperative pericardial effusion after day 15: the problem of the late tamponade. *Chest*, Vol.125, No.6, (Jun 2004), pp. 2182-2187, ISSN 0012-3692

[39] Min JK.; Swaminathan RV.; Vass M.; Gallagher S.; Weinsaft JW. (2009). High-definition multidetector computed tomography for evaluation of coronary artery stents: comparison to standard-definition 64-detector row computed tomography. *J Cardiovasc Comput Tomogr*, Vol.3, No.4, (Jul-Aug 2009), pp. 246-251, ISSN 1876-861X

[40] Mohara, J.; Konishi, H.; Kato, M.; Misawa, Y.; Kamisawa, O. & Fuse, K. (1998). Saphenous vein graft pseudoaneurysm rupture after coronary artery bypass grafting. *Annals of Thoracic Surgery*, Vol.65, No.3, (Mar 1998), pp. 831-832, ISSN 0003-4975

[41] Motwani, J. G. & Topol, E. J. (1998). Aortocoronary saphenous vein graft disease: pathogenesis, predisposition, and prevention. *Circulation*, Vol.97, No.9, (Mar 10 1998), pp. 916-931, ISSN 0009-7322

[42] Mueller, J.; Jeudy, J.; Poston, R. & White, C. S. (2007). Cardiac CT angiography after coronary bypass surgery: prevalence of incidental findings. *AJR. American Journal of Roentgenology*, Vol.189, No.2, (Aug 2007), pp. 414-419, ISSN 1546-3141

[43] Muneretto, C.; Bisleri, G.; Negri, A.; Manfredi, J.; Metra, M.; Nodari, S.; Culot, L. & Dei Cas, L. (2003). Total arterial myocardial revascularization with composite grafts improves results of coronary surgery in elderly: a prospective randomized comparison with conventional coronary artery bypass surgery. *Circulation*, Vol.108 Suppl 1, (Sep 2003), pp. II29-33, ISSN 1524-4539

[44] Myers, M. G. & Fremes, S. E. (2003). Prevention of radial artery graft spasm: a survey of Canadian surgical centres. *Canadian Journal of Cardiology*, Vol.19, No.6, (May 2003), pp. 677-681, ISSN 0828-282X

[45] Nakazawa G.; Finn AV.; Vorpahl M.; Ladich E.; Kutys R.; Balazs I.; Kolodgie FD.; Virmani R. (2009). Incidence and predictors of drug-eluting stent fracture in human coronary artery a pathologic analysis. *J Am Coll Cardiol*, Vol.54, No.21, (Nov 2009), pp.1924-1931, ISSN 1558-3597

[46] Nieman K.; Pattynama PM.; Rensing BJ.; Van Geuns RJ.; De Feyter PJ. (2003). Evaluation of patients after coronary artery bypass surgery: CT angiographic assessment of grafts and coronary arteries. *Radiology*, Vol.229, No.3, (Dec 2003), pp.749-756, ISSN 0033-8419

[47] Ohtsuka, T.; Akahane, M.; Ohtomo, K.; Kotsuka, Y. & Takamoto, S. (2000). Three-dimensional computed tomography for reoperative minimally invasive coronary artery bypass. *Annals of Thoracic Surgery*, Vol.70, No.5, (Nov 2000), pp. 1734-1735, ISSN 0003-4975

[48] Pang JH.; Kim D.; Beohar N.; Meyers SN.; Lloyd-Jones D.; Yaghmai V. (2009). Detection of stent fractures: a comparison of 64-slice CT, conventional cine-angiography, and intravascular ultrasonography. *Acad Radiol*, Vol.16, No.4, (Apr 2009), pp.412-417, ISSN 1878-4046

[49] Peng, M. J.; Vargas, F. S.; Cukier, A.; Terra-Filho, M.; Teixeira, L. R. & Light, R. W. (1992). Postoperative pleural changes after coronary revascularization. Comparison

between saphenous vein and internal mammary artery grafting. *Chest,* Vol.101, No.2, (Feb 1992), pp. 327-330, ISSN 0012-3692

[50] Pepi, M.; Muratori, M.; Barbier, P.; Doria, E.; Arena, V.; Berti, M.; Celeste, F.; Guazzi, M. & Tamborini, G. (1994). Pericardial effusion after cardiac surgery: incidence, site, size, and haemodynamic consequences. *British Heart Journal,* Vol.72, No.4, (Oct 1994), pp. 327-331, ISSN 0007-0769

[51] Possati, G.; Gaudino, M.; Prati, F.; Alessandrini, F.; Trani, C.; Glieca, F.; Mazzari, M. A.; Luciani, N. & Schiavoni, G. (2003). Long-term results of the radial artery used for myocardial revascularization. *Circulation,* Vol.108, No.11, (Sep 2003), pp. 1350-1354, ISSN 1524-4539

[52] Poston, R.; White, C.; Read, K.; Gu, J.; Lee, A.; Avari, T. & Griffith, B. (2004). Virchow triad, but not use of an aortic connector device, predicts early graft failure after off-pump coronary bypass. *Heart Surg Forum,* Vol.7, No.5, pp. E428-433, ISSN 1522-6662

[53] Pugliese F.; Cademartiri F.; van Mieghem C.; Meijboom WB.; Malagutti P.; Mollet NR.; Martinoli C.; de Feyter PJ.; Krestin GP. (2006). Multidetector CT for visualization of coronary stents. *Radiographics*, Vol.26, No.3, (May-Jun 2006), pp.887-904,

[54] Pym, J.; Brown, P. M.; Charrette, E. J.; Parker, J. O. & West, R. O. (1987). Gastroepiploic-coronary anastomosis. A viable alternative bypass graft. *Journal of Thoracic and Cardiovascular Surgery,* Vol.94, No.2, (Aug 1987), pp. 256-259, ISSN 0022-5223

[55] Rajiah P.; Schoenhagen P.; Mehta D.; Ivanc T.; Lieber M.; Soufan K.; Desai M.; Flamm SD.; Halliburton S. (2012). Low-dose, wide-detector array thoracic aortic CT angiography using an iterative reconstruction technique results in improved image quality with lower noise and fewer artifacts. *J Cardiovasc Comput Tomogr,* Vol.6, No.3, (May 2012), pp.205-213, ISSN 1876-861X

[56] Ricci, M.; Karamanoukian, H. L.; D'Ancona, G.; Salerno, T. A. & Bergsland, J. (2000). Reoperative "off-pump" circumflex revascularization via left thoracotomy: how to prevent graft kinking. *Annals of Thoracic Surgery,* Vol.70, No.1, (Jul 2000), pp. 309-310, ISSN 0003-4975

[57] Ropers, D.; Pohle, F. K.; Kuettner, A.; Pflederer, T.; Anders, K.; Daniel, W. G.; Bautz, W.; Baum, U. & Achenbach, S. (2006). Diagnostic accuracy of noninvasive coronary angiography in patients after bypass surgery using 64-slice spiral computed tomography with 330-ms gantry rotation. *Circulation,* Vol.114, No.22, (Nov 2006), pp. 2334-2341; quiz 2334, ISSN 1524-4539

[58] Ropers, D.; Ulzheimer, S.; Wenkel, E.; Baum, U.; Giesler, T.; Derlien, H.; Moshage, W.; Bautz, W. A.; Daniel, W. G.; Kalender, W. A. & Achenbach, S. (2001). Investigation of aortocoronary artery bypass grafts by multislice spiral computed tomography with electrocardiographic-gated image reconstruction. *American Journal of Cardiology,* Vol.88, No.7, (Oct 2001), pp. 792-795, ISSN 0002-9149

[59] Roy, M. C. (1998). Surgical-site infections after coronary artery bypass graft surgery: discriminating site-specific risk factors to improve prevention efforts. *Infection Control and Hospital Epidemiology*, Vol.19, No.4, (Apr 1998), pp. 229-233, ISSN 0899-823X

[60] Sarr, M. G.; Gott, V. L. & Townsend, T. R. (1984). Mediastinal infection after cardiac surgery. *Annals of Thoracic Surgery*, Vol.38, No.4, (Oct 1984), pp. 415-423, ISSN 0003-4975

[61] Schlosser, T.; Konorza, T.; Hunold, P.; Kuhl, H.; Schmermund, A. & Barkhausen, J. (2004). Noninvasive visualization of coronary artery bypass grafts using 16-detector row computed tomography. *Journal of the American College of Cardiology*, Vol.44, No.6, (Sep 2004), pp. 1224-1229, ISSN 0735-1097

[62] Seifarth, H.; Raupach, R.; Schaller, S.; Fallenberg, E. M.; Flohr, T.; Heindel, W.; Fischbach, R. & Maintz, D. (2005). Assessment of coronary artery stents using 16-slice MDCT angiography: evaluation of a dedicated reconstruction kernel and a noise reduction filter. *European Radiology*, Vol.15, No.4, (Apr 2005), pp. 721-726, ISSN 0938-7994

[63] Seifarth H.; Ozgün M.; Raupach R.; Flohr T.; Heindel W.; Fischbach R.; Maintz D. (2006). 64- Versus 16-slice CT angiography for coronary artery stent assessment: in vitro experience. *Invest Radiol*, Vol.41, No.1, (Jan 2006), pp.22-27, ISSN 0020-9996

[64] Shammas, N. W. (2000). Pulmonary embolus after coronary artery bypass surgery: a review of the literature. *Clinical Cardiology*, Vol.23, No.9, (Sep 2000), pp. 637-644, ISSN 0160-9289

[65] Song, B. G.; Choi, J. H.; Choi, S. M.; Park, J. H.; Park, Y. H. & Choe, Y. H. (2010). Coronary artery graft dilatation aided by multidetector computed tomography. *Asian Cardiovascular and Thoracic Annals*, Vol.18, No.2, (Feb 2010), pp. 177-179, ISSN 1816-5370

[66] Tochii, M.; Takagi, Y.; Anno, H.; Hoshino, R.; Akita, K.; Kondo, H. & Ando, M. (2010). Accuracy of 64-slice multidetector computed tomography for diseased coronary artery graft detection. *Annals of Thoracic Surgery*, Vol.89, No.6, (Jun 2010), pp. 1906-1911, ISSN 1552-6259

[67] Traverse, J. H.; Mooney, M. R.; Pedersen, W. R.; Madison, J. D.; Flavin, T. F.; Kshettry, V. R.; Henry, T. D.; Eales, F.; Joyce, L. D. & Emery, R. W. (2003). Clinical, angiographic, and interventional follow-up of patients with aortic-saphenous vein graft connectors. *Circulation*, Vol.108, No.4, (Jul 2003), pp. 452-456, ISSN 1524-4539

[68] Ueyama, K.; Ohashi, H.; Tsutsumi, Y.; Kawai, T.; Ueda, T. & Ohnaka, M. (1999). Evaluation of coronary artery bypass grafts using helical scan computed tomography. *Catheterization and Cardiovascular Interventions*, Vol.46, No.3, (Mar 1999), pp. 322-326, ISSN 1522-1946

[69] Vargas, F. S.; Cukier, A.; Hueb, W.; Teixeira, L. R. & Light, R. W. (1994). Relationship between pleural effusion and pericardial involvement after myocardial revascularization. *Chest*, Vol.105, No.6, (Jun 1994), pp. 1748-1752, ISSN 0012-3692

[70] Vembar, M.; Garcia, M. J.; Heuscher, D. J.; Haberl, R.; Matthews, D.; Bohme, G. E. & Greenberg, N. L. (2003). A dynamic approach to identifying desired physiological phases for cardiac imaging using multislice spiral CT. *Medical Physics*, Vol.30, No.7, (Jul 2003), pp. 1683-1693, ISSN 0094-2405

[71] Wiklund, L.; Bugge, M. & Berglin, E. (2002). Angiographic results after the use of a sutureless aortic connector for proximal vein graft anastomoses. *Annals of Thoracic Surgery*, Vol.73, No.6, (Jun 2002), pp. 1993-1994, ISSN 0003-4975

A Noninvasive Alternative to Coronary Angiography: Myocardial Contrast Echocardiography Following Strain Map as a Gate Way to Myocardial Contrast Echocardiography Map

Ri-ichiro Kakihara

Additional information is available at the end of the chapter

http://dx.doi.org/10.5772/45953

1. Introduction

[Background] Segmental left ventricular (LV) wall systolic dysfunction has been considered a significant sign of coronary artery disease (CAD) for many years. However, it is well known that many heart diseases besides CAD cause abnormal LV wall motion. Therefore, it is essential to verify that segmental LV wall systolic dysfunction is due to myocardial ischemia. Although coronary angiography is typically used to determine the clinical significance of CAD, it is also possible to visualize areas of ischemic myocardium noninvasively by echocardiography using microbubble contrast agents. Perfluorobutane microbubbles, consisting of a hydrogenated egg-phosphatidylserine shell encapsulating perfluorobutane gas, offers the advantage of resistance to destruction by ultrasound, thus enabling repeated scans per injection.

[Methods] We used phase-inversion harmonic ultrasonography to assess the ability of perfluorobutane microbubbles to detect ischemic myocardial areas due to coronary artery stenosis in 66 patients who had undergone coronary angiography (CAG). Abnormal LV wall motion was detected by longitudinal strain before CAG. Pre and post-injection images were evaluated from late-diastolic points along the time-intensity curve.

[Results] The injection of perfluorobutane microbubbles caused a significant change in intensity in the left ventricular wall in the AP and SAX views in segments perfused by normal coronary arteries ($p<0.0001$), but not in segments perfused by arteries with significant ($\geq$ 75%) stenosis. Receiver operating characteristic curve analysis showed that an intensity difference ≤ 6.3 dB in the AP view could detect ≥ 75% stenosis with a sensitivity of 98%, specificity of 94% and accuracy of 97%. An intensity difference ≤ 5.1 dB in the SAX view could detect ≥ 75% stenosis with a sensitivity of 97%, specificity of 96% and accuracy of 97%.

[Conclusions] These data indicate that when optimal signal intensity difference parameters have been accurately defined, perfluorobutane microbubbles can be used safely for highly sensitive, specific and accurate visualization of ischemic myocardial areas due to coronary artery stenosis.

2. Background

The ability to prevent, diagnosis and treat cardiac disease has improved over the last two decades due to the remarkable and seemingly exponential advances in imaging technology [1,2,3,4]. Ironically, the surprising increases in computing power and software design now at the physician's disposal have been greatly enhanced by the advent of a relatively uncomplicated and a readily-synthesized molecule, the microbubble. Perfluorobutane microbubbles consist of a macromolecular shell encapsulating a high molecular weight gas [5] and are typically 1 to 10 μ in diameter. Their small size allows them to be introduced safely into the circulatory system where they enhance ultrasonic wave scattering by blood, thereby providing higher contrast to ultrasound images of the left ventricular myocardial wall. Ultrascanners operating at frequencies < 15 MHz oscillate the microbubbles, which results in increased echo contrast. The vibrating microbubbles also emit harmonic signals that can preferentially enhance the signal-to-noise ratio. In addition to their diagnostic advantages, microbubbles also avoid the use of radiation and are generally more economical to use. Microbubble ultrasound technology has been used to image other organs besides the heart (liver, pancreas, breast and kidney, in particular), and can be used to target drug-delivery vehicles to different organs [6]. Basic biomedical researchers are also benefitting from microbubble reagents for delivering macromolecules, such as plasmid DNAs, into cells [7].

Two microbubble contrast agents for cardiac echocardiography, OPTISON™ and Definity™, are approved for use in the United States, SonoVue™ is approved in Europe and China, and Levovist in Japan. But OPTISON™ and Definity™ are used for opacification of the left ventricular cavity and endocardial border definition only. Levovist is used for myocardial contrast echocardiography (MCE). Safety problems occurred initially with each agent, but continuing clinical studies overwhelmingly indicated their efficacy and safety [8,9]. More recently, contrast-enhanced ultrasound (CEUS) has been found safe for pediatric use in subjects as young as two years old [10]. Furthermore, at the recent *16th European Symposium on Ultrasound Contrast Imaging in Rotterdam*, Porter (USA) presented highly compelling evidence that CEUS improved the prediction of patient outcomes when compared with nuclear imaging or non-contrast ultrasound. He also pointed out that contrast imaging avoids subjecting patients to the ionizing radiation inherent in nuclear techniques and suggested that there was significant underutilization of CEUS.

Because of these findings and our own clinical experience, we have persisted in our studies on perfluorobutane microbubbles for coronary artery disease. However, at the present time, this contrast agent has only been approved for hepatic diseases in Japan [11]. Here, we report our experience with the use of perfluorobutane microbubbles to perform MCE in 66 patients who had undergone coronary angiography. Our data showed that perfluorobutane microbubbles markedly and stably enhance visualization of ischemic myocardial areas due to significant coronary artery stenosis and provided superior images compared with Levovist™, but with the caveat that imaging parameters require careful optimization.

3. Materials and Methods

3.1. Patients

Sixty-six patients with a history of coronary angiography (CAG) within the last three months were enrolled in this study, and informed consent was obtained. The study was approved by the clinic's ethics committee. All procedures were performed in accordance with The Code of Ethics of the World Medical Association (Declaration of Helsinki) for experiments involving humans. The following aspects of the consent form were explained to the patients: 1) the advantages, benefits, risks and possible side effects of the procedure to them specifically as well as to patients with coronary artery disease in general, 2) the cost of the procedure according to the regulations of the National Health Service, 3) the approximate time of the procedure, and 4) the clinic staff and specialists that would be present during the procedure. In addition, the approval of the ethics committee required that the procedure be performed by a special team that included the following personnel: Dr. R. Kakihara since he was in charge of the study, the nurses and echocardiographers who had experience with MCE, at least one specialist in the use of Sonazoid™ from Daiichi Sankyo Co. Ltd, and a mechanical engineer and a technical specialist to operate the Vivid 7 Ultrasound System. All 24 patients enrolled had ≥ 75% significant coronary artery stenosis (significant stenosis). Among them, single vessel disease was present in 11 patients, double vessel disease in 9 and triple vessel disease in 4. No subject had a history of previous myocardial infarction. The following patient data were obtained: age, 69.9±11.4 y/o; body weight, 60.5±12.1 kg; body surface area, 1.61±4.3 m^2; blood pressure, 128.6±15.3/ 67.7±9.9 mmHg; heart rate, 65.3±9.0 beats/min; LVEF (by angiography), 60.5±4.3%; LDL-cholesterol, 125.6±38.1 mg/dl; and triglyceride, 193.1±134.1 mg/dl. Six patients were treated for diabetes mellitus by oral medication and their average HbA1c was 6.3±1.5%.

3.2. Instrumentation

Phase-inversion harmonic ultrasonography was performed using the Vivid 7 Dimension digital ultrasound system, Version 7.0.3 (General Electric Healthcare, Inc., U.S.A.), and a 1.5/4.0 MHz active-matrix array (AMA) probe. The images were analyzed offline using EchoPAC PC Version 108.1.4. Phase inversion harmonic sonography is two phase-inverted but otherwise identical sonographic pulses are transmitted. Summing the returning echoes in a buffer cancels most of the fundamental and odd harmonic echoes and effectively amplifies the second harmonic. [12]

3.3. The first step

A longitudinal peak systolic strain map (LPSSM) has high diagnostic reliability to detect segmental left ventricular wall abnormalities. [13,14] Thus, an LPSSM was created on any patient with coronary artery disease (CAD) risk factors. When the LPSSM showed abnormal left ventricular segmental wall systolic function, myocardial contrast echocardiography (MCE) was done using Sonazoid™ to confirm whether the dysfunction was due to myocardial ischemia.

3.4. The second step

Materials: Sonazoid™ was obtained from Daiichi Sankyo Co. Ltd. (Tokyo, Japan).

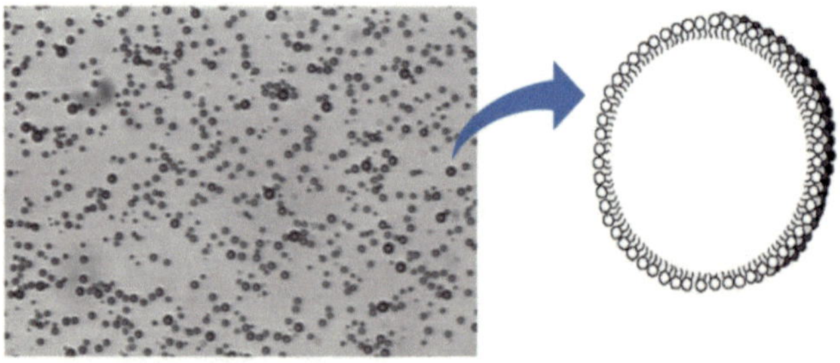

Figure 1. Magnified reconstituted Sonazoid solution. A macromolecular shell is encapsulated by a high molecular weight gas. The microbubbles are very weak and are destroyed easily by usual physical pressure and MI (mechanical index). Sonazoid reconstituted in saline for injection of 2.5mL: Volume concentration: 6.9μL MB/mL Particle size: 2.3~2.9μm (median diameter) Involving gas: Perflubutane (C_4F_{10}) Membrane element: Hydrogenated egg phosphatidyl serine (sodium) pH: 5.7~7.0 Osmotic pressure ratio: 0.9~1.1

Any remaining Sonazoid should be stored at room temperature and used within 2 hours.

Because Sonazoid™ microbubbles are susceptible to destruction by physical pressure, 2.5 ml were injected over at least 20 sec, not less than the systemic circulation time under the stress of low dose ATP (0.15 mg/kg/min of Adenosine 5- Triphosphate Disodium) Figure 1, Figure 2, Figure 3, Figure 4.

Measurements: The echocardiographer was blinded to the results of CAG in the patients enrolled. Three apex approach (AP) views and one parasternal short axis (SAX) view were recorded per injection. The instrument settings were as follows: mechanical index (MI), 0.4-0.6 for the AP and 0.22 for the SAX views; frame rate, 21.2; and frequency, 1.5/3.0 MHz. These were selected based on the recommendations of the specialist from Daiichi Sankyo Co. Ltd who had experience with liver imaging. The MI was very low so as not to destroy the microbubbles but high enough to vibrate them. This vibration energy is necessary to create ultrasonic cardiac images. The images taken were clear and of sufficient quality to be analyzed at

http://dx.doi.org/10.5772/45953

these settings. The images were acquired from the time-intensity curve in late diastole just before the P wave. Intensity differences before and after Sonazoid™ injection were measured at the same site. The intensity data were automatically shown on the upper right part of the screen. We examined 3 AP views (APLAX: mid-anterior septum & mid-posterior segment; AP2ch: mid-anterior and mid-inferior segment; AP4ch: mid lateral and mid-septal segments) and mid-papillary muscle level SAX views (mid-anterior, mid-lateral, mid-posterior, mid-inferior, mid-septal a mid-anterior septal segments). The segments in the 3 AP views that were perfused by coronary arteries with significant stenosis were designated as Group A and the segments in the SAX views were designated as Group B. The segments in the AP views that were perfused by normal or coronary arteries without significant stenosis were designated as Group C and the segments in the SAX views were designated as Group D. We compared the intensities of all four groups before and after Sonazoidinjection using a paired t-test.

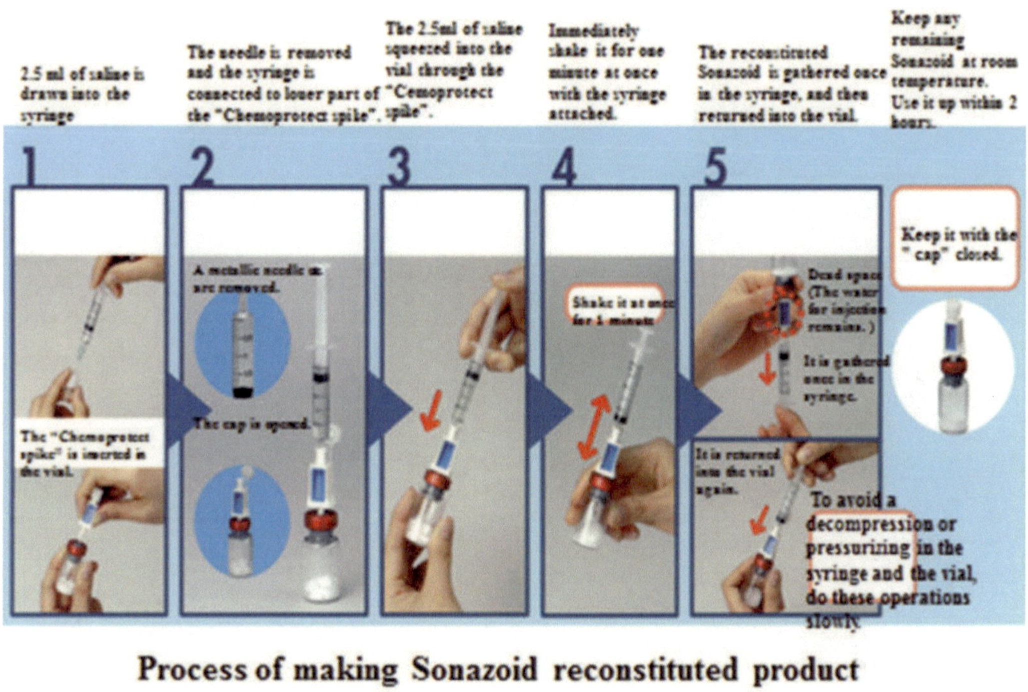

Figure 2. Process of making the Sonazoid reconstituted product. The "Chemoprotect spike" is inserted in the vial to keep the pressure in the vial unchanged. Then, 2.5 ml of saline is drawn into the syringe. Then the needle is removed and the syringe is connected to the luer part of the "Chemoprotect spike".Then, 2.5 ml of saline is squeezed into the vial through the "Chemoprotect spike". The solution is shaken for one minute with the syringe attached. The reconstituted Sonazoid is gathered once in the syringe, and then returned into the vial. To avoid decompression or pressurization in the syringe and vial, these procedures should be performed slowly.

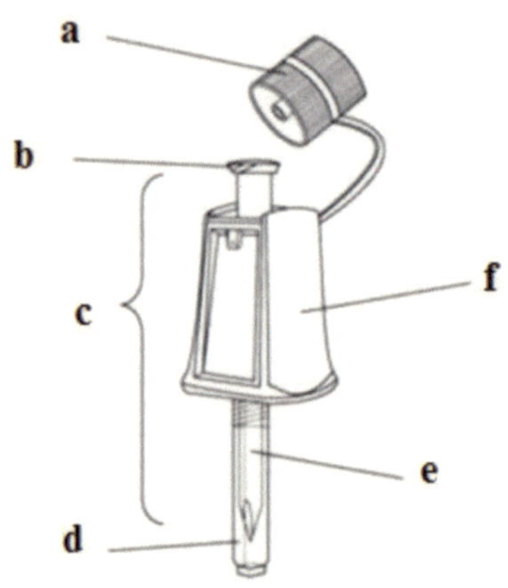

Figure 3. Chemoprotect Spike. This reconstituted Sonazoid production adjustment device consists of a main body, a luer portion, filter housing, spike part, built in liquid filter for drug solution filtration, and an air filter for ventilation. a : Cap, b : Luer portion, c : Spike (Main body), d : Protective cap, e : Protective cap, f : Filter housing, Fluid filter, Air filter

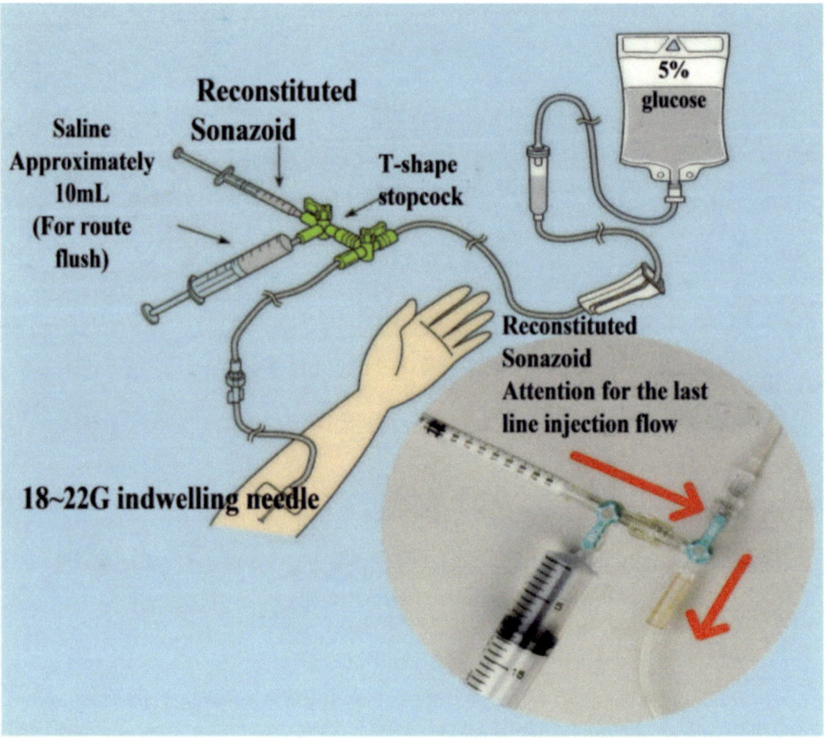

Figure 4. Method and route of injection of reconstituted Sonazoid. Sonazoid (2.5 ml) was injected slowly over 20 seconds. After finishing the injection of Sonazoid, saline (approximately 10 ml) was injected to flush the delivery route

http://dx.doi.org/10.5772/45953

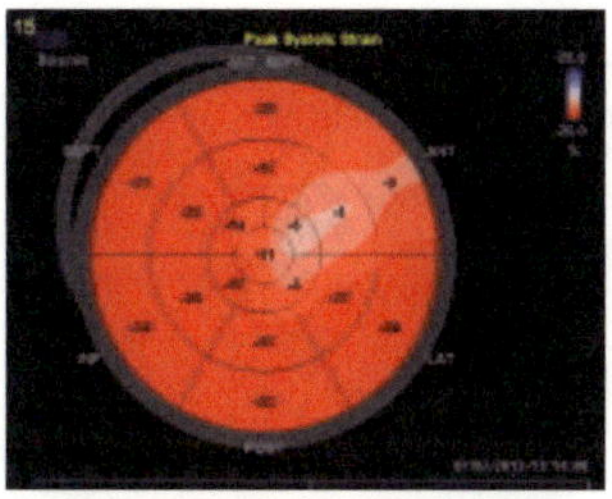

Figure 5. Longitudinal peak systolic strain map. This shows abnormal LV wall motion area, does not show ischemic area. Therefore coronary artery disease is not diagnosis by this map.

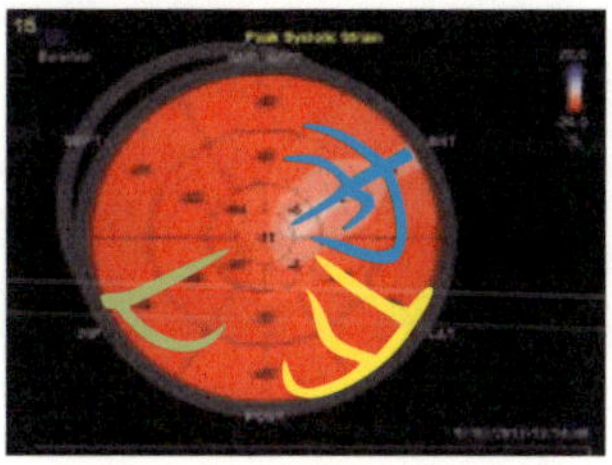

Figure 6. The picture of coronary arteries is superimposed on the strain map. By this method the relation between coronary arteries and the area of abnormal LV wall motion is confirmed.

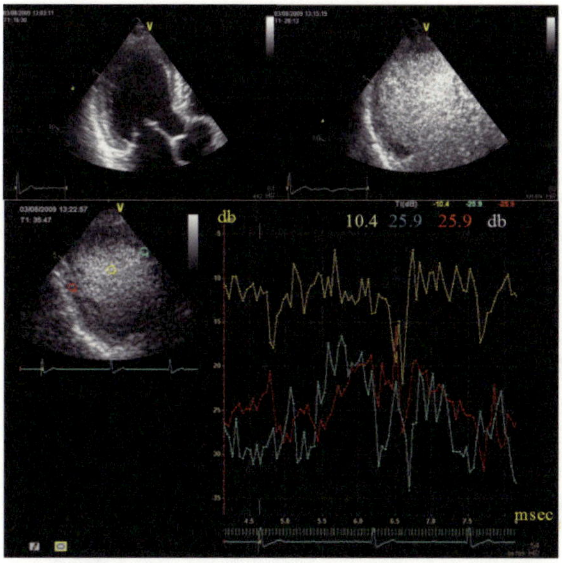

Figure 7. Sonazoid myocardial contrast echocardiography, APLAX views. The patient #7 (see Figure 3 for CAG images) was examined before and after Sonazoid injection. The instrument was set to MI = 0.4. APLAX views before (A) and after (B) Sonazoid. Intensity curves (C). Yellow, LV cavity; red, posterior wall (LCX area); and blue, interventricular septum (LAD #6 area)

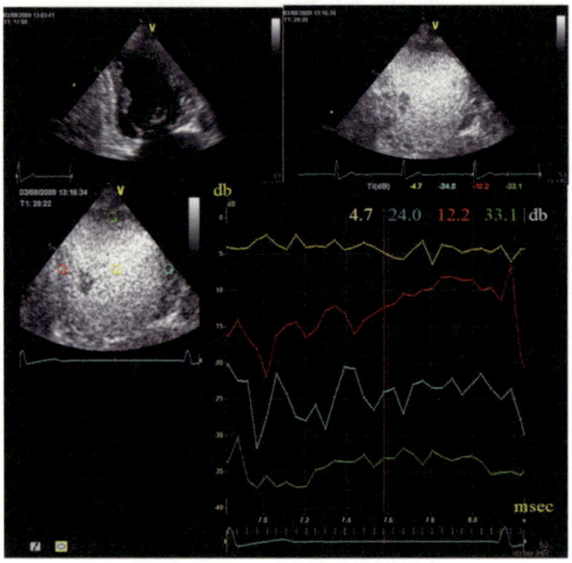

Figure 8. Sonazoid myocardial contrast echocardiography, AP 2-chamber views. The instrument was set to MI = 0.4. AP 2-chamber views before (A) and after (B) Sonazoid injection. Time-intensity curves (C). Yellow, LV cavity; red, inferior wall (RCA area); and blue, anterior wall (LAD area).

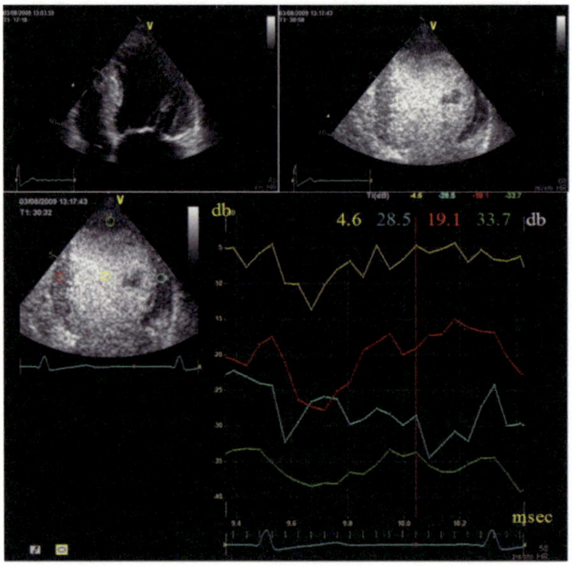

Figure 9. Sonazoid myocardial contrast echocardiography, AP-4 chamber views. The instrument was set to MI = 0.4. AP 4 chamber views before (A) and after (B) Sonazoid injection. Time-intensity curves (C). Yellow, LV cavity; red, interventricular septum (LAD #6 area); blue, lateral wall and apex (LAD #7 area).

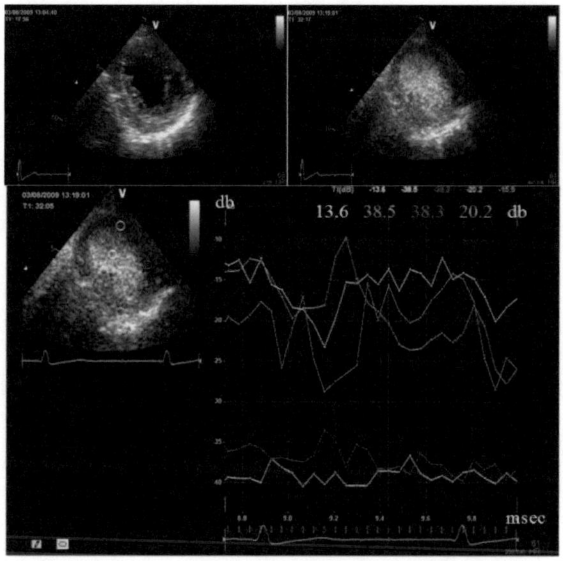

Figure 10. Sonazoid myocardial contrast echocardiography, SAX- pm views. The instrument was set to MI = 0.22. SAXpm views before (A) and after (B, C) Sonzaoid injection. Time-intensity curves (D). Yellow, LV cavity; blue, anterior wall; red, lateral wall (both are LAD #7 area); orange, posterior wall; green, inferior wall.

None of the patients experienced adverse affects of this procedure. Each of the 66 patients enrolled in the study had undergone CAG and was diagnosed with significant coronary artery stenosis. Patients were divided into four groups as described above, and myocardial segments perfused by the stenotic and normal vasculatures were examined by ultrasonography before and after Sonazoid administration. The data for one patient (#7) are presented in Figures 5 through Figure 10. Ultrasound images taken before and after Sonazoid administration are shown in 6 Figures, which represent the strain maps and APLAX, AP2ch, AP4ch and SAX-papillary muscle (pm) views, respectively. Figure 5 and Figure 6 show the longitudinal peak systolic strain map and Figure 6 which is superimposed coronary arteries on the map strongly implys this patient experienced no adverse affect and had LAD single vessel disease. Figure 11 shows an angiogram of the left and right coronary arteries. In the left panel, the angiogram (left coronary artery) clearly reveals left anterior descending coronary artery stenosis obstructing 75% of the vessel's normal diameter. Stenotic regions are indicated by the arrows.In contrast, no involvement of the right coronary artery could be discerned.

The data from 100 myocardial segments (16 patients) perfused by normal coronary arteries and from 283 myocardial segments (50 patients) perfused by stenotic coronary arteries in 66 patients with coronary artery disease were grouped into A, B, C and D as designated above and are summarized in Tables 1 and Table 2. Specifically, the intensity difference between A-pre-injection (A-pre) and A–post-injection (A-post) was 1.3 ± 3.5 dB; the intensity difference between B-pre and B-post was 0.9 ± 3.3 dB. The intensity differences in groups A and B were not significant. For C-pre and C-post, the intensities were -33.4 ± 5.1 dB and -22.3 ± 6.8

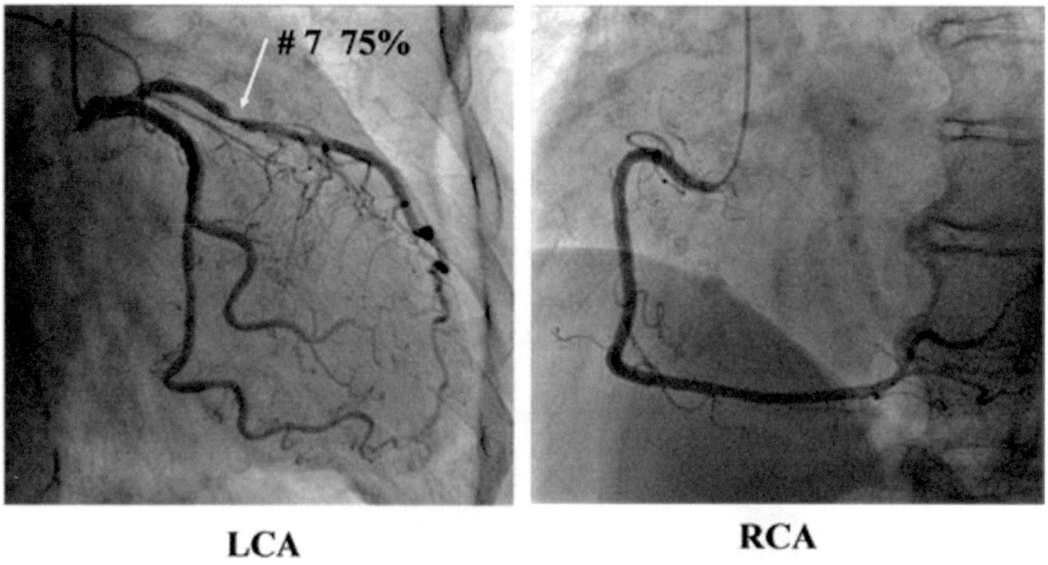

Figure 11. Coronary artery angiography. Left: left coronary artery. Left anterior descending artery had 75% stenosis at #7. Right: Right coronary artery was normal.

dB, respectively; and D-pre and D-post were -36.2 ± 4.8 dB and -22.6 ± 10.7 dB, respectively. The intensity differences in groups C (14.1 ± 5.8 dB) and D (11.5 ± 4.3 dB) were both significant (p < 0.001). By ROC (receiver operating characteristic curve) analysis, intensity differences ≤ 6.3 dB in the AP views could detect ≥ 75% stenosis with a sensitivity of 98%, specificity of 94% and accuracy of 97%. An intensity difference ≤ 5.1 dB in the SAX view could detect ≥ 75% stenosis with a sensitivity of 97%, specificity of 96% and accuracy of 97%. These data indicate the sensitivity, specificity and diagnostic accuracy of MCE using Sonazoid to detect ≥ 75% stenosis.

Stenotic Groups	
Group/View	Intensity difference
A/AP	1.3 ± 3.5 dB (N.S.)
B/SAX	0.9 ± 3.3 dB (N.S)
Normal Groups	
Group/View	Intensity difference
C/AP	14.1 ± 5.8 dB (*P* < .001)
D/SAX	11.5 ± 4.3 dB (*P* < .001)

Table 1. Intensity differences before and after Sonazoid administration. A-pre-injection (A-pre) and –post-injection (A-post): 1.3 ± 3.5 dB. B-pre and B-post: 0.9 ± 3.3 dB. The intensity differences for each pair were not significantly different. C-pre and C-post: -33.4 ± 5.1 dB and -22.3 ± 6.8 dB; D-pre and D-post: -36.2 ± 4.8 dB and -22.6 ± 10.7 dB. The differences between C (14.1 ± 5.8 dB) and D (11.5 ± 4.3 dB) were judged significant (P < 0.001)

http://dx.doi.org/10.5772/45953

View	Sensitivity	Specificity	Accuracy
AP (Δ ≤ 6.3 dB)	0.98	0.94	0.97
SAXpm (Δ ≤ 5.1 dB)	0.97	0.96	0.97

Table 2. Sonazoid's detection parameters for coronary artery stenosis. The optimal dB cut-off vales were selected that gave the highest sensitivity and specificity. By ROC, intensity differences ≤ 6.3 dB in AP views detects ≥ 75% stenosis with a sensitivity: 0.98, specificity: 0.94, accuracy: 0.97. In the SAX view an intensity difference ≤ 5.1 dB detects ≥ 75% stenosis with a sensitivity: 0.97, specificity: 0.96, accuracy: 0.97.

The intraobserver reproducibility was determined by imaging the same patients after a four-week interval and then calculating Cohen's kappa (κ= 0.76, $p < 0.001$). To obtain the four-week interval and then calculating Cohen's kappa (κ= 0.76, $p < 0.001$). To obtain the interobserver reproducibility, the same images were evaluated by another echocardiographer who was employed at a different medical institute and had no knowledge of the protocol. The interobserver reproducibility was excellent (κ= 0.98, $p < 0.001$). These two results indicate that the reproducibly of Sonazoid MCE is sufficient for the use of this agent in the clinical setting.

4. Discussion

Remarkable progress has been made over the last decade in medical imaging of the heart and other organs. However, there is still an enormous worldwide mortality and morbidity from coronary artery disease. A major hurdle in overcoming this situation is the inability to make a definite diagnosis of coronary artery stenosis or to screen coronary artery disease easily and inexpensively. Although myocardial ischemia it thought to start from 75% stenosis, patients usually have no symptoms with normal daily activities. When the stenosis is ≥ 90%, patients may become symptomatic with normal daily activities. Presently, CAG is only one diagnostic method, but it is invasive and expensive. Routine preventative cardiac imaging that would be safe (no ionizing radiation or allergenic contrast dyes), highly sensitive, specific and economical would obviously help mitigate this ongoing public health burden.

Echocardiography is one of the areas in which the most exciting advances have been made, and it is especially attractive because it is becoming progressively more miniaturized and can be used in a typical office setting rather than a dedicated imaging center. Current modalities include real-time three-dimensional echocardiography, speckle tracking, contrast echocardiography, intracardiac echocardiography and hand-held echocardiography.

Here, we show that Sonazoid can be successfully used in a local clinical setting and this contrast agent allows the accurate detection of coronary artery stenosis ≥ 75%. This may be accounted for by Sonazoid's resistance to acoustic pressure and its long half-life compared to other microbubble-based contrast agents [15]. Our patients did not experience adverse effects during or after the procedure. This is likely due to Sonazoid's intrinsic nontoxicity, but also by the rapid metabolism of microbubbles via the respiratory system. We compared our results with those of other studies [16, 17] and found similar accuracy for the detection of significant (≥ 75%) coronary artery stenosis. Thus, our data argue for continued investigations into its suitability for MCE and ultimate approval for this purpose, especially in view of the limited number of microbubble-based contrast agents now available to cardiologists. In future studies, it will be of great interest to determine whether Sonazoid is capable of detecting less significant degrees of stenosis.

5. Limitations

The limitations of this method are the same as the limitations of echocardiography. It is difficult to obtain good B-mode images in patients with a thick subcutaneous fatty layer or emphysematous lung. The reliability of MCE to detect ischemia is clearly dependent on the quality of the B-mode images. Another limitation is the process of making Sonazoid™ since the solution is somewhat complex compared with Levovist™. In addition, the detection of ischemic myocardial areas requires the ability to make and read time-intensity graphs. However, we learned to overcome these limitations after four or five subjects.

6. Conclusions

This study showed that Sonazoid™ has good clinical utility and better diagnostic accuracy to detect significant coronary artery stenosis than other contrast agents. This is because the concentration of Sonazoid™ in circulating blood is more stable, and the agent has a longer half-life than other contrast agents.

Comparisons between myocardial regions of affected and normal arteries in these patients before and after Sonazoid™ administration under low-dose ATP stress showed that MCE could detect ≥75% stenosis with a sensitivity of 97%, specificity of 96% and accuracy of 97%. An important factor in achieving these results was the optimization of the MI settings. We believe that these data, taken together with patients not experiencing adverse effects during or after the procedure, provide a compelling argument for extending these studies, with the ultimate goal of providing cardiologists a powerful new tool for routine echocardiography.

The ability of this MCE method to identify various degrees of coronary artery stenosis needs to be confirmed in larger, randomized trials. Although conventional echocardiography cannot detect the extent of myocardial tissue ischemia due to coronary artery stenosis, it can detect LV wall systolic dysfunction due to myocardial ischemia by strain mapping. By applying these two methods, we could develop a new and more accurate diagnostic method. The creation of an MCE map along with a strain map might be used to directly diagnose the severity of coronary artery stenosis and extent of the ischemic myocardial area.

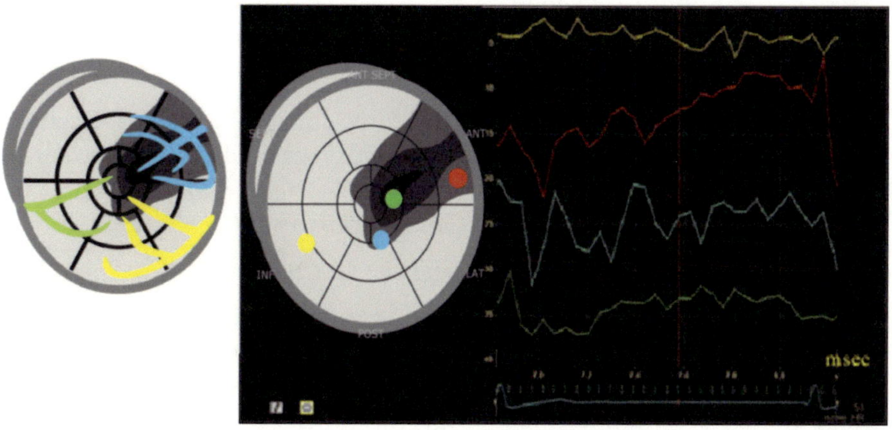

Figure 12. The image of myocardial contrast echocardiography map (MCE Map: left) and the time-intensity curve of the MCE of the patient by MCE MAP.

The extent of the ischemic myocardial area surely play a more leading and important role as an index more than the severity of coronary artery stenosis to decide the indication of coronary artery intervention.

Acknowledgements

The authors heartedly express our thanks to Mr. Yoshio Oonishi (Daiichi Sankyo Co. Ltd, Tokyo, Japan) who kindly provided us with Figures 1, 2, 3 and 4, and also to Mr Kenichiro Morinaga and Mr. Eiji Aoki (SEIKOTEC Co.,Ltd.) who helped me by drawing coronary arteries on strain maps (http://seikotec.com/). In addition I deeply appreciate Mr. Hisashi Koumyou's personal advice to edit this thesis.

Author details

Ri-ichiro Kakihara

Address all correspondence to: ri-ichiro.k@adagio.ocn.ne.jp

Department of Cardiology, Private Kakihara Clinic, Toyohashi, Japan

References

[1] Chelliah RK, Senior R. Contrast echocardiography: an update. Curr Cardiol Rep. 2009; 11(3) 216-224.

[2] Platts D, West C, Boga T, Hamilton-Craig C, Burstow D. Direct visualization of septal perforator coronary arterial blood flow during perflutren microsphere contrast echocardiography. Eur J Echocardiogr. 2009;10(6) 808-810.

[3] Cheng AS, Pegg TJ, Karamitsos TD, Searle N, Jerosch-Herold M, Choudhury RP, Banning AP, Neubauer S, Robson MD, Selvanayagam JB. Cardiovascular magnetic resonance perfusion imaging at 3-tesla for the detection of coronary artery disease: a comparison with 1.5-tesla. J Am Coll Cardiol. 2007; 49(25) 2440-2449.

[4] Schwarz F, Ruzsics B, Schoepf UJ, Bastarrika G, Chiaramida SA, Abro JA, Brothers RL, Vogt S, Schmidt B, Costello P, Zwerner PL. Dual-energy CT of the heart--principles and protocols. Eur J Radiol. 2008;68(3) 423-433.

[5] Schutt EG, Klein DH, Mattrey RM, Riess JG. Injectable microbubbles as contrast agents for diagnostic ultrasound imaging: the key role of perfluorochemicals. Angew Chem Int Ed Engl. 2003;42(28) 3218-3235.

[6] Klibanov AL. Microbubble contrast agents: targeted ultrasound imaging and ultrasound-assisted drug-delivery applications. Invest Radiol. 2006;41(3) 354-362.

[7] Hernot S, Klibanov AL. Microbubbles in ultrasound-triggered drug and gene delivery. Adv Drug Deliv Rev. 2008;60(10) 1153-1166.

[8] Dijkmans PA, Juffermans LJ, van Dijk J, Musters RJ, Spreeuwenberg, Kamp O. Safety and feasibility of real time adenosine myocardial contrast echocardiography with emphasis on induction of arrhythmias: a study in healthy volunteers and patients with stable coronary artery disease. Echocardiography. 2009;26(7) 807-814.

[9] Abdelmoneim SS, Bernier M, Scott CG, Dhoble A, Ness SA, Hagen ME, et al. Safety of contrast agent use during stress echocardiography: a 4-year experience from a single-center cohort study of 26,774 patients. JACC Cardiovasc Imaging. 2009 Sep;2(9): 1048-1056.

[10] McMahon CJ, Ayres NA, Bezold LI, Lewin MB, Alonzo M, Altman CA, et al. Safety and efficacy of intravenous contrast imaging in pediatric echocardiography. Pediatr Cardiol. 2005 26(4) 413-417.

[11] Moriyasu F, Itoh K. Efficacy of perflubutane microbubble-enhanced ultrasound in the characterization and detection of focal liver lesions: phase 3 multicenter clinical trial. Am J Roentgenology. 2009;193(1) 86-95.

[12] Stanton J. Rosenthal, Paul H. Jones, Louis H. Wetzel Phase Inversion Tissue Harmonic Sonographic Imaging: A Clinical Utility Study. Am J Roentgenology. 2001; 176(6) 1393-1398.

[13] Reisner SA, Lysyansky P, AgmonY, Mutlak D, Lessick J, Friedman Z. Global longitudinal strain: a novel index of left ventricular systolic function : J Am Soc Echocardiogr. 2004 June; 17(6) 630-633.

[14] Shimoni S, Gendelman G, Ayzenberg O, Smirin N, Lysyansky P, Edri O, Deutsch L, Caspi A, Friedman Z. Differential Effects of Coronary Artery Stenosis on Myocardial

Function: The Value of Myocardial Strain Analysis for the Detection of Coronary Artery Disease : J Am Soc Echocardiogr. 2011; 24(7) 748-757.

[15] Sontum PC. Physicochemical characteristics of Sonazoid, a new contrast agent for ultrasound imaging. Ultrasound Med Biol. 2008;34(5) 824-833.

[16] I Jucquois, P Nihoyannopoulos, A D'Hondt, V Roelants, A Robert, J Melin, D Glass, and J Vanoverschelde. Comparison of myocardial contrast echocardiography with NC100100 and 99mTc sestamibi SPECT for detection of resting myocardial perfusion abnormalities in patients with previous myocardial infarction. Heart. 2000; 83(5) 518–524.

[17] Binder T, Assayag P, Baer F, Flachskampf F, Kamp O, Nienaber C, Nihoyannopoulos P, Piérard L, Steg G, Vanoverschelde JL, Van der Wouw P, Meland N, Marelli C, Lindvall K. NC100100, a new echo contrast agent for the assessment of myocardial perfusion--safety and comparison with technetium-99m sestamibi single-photon emission computed tomography in a randomized multicenter study. Clin Cardiol. 1999;22(4) 273-282.

Chapter 10

Nuclear Cardiology — In the Era of the Interventional Cardiology

Branislav Baskot, Igor Ivanov, Dragan Kovacevic, Slobodan Obradovic, Nenad Ratkovic and Miodrag Zivkovic

Additional information is available at the end of the chapter

http://dx.doi.org/10.5772/55484

1. Introduction

The strength and breadth of nuclear cardiology lie in its great potential for future creative growth. This growth involves the development of new biologically derived radiopharmaceuticals, avdanced imaging techologies, and a broad/based set of research and clinical aplications involving diagnosis, functional categorization, prognosis, evaluation of therapeutic interventions, and the ability to deal with many of the major investigative issues in contemporary cardiology such as myocardial hibernation, stunning, and viability. The past decade has been caracteriyed by major advances in nuclear cardiology that have greatly enhanced the clinical utility of the various radionuclide techniques used for the assessment of regional myocardial perfusion and regional and global left ventricular function under resting and stress condotions. Despite the emergence of alternative noninvasive techniques for the diagnosis of coronary aretry disease (CAD) and the assessment of prognosis of viability, such as ergo- stress tests, stress echocardiography, the use and application of nuclear cardiology techniques have continued to increase. The establishment of the American Society of Nuclear Cardiology (ASNC) and its educational programs has led to a greater diffusion on nuclear cardiology technology in the community hospital setings and has promoted the emergence and dissemination of imaging and procedural guidelines for nuclear cardiology methods. The establishment of the Journal of Nuclear Cardiology, the official journal of ASNC, allowed a greater number of manuscript to be published in the field [1, 2, 3]

In the few past decade, significant advances have been made in the ability to image the heart with radionuclide tracers under stress and resting conditions in patientse with suspected or known coronary aretry disease (CAD) for the detection of ischemia, determination of prognosis, assessment of myocardial viability, preoperative risk assessment for patients undergoing noncardiac surgery, mand evaluation of the efficacy of revasculariyation in patients undergoing coronary artery bypass surgery or an interventional procedure [1, 2, 3].

For many years, planar imaging and SPECT with 201Tl (201 Talium) constituted the only scintigrafic techniques available for detecting CAD and assessing prognosis in patients undergoing stress perfusion imaging. The major limitation of 201Tl scintigraphy is the high false/positive rate observed in many laboratories, wich is attributed predominantly to image attenuation aretfact and variants of normal that are interpreted as defects consequent to a significant coronary artery stenoses. Although quantification of 201Tl images improves specificity, the false/positive rate remains problematic, particulary in the women and in obese patients. Breast attenuation artifact in women are sometimes difficult to distiguish from perfusion abnormalities secondary to inducible ischemia or myocardial scar.

In recent years, new 99mTc (technetium) labeled perfusion agents have been introduced into clinical practice to enhance the specificity of Single Photon Emission Cumputed Tomography (SPECT) and to provide additional information regarding and global left ventricular systolic function via ECG gating of images [3, 4, 8]. It was immadiately apparent that the quality of images obtained with these 99mTc-labeled radionuclides was superior to that images obtained with 201Tl because of the more favorable psysical characteristic of 99mTc imaging with gamma camera. Perhaps most importantly, 99mTc imaging allows easy gated acqusition, permiting simulateous evaluation of regional systolic thickening, global left ventricular function (LVEF), and myocardial perfusion. One the most significant avdances in myocardial perfusion imaging in the past decade is the development of quantitative SPECT perfusion imaging. Radionuclide imaging is an intrinsically digital technique that is ideally suited for quantification. A number of validated software packages are commercially available for quantification of SPECT myocardial perfusion and function (Auto Quant; Emory Toolbox; 4D/MSPECT; and Wackers Liu CQ), and are carried by the major vendors of nuclear medicine imaging equipment. The basic principles of SPECTR quantification are similar for each of these software packages. Each commercially available package also includes software for computation of LVEF and left ventricular volumes from ECG-gated SPECT images [7, 9, 10, 11].

2. Indications for nuclear cardiology procedures

2.1. Suspected coronary artery disease

CAD is still the single greatest cause of death of men and women in the world, despite a declining total death rate. Using USA data over 459.000 deaths were due to CAD -1 of every deaths. There are aproximatelly 2.2 million hospital discharges with CAD as the diagnosis annually.

The reduction of the morbidity and mortality due to CAD is thus primary importance to physicians and patients. Stress myocardial perfusion imaging (MPI) has emerged as an

http://dx.doi.org/10.5772/55484

important noninvasive means of evaluating patients with suspected CAD, with over than 10 millions studies performed in USA annually [1, 2, 16, 17, 18].

Risk factor assessment

The first step in evaluating patients for CAD involves the assessment of the presence of traditional risk factors. Modifiable risks include hypercholesterolemia, hypertension, diabetes mellitus, obesity, tobacco use, and physical inactivity. Nonmodifiable risk factor includes a family history of CAD in first-degree relatives under the age of 60, advanced age, and gender? Once risk factors associated with CAD are evaluated, a patient's risk for having CAD should be assessed. This is often performed by taking symptoms such as a chest pain, age, and gender into account. Symptoms suggestive of CAD, in addition to other risk factors, drive decisions for further testing [2, 12, 17, 18].

A cornerstone of the diagnosis of CAD has been exercise tolerance testing (ETT). The ETT is the safe and easily performed, usually in an office setting. But generally, ETT electrocardiography (ECG) has a sensitivity of 50 to 70%, and a specificity of 60 to 80%.

Thus, the major limitation of the ETT is its diagnostic accuracy for the detection of significant CAD. In patients able to exercise, the diagnostic accuracy of stress myocardial perfusion imaging (MPI) is significantly higher than the ETT alone and provides greater risk stratification for predicting the future cardiac events.

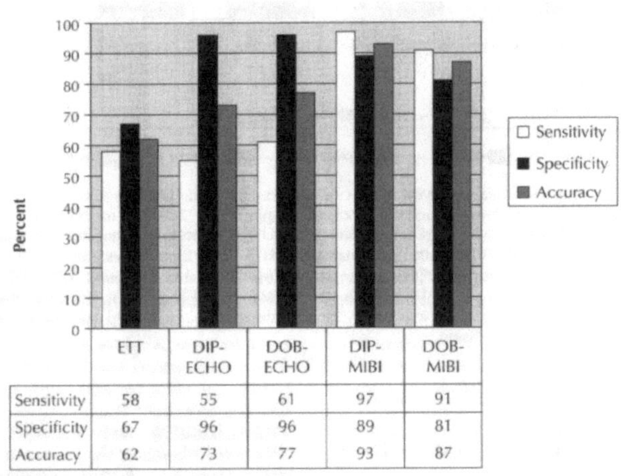

	ETT	DIP-ECHO	DOB-ECHO	DIP-MIBI	DOB-MIBI
Sensitivity	58	55	61	97	91
Specificity	67	96	96	89	81
Accuracy	62	73	77	93	87

Test

(Nuclear cardiology –practical applications)
ETT exercise treadmill test
DIP-ECHO dipyridamole echocardiography
DOB-ECHO dobutamine echocardiography
DIP- MIBI dipyridamole myocardial perfusion imaging with Tc-99m MIBI
DOB-MIBI dobutamine myocardial perfusion imaging with Tc-99m MIBI

Figure 1. Diagnostic accuracy of various tests of CAD

Because of limitation to performed exercise test (patients with medical illness, debilitation, musculoskeletal problems, and the older who can't reach a predicted maximum heart rate) MPI with pharmacologic stress using vasodilators (dipyridamole, and adenosine) or dobutamine can be implemented in such patients. In this moment, it has been estimated that 48% to 50% of all stress MPI is performed with pharmacologic agent. Briefly, dipyridamole and adenosine are potent coronary vasodilators that markedly increase coronary blood flow. This increased flow is less pronounced in arteries that are stenotic (flow restricted) due to atherosclerosis. This causes heterogeneous myocardial perfusion, which can be observed using that follows coronary blood flow as an alternative to vasodilator stress. Dobutamine works by increasing myocardial oxygen demand (through increased heart rate, systolic blood pressure, and myocardial contractility) [5, 6, 7, 8, 9]. As in exercise MPI scintigraphic images obtained at rest compared to those obtained during peak pharmacologic stress to distinguish myocardial ischemia from scar tissue (infarct area).

The diagnostic accuracy of Tc-99m imaging with pharmacologic stress test for angiographically significant CAD has been evaluated in numerous study.

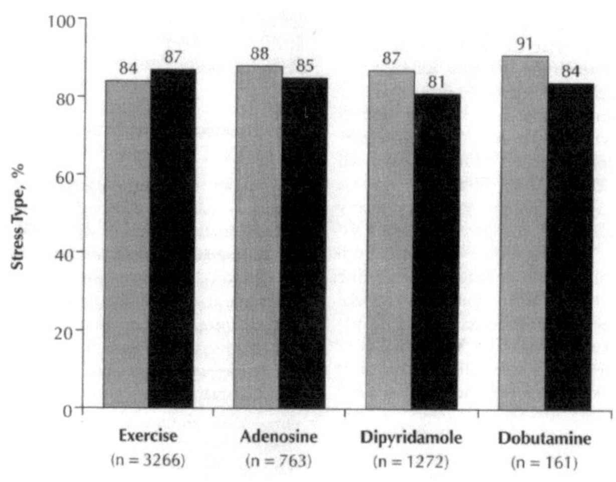

(Nuclear cardiology –practical applications)

Figure 2. Diagnostic accuracy of stress myocardial perfusion imaging.

2.2. Evaluating and determination CULPRIT lesion, in indication for interventional cardiology

One of the most powerfull uses of MPI is the evaluation of the risk for future events in patients with suspected or known CAD. Over the years, MPI has evolved as an essential tool in the evaluation and assessment of patient prior to coronary revascularization. It has a dual role. Prior to coronary angiography, MPI is extremly useful in documeting ischemia and determining the functional impact of single or multiple lesions indentified subsequently. After coronary anatomy is known, and despite some limitations in the setting of multivessel disease, MPI remains the test of choise for indentifying the lesion responsible for the ischemic symptoms, or so colled culprit lesion. That is extremly useful for futher management decisions with respect to percutaneous interventions. In compare, the absence of reversible ischemia in patients with known CAD is an excellent prognostic marker and predicts a low annual event rate.

The current definition of culprit lesion that is zone of ischemia under the coronary stenoses is not quite wright, because that is not definy two pathophysiologic aspects of ischemia; severity and extent. The primary objective of those study was to determinate and localizes culprit lesion by newly introduce parameters SRS (*summary reversible score*) and ISRS (*index of summary reversible score*), under the angiographically detected coronary narrowing ≥75% for the least one coronary artery [2, 6, 9, 11, 15].

In the past two decades, a great body of literature has established the use of nuclear imaging for risk stratification in patients with known or suspected coronary artery disease (CAD). Risk stratification is of crucial importance for the practice of contemporary medicine. Extending the paradigm of noninvasive cardiac testing beyond the detection of disease is especially important, may risk assessment permits patients who are identified as being at a high risk for subsequent cardiac events should receive aggressive management, possibly including cardiac catheterization for potential revascularization procedures that may improve their outcome. CAD is disease with a wide spectrum of severity and extent with outcome, such as nonfatal myocardial infarction (MI) or cardiac death being related to the severity of disease. Clinical trials have shown that patients with severe CAD as left main coronary artery disease, especially those with left ventricular dysfunction, can benefit from coronary artery bypass graft surgery (CABG) with significant reduction in their mortality rate. Whereas patients with single-vessel or with two-vessel disease (without proximal left anterior descending artery involvement) would have improved symptoms of angina following CABG and percutaneous transluminal coronary angioplasty with or without stent implantation, without any effect on their mortality rate.

Coronary angiography, considered the "gold standard" for the diagnosis of CAD, often does not provide information about the physiologic significance of atherosclerotic lesions, especially in borderline lesions. More importantly, it does not provide a clear marker of risk of adverse events, especially in patients with moderate disease severity. Andreas Gruentzig said; *"When coronary angiography founded coronary artery disease, I would like to have diagnostic procedure who will give me functional significance that lesion."* [2, 10, 12, 18].

The presence of normal scintigraphic MPI study at a high level of stress (≥ 85 % of maximum predicted heart rate) or proper pharmacologic stress carries a very benign prognosis, with mortality rate less than 0.5% per year. This finding has been reproduced in many studies. Iskander and Iskandiran, pooling the results of SPECT imaging from more than 12000 patients in 14 studies, demonstrated that the events rate (death/MI) for patients with normal MPI finding is 0.6%, whereas abnormal study carries 7.4% per year event rate, a 12-fold increase [2, 3, 14, 18]..

The current definition of culprit lesion; that is zone of ischemia under the coronary stenoses (what degree? That is not definition. Some autors ofer degree of stenoses ≤ 70 %, some ≤ 75%, even < 80-85%) is not quite wright, because that is not definy two pathophysiologic aspects of ischemia; severity and extent. Iskander and Iskadrian have also shown that defects reversibility is an important predictor of type of cardiac events, whereas reversible perfusion defects are associated with nonfatal MI. This is very important finding, since a reversible defect on MPI imaging is the only available diagnostic tool that can independently predict the risk of nonfatal MI. Therefore, stress perfusion studies should be reported documenting defect severity (mild, moderate, severe), size (small, moderate, large) and reversibility to provide essential risk stratification.[2, 3, 16].

The size and severity of the perfusion abnormality provide powerful prognostic information and has been shown to directly relate to outcome. MPI perfusion imaging and determination of culprit lesion is more predicitble of cardiac events than coronary angiography. As MPI imaging may identify those patients at high risk for subsequent cardiac events, perfusion imaging may be used to help guide further testing and revascularization procedures, and this obviously has important cost-effectiveness ramifications.

The primary objective of this study was to determinate and localizes culprit lesion by newly introduce parameters SRS (*summary reversible score*) and ISRS (*index of summary reversible score*), under the angiographically detected coronary narrowing ≥75% for the least one coronary artery [2].

The rapid rates of technical advances and improved operator expertise have enabled this technique to gain more widespread application. Despite the large number of PTCA-s performed yearly, preprocedure documentation of myocardial ischemia is uncommon, occurring in only 29% of patients.

Myocardial perfusion imaging provides information on the extent and location of myocardial ischemia. The assessment of jeopardized myocardium may be performed and provides a measure of the relative value of PTCA in terms of the amount of jeopardized myocardium. The location of the stenosis may dictate the area at risk: extent and severity of perfusion defects were significantly smaller in patients with proximal compared with distal coronary artery occlusions.

Before revascularization is performed, myocardial perfusion imaging may assist in management decisions by demonstrating the presence of myocardial ischemia, viability and delineating the severity and extent of coronary artery disease. The significance of equivocal lesions may be determined and culprit vessel may be successfully defined by SPECT imaging before angioplasty [2, 3, 10, 18].

The coronary angiography provides information on the anatomical state of the coronary tree and, specifically, on the large epicardial arteries, while perfusion SPECT facilitates the evaluation of the grade of ischemia that a particular stenosis produces. MPI SPECT is of considerable use in the procedural indications of partial revascularization in patients with chronic coronary artery disease (CAD). In these cases the purpose is to detect the coronary stenosis that provokes the ischemia and is termed the "culprit lesion".

http://dx.doi.org/10.5772/55484

The aim of the study Baskot at all. [2] was to determine and localize culprit lesion by MPI in cases of angiographically detected coronary narrowing ≥ 75% of at least one coronary artery.

In the study four hundred and thirty-seven [437] patients were studied. In all of them angiographically detected significant coronary narrowing (≥ 75% luminal stenosis) before PCI. All the patients were submitted to MPI ^{99m}Tc-MIBI, with pharmacologic dipyridamole stress protocol with concomitant low level bicycle exercise 50 W (DipyEX). We measured relative uptake ^{99m}Tc-MIBI for each myocardial segment using short-axis tomogram study. A 5-point scoring system was used to assess the difference between uptake degree in stress and rest studies for the same segment, and we created two indices: Sum reversible score (SRS), Index of sum reversibility score (ISRS). In the results a total 1311 vascular territories (7429 segments) were analyzed before elective percutaneous coronary intervention (ePCI). Overall sensitivity, specificity and accuracy using SRS were 89.7%, 86, 7%, and 88, 2%, with a positive predictive value of 92, 7%. Overall sensitivity, specificity and accuracy using ISRS were 92.8%, 89.1%, and 92.3%, and the positive predictive value was 93.7%. Conclusion this work that is DipyEX MPI with two indices created SRS and ISRS significantly improves sensitivity, specificity and accuracy in the determination and localization of culprit lesion in patients undergoing elective PCI. In this work author defined culprit lesion using two physiological aspects; severity of ischemia and extension zone of ischemia. With quantification of these two parameters of culprit lesion, the author determined patients who underwent ePCI with stent implantation, and who had the best therapy effects with PCI therapy.

Case 1.

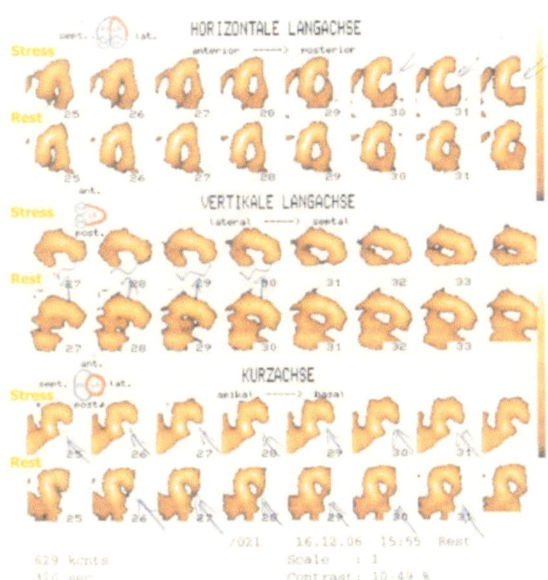

Figure showed culprit lesion in the inferolateral segments in the AdenoEx (up line slices) MPI study

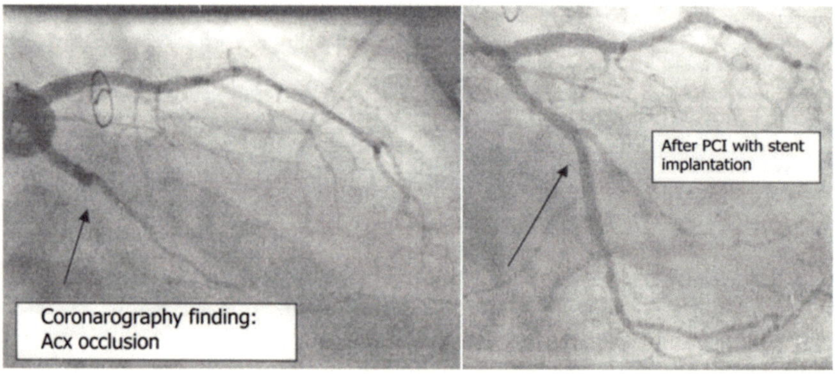

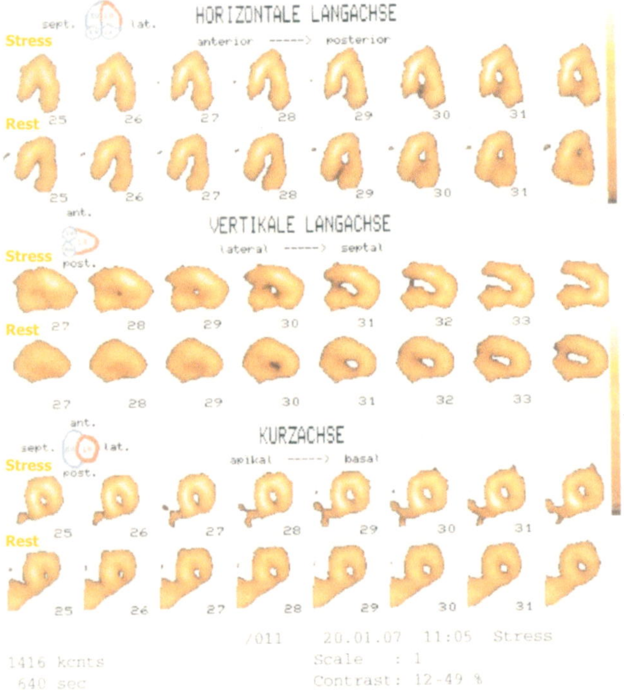

Nearly after elective PCI intervention we performed MPI with normal finding of perfusion

Case 2.

- Patient male 61 year old. St post IM with revascularization 1996 triple ACB (LIMA – LAD; venous graft on the D1 and
- In April 2010 performed SPECT MPI, finding sugested invasive intervention.
- Coronarography finding ;LM 90%, LAD occluded, LIMA graft wide open. Venous graft on the D1 occluded.

- ACx stenoses 90%, OM with tubular stenosis 50 -70%
- RCA dominant, occluded ostial, venous graft occluded okludiran.
- Performed PCI with stent implantation (Tsunami gold 3.5 x 15) on LM and ACX
- After four month MPI control when we founded in stent stenosis.

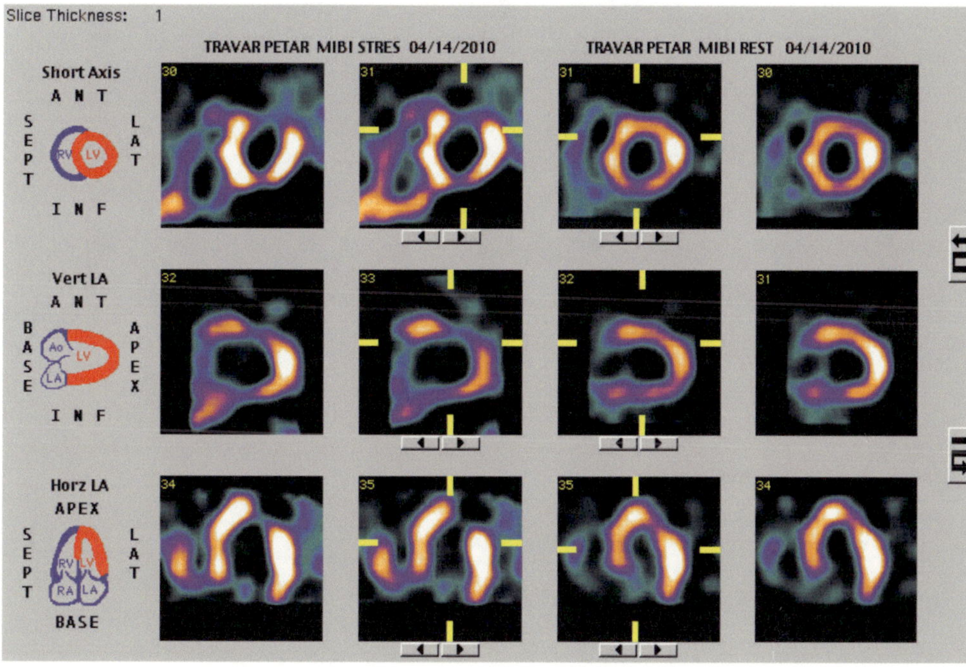

Culprit lesion

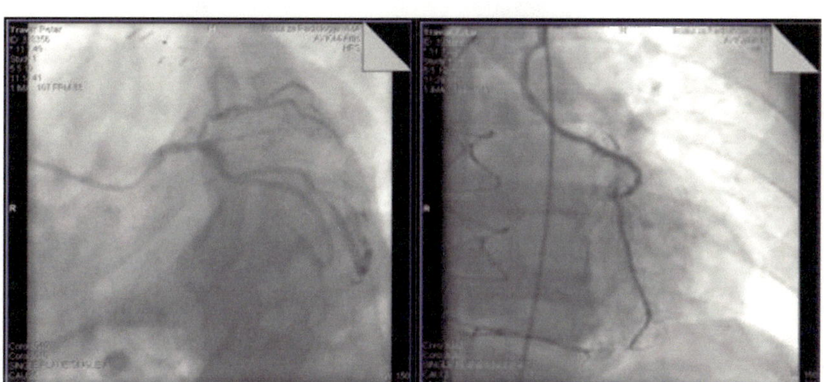

Coronarography finding

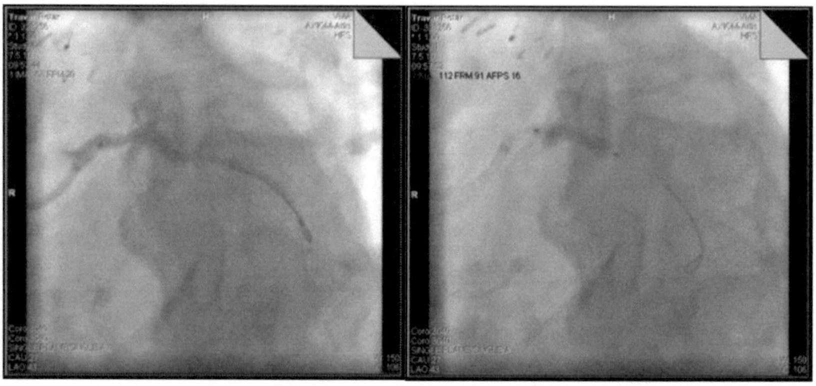

In the same act PCI with stent implantation

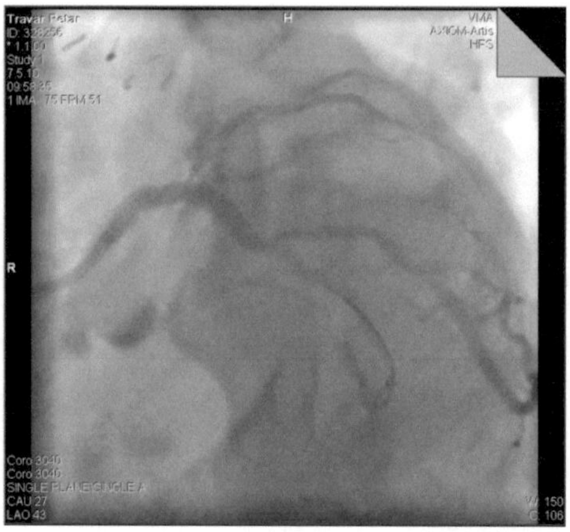

Final effect PCI

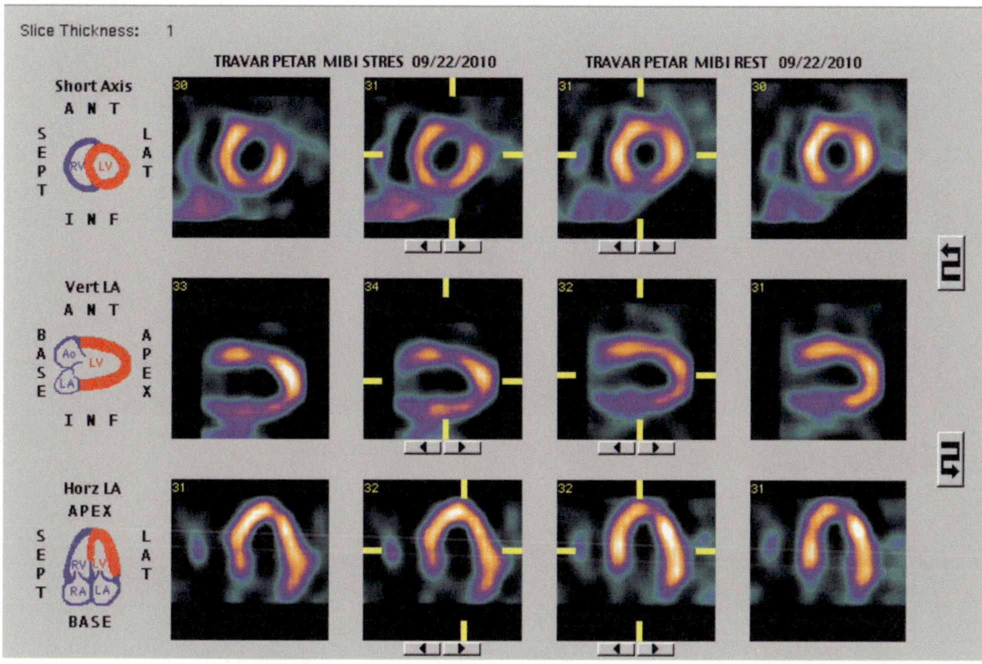

Control MPI after four month after PCI

We finding zone of reversible ischemia in the same area, suggest restenosis

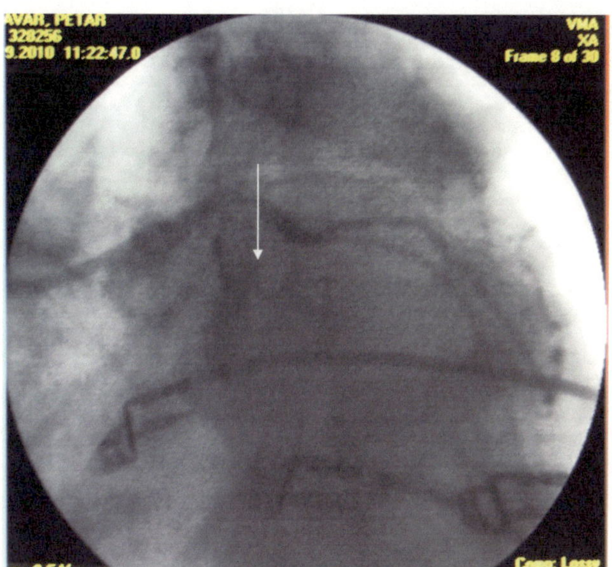

Control Coronarography - fidning in stent stenonis

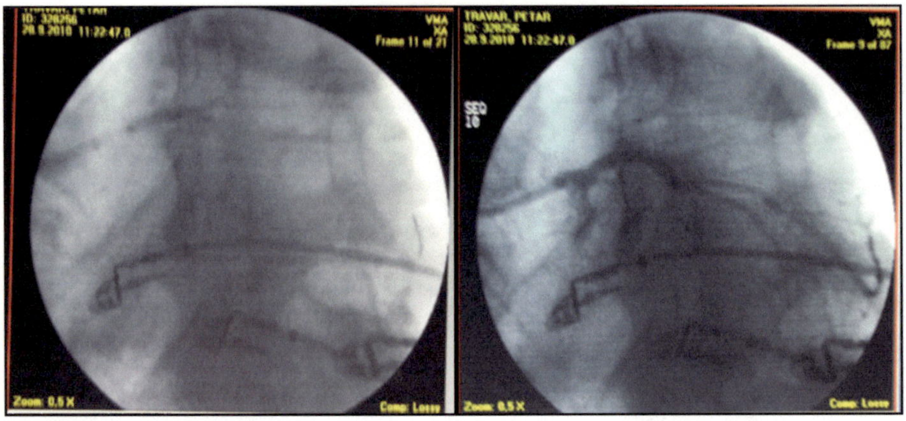

Re PCI with stent implantation

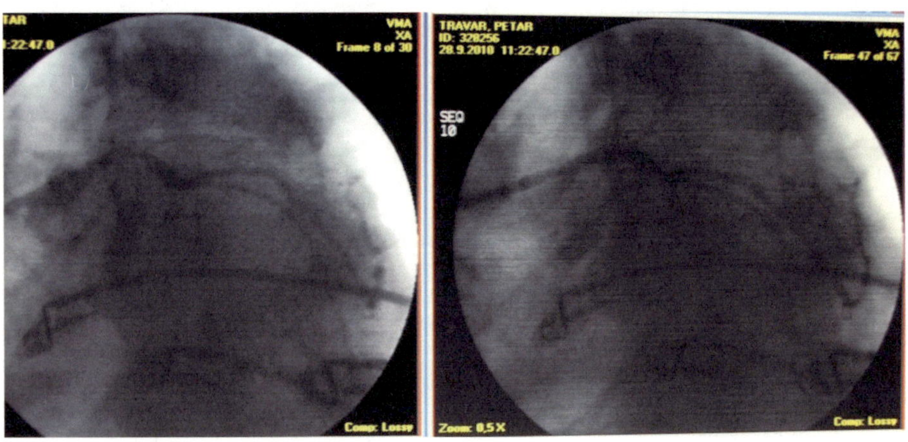

Final effect

Conversely, patients with high-risk scans may benefit from an early invasive strategy with a view toward revascularization depending on coronary anatomical finding. A substantial number of patients undergoing SPECT perfusion imaging will have mild ischemia without a multi-vessel disease scan pattern. If patients with mild ischemia have good exercise tolerance, they should be considered as candidates for intense medical therapy with follow-up exercise SPECT imaging possibly at 1 year. Unpublished data from the Clinical Outcomes Utilizing Revascularization and Aggressive Drug Evaluations (COURAGE) trial seem to indicate that many ischemic defects may markedly improve with aggressive lowering of abnormal lipids an the other pharmacological interventions. Hachamovitch and colleagues reported patients with the mildly abnormal scan had a 0.8% annual cardiac death rate compared with 0.9% for those who underwent revascularization. The death rate in medically treated patients who had moderately abnormal scans was 2.3% versus 1.1% for such patients undergoing revascularization. Finally, patients with a severely abnormal scan treated medically had an annual cardiac death rate of 4.6% versus 1.3% for such patients who were revascularized. In the second study, these investigators showed that medically treated patients who had greater than 20% of the total myocardium rendered ischemic had higher annual cardiac death rate (6.7%) compared with 2.0% for patients with this degree of extensive ischemia who underwent revascularization. For patients with 10% or less of the total myocardium rendered ischemic, there was no difference in outcome between medical therapy and revascularization.

Exercise myocardial perfusion imaging is a valuable adjunct for separating high to low risk patients who present symptoms consistent with stable CAD, or in patients who have known disease and in whom further prognostication is warranted. Multiple high-risk nuclear imaging variables can be identified, and the greater the extent of exercise/induced ischemia, the greater the risk of cardiac events. Adjunctive variables, such as transient ischemic cavity dilatation and functional assessment with evaluation of regional wall thickening or wall motion and left ventricular ejection fraction greatly assist in the risk stratification process [1, 3, 16, 18].

Nuclear cardiology is uniquely placed to address all the major determinants of prognosis in CAD can be assessed by measurements of stress-induced perfusion or function. These measurements include the amount of infarcted myocardium, the amount of jeopardized myocardium (supplied by vessels with hemodynamically significant stenosis), and the degree of jeopardy (tightness of the individual coronary stenosis). Recent evidence in large patient cohorts has revealed that factor estimating the extent of left ventricular dysfunction (left ventricular ejection fraction, extent of infarcted myocardium, transient ischemic dilatation of the left ventricle and increasing lung uptake) are excellent predictors of cardiac mortality. However, measurements of inducible ischemia are the best predictors of the development of acute coronary syndromes. Several reports have shown that nuclear testing yields incremental prognostic value over clinical information with respect to cardiac death, or the combination of cardiac death and nonfatal myocardial infarction as isolated endpoints. Now it is possible to tailor therapeutic decision making for an individual patient based upon combination of clinical factors and nuclear scan results. Patients with severe perfusion abnormalities on their stress image may have a five- to ten-fold higher likelihood of cardiac death versus patient with a normal myocardial perfusion SPECT. If the defects perfusion determined as a culprit lesion, invasive therapy (PCI) is an optimized outcome for that patient [2, 12, 13, 15].

The explosion of PTCA and stent placement in patients with single or multi-vessel disease has created a necessity for early detection of restenosis. A number of clinical studies have documented the usefulness of stress MPI for identifying restenosis in patients after PCI. One point of controversy is the optimal time to performing SPECT imaging after coronary intervention. Although current consensus in to obtain an exercise MPI study 4 to 6 weeks post intervention, whenever indicated, the proper timing for use of MPI remains to be determined. Based on existing knowledge about the timing interval of subacute thrombosis (< 4 weeks) and in-stent restenosis (3-6 month), we purpose the algorithm as a guide for the management of patients with known CAD after PCI [2, 15, 16, 18].

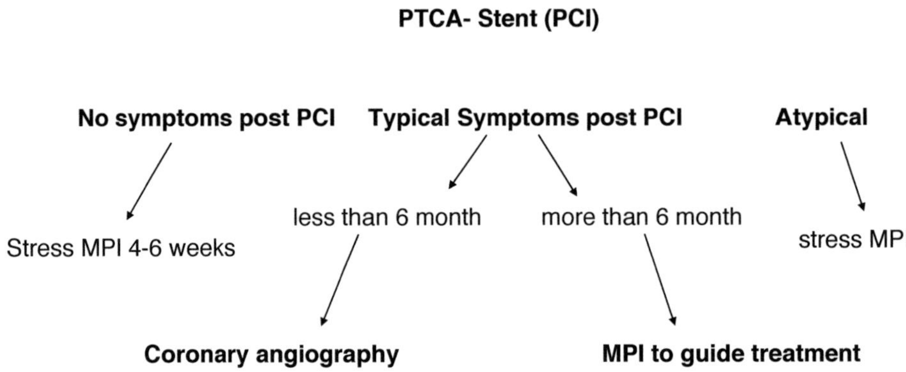

Figure 3. Recommendation for the diagnostic treatment after PCI.

Asymptomatic patients may be considered for stress MPI 4 to 6 weeks post intervention in order to assess the functional results of PCI and established a new baseline. Subsets of patients that benefit from this approach include those at high risk post PCI (patients with decreased LV function, proximal left anterior descending artery disease, previous sudden death, diabetes mellitus, hazardous occupations, and suboptimal PCI results). Stress MPI is also recommended in patients who develop atypical symptoms after PCI and there is necessity to assess whether these symptoms represent ischemia. Patient with symptoms typical of ischemia < 6 months post intervention should proceed with coronary angiography as a first step, unless contraindicated. If angina occurs later (> 6 months post PCI), stress/pharmacologic MPI can be used to assess degree and area of ischemia, since progression of native coronary disease rather than in-stent restenosis is more likely.

Incremental prognostic value of MPI; Because nuclear test are expensive the cost-effectiveness of these tests should demonstrate incremental prognostic information that cannot be derived from less expensive modalities such as clinical patient history and risks factors, standard ECG, and exercise ECG.

The combination clinical and exercise MPI variables provided greater prognostic information than the combination of clinical and angiographic data. Iskandrian et al showed that in medically treated patients with CAD, exercise SPECT imaging provided independent and incremental prognostic information even when catheterization data are available. The extent of perfusion abnormality was the single best predictor of prognosis. MPI added incremental prognostic information and risk-stratified patient even after clinical and exercise information were known. The incremental prognostic information about prognosis and need for coronary angiography provided by MPI has additionally been demonstrated for specific patients subsets: women, patient following coronary angioplasty or CABG, after MI, and with unstable angina. Hachamovitch et al demonstrated the use of MPI to yield incremental prognostic information toward the identification of cardiac death. Patient with a mildly abnormal scan after exercise stress are at low risk for cardiac death, but intermediate risk for nonfatal MI. A noninvasive strategy of optimizing medical therapy in this patient subgroup may result in significant cost saving when compared with invasive management strategy [1, 2, 3, 12, 18].

http://dx.doi.org/10.5772/55484

The prognostic efficacy of MPI is well established. Subsequent data have demonstrated in various patient subsets that nuclear tests add significant and incremental predictive value to less expensive clinical and exercise testing data. Angiographic data obtained from more expensive cardiac catheterization procedures add little or no significant incremental prognostic value when added to the results of MPI.

The introduction of new drugs and interventional devices to treat CAD, coupled with the arrival of manage care, has led to era of cost-containment within the practice of cardiology. Stress MPI is increasingly seen as a gatekeeper for more costly diagnosis and interventional procedures. Steingart et al evaluated 378 patients with a full range of pretest probabilities for CAD, and demonstrated that the results of MPI significantly reduced referring physicians' likelihood of recommending cardiac catheterization, on average by 49%.

Under managed care health systems that operate under cost-containment and capitation, MPI will continue to impact significantly on the decision to perform cardiac catheterization and to refer patients for coronary revascurization. Recommendations for invasive and interventional procedures are often coupled with an appropriate understanding of the prognostic value of MPI. Patients with the normal stress radionuclide study do not generally require referral for additional procedures, even when the likelihood of underlying CAD is high, as based on clinical and stress ECG data. The need for cardiac catheterization and coronary revascularization rates should be based on the degree of abnormality as detected by MPI. Thus, there is an increasing role of MPI to play an important gatekeeper function in the current era of managed care and emphasis on cost-containment [2, 3, 8, 12, 18].

Stress MPI has became a central guide in decision making with regard to CAD patients. Stress MPI is commonly used either before consideration of coronary revascularization or after its performance, to optimize decision making for CAD patients. Stress MPI is also used after myocardial revascularization procedures, to evaluate therapeutic efficacy; following the stabilization of acute ischemic syndromes; to determine subsequent risk; and before the performance of elective non-cardiac surgery, to identify the high-risk subsets of CAD patients who will require coronary revascularization prior to elective surgery.

After all, MPI has became an important instrument in defining cardiac risk and in identifying patients who are most likely to benefit from additional invasive diagnostic testing and potential coronary revascularization. MPI demonstrated significant incremental prognostic

3. Heart failure — New approach of therapy and diagnostic evaluation of therapy effect[1]

Heart failure (HF) is becoming the main clinical challenge in cardiology in the twenty - first century and is associated with high morbidity and mortality. Heart failure is the third most

1 Zivkovic Miodrag, Baskot Branislav

prevalent cardiovascular disease in the United States. An estimated 5 million people in the USA have heart failure, and the prevalence of the condition increase to 10 million by 2040, according to prediction. The prevalence of heart failure increase with age from less than 1% in the 20 – 30-year-old age group to over 20% in people age 80 years and older. The diagnostic and therapeutic costs involved are estimated to have exceeded $34 billion in only one year. Despite advances in therapies, the long-term prognosis from patients with heart failure remain poor; 80% of men and 70% of women greater than 65 years of age with heart failure die within 8 years [1, 2, 19, 20, 21].

3.1. What we need for good and quality therapy

The underllying etiology of HF needs to be determined; most patients have CAD (approximately 70% - 80%). Nuclear imaging can help in the differentiation between patients with ischemic and non-ischemic HF. In patients with ischemic cardiomiopathy, the precise coronary anatomy is also needed to determinate if revascularization needs to be considered. At present, invasive angiography is performed to obtain the coronary anatomy, but multi-slice CT (MSCT) may also provide this information. The presence of ischemia and viability needs to be determined to decide further if revascularization is indicated.

Nuclear imaging is considered the first choice technique for assessment of ischemia and viability; booth single-photon emission CT (SPECT), and positron emission tomography (PET) can provide this information.

Nuclear imaging can provide some indirect evidence in the differentiation between ischemic and non-ischemic HF. With stress,-rest SPECT study, reversible defects indicate ischemia and fixed defects of perfusion indicates scar tissue; booth this findings are markers of coronary artery disease. Moreover, lot of studies with nuclear perfusion imaging demonstrated that patients with ischemic HF had extensive and diffuse perfusion defects, whereas tracer uptake (myocardial perfusion) was mostly homogeneous (ischemic) in patients with non-ischemic HF.

Similarly, PET studies also demonstrated that patients with non-ischemic HF had more homogeneous tracer uptake, whereas patients with ischemic HF had areas of severely reduced uptake (reflecting scar formation). Accordingly, nuclear imaging can help in the differentiation between ischemic and non-ischemic cardiomyopathy, but for the diagnosis of underlying coronary artery disease, visualization of the coronary artery is needed. Invasive angiography is the technique of choice, but recently MSCT has been introduced for noninvasive angiography. With 64-slice MSCT and dual-source slice MSCT, we obtained more consistent image quality with improve visualization of the coronary artery tree. In the presence of a flow-limiting stenosis, resting myocardial is preserved, but once an increased myocardial oxygen demand occurs, a perfusion demand-supply mismatch follows, resulting in myocardial ischemia. Then, a sequence of events is initiated, which is referred to as the "ischemic cascade". Perfusion abnormalities occur at an early stage, whereas diastolic and systolic left ventricular dysfunction occur later. Accordingly, such techniques as nuclear imaging that defect perfusion abnormalities should have a high sensitivity for detection of ischemia, because these abnormalities occur early in the cascade [19, 20, 21].

In the heart failure patients, the combination between the coronary anatomy and the presence of ischemia in the territories of the stenotic vessels determines the need for revascularization. In the absence of ischemia, the presence of viability needs to evaluation.

Another nuclear study performed in the evaluating of therapy effects in HF, is radionuclide angiography (RNV). That is the most reproducible, accurate, and simple method for noninvasively assessing left ventricular ejection fraction (LVEF). RNV are now most often used for serial assessment of LVEF in patients who undergo chemotherapy, assessment of global regional wall motion in patients with recent or old myocardial infarction, and in patients with congestive heart failure. In the patients with heart failure, evaluation of left ventricular systolic function is essential to plan management and determine prognosis. At the present time most RNV are acquired by multiple – view planar image technique. In this moment SPECT RNV is not routinely performed in most nuclear cardiology laboratories. The greatest attraction of SPECT RNV is the ability to evaluate cardiac chambers and regional wall motion without overlap of other structures. LVEF may be calculated based on count changes from either a conventional planar image (*best septal*) or from SPECT RNV.

In the pilot study Zivkovic, Baskot at all. We introduced new therapy, hyperbaric oxygenation (HBO) and erythropoietin (EPO) in the treatment of heart failure. The aim of this study is to show positive therapeutic effects of synergistic applications of HBO as a strong generator of regenerator activities in human tissues, and recombinant EPO as a general growth factor, in the treatment HF ischemic and non-ischemic origin [19, 20, 21].

HBO is medical procedure of breathing the 100% oxygen under pressures higher than atmospheric pressure is and it carries out into hyperbaric chambers. Contemporary, HBO changes the rheological blood characteristic, recovers the function of blood vessels endothelium and it has good antiaggregation effects. The oxygen's pharmacokinetic and neo-angiogenesis effects and its effect on oxygen-dependent reactions inside the mitochondria's and homeopathy effect on the other organs are the reasons to use HBO in the treatment of HF. Nuclear imaging by SPECT imaging in the evaluation between ischemic and non-ischemic HF we performed, and followed with quantification per segments before and after therapy in the evaluation positive therapeutic effect. We also performed RNV like gold standard in the evaluation global and regional LVEF before and after the therapy. In the pilot study with 18 patients, we had recovery perfusion in all patients with non-ischemic HF. Before therapy we finding with RNV average measured LVEF was 23.4%. After treatment LVEF measured average 34, 3%. The results was increase by 10, 9% (from 5% to 20% measured individually).

Conclusion of this pilot study was that diagnostic information finding by nuclear cardiology (perfusion and function) suggested significantly positive therapy effects HBO and Erythropoietin in the therapy of heart failure ischemic and non-ischemic origin.

Case report 1. Patient female with multi vessel disease by coronarography

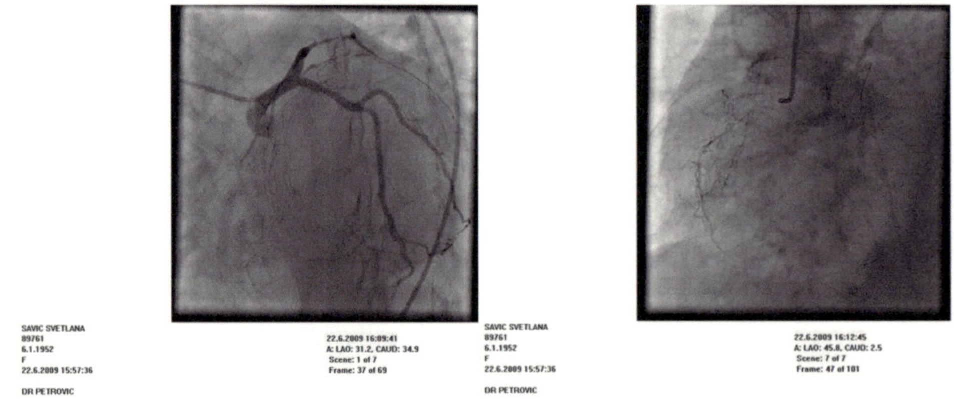

SPECT with DipyEX (dipyridamole = concomitant low level exercise 50W) performed and evaluated before and after HBO + EPO therapy

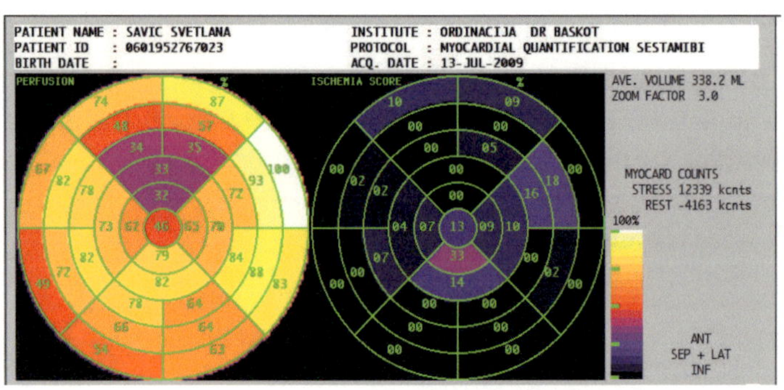

quantification of perfusion by Stierner
- segments quantification 07.13.2009

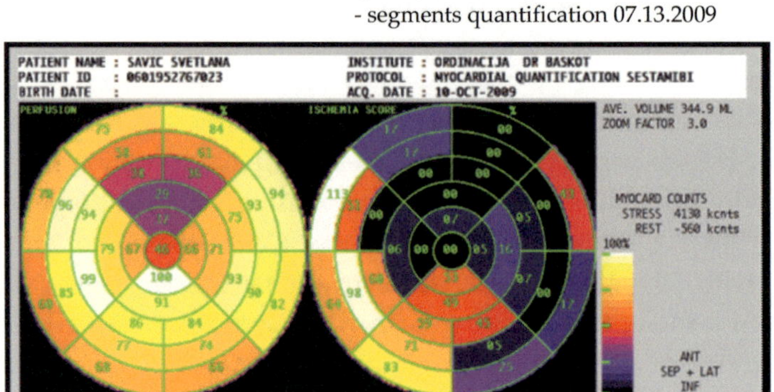

quantification of perfusion by Stierner
- segments quantification 10/10/2009

Radonuclide ventriculography for evaluating global ejection fraction Performed before and after HBO = EPO therapy

http://dx.doi.org/10.5772/55484

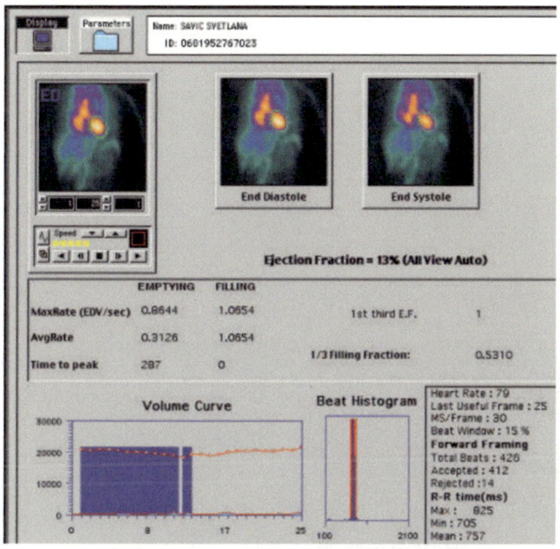

radionuclide ventriculography (RNV) performed 07.17. 2009 before therapy

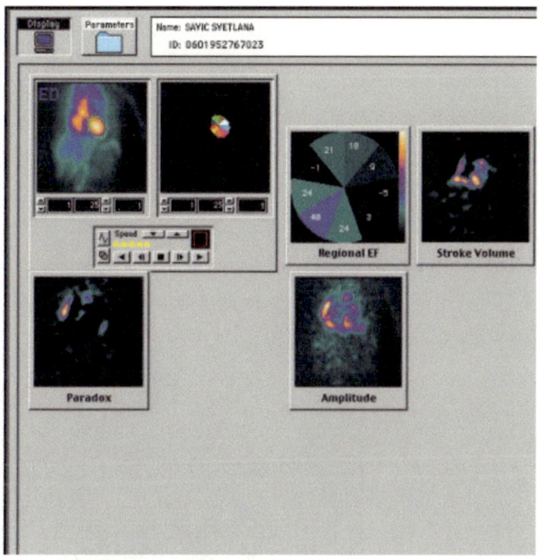

radionuclide ventriculography (RNV) regional ejection fraction

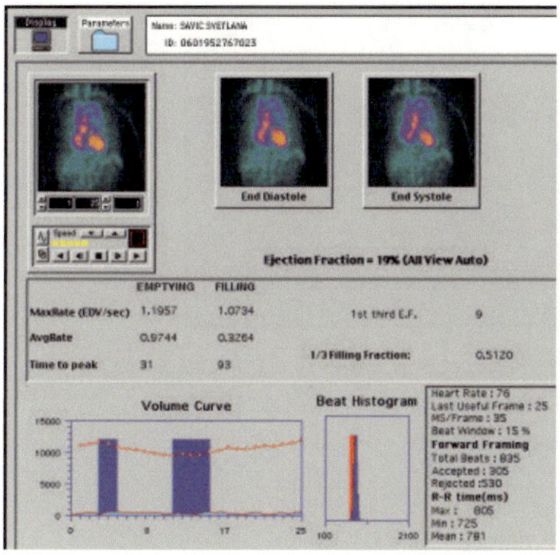

radionuclide ventriculography (RNV) performed 10.12.2009 after therapy

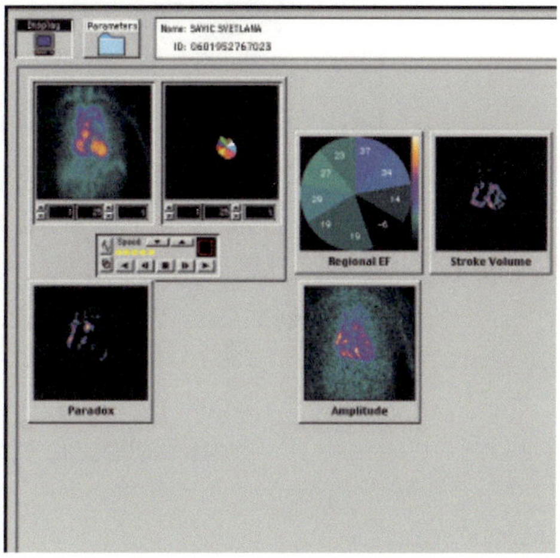

radionuclide ventriculography (RNV) regional ejection fraction

Case report 2. Male with non-ischemic heart failure

SPECT scan performed before HBO = EPO therapy

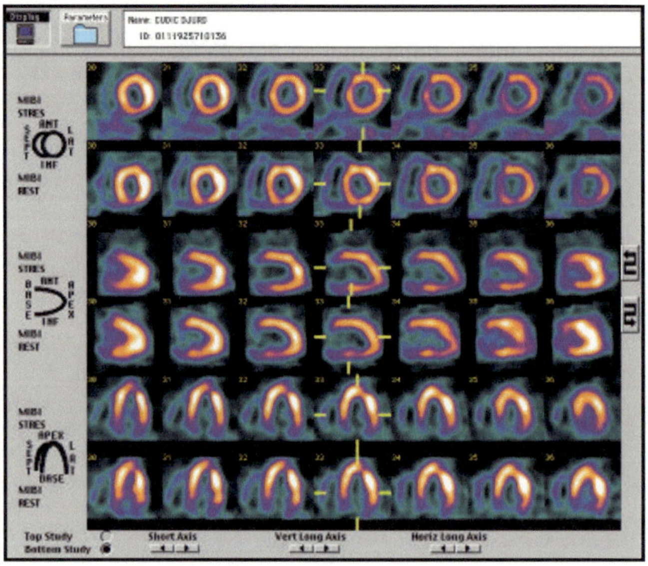

SPECT MPI performed 13.01.2011
Scan pattern - dilatative myocardiopathy
non-ischemic type

Radionuclide venticulography performed before and after HBO = EPO therapy when we seen the greatest increase of LVEF with improve wall motion and regional kinetics

http://dx.doi.org/10.5772/55484

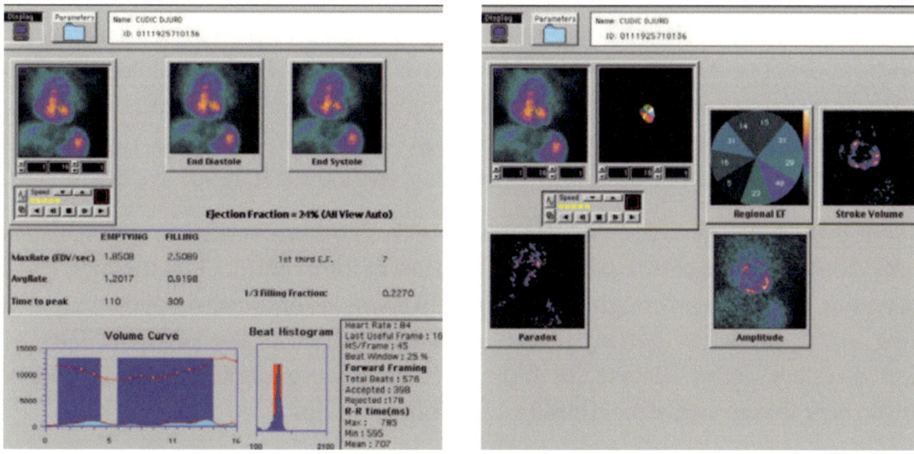

RNV with global and regional ejection fraction performed 01.17. 2011 – before therapy

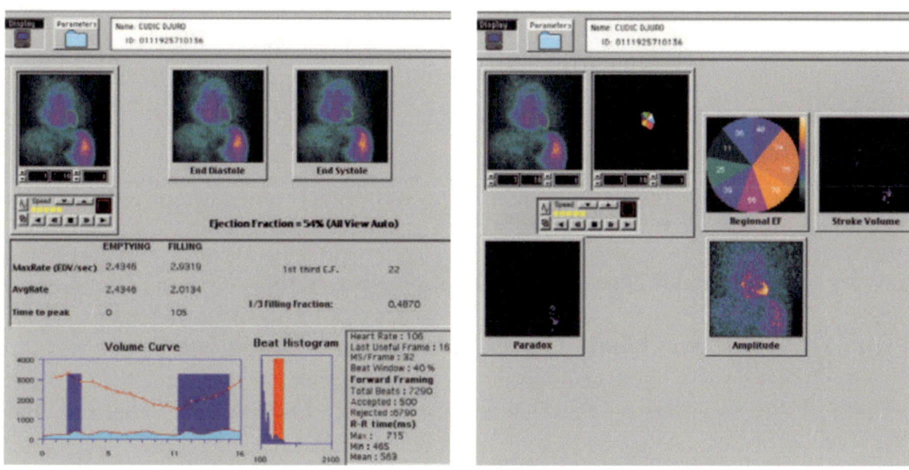

RNV with global and regional ejection fraction performed 03.23. 2011 – after therapy

Summary

The field of cardiovascular imaging is changing. In one hand, myocardial perfusion imaging is a well/established clinical technique for the diagnostic and prognostic workup of coronary artery disease. It has been the mainstay of nuclear cardiology for decades. On the other hand, several alternative imaging methodologies for noninvasive functional assessment of ischemic heart disease have emerged, and noninvasive coronary angiography is becoming a clinical reality. Nuclear imaging technology has progressed significantly toward higher sensitivity and resolution, and novel, highly specific radiotracers have been introduced. These developments are indicator of steady evolution of nuclear cardiology beyond the assessment of myocardial perfusion and toward characterization of biologic events on the tissue level. It is hoped that radiotracers techniques, with their unique translational potential and their superior detection sensitivity, will take a leading role in personalized cardiovascular medicine, in which therapeutic and/or preventive strategies are based on individual disease biology. The value of more specific imaging targets, which are increasingly entering clinical practice. This includes imaging of heart failure, absolute quantification of myocardial blood flow, imaging of myocardial metabolism, and imaging of the cardiac autonomic nervous system.

The goal of this chapter is to provide the reader with a comprehensive overview of the most recent development in nuclear cardiology, in the era of interventional cardiology. It is hoped that the reader, after going through this article, will share the enthusiasm of the author for this discipline, which holds the potential to be a key component in the new paradigm of early detection coronary artery disease for indication for interventional cardiology, as well as assessment new therapeutic effect (HBO + EPO) of heart failure.

Author details

Branislav Baskot[1], Igor Ivanov[2], Dragan Kovacevic[2], Slobodan Obradovic[3], Nenad Ratkovic[3] and Miodrag Zivkovic[4]

1 Private "Clinic Dr Baskot", Belgrade, Serbia

2 Institute for Cardiovascular Disease Sremska Kamenica, Serbia

3 Clinic for Urgent Medicine, Medical Military Academy, Belgrade, Serbia

4 HBO Medical Center, Medical Practice for Hyperbaric Oxygenation Therapy, Belgrade, Serbia

References

[1] ACC/AHA/ASNC Guidelines for the Clinical Use of Cardiac Radionuclide Imaging. A Report of the American College of Cardiology/American Heart Association Task Force on Practice Guidelines (ACC/AHA/ASNC Committee to Revise the 1995 Guidelines for the Clinical Use of cardiac Radionuclide Imaging). Journal of the American Coll Cardiol October. 1. 2003. ACC/AHA/ASNC Practice Guidelines 01–69.

[2] Branislav Baskot: Nuclear cardiology - determination of culprit lesion. Belgrade: Andrejevic foundation; 2006.

[3] Garry V. Heller, Robert C. Hendel: Nuclear Cardiology – practical application 259-71 The McGroaw-Hill Companies, Inc. 2004

[4] Masud H. Khandaker, Tod D. Miller, Panithaya Chateronthaitawee, J. Wells Askew, David O. Hodge, Raymond J. Gibbons: Stress single photon emission computed tomography for detection of coronary artery disease and risk stratification of asymptomatic patients at moderate risk. Journal of Nuclear Cardiology Vol 16, No 4;516-23 July/August 2009

[5] Shaw LJ, Hendel R., Borges-Neto S. Lauer MS: Prognostic value of normal exercise and adenosine (99m) Tc-tetrofosmine SPECT imaging; results from the multicenter registry of 4,728 patients. J Nucl Med 44: 134, 2003

[6] Baskot B, Rafajlovski S, Ristić-Angelkov A, Obradović S, Gligić B, Orozović V, Agbaba N.: Study of efficacy and safety of pharmacological stress tests in nuclear cardiology. Vojnosanit Pregl. 2009 Mar;66(3):193-8. Serbian.

[7] Michael I. Miyamoto, Sharon L. Vernicoto, Haresh Majmundar, Gregory S. Thomas: Pharmacological stress myocardial perfusion imaging: A practical approach. Journal of Nuclear Cardiology 2007; vol 14 No 2, 250-55

[8] Georg A. Beller: Compliance with appropriate use criteria for cardiac radionuclide imaging. Journal of Nuclear Cardiology vol 17; No 2;165-67 March/April 2010

[9] Tim J.F., Johannes C. Kelder, Herbert W.M. Plokker, J. Fred Verzijlbergen, Norbert M. van Hemel: Myocardial perfusion SPECT identifies patients with left bundle branch block patterns at high risk for future cardiac events. Journal of Nuclear Cardiology vol 17; No 2;216-24 March/April 2010

[10] Georg A. Beller; Implications of randomized studies of medical therapy vs revascularization for reducing rising costs of helth care. Journal of Nuclear Cradiology vol 16. No 4;483-85 July/August 2009

[11] American Heart Association Writing Group on Myocardial Segmentation and Registration for Cardiac Imaging. Standardized myocardial segmentation and nomenclature for tomographic imaging of the heart: A statement for healthcare professionals from the Cardiac Imaging Committee of the Council on Clinical Cardiology of the American Heart Association. Circulation 2002; 105:539–42.

[12] Gary V. Heller, Robert C. Hendel.: Nuclear Cardiology Practical Applications. McGraw-Hill medical Publishing divison. The McGraw-Hill Companies, Inc. Copyright 2004; 193-243

[13] Udelson JE., Beshansky JR., Ballin DS.: Myocardial perfusion imaging for evaluation and triage of patients with suspected acute cardiac ischemia: a randomized controlled trial. JAMA 2002; 288:2693-2700

[14] Baskot B., Jankovic Z., Obradovic S., Rusovic S., Orozovic V., Gligic B., Jung R., Ivanovic V., Pavlovic M., Ratkovic N.,: Diagnostic significance of myocardial perfusion scintigraphy in identification and localization of culprit lesions in patients undergoing elective PTCA. VSP vol 65; No 2 (158-62) ; 2008

[15] Leslee J Shaw, Allen Taylor, Paolo Raggi, Daniel S Berman: Role of noninvasive imaging in asymptomatic high/risk patients. J Nucl Cardiol 2006; vol 13 No2(156-62).

[16] AN Clarc, GA Beller: The present role of nuclear cardiology in clinical practice. The quarterly journal of Nuclear Medicine and Molecular Imaging. vol. 49 No 1(43-58) March 2005.

[17] Barry L. Zaret, George A. Beller: Clinical Nuclear Cardiology; state of the art and future directions. Elsevier Mosby. 2005.

[18] Vasken Dilsizian, Jagat Narula; Atlas of Nuclear Cardiology – second edition. Current medicine LLC 2006.

[19] Baskot B, Zivković M, Tepić S, Obradović S.: Evaluation of the therapeutic effect of hyperbaric oxygenation and erithropoietin in the treatment of chronic heart failure using myocardial perfusion scintigraphy G/SPECT. Vojnosanit Pregl. 2009 May;66(5): 399-402.

[20] Zivkovic Miodrag: Guide for Hyperbaric Medicine. Serbian Health Organization, Belgrade, Serbia. - 2010.

[21] Zivkovic M., Todorovic V., Tepic S., Jakovljevic V. Synergistic application of hyperbaric oxygenation therapy and erythropoietin in treatment of ch ronic heart failure. Medical review, No. 1-2, pp. 19/24. Novi Sad Serbia, 2007

Section 3

Invasive Approach and Interventional Cardiology

Chapter 11

Coronary Angiography

Azarisman Mohd Shah

Additional information is available at the end of the chapter

http://dx.doi.org/10.5772/54043

1. Introduction

Our understanding of the concept of cardiac anatomy and physiology has been greatly enhanced in the last 70 years due to tremendous advances in the field of cardiac catheterization. Cardiac catheterization was first performed methodically and with careful application of scientific methods, by Claude Bernard in 1844. He entered both the left and right ventricles of a horse through the retrograde approach via the carotid artery and jugular vein.[1] This led to a period of intense investigation into the cardiac physiology of animals.

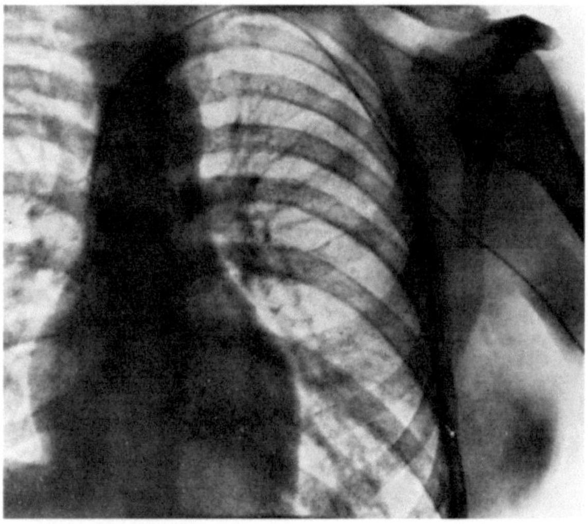

Figure 1. The first fluoroscopic guided view of the right heart catheterization. Klin Wochenschr 1929; 8:2085-87. Springer-Verlag, Berlin, Heidelberg, New York.

The next step into investigating human physiology was aided greatly by Werner Forssmann who performed the first cardiac catheterization on a living person, having passed a 65 cm catheter through his left antecubital vein and into his right atrium under fluoroscopic guidance in 1929 (Figure 1).[2] Further development in selective coronary arteriography was generated by Sones and others by 1959 with greater emphasis on better catheterization techniques, improved radiographic images and less toxic radio-contrast agents. Cumulatively, these developments led to marked improvement in the adoption of cardiac catheterization as an important diagnostic tool.

Andreas Grüntzig then heralded the next great step in cardiac catheterization when he introduced balloon angioplasty of the coronary arteries in 1977.[3-5] This led to the mushrooming of cardiac catheterization into the new field of interventional cardiology with ever expanding indications and improved results.[6]

2. Coronary angiographic views

Accurate diagnosis of a coronary stenosis is dependent on acquiring multiple views to enable accurate visualization of all the coronary segments without foreshortening or overlap. This is achieved by maneuvering the image intensifier into the right and left anterior oblique planes and either the cranial or caudal projections as is seen in Figures 2 and 3 below.

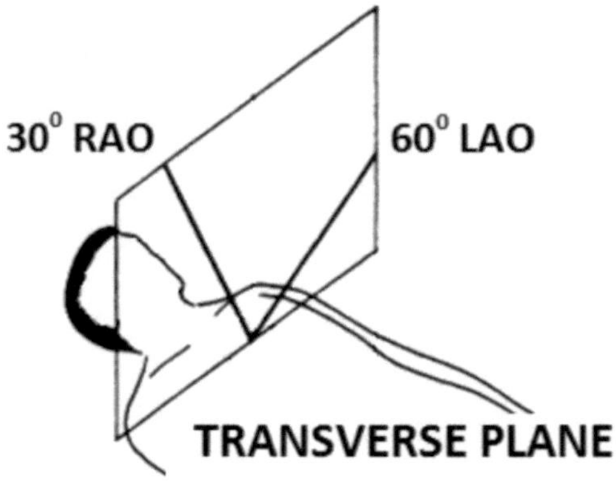

Figure 2. The right and left anterior oblique planes corresponding to the planes of the AV valves and the interventricular septum respectively.

http://dx.doi.org/10.5772/54043

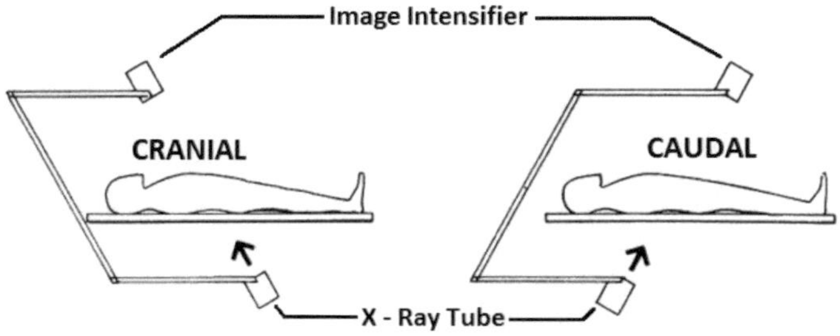

Figure 3. The cranial and caudal projections which when combined with the oblique planes, ensures the capture of most normal segments.

3. Viewing the LAD and LCx

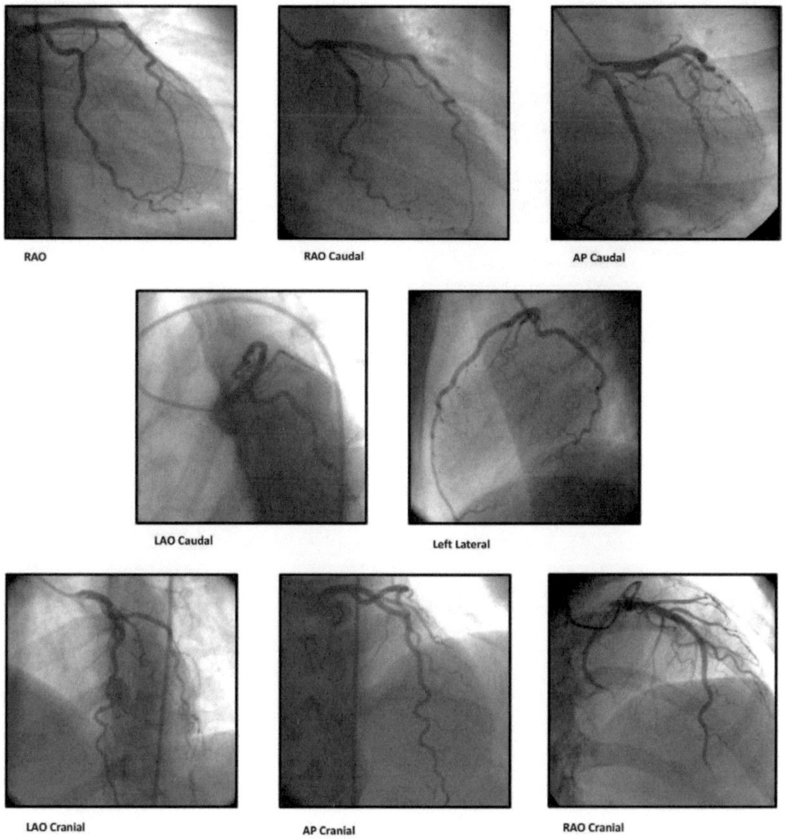

Figure 4.

4. Viewing the RCA

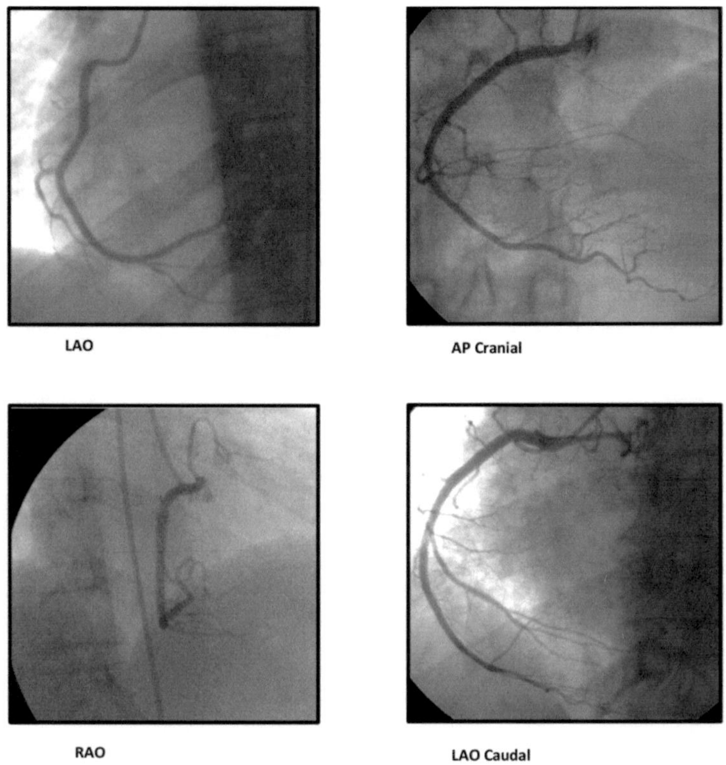

Figure 5.

Author details

Azarisman Mohd Shah

Department of Internal Medicine, Faculty of Medicine, International Islamic University Malaysia, Pahang, Malaysia

References

[1] Cournand A. Cardiac catheterization; development of the technique, its contributions to experimental medicine, and its initial applications in man. Acta Med Scand Suppl. 1975; 579:3-32

http://dx.doi.org/10.5772/54043

[2] Forssmann W. Die Sondierung des rechten Herzens [Probing of the right heart]. Klin Wochenschr 1929; 8:2085-87

[3] Sones FM, Shirley EK, Proudfit WL, Wescott RN. Cine coronary arteriography. Circulation 1959; 20:773 (abstract)

[4] Ryan TJ. The coronary angiogram and its seminal contribution to cardiovascular medicine over five decades. Circulation 2002; 106: 752–56

[5] Grüntzig A, et al. Coronary transluminal angioplasty. Circulation 1977; 56(II):319 (abstract)

[6] King SB 3rd. The development of interventional cardiology. J Am Coll Cardiol 1998; 15:31(4 Suppl B):64B-88B

Chapter 12

Coronary Angiography (IJECCE)

Chiu-Lung Wu and Chi-Wen Juan

Additional information is available at the end of the chapter

http://dx.doi.org/10.5772/54080

1. Introduction

The ACC/AHA Task Force on Practice Guidelines herein revises and updates the original "Guidelines for Coronary Angiography," published in 1987 The frequent and still-growing use of coronary angiography, its relatively high costs, its inherent risks and the ongoing evolution of its indications have given this revision urgency and priority.

The expert committee appointed included private practitioners and academicians. Committee members were selected to represent both experts in coronary angiography and senior clinician consultants. Representatives from the family practice and internal medicine professions were also included on the committee [1].

1.1. Definitions

Coronary angiography is defined as the radiographic visualization of the coronary vessels after the injection of radiopaque contrast media. The radiographic images are permanently recorded for future review with either 35 mm cine film or digital recording. Percutaneous or cutdown techniques, usually from the femoral or brachial artery, are used for insertion of special intravascular catheters. Coronary angiography further requires selective cannulation of the ostium of the left and right coronary arteries and, if present, each saphenous vein graft or internal mammary artery graft to obtain optimal selective contrast injection and imaging. Numerous specialized catheters have been designed for this purpose. Physicians performing these procedures must be technically proficient in all aspects of the procedure and have a complete understanding of the clinical indications and risks of the procedure and of coronary anatomy, physiology and pathology. It is also important that these physicians understand the fundamentals of optimal radiographic imaging and radiation safety. Coronary angiography is usually performed as part of cardiac catheterization, which may also involve angiography of other vessels or cardiac chambers, and hemodynamic assessment as needed for a complete invasive diagnostic evaluation of the individual patient's cardiovascular condition[2,3].

1.2. Purpose

The purpose of coronary angiography is to define coronary anatomy and the degree of luminal obstruction of the coronary arteries. Information obtained from the procedure includes identification of the location, length, diameter, and contour of the coronary arteries; the presence and severity of coronary luminal obstruction(s); characterization of the nature of the obstruction (including the presence of atheroma, thrombus, dissection, spasm, or myocardial bridging), and an assessment of blood flow. In addition, the presence and extent of coronary collateral vessels can be assessed.

Coronary angiography remains the standard for assessment of anatomic coronary disease, because no other currently available test can accurately define the extent of coronary luminal obstruction. Because the technique can only provide information about abnormalities that narrow the lumen, it is limited in its ability to accurately define the etiology of the obstruction or detect the presence of nonobstructive atherosclerotic disease.A coronary angiography, which can help diagnose heart conditions, is the most common type of heart catheter procedure. [2,3]

2. Coronary angiography for specific conditions

2.1. General considerations

Coronary atherosclerosis is a slowly progressive process that can be clinically inapparent for long periods of time [78–80]. Coronary disease often becomes clinically evident because of the occurrence of symptoms, such as angina or those associated with MI. Patients with known CAD are those in whom the disease has been documented by either angiography or MI. "Suspected coronary disease" means that a patient's symptoms or other clinical characteristics suggest a high likelihood for significant CAD and its related adverse outcomes but that evidence of CAD has not yet been documented as defined above.

Patients may develop symptoms at one point in time but may become asymptomatic thereafter as the result of a change in the disease or as the result of therapy. For instance, many patients are symptomatic after an uncomplicated MI, as are patients with mild angina, who can be rendered asymptomatic by medications. The severity of clinical presentations and the degree of provocable ischemia on noninvasive testing are the principal factors used in determining the appropriateness of coronary angiography.

2.2. Stable angina

Patients with CAD may become symptomatic in many different ways but most commonly develop angina pectoris. In this document, angina pectoris (or simply angina) means a chest

http://dx.doi.org/10.5772/54080

discomfort due to myocardial ischemia, often described as a transient squeezing, pressure-like precordial discomfort. Angina is generally provoked by physical effort (particularly during the postprandial state), with exposure to cold environment or by emotional stress. The discomfort on effort is relieved by rest, its duration being a matter of minutes. The ease of provocation, frequency and duration of episodes may remain relatively unchanged in individuals for extended time periods, leading to the term "stable angina pectoris."

Recommendations for Coronary Angiography in Patients With Nonspecific Chest Pain Class I

High-risk findings on noninvasive testing. *(Level of Evidence: B)*

Class IIa: None.

Class IIb:

Patients with recurrent hospitalizations for chest pain who have abnormal (but not high-risk) or equivocal findings on noninvasive testing. *(Level of Evidence: B)*

Class III:

All other patients with nonspecific chest pain. *(Level of Evidence: C)*

2.3. Unstable angina

The acute coronary syndromes include unstable angina, non–Q-wave MI, and acute Q-wave MI. The diagnosis of unstable angina has been complicated by a broad range of presentations that can vary between atypical chest pain and acute MI. An expert panel of clinicians attempted to clarify the definition of unstable angina in the recently published "Clinical Practice Guideline for Unstable Angina"[129,130]. Three possible presentations are described:

- Symptoms of angina at rest (usually prolonged 20 minutes);
- New-onset (<2 months) exertional angina of at least CCS class III in severity;
- Recent (<2 months) acceleration of angina as reflected by an increase in severity of at least one CCS class to at least CCS class III.[4,5]

Variant angina, non–Q-wave MI and recurrent angina24 hours after MI are considered part of the spectrum of unstable angina. However, in this document, non–Q-wave MI is discussed in the section on acute MI. [4,5]

Recommendations for Coronary Angiography in Patients With Postrevascularization Ischemia

Class I

1. Suspected abrupt closure or subacute stent thrombosis after percutaneous revascularization. *(Level of Evidence: B)*

2. Recurrent angina or high-risk criteria on noninvasive evaluation (Table 5) within nine months of percutaneous revascularization. *(Level of Evidence: C)*

Class IIa

1. Recurrent symptomatic ischemia within 12 months of CABG. (Level of Evidence: B)

2. Noninvasive evidence of high-risk criteria occurring at any time postoperatively. (Level of Evidence:B)

3. Recurrent angina inadequately controlled by medical means after revascularization. (Level of Evidence: C)

Class IIb

1. Asymptomatic post-PTCA patient suspected of having restenosis within the first months after angioplasty because of an abnormal noninvasive test but without noninvasive high-risk criteria. *(Level of Evidence: B)*

2. Recurrent angina without high-risk criteria on noninvasive testing occurring >1 year postoperatively. *(Level of Evidence: C)*

3. Asymptomatic postbypass patient in whom a deterioration in serial noninvasive testing has been documented but who is not high risk on noninvasive testing. *(Level of Evidence: C)*

Class III

1. Symptoms in a postbypass patient who is not a candidate for repeat revascularization. *(Level of Evidence: C)*

2. Routine angiography in asymptomatic patients after PTCA or other surgery, unless as part of an approved research protocol. *(Level of Evidence: C)*

Coronary angiography during the initial management of patients in the emergency department

Patients Presenting With Suspected MI and ST- segment Elevation or Bundle-Branch Block Of all patients who ultimately are diagnosed with acute MI, those resenting with ST-segment elevation have been studied most extensively. Patients with ST-segment elevation have a high likelihood of thrombus occluding the infarct-related artery [6,7]. Considerable data exist showing that coronary reperfusion can be accomplished either by intravenous thrombolytic therapy or direct mechanical intervention within the infarct-related artery. Because the benefit obtained is directly linked to the time required to reestablish normal distal blood flow [8–10], rapid triage decisions are mandatory, and delays in instituting reperfusion therapy must be minimized. The "ACC/AHA Guidelines for the Management of Patients with Acute Myocardial Infarction" provide a comprehensive discussion of the indications, contraindications, advantages, and disadvantages of thrombolytic therapy and direct coronary angioplasty [11]. Although it is not the purpose of these guidelines to re-ex-

http://dx.doi.org/10.5772/54080

amine in detail the merits of these two reperfusion strategies, this is a rapidly evolving area, and some new information exists.

Recommendations for coronary angiography during the initial management of acute MI (MI suspected and ST-segment elevation or bundle-branch block present)

Coronary angiography coupled with the intent to perform primary PTCA

Class I

1. As an alternative to thrombolytic therapy in patients who can undergo angioplasty of the infarct artery within 12 hours of the onset of symptoms or beyond 12 hours if ischemic symptoms persist.
2. In patients who are within 36 hours of an acute ST elevation/Q-wave or new LBBB MI who develop cardiogenic shock, are less than 75 years of age and revascularization can be performed within 18 hours of the onset of shock

Class IIa

1. As a reperfusion strategy in patients who are candidates for reperfusion but who have a contraindication to fibrinolytic therapy, if angioplasty can be performed as outlined above in class I. (Level of Evidence: C)

Class III

1. In patients who are beyond 12 hours from onset of symptoms and who have no evidence of myocardial ischemia. (Level of Evidence: A)
2. In patients who are eligible for thrombolytic therapy and are undergoing primary angioplasty by an unskilled operator in a laboratory that does not have surgical capability. (Level of Evidence: B)

Recommendations for early coronary angiography in the patient with suspected MI (ST-segment elevation or BBB present) who has not undergone primary PTCA

Class I: None.

Class IIa: Cardiogenic shock or persistent hemodynamic instability.*(Level of Evidence: B)*

Class IIb:

1. Evolving large or anterior infarction after Thrombolytic treatment when it is believed that reperfusion has not occurred and rescue PTCA is planned. (Level of Evidence: B)
2. Marginal hemodynamic status but not actual cardiogenic shock.(Level of Evidence: C)

Class III

1. In patients who have received thrombolytic therapy and have no symptoms of ischemia. *(Level of Evidence:A)*
2. Routine use of angiography and subsequent PTCA within 24 hours of administration of thrombolytic agents. *(Level of Evidence: A)*

Recommendations for early coronary angiography in acute MI (MI suspected but no st-segment elevation)

Class I

1. Persistent or recurrent (stuttering) episodes of symptomatic ischemia, spontaneous or induced, with or without associated ECG changes. (Level of Evidence:A)
2. The presence of shock, severe pulmonary congestion,or continuing hypotension. (Level of Evidence: B)

Class II: None.

Class III: None.

Hospital-management phase of acute MI

The hospital-management phase of acute MI can encompass several clinical situations. Some patients with acute MI present too late in their course to be candidates for reperfusion therapy, and in others, the occurrence of infarction may not be appreciated at he time of presentation. These groups skip the acute-treatment phase of MI and enter the hospital-management phase directly. During the hospital management phase, the actions of the clinician are driven by the consequences of the infarction, such as congestive heart failure, hemodynamic instability, recurrent ischemia or arrhythmias. Although it is still convenient to divide patients into those with Q-wave and non–Q-wave infarctions, some indications for coronary angiography are common to all patients with MI regardless of how they have been treated initially and whether or not Q waves ultimately develop.

Recommendations for use of coronary angiography in patients with valvular heart disease Class I

1. Before valve surgery or balloon valvotomy in an adult with chest discomfort, ischemia by noninvasive imaging, or both. (Level of Evidence: B)
2. Before valve surgery in an adult free of chest pain but with multiple risk factors for coronary disease. (Level of Evidence: C)
3. Infective endocarditis with evidence of coronary embolization. (Level of Evidence: C)

Class IIa

None.

Class IIb

During left-heart catheterization performed for hemodynamic evaluation before aortic or mitral valve surgery in patients without preexisting evidence of coronary disease, multiple CAD risk factors or advanced age. (Level of Evidence: C)

Class III

1. Before cardiac surgery for infective endocarditis when there are no risk factors for coronary disease and no evidence of coronary embolization. (Level of Evidence: C)

http://dx.doi.org/10.5772/54080

2. In asymptomatic patients when cardiac surgery is not being considered. (Level of Evidence: C)

3. Before cardiac surgery when preoperative hemodynamic assessment by catheterization is unnecessary, and there is neither preexisting evidence for coronary disease, nor risk factors for CAD. (Level of Evidence: C)

Congenital heart disease

Although there are no large trials to support its use, coronary angiography is performed in congenital heart disease for two broad categorical indications. The first indication is to assess the hemodynamic impact of congenital coronary lesions (375). The second is to assess the presence of coronary anomalies, which by themselves may be innocent but whose presence, if unrecognized, may lead to coronary injury during the correction of other congenital heart lesions. Congenital anomalies with hemodynamic significance include congenital coronary artery stenosis or atresia, coronary artery fistula [11], anomalous left coronary artery arising from the pulmonary artery [12], and anomalous left coronary artery arising from the right coronary artery or right sinus of Valsalva and passing between the aorta and right ventricular outflow tract [13]. Patients with congenital coronary stenosis may present with angina or unexplained sudden death in childhood, whereas patients whose left coronary passes between the pulmonary artery and aorta often have the same symptoms later in life. Patients with a coronary arteriovenous fistula often present with a continuous murmur or may have unexplained angina or congestive heart failure. Anomalous origin of the left coronary artery from the pulmonary artery should be suspected when there is unexplained MI or heart failure in early childhood. Other coronary anomalies of position or origin may cause no physiologic abnormality by themselves. Some, such as origin of the circumflex artery from the right sinus of Valsalva, are not associated with other congenital anomalies and present only as incidental findings and are significant only because they complicate the performance and interpretation of coronary angiograms.

Recommendations for use of coronary angiography in patients with congenital heart disease

Class I

1. Before surgical correction of congenital heart disease when chest discomfort or noninvasive evidence is suggestive of associated CAD. (Level of Evidence: C)

2. Before surgical correction of suspected congenital coronary anomalies such as congenital coronary artery stenosis, coronary arteriovenous fistula and anomalous origin of left coronary artery. (Level of Evidence: C)

3. Forms of congenital heart disease frequently associated with coronary artery anomalies that may complicate surgical management. (Level of Evidence: C)

4. Unexplained cardiac arrest in a young patient. (Level of Evidence: B)

Class IIa

Before corrective open heart surgery for congenital heart disease in an adult whose risk profile increases the likelihood of coexisting coronary disease. (Level of Evidence: C)

Class IIb

During left-heart catheterization for hemodynamic assessment of congenital heart disease in an adult in whom the risk of coronary disease is not high. (Level of Evidence: C)

Class III

In the routine evaluation of congenital heart disease in asymptomatic patients for whom heart surgery is not planned. (Level of Evidence: C)

Congestive heart failure

1. Systolic dysfunction

Although it was once believed that myocardial ischemia was either short-lived and resulted in little or no muscle dysfunction or resulted in infarction with permanent damage, it is now clear that a middle state may exist in which chronic ischemic nonfunctioning myocardium is present, to which function may return after myocardial revascularizations [15,16]. This intermediate state has been termed "myocardial hibernation." Although most cases of myocardial dysfunction resulting from CAD are probably irreversible when due to infarction and subsequent deleterious ventricular remodeling (ischemic cardiomyopathy) [17], some patients with hibernating myocardium have been shown to experience a doubling of resting ejection fraction with resolution of congestive heart failure after coronary revascularization [18,19]. However, in most cases of hibernation, a more modest improvement in ejection fraction of 5% occurs after revascularization [20].

2. Diastolic dysfunction

Isolated diastolic dysfunction is the cause of heart failure in 10% to 30% of affected patients. This disorder is common in older patients with hypertension and often is suspected because of echocardiographically detected concentric left ventricular hypertrophy, normal systolic function and abnormal transmitral flow velocity patterns [21]. However, in some patients with normal systolic function, the abrupt onset of pulmonary edema raises the suspicion that transient ischemia was the cause of decompensation, because elderly patients with hypertension have, by definition, at least two risk factors for coronary disease. In these patients, who are often too ill to undergo stress testing, coronary angiography may be necessary to establish or rule out the diagnosis of ischemically related diastolic dysfunction and heart failure.

Recommendations for use of coronary angiography in patients with congestive heart failure

Class I

1. Congestive heart failure due to systolic dysfunction with angina or with regional wall motion abnormalities and/or scintigraphic evidence of reversible myocardial ischemia when revascularization is being considered. (Level of Evidence: B)

http://dx.doi.org/10.5772/54080

2. Before cardiac transplantation. (Level of Evidence: C)

3. Congestive heart failure secondary to postinfarction ventricular aneurysm or other mechanical complications of MI. (Level of Evidence: C)

Class IIa

1. Systolic dysfunction with unexplained cause despite noninvasive testing. (Level of Evidence: C)

2. Normal systolic function, but episodic heart failure raises suspicion of ischemically mediated left ventricular dysfunction. (Level of Evidence: C)

Class III

Congestive heart failure with previous coronary angiograms showing normal coronary arteries, with no new evidence to suggest ischemic heart disease. (Level of Evidence: C)

1. Aortic dissection

The need for coronary angiography before surgical treatment for aortic dissection remains controversial because there are no large trials to support its use. In young patients with dissection due to Marfan syndrome or in dissection in peripartum females, coronary angiography is unnecessary unless there is suspicion that the dissection has affected one or both coronary ostia. In older patients, in whom dissection is usually related to hypertension, coronary angiography is often necessary, especially if patients are suspected of having coronary disease because of a history of angina or objective evidence of myocardial ischemia. In patients who have no history of coronary disease, the indications for coronary angiography are much less certain. Because of the high incidence of coronary disease in older patients with dissection, some studies have advocated routine coronary angiography [22], whereas others have found increased mortality when angiography is performed [23].

2. Hypertrophic cardiomyopathy

Significant CAD due to atherosclerosis is found in 25% of patients aged >45 years with hypertrophic cardiomyopathy [26]. Because symptoms due to CAD and hypertrophic cardiomyopathy are similar, patients with ischemic symptoms not well controlled with medical therapy may require coronary angiography to resolve the cause of chest pain. Coronary angiography also is indicated in patients with chest discomfort and hypertrophic cardiomyopathy in whom a surgical procedure is planned to correct outflow tract obstruction.

3. Arteritis

Some patients with inflammatory processes affecting the aorta, such as Takayasu arteritis, may have coronary artery involvement requiring coronary artery revascularization. In such patients, coronary angiography is required before the surgical procedure. Kawasaki disease can result in coronary artery aneurysm and coronary artery stenosis producing myocardial ischemia or silent occlusion and may require coronary angiographic assessment [24,25].

4. Chest trauma

Patients who have an acute MI shortly after blunt or penetrating chest trauma may have atherosclerotic CAD, but coronary artery obstruction or damage has been reported in the absence of coronary atherosclerosis [27]. Furthermore, myocardial contusion may simulate acute MI. Infrequently, coronary angiography is indicated in the management of such patients.

Recommendations for use of coronary angiography in other conditions

Class I

1. Diseases affecting the aorta when knowledge of the presence or extent of coronary artery involvement is necessary for management (e.g., aortic dissection or aneurysm with known coronary disease). (Level of Evidence: B)
2. Hypertrophic cardiomyopathy with angina despite medical therapy when knowledge of coronary anatomy might affect therapy. (Level of Evidence: C)
3. Hypertrophic cardiomyopathy with angina when heart surgery is planned. (Level of Evidence: B)

Class IIa

1. High risk for coronary disease when other cardiac surgical procedures are planned (e.g., pericardiectomy or removal of chronic pulmonary emboli). (Level of Evidence: C)
2. Prospective immediate cardiac transplant donors whose risk profile increases the likelihood of coronary disease. (Level of Evidence: B)
3. Asymptomatic patients with Kawasaki disease who have coronary artery aneurysms on echocardiography. (Level of Evidence: B)
4. Before surgery for aortic aneurysm/dissection in patients without known coronary disease.
5. Recent blunt chest trauma and suspicion of acute MI, without evidence of preexisting CAD. (Level of Evidence: C)

3. Special considerations regarding coronary angiography

3.1. Accuracy

Cineangiographic images of coronary arteries have been the principal clinical tool for determining the severity of coronary luminal stenosis. Modern angiographic equipment has a resolution of four to five line pairs per millimeter with a six-inch field of view, the usual image magnification for coronary angiography [28]. Validation studies that use known phantoms show a high correlation between actual size and that measured by quantitative coronary angiography (QCA) ($r = 0.95$) [29–32]. The resolution of these phantom studies indicates the precision of coronary angiography to be 0.02 to 0.04 mm. Factors that limit resolution in the clinical setting include grainy films from "quantum mottling" and motion artifact that, in a clinical setting, limit resolution to 0.2 mm, far less than that realized from static images of known phantoms. Other factors, such as angulation, overlap of vessels and image tube resolution can also influence accuracy in the clinical setting. Nevertheless, the accuracy of coronary angiography does allow for anatomic detail that is not obtainable by current noninvasive or other invasive technology. Only intravascular ultrasound, which is discussed in Appendix C, has an image resolution greater than that of coronary angiography. However, intravascular ultrasound cannot visualize the entire coronary tree nor define the anatomic course of the coronary vessels. It is also limited by shadowing from heavy calcification and by its inability to image very small vessels or very severe stenosis.

3.2. Digital imaging of coronary angiography

Recent advances in computer storage technology have made feasible digital acquisition, processing and archival storage of angiographic images obtained during cardiac catheterization. Widespread conversion from cineangiographic film to digital archiving and storage is anticipated during the next decade. Analog storage technologies such as super VHS videotape and analog optical disks have inadequate resolution to faithfully record coronary angiography. Digital storage methods are generally adequate but until recently have lacked standardization, which precluded easy exchange of digital angiograms between centers with different equipment. The development of the Digital Imaging and Communication standard (DICOM) for cardiac angiography ensures compatibility between equipment from participating vendors.

In the interventional era, the advantages of digital angiography are important. The image quality provided by digital angiography is better than any common videotape format. Improvements in computer speed and processing capability enable rapid replay of coronary injection sequences, as well as evaluation of the results of each intervention and identification of complications such as intraluminal thrombus and dissection. In many laboratories, the availability of high-quality images during catheterization permits diagnostic and therapeutic catheterization to consist of a single procedure, a capability with significant implications for the cost of interventional procedures. Industry sources now estimate that >75% of existing laboratories are equipped with digital imaging capability.

The ACC Cardiac Catheterization Committee is coordinating efforts to develop and promote a standard for archival storage and exchange of digital cardiac angiography. The committee has joined in this common cause with an industry organization, the National Electrical Manufacturers Association (NEMA), and representatives of the American College of Radiology (ACR). The ACR and NEMA have recently released an interim standard known as Digital Imaging Communication in Medicine (DICOM version 3.0).

The initial efforts of the standards committee have focused on adoption of a file format and physical medium for interchange of digital angiographic studies. To transfer images between medical centers, the sender would generate a DICOM-compatible file for review by the receiver. Recently, this working group has chosen a recordable form of the common CD-

ROM, termed CD-R, as the official exchange medium. Nearly all equipment vendors have announced support for this format.

3.3. Reproducibility

In clinical practice, the degree of coronary artery obstruction is commonly expressed as the percent diameter stenosis. This is done by comparing the diameter of the site of greatest narrowing (minimal lumen diameter) to an adjacent segment assumed to be free of disease. In clinical practice, the most common method used to estimate the percent diameter narrowing is subjective visual assessment. Because vasomotor tone can alter the reference diameter, nitroglycerin is frequently administered before angiography to improve the reproducibility of the measurement. Several studies have shown that measurement of the degree and extent of luminal narrowing correlates with symptoms as well as with assessments of coronary flow reserve (CFR) and abnormalities on treadmill exercise testing, perfusion imaging with Tl or sestamibi, stress echocardiography and fast computerized tomography [33– 37]. In addition, the percent diameter reduction and the number of stenosis of >50% to 70% correlate with long-term outcome [33–37].

3.4. Limitations

Although coronary angiography is considered the reference standard for anatomic assessment of coronary obstructions, there are limitations to the technique. When luminal narrowings are present on coronary angiography (in the absence of spasm), pathological analyses almost always demonstrate severe atherosclerotic obstruction. Even minor angiographic abnormalities are associated with a poorer long-term outcome than are completely normal appearing angiograms. Coronary angiography has a high predictive value for the presence of CAD when abnormalities are present. However, the converse is not true. A normal coronary angiogram does not exclude atherosclerosis, and in fact, most pathological studies suggest that angiography grossly underestimates the extent and severity of atherosclerosis [38–42]. Several factors contribute to this discrepancy.

First, angiography depicts coronary anatomy from a planar two-dimensional silhouette of the contrast-filled vessel lumen. However, coronary lesions are often geometrically complex, with an eccentric luminal shape such that one angle of view may misrepresent the extent of narrowing [39]. Two orthogonal angiograms should demonstrate more correctly the severity of most lesions, but adequate orthogonal views are frequently unobtainable because the stenosis may be obscured by overlapping side branches, disease at bifurcation sites, diographic foreshortening or tortuosity. This can be especially difficult in the left main coronary artery, where identifying a significant stenosis is of utmost clinical importance [43].

Second, an adaptive phenomenon, coronary remodeling," contributes to the inability of coronary angiography to identify mild atherosclerosis [44]. Remodeling was initially observed on histology as the outward displacement of the external vessel wall in vascular segments with significant atherosclerosis. In the early phases of atherosclerosis, this vessel enlargement "compensates" for luminal encroachment, thereby concealing the atheroma from the angiogram. When the atherosclerotic plaque becomes severe, luminal encroachment becomes evident. Although such mild lesions do not restrict blood flow, clinical studies have demonstrated that these minimal or even unseen angiographic lesions represent an important predisposing cause of acute coronary syndromes, including MI [55].

Third, assessment of luminal diameter narrowing is complicated by the frequent absence of a normal reference segment[56]. Angiography visualizes only the lumen of the vessel and cannot determine if the wall of the reference segment has atherosclerosis [38–42]. In the presence of diffuse reference segment disease, percent stenosis will predictably underestimate the true amount of diameter narrowing.

Finally, in the setting of percutaneous intervention, the assumptions underlying simple projection imaging of the lumen are further impaired. Necropsy studies and intravascular ultrasound demonstrate that most mechanical coronary interventions exaggerate the extent of luminal eccentricity by fracturing or dissecting the atheroma within the lesion [45– 49]. The angiographic appearance of the postintervention vessel often consists of an enlarged, although frequently "hazy" lumen [46]. In this setting, the lumen size on angiography may overestimate the vessel cross-sectional area and misrepresent the actual gain in lumen size.

Experimental and clinical studies have shown that when percent stenosis is >50%, the ability to increase blood flow in response to metabolic demands is impaired [50]. This augmentation of coronary blood flow to demand is termed the coronary flow reserve. Determination of CFR requires measurement of blood flow at rest and after induction of reactive hyperemia, usually by administration of a coronary vasodilator. Several methods for measurement of CFR in patients have been developed, including intracoronary Doppler flow probes, digital angiography and quantitative PET [51– 54].

Coronary collaterals can provide significant additional blood flow to territories served by stenotic vessels [58]. In general, collaterals are not evident unless resting ischemia is present, such as that which occurs with a stenosis.90%. In many patients, collateral flow merely restores normal resting blood flow but does not provide adequate flow when metabolic demand increases. The presence of collaterals, however, is associated with preservation of myocardial function after MI, reduced myocardial ischemia on noninvasive stress testing, and reduced ischemia during angioplasty [59,60]. Paradoxically, a greater ischemic response on noninvasive functional testing with adenosine than with exercise has been reported in the presence of collaterals, presumably due to an increase in the coronary steal phenomenon [61]. Collateral blood flow can only be semiquantified by angiography [62], and precise assessment of perfusion by angiography is poor. This inability to adequately measure collateral flow is one of the factors that prevent accurate assessment of the functional significance of coronary stenosis by angiography alone [57].

3.5. Contrast agents

For an understanding of the pharmacologic properties and adverse effects of contrast agents, the reader is referred to the 1993 review of the subject by the ACC Cardiovascular Imaging Committee [63] and the 1996 review by Hirshfeld [64].

Except for a less potent anticoagulant effect, nonionic agents are better tolerated and have fewer side effects than ionic agents [63]. Several randomized trials have compared their use during cardiac angiography. Barrett et al. [65] compared a nonionic low-osmolar contrast agent with an ionic high-osmolar contrast agent. Although adverse events were reduced, severe reactions were confined to patients with underlying severe cardiac disease. These authors supported the use of nonionic low-osmolar agents in these high-risk patients. Steinberg et al. [66]

The difference in the incidence of any major contrast reaction is proportional to the New York Heart Association clinical function class, rising from 0.5% for class I patients to 3.6% for class IV patients [68]. Given these observations, it has been suggested that nonionic agents should be reserved for patients who are at high risk for adverse reactions and that ionic agents should be used for all other patients [64].

Factors that have been associated with high risk of adverse reactions to contrast media include prior adverse reaction to contrast agents, age >65 years, New York Heart Association functional class IV (or hemodynamic evidence of congestive heart failure), impaired renal function (creatinine >2.0 mg/dL), acute coronary syndromes (unstable angina or acute MI) and severe valvular disease (aortic valve area <0.7 cm^2 or mitral valve area <1.25 cm^2) [64]. It is recommended that the individual practitioner appropriately assess the cost and benefit relationship when selecting contrast agents in any individual patient and that a strategy of reserving nonionic agents for patients who are at high risk of adverse reactions is prudent and cost-effective.[69]

ACC/AHA classifications of class I, II, and III. These classes summarize the indications for coronary angiography as follows:

Class I: Conditions for which there is evidence and/or general agreement that this procedure is useful and effective.

Class II: Conditions for which there is conflicting evidence and/or a divergence of opinion about the usefulness/efficacy of performing the procedure. *Class IIa:* Weight of evidence/opinion is in favor of usefulness/ efficacy. *Class IIb:* Usefulness/efficacy is less well established by evidence/opinion. *Class III:* Conditions for which there is evidence and/or general agreement that the procedure is not useful/effective and in some cases may be harmful.[70,71]

Coronary angiography indications

- Unstable angina or Chest pain [uncontrolled with medications or after a heart attack]
- Heart attack
- Aortic Stenosis
- Before a bypass surgery
- Abnormal treadmill test results
- Determine the extent of coronary artery disease

http://dx.doi.org/10.5772/54080

- Disease of the heart valve causing symptoms (syncope, shortness of breath)
- To monitor rejection in heart transplant patients
- Syncope or loss of consciousness in patients with aortic valve disease
- Pain in the Jaw,Neck or Arm

Risks

- Generally the risk of serious complications ranges from 1 in 1,000 to 1 in 500. Risks of the procedure include the following :
- Stroke
- Heart attack
- Irregular heart beats
- Low blood pressure
- Injury to the coronary artery
- Allergic reaction to contrast dye[3]

Rare risks and complications include:

- Need for emergency heart surgery or angioplasty.
- A stroke.
- Heart attack.
- Surgical repair of the groin/arm puncture site or blood vessel.
- Abnormal heart rhythm that continues for a long time. This may need an electric shock to correct.
- An allergic reaction to the x-ray dye.[2]

Other, less common complications include:

- Arrhythmias. These irregular heartbeats often go away on their own. However, your doctor may recommend treatment if they persist.
- Kidney damage caused by the dye that's used during the test.
- Blood clots that can trigger a stroke,heart stroke, or other serious problems.
- Low blood pressure.[2]

Coronary angiography contraindications

- Fever
- Kidney failure or dysfunction
- Problems with blood coagulation (Coagulopathy)

- Active systemic infection
- Uncontrolled Blood Pressure (Hypertension)
- Allergy to contrast (dye) medium
- Transient Ischemic attack
- Severe anemia
- Electrolyte imbalance
- Uncontrolled rhythm disturbances (arrhythmias)
- Uncompensated heart failure[4]

Author details

Chiu-Lung Wu[1] and Chi-Wen Juan[1,2]

*Address all correspondence to: juanchiwen@yahoo.com.tw

1 Department of Emergency Medicine, Kuang Tien General Hospital, Sha-Lu,Taichung, Taiwan, R.O.C.

2 Department of Nursing,Hungkuang University, Taichung, Taiwan, R.O.C.

References

[1] Ross J Jr, Brandenburg RO, Dinsmore RE, et al. ACC/AHA Guidelines for coronary angiography. A report of the American College of Cardiology/American Heart Association Task Force on Assessment of Diagnostic and Therapeutic Cardiovascular Procedures (Subcommittee on Coronary Angiography). J Am Coll Cardiol 1987;10:935–50.

[2] Marcus ML, Schelbert HR, Skorton DJ, et al, editors. *Cardiac Imaging: A Companion to Braunwald's Heart Disease.* Philadelphia, Pa: WB Saunders, 1991.

[3] Grossman WB, Baim DS, editors. *Cardiac Catheterization, Angiography and Intervention.* Philadelphia, Pa: Lea & Febiger, 1991.

[4] Braunwald E, Mark DB, Jones RH, et al. Clinical Practice Guideline Number 10: Unstable Angina: Diagnosis and Management. 86th ed. Rockville, Md: US Dept of Health and Human Services, Agency for Health Care Policy and Research, 1994. AHCPR publication 94-0602.

[5] Braunwald E, Jones RH, Mark DB, et al. Diagnosing and managing unstable angina: Agency for Health Care Policy and Research.Circulation 1994;90:613–22.

[6] DeWood MA, Spores J, Notske R, et al. Prevalence of total coronary occlusion during the early hours of transmural myocardial infarction. N Engl J Med 1980;303:897–902.

[7] de Feyter PJ, van den Brand M, Serruys PW, Wijns W. Early angiography after myocardial infarction: what have we learned? Am Heart J 1985;109:194 –9.

[8] Lincoff AM, Topol EJ. Illusion of reperfusion: does anyone achieve optimal reperfusion during acute myocardial infarction? Circulation 1993;88:1361–74.

[9] Lincoff AM, Topol EJ, Califf RM, et al. Significance of a coronary artery with thrombolysis in myocardial infarction grade 2 flow "patency" (outcome in the thrombolysis and angioplasty in myocardial infarction trials): Thrombolysis and Angioplasty in Myocardial Infarction Study Group. Am J Cardiol 1995;75:871– 6.

[10] Simes RJ, Topol EJ, Holmes DR Jr, et al. Link between the angiographic substudy and mortality outcomes in a large randomized trial of myocardial reperfusion: importance of early and complete infarct artery reperfusion. GUSTO-I Investigators. Circulation 1995;91:1923– 8.

[11] Vavuranakis M, Bush CA, Boudoulas H. Coronary artery fistulas in adults: incidence, angiographic characteristics, natural history. Cathet Cardiovasc Diagn 1995;35:116 –120.

[12] Carvalho JS, Redington AN, Oldershaw PJ, Shinebourne EA, Lincoln CR, Gibson DG. Analysis of left ventricular wall movement before and after reimplantation of anomalous left coronary artery in infancy. Br Heart J 1991;65:218 –22.

[13] Leberthson RR, Dinsmore RE, Bharati S, et al. Aberrant coronary artery origin from the aorta: diagnosis and clinical significance. Circulation 1974;50:774 –9.

[14] Levin DC, Fellows KE, Abrams HL. Hemodynamically significant primary anomalies of the coronary arteries: angiographic aspects. Circulation 1978;58:25–34.

[15] Dilsizian V, Bonow RO. Current diagnostic techniques of assessing myocardial viability in patients with hibernating and stunned myocardium. Circulation 1993;87:1–20.

[16] Braunwald E, Rutherford JD. Reversible ischemic left ventricular dysfunction: evidence for the "hibernating myocardium." J Am Coll Cardiol 1986;8:1467–70.

[17] Greenberg B, Quinones MA, Koilpillai C, et al. Effects of long-term enalapril therapy on cardiac structure and function in patients with left ventricular dysfunction: results of the SOLVD echocardiography substudy. Circulation 1995;91:2573– 81.

[18] Akins CW, Pohost GM, Desanctis RW, Block PC. Selection of angina-free patients with severe left ventricular dysfunction for myocardial revascularization. Am J Cardiol 1980;46:695–700.

[19] Rankin JS, Newman GE, Muhbaier LH, Behar VS, Fedor JM, Sabiston DC Jr. The effects of coronary revascularization on left ventricular function in ischemic heart disease. J Thorac Cardiovasc Surg 1985;90:818 –32.

[20] Dilsizian V, Bonow RO, Cannon RO III, et al. The effect of coronary artery bypass grafting on left ventricular systolic function at rest: evidence for preoperative subclinical myocardial ischemia. Am J Cardiol 1988;61:1248 –54.

[21] Bonow RO, Udelson JE. Left ventricular diastolic dysfunction as a cause of congestive heart failure: mechanisms and management. AnnIntern Med 1992;117:502–10.

[22] Creswell LL, Kouchoukos NT, Cox JL, Rosenbloom M. Coronary artery disease in patients with type A aortic dissection. Ann Thorac Surg 1995;59:585–90.

[23] Rizzo RJ, Aranki SF, Aklog L, et al. Rapid noninvasive diagnosis and surgical repair of acute ascending aortic dissection: improved survival with less angiography. J Thorac Cardiovasc Surg 1994;108:567–74.

[24] Kato H, Ichinose E, Yoshioka F, et al. Fate of coronary aneurysms in Kawasaki disease: serial coronary angiography and long-term follow-up study. Am J Cardiol 1982;49:1758–66.

[25] Suzuki A, Kamiya T, Kuwahara N, et al. Coronary arterial lesions of Kawasaki disease: cardiac catheterization findings of 1,100 cases. Pediatr Cardiol 1986;7:3–9.

[26] Walston A II, Behar VS. Spectrum of coronary artery disease in idiopathic hypertrophic subaortic stenosis. Am J Cardiol 1976;38: 12–6.

[27] Oren A, Bar-Shlomo B, Stern S. Acute coronary occlusion following blunt injury to the chest in the absence of coronary atherosclerosis. Am Heart J 1976;92:501–5.

[28] Nissen SE, Gurley GL. Assessment of coronary angioplasty results by intravascular ultrasound. In: Serruys PW, Straus BH, King SB III, editors. Restenosis After Intervention With New Mechanical Devices. Dordrecht, Netherlands: Kluwer 1992:73–96.

[29] Keane D, Haase J, Slager CJ, et al. Comparative validation of quantitative coronary angiography systems: results and implications from a multicenter study using a standardized approach. Circulation 1995;91:2174–83.

[30] Reiber JH, Serruys PW, Kooijman CJ, et al. Assessment of short-, medium-, and long-term variations in arterial dimensions from computer-assisted quantitation of coronary cineangiograms. Circulation 1985;71:280–8.

[31] Reiber JH, van der Zwet PM, Koning G, et al. Accuracy and precision of quantitative digital coronary arteriography: observer-, short-, and medium-term variabilities. Cathet Cardiovasc Diagn 1993;28:187–98.

[32] Reiber JHC, Reiber JC, Serruys PW, editors. Advances in QuantiQuantitative Coronary Arteriography. Dordrecht, Netherlands: Kluwer,1993:55–132.

[33] Amanullah AM, Aasa M. Significance of ST segment depression during adenosine-induced coronary hyperemia in angina pectoris and correlation with angiographic,

http://dx.doi.org/10.5772/54080

scintigraphic, hemodynamic, and echocardiographic variables. Int J Cardiol 1995;48:167–76.

[34] Arnese M, Salustri A, Fioretti PM, et al. Quantitative angiographic measurements of isolated left anterior descending coronary artery stenosis: correlation with exercise echocardiography and technetium- 99m 2-methoxy isobutyl isonitrile single-photon emission computed tomography. J Am Coll Cardiol 1995;25:1486 –91.

[35] Fallavollita JA, Brody AS, Bunnell IL, Kumar K, Canty JM Jr. Fast computed tomography detection of coronary calcification in the diagnosis of coronary artery disease: comparison with angiography in patients ,50 years old. Circulation 1994;89:285–90.

[36] Salustri A, Arnese M, Boersma E, et al. Correlation of coronary stenosis by quantitative coronary arteriography with exercise echocardiography. Am J Cardiol 1995;75:287–90.

[37] Tron C, Kern MJ, Donohue TJ, et al. Comparison of quantitative angiographically derived and measured translesion pressure and flow velocity in coronary artery disease. Am J Cardiol 1995;75:111–7.

[38] Arnett EN, Isner JM, Redwood DR, et al. Coronary artery narrowing in coronary heart disease: comparison of cineangiographic and necropsy findings. Ann Intern Med 1979;91:350–6.

[39] Blankenhorn DH, Curry PJ. The accuracy of arteriography and ultrasound imaging for atherosclerosis measurement: a review. Arch Pathol Lab Med 1982;106:483–9.

[40] Grondin CM, Dyrda I, Pasternac A, Campeau L, Bourassa MG, Lesperance J. Discrepancies between cineangiographic and postmortem findings in patients with coronary artery disease and recent myocardial revascularization. Circulation 1974;49:703–8.

[41] Vlodaver Z, Frech R, Van Tassel RA, Edwards JE. Correlation of the antemortem coronary arteriogram and the postmortem specimen. Circulation 1973;47:162–9.

[42] Roberts WC, Jones AA. Quantitation of coronary arterial narrowing at necropsy in sudden coronary death: analysis of 31 patients and comparison with 25 control subjects. Am J Cardiol 1979;44:39–45.

[43] Isner JM, Kishel J, Kent KM, Ronan JA Jr, Ross AM, Roberts WC. Accuracy of angiographic determination of left main coronary arterial narrowing: angiographic-histologic correlative analysis in 28 patients. Circulation 1981;63:1056–64.

[44] Glagov S, Weisenberg E, Zarins CK, Stankunavicius R, Kolettis GJ. Compensatory enlargement of human atherosclerotic coronary arteries. N Engl J Med 1987;316:1371–5.

[45] Keeley EC, Lange RA, Landau C, Willard JE, Hillis LD. Quantitative assessment of coronary arterial diameter before and after balloon angioplasty of severe stenoses. Am J Cardiol 1995;75:939–40.

[46] Waller BF. "Crackers, breakers, stretchers, drillers, scrapers, shavers, burners, welders and melters:" the future treatment of atherosclerotic coronary artery disease? A clinical-morphologic assessment. J Am Coll Cardiol 1989;13:969–87.

[47] Tenaglia AN, Buller CE, Kisslo KB, Stack RS, Davidson CJ. Mechanisms of balloon angioplasty and directional coronary atherectomy as assessed by intracoronary ultrasound. J Am Coll Cardiol 1992;20:685–91.

[48] Berkalp B, Nissen SE, De Franco AC, et al. Intravascular ultrasound demonstrates marked differences in surface and lumen shape following interventional devices (abstr). Circulation 1994;90:I-58.

[49] DeFranco AC, Tuzcu EM, Moliterno DJ, et al. Overestimation of lumen size after coronary interventions: implications for andomized trials of new devices (abstr). Circulation 1994;90(pt 2):I-550.

[50] Gould KL, Lipscomb K, Hamilton GW. Physiologic basis for assessing critical coronary stenosis: instantaneous flow response and regional distribution during coronary hyperemia as measures of coronary flow reserve. Am J Cardiol 1974;33:87–94.

[51] Kern MJ, Donohue TJ, Aguirre FV, et al. Assessment of angiographically intermediate coronary artery stenosis using the Doppler flowire. Am J Cardiol 1993;71:26–33D.

[52] Lamm C, Dohnal M, Serruys PW, Emanuelsson H. High-fidelity translesional pressure gradients during percutaneous transluminalcoronary angioplasty: correlation with quantitative coronary angiography. Am Heart J 1993;126:66 –75.

[53] Nissen SE, Elion JL, Booth DC, Evans J, DeMaria AN. Value and limitations of computer analysis of digital subtraction angiography in the assessment of coronary flow reserve. Circulation 1986;73:562–71.

[54] Nissen SE. Radiographic principles in cardiac catheterization. In: Roubin GS, Califf RM, O'Neill W, Phillips H, Stack R, editors. Interventional Cardiac Catheterization: Principles and Practice. New York: Churchill Livingstone, 1993:409 –25.

[55] Little WC, Constantinescu M, Applegate RJ, et al. Can coronary angiography predict the site of a subsequent myocardial infarction in patients with mild-to-moderate coronary artery disease? Circulation 1988;78:1157– 66.

[56] Leung WH, Alderman EL, Lee TC, Stadius ML. Quantitative arteriography of apparently normal coronary segments with nearby or distant disease suggests presence of occult, nonvisualized atherosclerosis. J Am Coll Cardiol 1995;25:311–7.

[57] Sambuceti G, Parodi O, Giorgetti A, et al. Microvascular dysfunction in collateral-dependent myocardium. J Am Coll Cardiol 1995; 26:615–23.

[58] Sasayama S. Effect of coronary collateral circulation on myocardial ischemia and ventricular dysfunction. Cardiovasc Drugs Ther 1994; 8:327–34.

[59] Dacanay S, Kennedy HL, Uretz E, Parrillo JE, Klein LW. Morphological and quantitative angiographic analyses of progression of coronary stenoses: a comparison of Q-wave and non-Q-wave myocardial infarction. Circulation 1994;90:1739–46.

[60] Dellborg M, Emanuelsson H, Swedberg K. Silent myocardial ischemia during coronary angioplasty. Cardiology 1993;82:325–34.

[61] Akutsu Y, Hara T, Michihata T, et al. Functional role of coronary collaterals with exercise in infarct-related myocardium. Int J Cardiol 1995;51:47–55.

[62] Nishimura S, Kimball KT, Mahmarian JJ, Verani MS. Angiographic and hemodynamic determinants of myocardial ischemia during adenosine thallium-201 scintigraphy in coronary artery disease. Circulation 1993;87:1211–9.

[63] Ritchie JL, Nissen SE, Douglas JS Jr, et al. Use of nonionic or low osmolar contrast agents in cardiovascular procedures: American College of Cardiology Cardiovascular Imaging Committee. J Am Coll Cardiol 1993;21:269 –73.

[64] Hirshfeld JW. Radiographic contrast agents. In: Marcus ML, editor. Cardiac Imaging: A Companion to Braunwald's Heart Disease. Philadelphia, PA: WB Saunders, 1996.

[65] Barrett BJ, Parfrey PS, Vavasour HM, O'Dea F, Kent G, Stone E. A comparison of nonionic, low-osmolality radiocontrast agents with ionic, high-osmolality agents during cardiac catheterization. N Engl J Med 1992;326:431– 6.

[66] Steinberg EP, Moore RD, Powe NR, et al. Safety and cost effectiveness of high-osmolality as compared with low-osmolality contrast material in patients undergoing cardiac angiography. N Engl J Med 1992;326:425–30.

[67] Jacobson PD, Rosenquist CJ. The introduction of low-osmolar contrast agents in radiology: medical, economic, legal, and public policy issues. JAMA 1988;260:1586 –92.

[68] Hirshfeld JW Jr, Kussmaul WG, DiBattiste PM, Investigators of the Philadelphia Area Contrast Agent Study. Safety of cardiac angiography with conventional ionic contrast agents. Am J Cardiol 1990; 66:355– 61.

[69] Patrick J. Scanlon, David P. Faxon, Anne-Marie Audet, et al. ACC/AHA guidelines for coronary angiography: A report of the American College of Cardiology/American Heart Association Task Force on Practice Guidelines (Committee on Coronary Angiography) developed in collaboration with the Society for Cardiac Angiography and Interventions J. Am. Coll. Cardiol. 1999;33;1756-1824.

[70] Ryan TJ, Anderson JL, Antman EM, et al. ACC/AHA guidelines for the management of patients with acute myocardial infarction: a report of the American College of Cardiology/American Heart Association Task Force on Practice Guidelines (Committee on the Management of Acute Myocardial Infarction). J Am Coll Cardiol 1996;28:1328–428.

[71] American Heart Association,ACC/AHA Guidelines for Coronary Angiography,(*Circulation*).1999;99:pp2345-2357.

[72] Simes RJ, Topol EJ, Holmes DR Jr, et al. Link between the angiographic substudy and mortality outcomes in a large randomized trial of myocardial reperfusion: importance of early and complete infarct artery reperfusion. GUSTO-I Investigators. Circulation 1995; 91:1923– 8.

Chapter 13

Improving the Utility of Coronary Angiography: The Use of Adjuvant Imaging and Physiological Assessment

Alexander Incani, Anthony C. Camuglia,
Karl K. Poon, O. Christopher Raffel and
Darren L. Walters

Additional information is available at the end of the chapter

http://dx.doi.org/10.5772/54041

1. Introduction

The most important role of coronary angiography is to delineate coronary lesions that cause inducible ischaemia. It remains the primary tool influencing the decision to undertake revascularization and patient outcomes [1] [2-4]. However, there are inherent limitations to diagnostic angiography. These pitfalls include difficulties delineating eccentric plaque (that can be underappreciated in the absence of multiple angiographic views), difficulty assessing lesions of moderate severity, the assessment of overall plaque burden and the composition, appreciation of ostial lesions, culprit lesion assessment in acute infarct patients and side branch analysis in bifurcation lesions. Heavily calcified lesions can also produce hazy angiographic appearances which often leaves the operator at a loss to determine the actual true lumen path and in some circumstances even misdiagnose calcification as "pseudothrombus" [5]. This latter phenomenon significantly changes the approach to intervention. The artery can be put at risk of perforation in the absence of adequate lesion preparation or wire induced dissection as calcified plaque is often undermined, complex and much more difficult to wire than soft thrombus.

Furthermore, angiography is usually used in isolation to guide intervention and ensure an adequate final stent result. FFR, IVUS and OCT can all be used to assess final PCI results and stent performance over time.

To aid decision making processes, adjunctive tools are becoming essential in "getting it right" in the catheterization laboratory. In this chapter, the use of FFR, IVUS and OCT for assessing left main and non left-main coronary artery disease will be discussed.

2. An overview of FFR

Fractional Flow Reserve (FFR) is the ratio of two flows - maximal flow in the diseased vessel expressed as a ratio to maximal flow if the vessel was theoretically normal[6]. During the procedure, a 0.014 inch pressure sensor coronary guide wire is advanced beyond a coronary stenosis and under conditions of maximal hyperaemia, distal pressure recorded and divided by guiding catheter pressure. The procedure requires routine anticoagulation, a calibration process [zeroing and equalization of the aortic (guiding catheter pressure Pa) with the pressure wire (Pd) and attainment of maximal hyperaemia (this is usually achieved by intravenous or intracoronary adenosine)[6]. FFR is a robust technique and reproducible which is remarkable in that the microcirculation is able to vasodilate to the same degree each time and is independent of heart rate and blood pressure [7,8]. It takes into account length of lesion, lesion severity, amount of myocardium supplied, viability and contribution of collateral blood flow [3,9,10]. It is now considered the gold standard for invasive functional assessment of the physiological significance of coronary stenosis. It has recently been given a Class Ia indication for guiding PCI in multivessel coronary disease by the European Society of Cardiology [6].

2.1. Practicalities of FFR

Pressure Transducers: The current pressure transducers usually comprise a regular transducer for aortic pressure (Pa) recorded through the guiding catheter and the second pressure (Pd beyond the stenosis) via a miniaturized sensor-tipped pressure wire that is connected to a small computerized interface. Of note, a new wireless system is also about to enter the commercial arena. Mean pressure recordings are essential as these form the numerator and denominator of the FFR formula, not peak systolic pressure. It is optional to record Pv (central venous or right atrial pressure) via a central line if the operator wishes to correct FFR for right atrial pressure – a concept that has been reborn in the modern FFR era whereby filling pressures in cardiac failure patients may be significantly elevated and can affect FFR recordings.

Medications: As is usual in any case where coronary wires are placed down coronary arteries, systemic anticoagulation (unfractionated heparin, low molecular weight heparin or bivalirudin) is essential to avoid wire induced coronary thrombus. At our institution, the usual practice is to administer heparin to achieve an ACT of at least 250 seconds. Intracoronary nitrate is then administered to overcome epicardial vessel vasospasm and for achieving hyperaemia, either intracoronary or intravenous adenosine. Our preference is for intravenous adenosine via a femoral venous sheath, although all that is required is to achieve hyperaemia – the route of administration is not as important. Intracoronary adenosine can also be given, however, this is not suitable when there are side holes in the guiding catheter, when ostial disease exists and when the aim of the study is to achieve a "pull-back" over the course of a coronary artery. Alternative agents for achieving maximal hyperaemia include intracoronary papaverine, intracoronary ATP, intravenous dipyridamole and intravenous dobutamine, however these have not been as widely adopted.

http://dx.doi.org/10.5772/54041

Catheters: In general, 5Fr or 6 Fr guiding catheters are used for performing FFR. This then allows the operator to immediately go on to perform an intervention based on the FFR result or indeed fix a wire induced dissection without needing to change catheters. The latter is a rare phenomenon in experienced hands and with modern steerable soft tip pressure wires. Larger French sizes are generally avoided on account of increased risk of catheter induced ostial spasm and the possibility of reducing proximal coronary artery pressure.

Basic Formula for FFR:

FFR = Qs/Qn

Qs = flow in diseased artery and Qn = flow in artery if theoretically normal

Therefore: FFR = [Pd-Pv/R] / [Pa-Pv/R]

Pd = pressure distal to stenosis; Pa = aortic or guiding catheter pressure

Pv = venous or right atrial pressure

R = resistance

Given Pv is assumed to be negligible equal and at maximal hyperaemia R (resistance) is minimal then FFR = Pd/Pa

---

2.2. Summary for the sequence of events for performing FFR

1. Systemic Heparin to achieve ACT of at least 250 sec
2. Guiding Catheter sitting at ostium of coronary artery without damping
3. Zero guide and pressure wire
4. Remove wire introducer
5. Intracoronary GTN to overcome epicardial conduit resistance
6. Flush with saline
7. Equalize pressure wire and guiding catheter transducers
8. Cross stenosis with the pressure wire (N.B. the pressure sensor is at the junction of the radiolucent and radio-opaque segments of the wire)
9. Run intravenous adenosine (our preferred method) to achieve maximal hyperaemia
10. Record FFR tracing with at least 2-3 min of adenosine
11. Remain vigilant for pressure signal drift and catheter damping
12. Pullback recording is reasonable across tandem stenoses or diffuse plaque

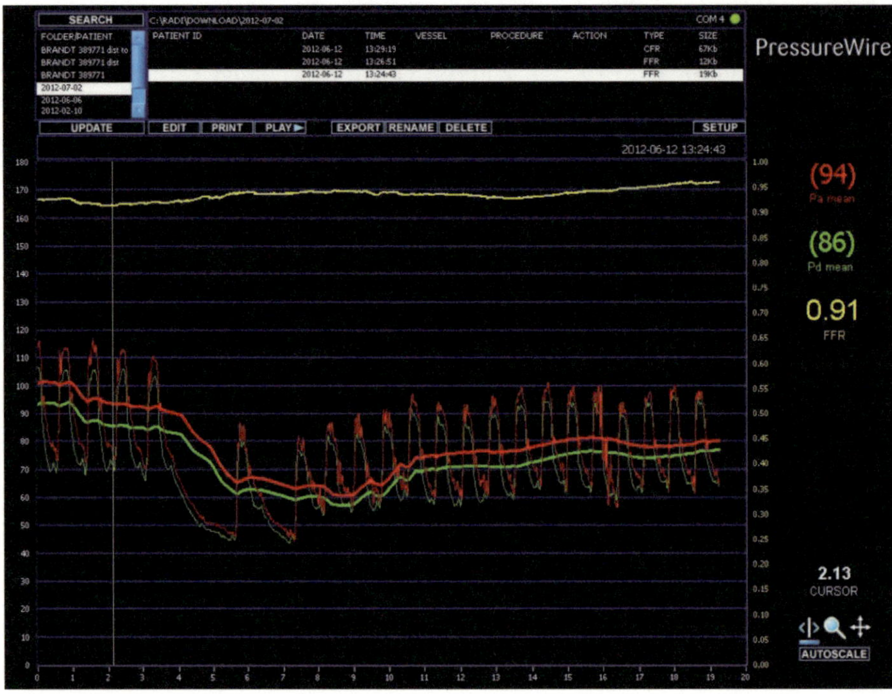

Figure 1. Typical Example of FFR Recording (n.b. mean Pd and Pa pressures and automatic FFR recording as well as transient bradycardia consistent with adenosine)

2.3. Pitfalls in FFR

Like most tools in coronary intervention, Fractional Flow Reserve is not immune to technical mistakes [11]. It is important to be aware of the following various pitfalls to ensure that the FFR measurement is both valid and reproducible.

a. **Use of a guide wire introducer:** when used through the Y connector, there is a subtle leak of aortic guiding catheter pressure. Although it tends to only be small (<10mmHg), when the FFR is near the ischemic zone, this small difference may have important implications. It is therefore recommended that when equalizing, measuring FFR and checking for drift at the end of the procedure, that the wire introducer be removed.

b. **Not clearing the catheter of contrast:** ensuring that the guiding catheter is cleared of contrast during equalization and FFR measurement is important to avoid subtle contrast induced damping of pressure waveform. To overcome this, the guiding catheter should be flushed with saline at the time of equalization and FFR measurement. It is important to note ST changes at this time as over-enthusiastic flushing of the guiding catheter can lead to ischaemia induced ventricular fibrillation. It is advisable to flush in stages giving the patient a break between 5-second flushes until the catheter is clear of contrast on fluoroscopy.

http://dx.doi.org/10.5772/54041

c. **Damping of pressure by the guiding catheter:** this is particularly true with diseased ostia and when using large guiding catheters. It creates a gradient between the guiding catheter and the proximal segment of the coronary artery and may only be unmasked during maximal hyperaemia. It is important to monitor the Pa waveform at baseline and during the FFR measurement and if indeed there is damping, the guiding catheter needs to be "backed out" over the wire to ensure the Pa measurement is valid. This usually necessitates the use of intravenous adenosine to maintain maximal hyperaemia during the FFR recording. If guiding catheter damping is not appreciated, the obtained FFR value will be artificially higher and the true severity of the stenosis underestimated.

d. **Guiding Catheter with Side Holes:** it is technically obvious to avoid intracoronary adenosine in this setting however it is also important to always disengage the guide because the side holes may actually confound true proximal coronary pressure measurement. Therefore, if side holes are used, intravenous adenosine and a guiding catheter sitting out of the ostium are imperative for an accurate FFR recording.

e. **Signal Drift:** High fidelity equipment make problems of signal drift less likely. However the problem can still occur. This issue is detected when an apparent gradient appears between Pd and Pa without a change in waveform of the distal pressure. It should be checked for at the end of the FFR procedure by ensuring that equalization still holds true when the coronary wire is withdrawn back into the guiding catheter. This is an internal check for the operator to ensure the final FFR reading is valid. In practical terms however, a pullback curve will also overcome this limitation.

f. **Maximal Hyperaemia:** It cannot be emphasized enough that there is no such thing as a resting FFR. It is only at maximal hyperaemia that resistance is minimal and that flow develops a linear relationship to pressure – a vital prerequisite for the FFR equation to hold true. Not achieving maximal hyperaemia will usually overestimate the FFR value and therefore underestimate the true severity of a coronary stenosis. At the usual dose of intravenous adenosine 140mcg/kg/min via a central sheath, all patients usually achieve maximal hyperaemia within 2 minutes. Patients will often complain of chest tightness and dyspnoea and there will be a transient rise in blood pressure before the Pd value reduces and adopts an ischaemic waveform with diastolic blunting. At this stage, increasing the dose of adenosine will not alter the FFR value and the clinician will be comfortable that maximal hyperaemia is achieved. It is not unusual for PR prolongation or transient heart block to occur which can also be used as surrogate measures of maximal hyperaemia [12].

3. An overview of IVUS

Intravascular ultrasound is a catheter based pullback technique that provides invasive cross-sectional tomographic imaging [13,14]. The ultrasound signal is produced by sending an electrical current through a crystal element on the transducer. Sound waves are reflected or pass through structures depending on their acoustic impedance. The scanning process provides both a qualitative and quantitative assessment of the artery. Vessel wall, atherosclerotic burden and plaque composition can all be assessed and with a well defined lumen-intima interface, measurements made of lesion severity such as minimum lumen area.

3.1. IVUS assessment of wall layers

The intima is a single layer of endothelial cells that is largely defined by its interface with blood in the lumen [15]. Saline or contrast flush can help delineate this interface in complex undermined plaque or when this interface may be ambiguous in cases such as lumen filling defects or intramural haematoma.

The media is composed of smooth muscle cells and does not reflect ultrasound and therefore appears as a dark ring during the pullback [15]. It is often used to help size stents along with reference lumen dimensions.

The adventitia is a matrix of collagen and elastin and reflects ultrasound markedly to give a whitish appearance on the outer segments of the vessel wall [15].

3.2. IVUS transducer type

There are two main types of transducers commercially available - a rotational single transducer and multiple stationary transducers in a phased array system [16]. The following table compares the current commercially available products.

Comparison	Boston Scientific	Volcano	Volcano
Commercial Name	iCross	Eagle Eye Platinum	Revolution
Imaging Method	IVUS	IVUS	IVUS
Scanning Design	Rotational	Phased Array	Rotational
Frequency	40 MHz	20 MHz	45 MHz
Overall Profile	3.2 Fr	3.5 Fr	3.2 Fr
Tip Entry Profile	0.022"	0.019"	
Guide Catheter	6Fr	5Fr	6Fr
Delivery	Monorail	Rapid Exchange	Monorail

Table 1.

The most commonly used device in our institution is the rotational system. There is a drive cable that rotates a single transducer element at the tip. The imaging system is located within a protective sheath that is very soft and creates a fluid interface for the imaging transducer. The two main artifacts that are encountered include wire artifact and occasionally NURD (Non-uniform Rotational Distortion) [16].

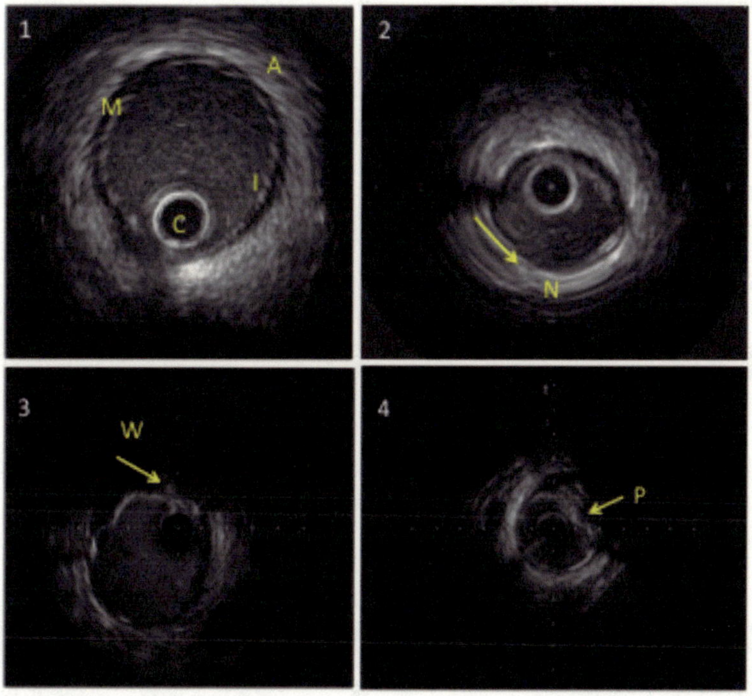

Figure 2. Panel 1: Adventitia (A), Media (M), Intima (I) and Catheter (C), Panel 2: NURD (N), Panel 3: Wire Artifact, Panel 4: Eccentric fibrous plaque (P)

3.3. Plaque morphology by IVUS

Calcified Plaque has marked acoustic shadowing with signal drop out and appears white on IVUS [15]. If circumferential calcification exists, this may prompt the operator to perform rotablation to ensure full stent expansion. Eccentric masses of bulky calcified plaque should also alert the operator to the potential risk of vessel perforation during percutaneous coronary intervention (particularly if a cutting balloon is used or if aggressive postdilation is performed) or focal stent under expansion. Generally, when only part of the vessel perimeter is rigid, aggressive postdilation will force stent expansion into the direction of least resistance.

IVUS is also able to detect soft plaque, fibrous tissue and in-stent restenosis. Positive and negative remodeling are also easily identified and generally best identified by IVUS.

Definition of diagnostic IVUS parameters for describing parameters of lesion significance as per the "JACC IVUS Consensus Document" [17]:

Term	Description
Lumen Cross-Sectional Area (CSA)	The area defined by the luminal border
Minimum Lumen Diameter (MLD)	The shortest diameter through the centre point of the lumen
Maximum Lumen Diameter	The maximum diameter through the centre point of the lumen
Lumen Eccentricity	(Maximum lumen – MLD)/Maximum Lumen Diameter
Lumen Area Stenosis	(Reference Lumen CSA – Minimum lumen CSA)/Reference Lumen CSA
Lumen Diameter Stenosis	(Reference Diameter – MLD)/Reference Diameter

Table 2.

Reference segments can be proximal and distal to the tightest point of the lesion and are usually arbitrarily defined to be within 10 mm of the MLA at a point with the least disease and not involving any side-branches.

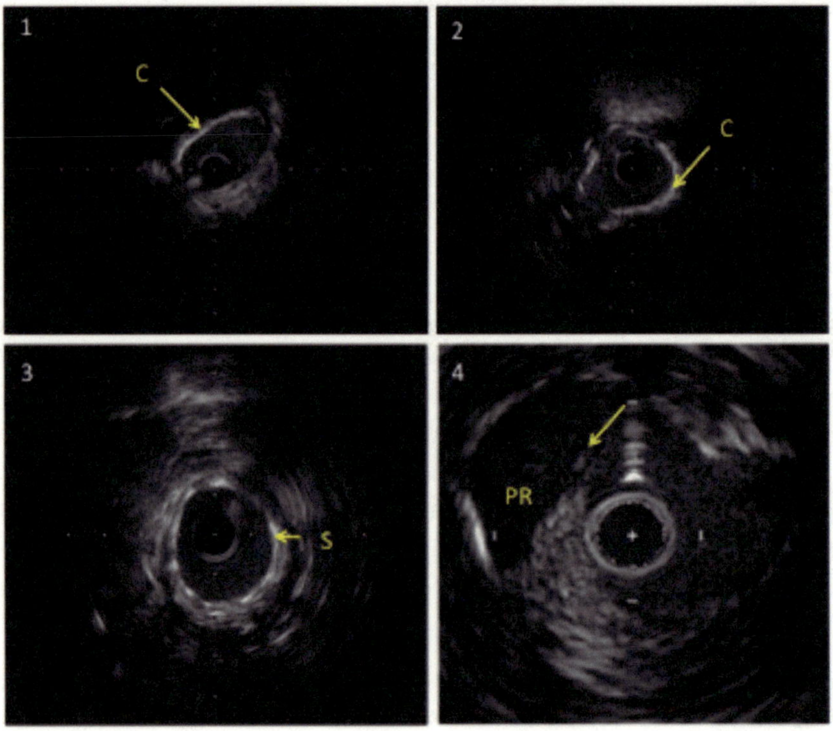

Figure 3. Panel 1: 180 degree arc of calcium (C), Panel 2: Near 360 degree ring of calcium (C) – this would warrant rotablator, Panel 3: Post Rota-PCI with full stent expansion (S), Panel 4: Plaque rupture (PR) – unstable plaque during ACS

http://dx.doi.org/10.5772/54041

3.4. IVUS to guide intervention

Despite the relatively attractive ability to size stents and ensure adequate apposition and full stent expansion, there is unfortunately a lack of evidence that IVUS improves the incidence of MACE in patients undergoing stenting although 6-month angiographic diameters may be improved (refer to table below). The exception to this however is in the left main interventional area whereby the use of IVUS improves outcomes [18].

Study	Number (N)	End Point	Result
Albiero et al [19]	312	6mth angio	IVUS better
Blasini et al [20]	212	6 mth angio	IVUS better
Choi et al [21]	278	Acute closure; 6 month angio	IVUS better
Gaster et al [22]	108	6 mth angio	IVUS better
AVID [23]	759	12 mth TLR	IVUS better
CRUISE [24]	499	9 mth TVR	IVUS better
OPTICUS [25]	550	6 mth angio; 12mth MACE	NO DIFFERENCE
PRESTO [26]	9070	9 mth MACE	NO DIFFERENCE
RESIST [27]	155	18mth MACE	NO SIGNIFICANT DIFFERENCE
SIPS [28]	269	2 year TLR	IVUS better
TULIP [29]	144	12 mth MACE	IVUS better

Table 3. IVUS vs Angiographic Guidance of Bare Metal Stent Implantation

The use of IVUS in elucidating the mechanism of instent restenosis is also important particularly given that it may not be as benign as initially thought. Walters et al. have described that an acute coronary syndrome is a common presentation for in-stent restenosis [30]. Angiography alone tends to overestimate the degree of restenosis and usually offers little information regarding the mechanism such as stent undersizing, incomplete expansion, strut fracture and geographic miss. Now that we have arrived in the OCT era, we may gain further insights into neoatherosclerosis as apposed to proliferative fibrous neointima as the pathology behind restenosis.

4. Overview of optical coherence tomography

OCT is an intravascular imaging modality akin to intravascular ultrasound (IVUS), however, where IVUS uses sound, OCT uses light. The use of near infrared frequency (1300 nm) light waves has remarkably increased resolution. OCT, unlike IVUS, requires a bloodless field. This was originally achieved with proximal occlusion (i.e. time-domain OCT) but in its most recent iteration, has been achieved by contrast injection with Fourier Domain OCT. This has significantly improved the user-friendliness of OCT. The characteristics of IVUS, TD-OCT and FD-OCT are detailed below:

	IVUS	TD-OCT	FD-OCT
Axial resolution, micron	100	10-15	10-15
Wavelength	Ultrasound	Near-infrared	Near-infrared
Frame rate, frames/sec	30	20	100
Maximum scan diameter, mm	10	6.8	9.7
Proximal occlusion	No	Yes	No
Pullback rate, mm/s	1	1-3	20

Table 4.

4.1. Procedural detail

The currently available OCT catheter is a rapid exchange catheter compatible with a 6Fr guiding catheter. The OCT catheter has several markers and the position of the imaging optical lens is noted to be 25 mm from the tip of the catheter and 5 mm proximal to the proximal marker. It appears as a radiolucent gap in the imaging catheter. It is thus important to note that a considerable length of catheter is needed to be placed beyond a stenosis and therefore a suitable landing zone is required that is of reasonable caliber and not excessively tortuous. A calibration process is performed prior to image acquisition – z offset or auto-calibration whereby marker fiducials are placed equidistant around the border of the catheter on the computer interface. With an automated injection system, we advocate a contrast injection of 4mL/sec, 14mL volume for the left coronary system; 3mL/sec, 12 mL for the right coronary system. For manual injection, usually 10mL contrast at reasonably sustained injection pressure will be sufficient to opacify the vessel. Ischemic electrocardiographic changes are not infrequent but almost always self-limiting; arrhythmia is rare and less frequent than with TD-OCT. REF Other complications such as those from guiding catheters and coronary wires are not attributable to OCT per se but are a part of the inherent risk of the procedure. The main advantages with the FD-OCT over TD-OCT are the faster pullback speed (20mm/sec) and the avoidance of proximal vessel occlusion, with potentially clearer images and larger reference segment dimensions [31]. The safety and feasibility of FD-OCT has been widely reported [32-34]. Slowing the pullback speed to 10 mm/sec can enhance the imaging detail particularly if imaging for stent complications at the end of a PCI.

4.2. Current uses of OCT

Sine 1996, a lot of work has been performed evaluating the correlation of OCT with histopathology – an essential prerequisite to describing vessel pathology. Exquisite images and detailed analysis of plaque composition [35] can be achieved including clarification of lipid

http://dx.doi.org/10.5772/54041

rich plaque, fibrous plaque, calcified nodules, macrophages, intimal disruption, red and white thrombus and thin capped fibroatheroma. OCT has revolutionized the assessment of stent performance with an unrivalled ability to detect malapposition, stent expansion, edge dissection, prolapse, filling defects, strut appearance and strut coverage. It can even discriminate between neointima and neo-atherosclerosis with regard to in-stent restenosis and detect neorevascularisation. OCT is in its infancy in its ability to define flow-limiting stenoses on the basis of lesion parameters for severity (akin to IVUS measurements).

Histopathological Features	OCT Features
Fibrous	Homogeneous, Signal Rich, Birefringent
Calcified	Heterogenous, Signal Poor, Sharp Border
Lipid Rich	Signal Rich at the Top; High attenuation regions
Macrophage Foam Cells	Heterogenous; lumpy; signal rich; high attenuation
Intima	Signal rich layer near the lumen
Media	Signal poor middle layer
Adventitia	Signal rich, heterogenous outer layer

Table 5.

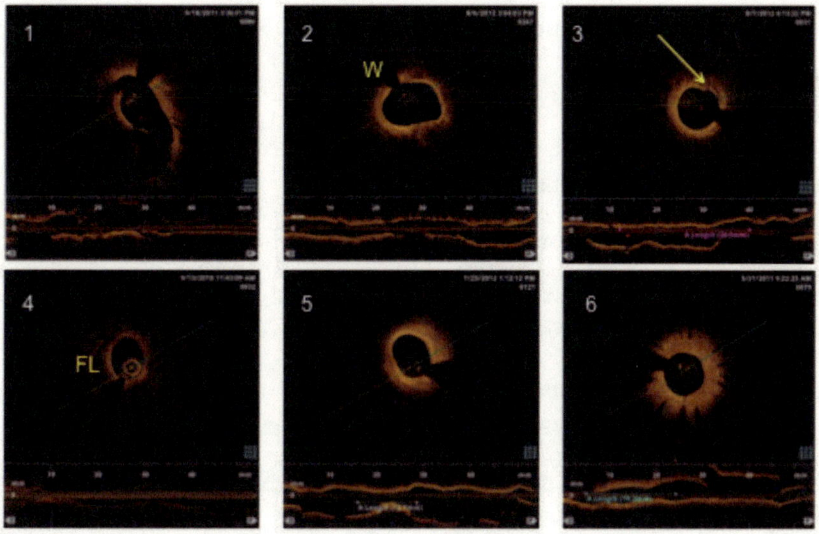

Figure 4. Panel 1: Blood swirl artifact ; Panel 2: Wire artifact (W) ; Panel 3: Stitch artifact from catheter movement (arrow) ; Panel 4: Spontaneous coronary dissection with visible false lumen (FL) ; Panel 5: Fibrous Plaque ; Panel 6: Proliferative neointima within a stent

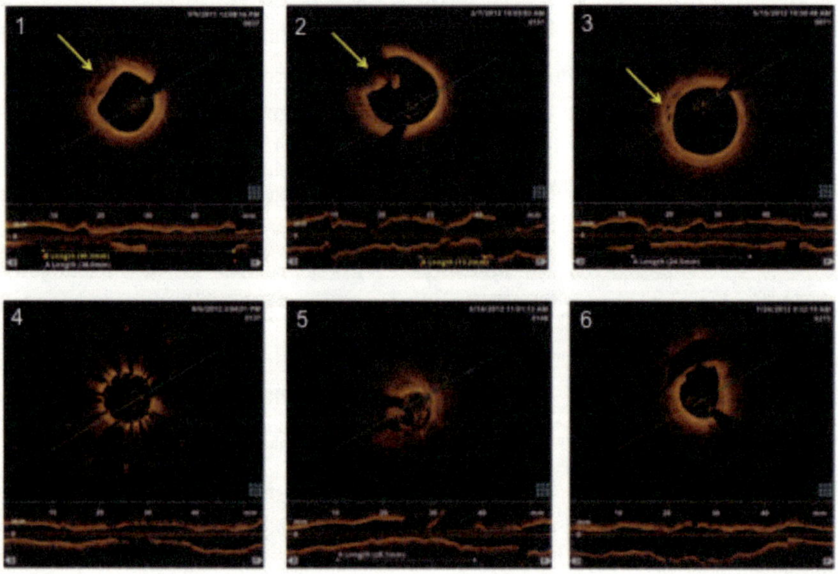

Figure 5. Panel 1: Calcified Nodule (arrow); Panel 2: Red thrombus (arrow) ; Panel 3: Vasa Vasorum (arrow) ; Panel 4: Covered stent – uncovered 7 years post deployment; Panel 5: Lipid rich plaque that is catheter hugging ; Panel 6: disrupted intima with a small cavity

4.3. Despite the overall attractiveness of OCT, some drawbacks include

- Need for extra contrast
- Limited ability to image very large vessels given limited depth of penetration (imaging >4.5 mm diameter vessels is difficult)
- Difficulty to image true aorto-ostial disease (IVUS is preferred in this scenario)
- Blood pool artifact (this occurs when the lumen is not devoid of blood because of inadequate contrast injection – the erythrocytes cause a severe scatter of light)
- Stitch artifact (usually only subtle and not a major issue; this artifact relates mostly to catheter movement within the vessel and appears as an abrupt step in the vessel wall)
- If the catheter does not sit coaxially within the vessel then an oblique cut may be made through the lumen and vessel wall
- Given the imaging catheter remains in the artery, there may be a tendency to straighten the vessel, cause vessel concertina and perhaps even distort stents of questionable longitudinal strength

- In the early phases of operator inexperience, there can be difficulty identifying calcium and differentiating it from lipid rich plaque

5. Assessment of moderate coronary artery disease – Non Left Main

The presence of myocardial ischemia is an important determinant of adverse cardiac outcome [36,37]. Revascularization of stenotic coronary lesions, by eliminating myocardial ischemia can improve patient symptoms, functional status and in patients with proven ischaemia, reduce death and major adverse cardiovascular events [38-40]. Importantly, for stenotic lesions that do not induce ischemia, medical therapy alone is likely to be equally effective with less benefit for revascularization [2,3,40]. While most patients undergo non-invasive testing to detect the presence of myocardial ischemia prior to consideration of angiography many patients with high clinical likelihood of CAD are catheterized without functional testing. Additionally, noninvasive stress imaging studies may be non-diagnostic and are limited in their ability to accurately localize culprit lesions in patients with multivessel CAD [41]. Ultimately where revascularization is considered, patients undergo coronary angiography.

Proving ischaemic burden in intermediate lesions requires invasive adjunctive tools – pressure derived measurements using FFR aim at functional evaluation whilst intravascular ultrasound (IVUS) and OCT provide anatomical clarification of the vessel anatomy and lesion dimensions. Both intracoronary IVUS and OCT can be used to measure lesion and vessel parameters such as minimum luminal area and diameter. Unlike IVUS, OCT has only just begun to be validated against FFR. Given FFR is now the gold standard of invasive physiological assessment of the stenosis functional significance, there are studies underway to validate lesion parameters for severity on OCT with the physiological information obtained by FFR.

5.1. Coronary angiography and stenosis significance

Coronary angiography is a 2-dimensional lumenogram of a 3-dimensional vascular lumen. It reports stenosis severity as a ratio of the lesion minimal lumen diameter to the adjacent "normal" reference segment. But, coronary atherosclerosis is a diffuse process and the accuracy of angiographic assessment is limited by the inability to identify both "diseased" and "normal" vessel segments. Histopathological studies have demonstrated that angiography fails to detect atheroma until the area stenosis approaches 40-50% as this is the approximate critical level at which further expansion of the external elastic membrane is not possible and so plaque begins to encroach upon the lumen. Furthermore, eccentric plaque produces an eccentric lumen that can give conflicting degrees of angiographic narrowing dependant on the viewing angulations. Despite improvements in quantitative coronary angiographic (QCA) techniques, coronary angiography frequently fails to identify the accurate hemodynamic significance of coronary stenoses, particularly those between 30% and 70% diameter stenosis [42-44]. The assessment and management of these "intermediate coronary lesions", then becomes a dilemma for the clinician. In this context, a more reliable technique at the time of angiography is vital to direct appropriate revascularization or medical therapy in a single setting. Fractional flow reserve (FFR) assessment and Intravascular ultrasound (IVUS) are two such techniques which are now part of standard clinical practice in guiding treatment of patients with intermediate coronary lesions [43,44] [45].

5.2. Fractional flow reserve and stenosis significance

Coronary pressure wire-derived FFR is now the technique of choice used in the cardiac catheterization laboratory to determine the functional significance of a coronary stenosis [45]. This method relies on the decrease in intra-arterial pressure induced by a stenosis to determine whether the lesion is producing physiologically significant ischemia. As described previously, Fractional flow reserve (FFR) is defined as the ratio of flow in the stenotic artery to the flow in the same artery in the theoretic absence of the stenosis [46]. Pressure is used as a surrogate of flow and FFR can be calculated by measuring the pressure difference across a stenosis under maximal hyperemia induced usually by adenosine. The pressure distal to the stenosis is accurately measured by a 0.014-inch pressure sensor angioplasty guidewire passed distal to the stenosis. FFR in a normal coronary artery = 1.0. FFR values of <0.75 (normal 1.0) are associated with positive functional stress tests in numerous comparative studies [sensitivity (88%), specificity (100%), positive predictive value (100%), and overall accuracy (93%)[45]. FFR values >0.80 are associated with negative ischemic results with a predictive accuracy of 95% [45]. Deferring revascularisation based on non-significant FFR values (>0.75) are associated with rates of death or myocardial infarction lower than that after routine stenting [3]. In patients with multivessel coronary artery disease FFR-guided PCI is associated with reduced major adverse cardiac events [40]. Furthermore, De Bruyne et al have recently demonstrated that managing patients medically (deferring PCI) with lesions that have documented ischaemic burden (defined as FFR < 0.80) have an increased risk of urgent revascularisation [47].

Author	Ref	Patients	No	Test	Threshold
De Bruyne	Circ 1995	1-VD	60	Bic ECG	0.72
Pijls	Circ 1995	1-VD (PCI)	60	Bic ECG	0.74
Pijls	NEJM 1996	1-VD	45	Bic ECG; Thallium; Dob ECHO	0.75
Bartunek	JACC 1996	1-VD	75	Dob ECHO	0.78
Chamuleau	JACC 2000	MVD	127	MIBI	0.74
Abe	Circ 2000	1-VD	46	Thallium	0.75
De Bruyne	Circ 2001	Post MI	57	MIBI	0.75-0.80

Table 6.

http://dx.doi.org/10.5772/54041

5.3. Fractional flow reserve corrected for right atrial pressure and stenosis significance

The original FFR calculation was derived from the following formula: FFR= (Pd-Pv)/(Pa-Pv) where Pd is distal mean pressure, Pa is aortic/guiding catheter mean pressure and Pv is central venous/RA (right atrial) pressure [48,49]. Effectively, this is an FFR corrected for right atrial pressure (FFR_{RA}). FFR_{RA} was used in some [49,50] but not all of the original validation studies to determine which FFR values best predicts an ischaemic burden [51-53]. In all recent studies validating IVUS with FFR and FFR with revascularisation/outcomes, FFR was never corrected for RA pressure. The simplified formula FFR = Pd/Pa was used largely based on the assumption that Pv was minimal and therefore did not greatly influence the final FFR result. Furthermore, previous data suggested that a correlation existed between FFR and positron emmission tomography (PET) derived myocardial blood flow indices even when RA pressure was ommitted [50]. However, this was a small series of low risk patients with a mean RA pressure of 5 mmHg. This does not necessarily reflect the cohort of patients coming through a high volume tertiary hospital with congestive cardiac failure patients in which filling pressure may not be insignificant. This lead Layland et al to compare FFR_{RA} with FFR in assessing coronary stenoses in a real world cohort. They demonstrated that right atrial pressure does in fact influence the FFR and tends to shift it downward into the ischaemic threshold [54]. It is not known however, whether FFR_{RA} (as opposed to FFR) can be used to guide intervention or whether it would better correlate with IVUS or OCT parameters for lesion severity.

5.4. Intravascular ultrasound (IVUS) and stenosis significance

As previously described, intravascular ultrasound is a catheter-based technique that provides high-resolution (up to 150microns) cross-sectional tomographic images of the coronary lumen and the coronary arterial wall that can be visualized in real time. It is currently the commonest intravascular imaging modality used as an adjunct to coronary angiography and PCI. Intravascular ultrasound is simple to perform, and its use is associated with very low complication rates [55]. IVUS does not provide direct hemodynamic data of a coronary lesion. However, several studies have demonstrated a strong correlation between IVUS lesion parameter and ischemia by myocardial perfusion imaging [56], and FFR [57,58]. Parameters that correlated with an FFR value ≤0.75 were area stenosis (>60-70%), minimal lumen cross-sectional area ≤3.0 - 4.0mm^2 and minimal lumen diameter ≤1.8 mm. IVUS is used in preference to FFR when:

1. Precise information on extent of the atherosclerosis, plaque characteristics including degree of calcification and accurate vessel size are required.
2. FFR assessment is contraindicated; significant conducting system disease or bradyarrhythmia or severe asthma precluding the use of adenosine.
3. Situations where FFR values may be misleading; previous MI with significant scar, diffuse coronary disease, microvascular disease, significant left ventricular hypertrophy.

The traditional cutoff of MLA <4 mm^2 on IVUS has been questioned in recent studies, and it is now thought that an MLA of <2.4 mm^2 may better predict a significant lesion [57-59]. Ultimately, it is still unclear which of the two MLA cuttoff's is more efficient in predicting sign-ficant stenoses, and future IVUS and OCT studies may also suffer from this "shifting goalpost" phenomenon. This reflects the need for more studies validating anatomical with physiological data.

In our catheterization laboratory about half of the stenosis assessments are done with IVUS. In some centers' it is the primary tool used [60]. There is a growing trend in our labarotory now for using OCT instead of IVUS for plaque characterisation and vessel dimensions.

5.5. Optical coherence tomography and stenosis significance

Optical coherence tomography (OCT) is a recently introduced medical imaging technology. It is an optical analogue of IVUS and measures the back-reflection of near-infrared light directed at tissues and generates images with a resolution close to 10micron; 10-15X greater than IVUS. With the current generation of FD-OCT imaging engines, it is also up to 20 times faster in imaging [35]. The safety of OCT imaging has been well described [61,62]. Given its significantly higher resolution, OCT has many advantages over IVUS both in atherosclerotic plaque assessment and in evaluating the acute and long-term effects of PCI [35]. It is likely to replace IVUS as the primary intravascular imaging modality.

Author	Year	Against	N	Cut-Off MLA (mm^2)	Ref Area
Nishioka	1999	SPECT	70	4.0	11.4+/-3.9
Takagi	1999	FFR 0.75	51	3.0	9.3+/-2.7
Lee	2010	FFR 0.75	94	2.0	5.7 +/- 2.0
Kang	2011	FFR 0.80	236	2.4	7.6 +/-2.5
Ben-Dor	2011	FFR 0.80	92	3.2	RVD >2.5
Koo	2011	FFR 0.80	267	2.8	6.8 +/- 2.5
F1RST	2011	FFR 0.80	320	3.0	RVD 2.9
Gonzalo	2012	FFR 0.80	56	OCT 1.95	6.5 +/- 2.7

Table 7.

With its better definition of the intimal-luminal interface and higher resolution compared to IVUS, OCT may improve accuracy and reduce observer variability in intravascular luminal cross-sectional measurements; in this context OCT may be particularly useful in assessing (intermediate) coronary stenosis severity. However, unlike IVUS which has many studies validating it against FFR albeit with differing MLA results, there has only been one such trial using OCT [59]. In this study, it was demonstrated that an MLA of 1.95 mm^2 was most efficient at predicting physiological significance. Gonzalo et al. [59] also demonstrated that OCT was more efficient than IVUS in predicting stenosis severity and that the geometric cutoff values for both

http://dx.doi.org/10.5772/54041

OCT and IVUS were indeed much smaller than the traditional 4 mm^2. However, this study did not correct FFR for right atrial pressure nor did it include OCT values indexed to the size of the patient or reference vessel (in a bid to roughly adjust for mass of myocardium supplied) – two corrections that may improve the correlation between OCT and FFR and affect the anatomical parameter and its value that best predicts an FFR ≤0.80. Further studies are therefore a vital pre-requisite before OCT can be validly used to establish stenosis significance.

In-vitro studies with a vascular phantom have shown that not only do OCT luminal measurements correlate strongly with IVUS but they are more accurate than IVUS [63]. Both in vitro and in vivo studies suggest, however, that OCT measurements tend to be smaller than IVUS measurements probably because of its better luminal definition [62,64]. Therefore, direct translation of IVUS parameters of stenosis significance to OCT is not appropriate or valid. Specific in vivo validation data against FFR is required.

6. Other uses for FFR

FFR can be used to guide PCI formally to ensure full stent expansion based on FFR >0.94 [65] and can also be used to evaluate side branch "pinching" post PCI. Koo et al demonstrated that when the side branch was <75% stenosed post PCI, the FFR was never in the ischaemic range and when it was >75% stenosed, it only fell into the ischaemic range approximately 1/3 of the time [66]. This emphasizes a common issue of over-interpreting the side branch appearance in PCI cases and vindicates bifurcation studies such as Nordic-Baltic Bifurcation Study III [67] whereby a simple approach to the side-branch is usually all that is required.

The use of FFR in vein grafts or in cases of severe left ventricular hypertrophy has not yet been validated. Nor, is it a useful tool in the acute setting such as a STEMI when the microvasculature pressures are high and thereby the FFR falsely elevated [6].

The pressure sensor wire also has a temperature sensing function that enables it to detect changes in temperature with saline flushes. Although beyond the scope of this chapter, it has allowed the FFR wire to also measure microcirculatory function (Index of Microcirculatory Resistance or IMR). The basic physiology behind IMR relates to transit time and temperature change detected by the wire sensor after flushing 3mls of saline via the guiding catheter. Ultimately, transit time is inversely proportional to microcirculatory resistance [68]. Although IMR is still largely a research tool, it has been shown to correlate with peak CK enzyme rise post STEMI and therefore offers a proof of concept that microvascular obstruction post ACS is detrimental [69].

7. Assessment of the ambiguous left main

7.1. Background

The accurate detection and description of disease of the left main coronary artery (LMCA) is of fundamental importance in the evaluation of patients in the catheterization laboratory.

Significant LMCA stenosis carries a poor prognosis without appropriate revascularization. [70-72] Therefore, the presence or absence of left main disease has a critical impact on therapeutic decision making following angiographic evaluation.

Angiographic assessment of the LMCA can be challenging. The anatomical plane of the LMCA, issues with vessel overlap, elliptical vessel configuration and plaque eccentricity all contribute to potential difficulty in accurately quantifying LMCA disease with conventional coronary angiography alone. In cases where LMCA disease severity is ambiguous, indeterminate or equivocal, adjunctive intravascular imaging or physiological assessment is of key importance.[18]

Fractional flow reserve (FFR) offers a real time stress physiological assessment of coronary pressure dynamics. Intravascular ultrasound (IVUS) is able to define the anatomy of the LMCA. Both of these technologies allow for the potential to improve LMCA assessment and attendant clinical outcomes and are discussed further below. Optical coherence tomography (OCT) has a limited role in LMCA assessment, especially for ostial LMCA disease, largely due to the dependence on having a contrast filled lumen to allow satisfactory imaging resolution to occur. [73]

7.2. Fractional flow reserve physiological assessment

FFR has been evaluated in several studies in the setting of LMCA disease. A cut off value for the Pd/Pa (pressure distal/pressure aortic) ratio, following induction of hyperaemia, of <0.75 – 0.8 has been demonstrated to safely discriminate between patients who should be referred for revascularization, usually coronary artery bypass grafting, as opposed to ongoing medical therapy and observation. [74-81] Patients with readings between 0.75 – 0.8 have physiology in a range that requires further study. In patients with intermediate readings of this kind the clinical context, as well consideration to additional evaluation with intravascular ultrasound become important.

The FFR technique involves the placement of a high fidelity pressure sensor beyond the left main plaque just as described in the "non left main" section previously. Consideration should be given to performing the procedure in both the left anterior descending and left circumflex artery to ensure concordance of results – this is particularly important if the circumflex is dominant [18]. Once the wire is in position and the catheter flushed with 100 – 200 mcg of intracoronary nitroglycerine followed by saline, hyperaemia is induced with the use of adenosine, 140 - 180 mcg/kg/min via intravenous infusion (central or peripheral). Higher doses may be required if a systemic response is not demonstrated. Venous infusion is preferred, however, adenosine can also be delivered by intracoronary bolus and studies in the area suggest no major difference between the three administration methods, [82,83] although intracoronary bolus doses of up to 720 mcg on each injection may be required.[84]

There are several potential pitfalls to FFR evaluation of the left main. Of utmost importance is the particular issue of guiding catheter damping and potential obstructive interference with coronary flow. Disengagement of the guide catheter is required for accurate evaluation in order to not underestimate the significance of the FFR. If a peripheral line is used for the adenosine infusion, care should be taken to ensure that the peripheral intravenous site is flushing normally and appropriately connected. Maximal hyperaemia will be achieved in most patients by two to three minutes, at which point the infusion can be ceased. An alternative to the infusion of adenosine is intracoronary bolus injection, but this is potentially a less robust [85] method and can be practically difficult if guide catheter pressure damping mandates catheter disengagement. A further potential confounder is the role of right atrial pressure in FFR assessment. Although FFR adjusted for right atrial pressure was tested by Layland et al in the non-left main subset, adjusting for assessment of left main has not been conducted although a similar phenomenon would be expected – that being as FFR approaches the ischaemic zone, right atrial pressure becomes increasingly important.[54] This is an area that requires further investigation.

7.3. Intravascular ultrasound assessment

Intravascular ultrasound (IVUS) of the LMCA provides sonographically derived images of the LMCA lumen and vessel wall. As a result, IVUS provides real time anatomical and pathological information in 2 dimensions. IVUS parameters have been evaluated in multiple studies in the setting of LMCA disease. Initial work that correlated IVUS data with clinical outcomes demonstrated a relationship between IVUS derived minimal luminal diameter (MLD) and minimal lumen area (MLA) at a lesion site with major adverse cardiovascular events (MACE).[86] [87]These initial studies, however, did not mandate any specific cut off values for treatment decisions. A clinical outcome based study by Fassa et al subsequently demonstrated that deferral of revascularization is the appropriate strategy where the LMCA MLA is ≥7.5 mm^2. [88]More recent work has revised this measurement down to ≥6 mm^2. [89]

Given the clinically validated findings for FFR, IVUS has also been investigated utilizing FFR as a gold standard comparator. In a cohort of 51 North American patients Jasti et al demonstrated that an MLD ≤2.8 mm^2 or an MLA ≤5.9 mm^2 correlated strongly with a FFR <0.75. This study also correlated FFR measurements with clinical outcomes and confirmed the appropriateness of an FFR cut off of <0.75. [90]Kang et al performed a similar correlation study in 55 South Korean patients. They found a MLA cut off of <4.1 mm^2 correlated well with a FFR <0.75 and a MLA cut off of <4.8 mm^2 correlated with a FFR of <0.8. However, evaluation of clinical outcomes was not performed as was done in the study by Jasti et al. In addition, the applicability of the study by Kang et al to patients of European ethnicity is unclear. Both studies also demonstrated that relative disease burden metrics such as plaque burden and area stenosis were insufficiently predictive of FFR measurements to be useful in clinical practice.

Based on the above data, a cut off of ≤5.9 mm^2 for MLA, if using IVUS alone, should be used in determining referral for LMCA revascularization following IVUS evaluation. Where there is uncertainty or ambiguity around measurements or their relevance in specific patients, strong consideration should be given to adjunctive FFR evaluation.

8. Case examples

Case #1: FFR and IVUS of Left Main

A 48 year-old gentleman presents with ischaemic sounding chest pain, troponin 1.3 ng/L and subtle precordial ST depression on his ECG. He has a background history of smoking, dyslipidaemia and a strong family history of premature coronary disease.

Angiography revealed an ambiguous left main with a complex hazy calcified roof. There was an impression of severe ostial plaque with only a narrow jet of contrast effluxing back into the left coronary cusp.

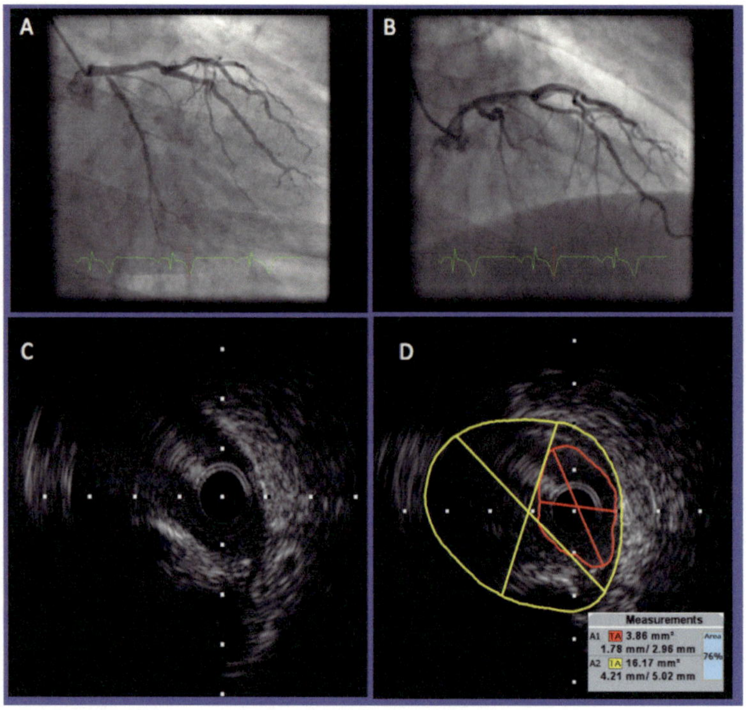

Figure 6. Angiographic (A and B) views and IVUS of left main (panels C and D)

The patient clearly had a left main lesion with an MLD < 2.8 mm and MLA < 5.9 mm^2 and an FFR <0.71 which was all consistent with a haemodynamically significant lesion. On the basis of physiological and anatomical confirmation of severity, the patient was sent for CABG and made an uneventful recovery. This case highlights the importance of careful inspection of the angiogram in multiple views, consideration of the pitfalls of angiography and the combined use of IVUS and FFR to assess ambiguous left main plaque.

Case #2: FFR and OCT of a moderate RCA lesion:

A 65 year old female presented with a long history of exertional chest discomfort and dyspnoea. A stress echocardiogram demonstrated possible mild exercise induced basal inferior wall hypokinesia. She had a background history of severe uncontrolled hypertension. Her left coronary tree was unremarkable. A 50% mid RCA lesion was interrogated by OCT and FFR – refer to figures 8 and 9.

Given an MLA > 1.95mm^2 on OCT and FFR > 0.80, the lesion was not stented. The recommendation was for improved blood pressure control. This case highlights the importance of thorough assessment of moderate lesions despite a typical symptom profile of angina. This patient almost certainly had hypertensive heart disease as a cause of her shortness of breath and chest discomfort.

Case #3: Use of IVUS and OCT to diagnose spontaneous coronary dissection:

A 37 year-old female with a family history of coronary disease presents with chest pain, elevated biomarkers and ST praecordial T wave inversion on her 12 lead ECG a few months postpartum.

Angiography revealed diffuse narrowing of distal left anterior descending artery (refer to figure 10).

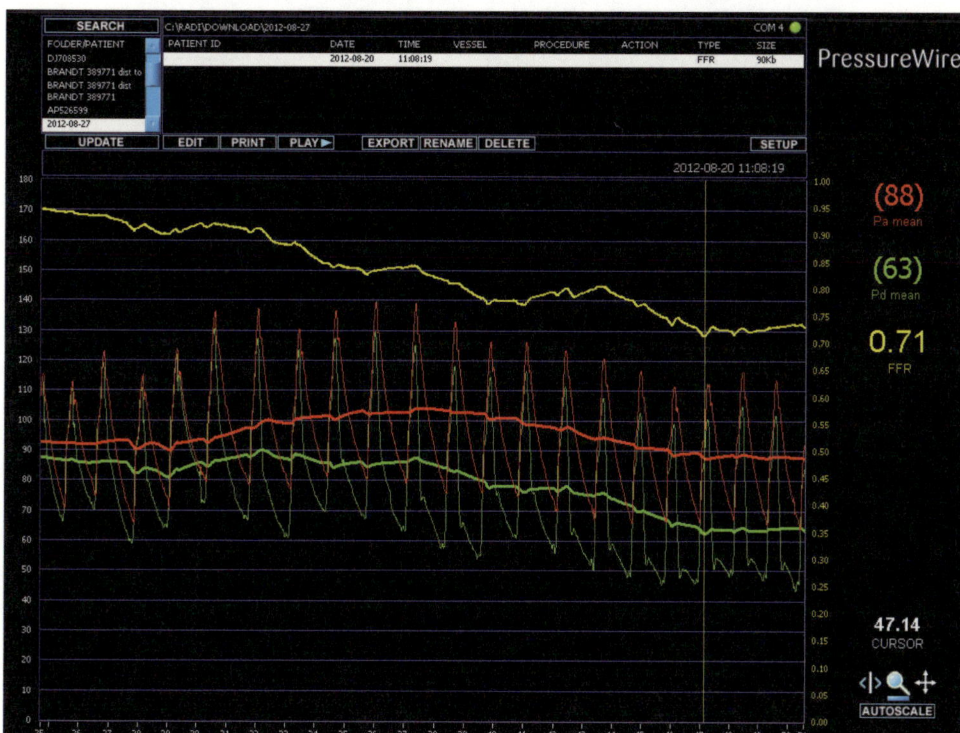

Figure 7. FFR of Left Main into LAD – dramatic drop in FFR to 0.71

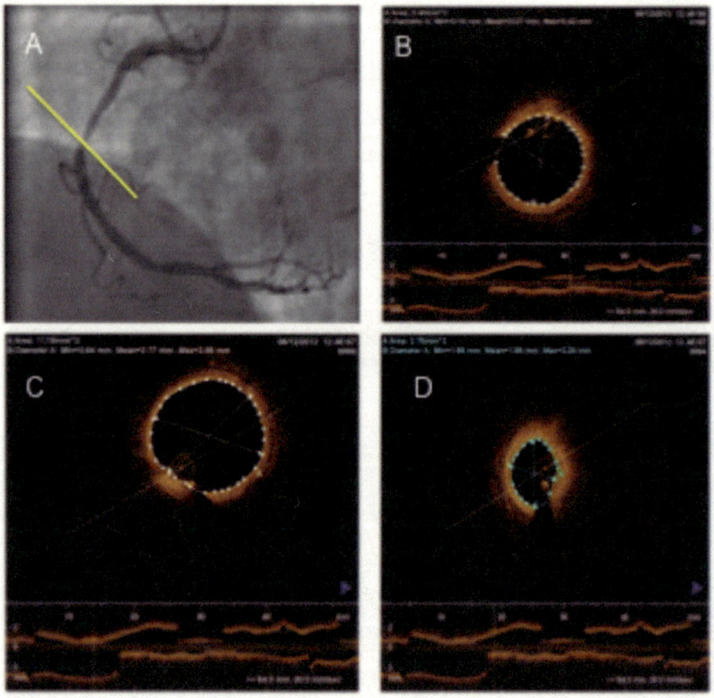

Figure 8. Panel A: Moderate RCA lesion with yellow line through the tightest point, Panel B: Proximal Reference Dimensions, Panel C: Distal Reference Dimensions, Panel D: MLA and MLD

http://dx.doi.org/10.5772/54041

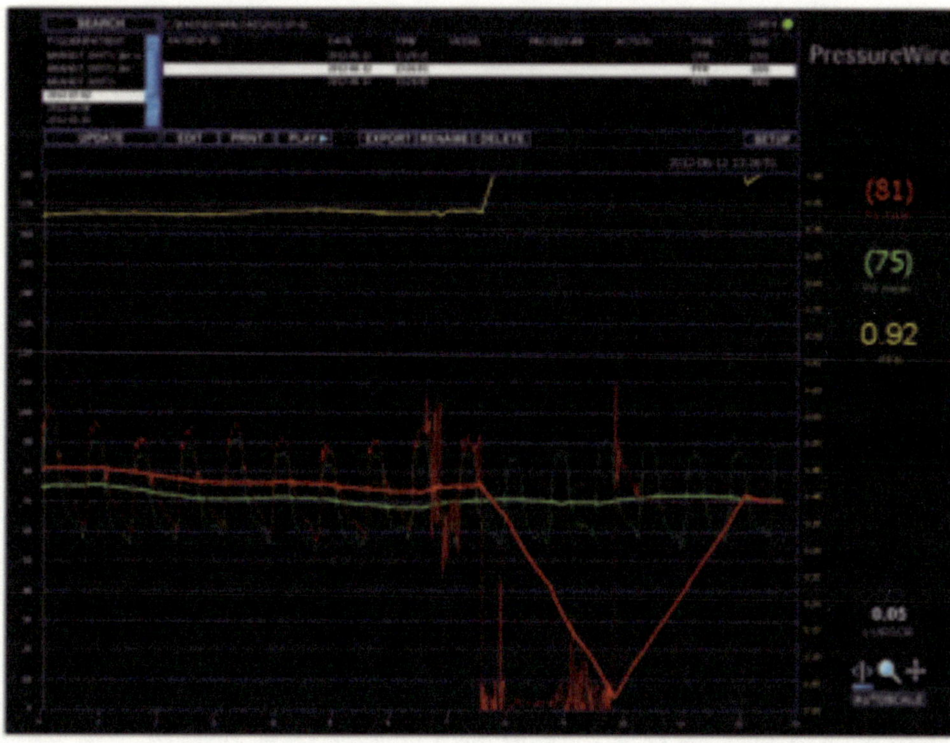

Figure 9. FFR clearly not in the ischaemic zone

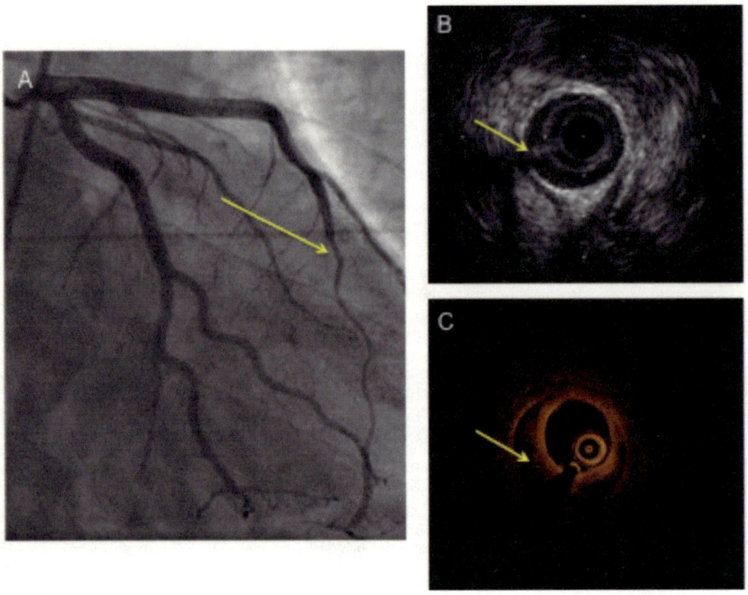

Figure 10. Angiogram, IVUS and OCT of the mid to distal LAD, Panel A: Arrow points to abrupt change in vessel caliber, Panel B: IVUS with intramural haematoma (arrow), Panel C: OCT with intramural haematoma (arrow)

IVUS and OCT both confirmed spontaneous coronary dissection as the cause of the angiographic appearance with clear evidence of intramural haematoma. The patient was managed conservatively and made an uneventful recovery.

9. Concluding statement

This chapter has highlighted some of the most important points regarding FFR, OCT and IVUS. In essence, these modalities are complimentary and it is up to the experienced operator to decide on when one modality may have a clear advantage over another (e.g. IVUS being more appropriate than OCT for imaging true aorto-ostial disease). It is generally accepted that FFR is the most useful tool to help decide when to revascularise and IVUS/OCT to help decide on pathology, guide the intervention and optimise the PCI result.

Author details

Alexander Incani[1], Anthony C. Camuglia[1], Karl K. Poon[1], O. Christopher Raffel[1] and Darren L. Walters[1]

1 The Prince Charles Hospital, Rode Rd, Chermside, Brisbane, Queensland, Australia

2 University of Queensland, St Lucia, Brisbane, Queensland, Australia

http://dx.doi.org/10.5772/54041

References

[1] Myers WOW, Schaff HVH, Gersh BJB, Fisher LDL, Kosinski ASA, Mock MBM, et al. Improved survival of surgically treated patients with triple vessel coronary artery disease and severe angina pectoris. A report from the Coronary Artery Surgery Study (CASS) registry. J Thorac Cardiovasc Surg. 1989 Mar. 31;97(4):487–495.

[2] Boden WE, O'Rourke RA, Teo KK, Hartigan PM, Maron DJ, Kostuk WJ, et al. Optimal medical therapy with or without PCI for stable coronary disease. N. Engl. J. Med. 2007 Apr. 12;356(15):1503–1516.

[3] Pijls NHJ, van Schaardenburgh P, Manoharan G, Boersma E, Bech J-W, van't Veer M, et al. Percutaneous coronary intervention of functionally nonsignificant stenosis: 5-year follow-up of the DEFER Study. J Am Coll Cardiol. 2007 May 29;49(21):2105–2111.

[4] Serruys PWP, Morice M-CM, Kappetein APA, Colombo AA, Holmes DRD, Mack MJM, et al. Percutaneous coronary intervention versus coronary-artery bypass grafting for severe coronary artery disease. CORD Conference Proceedings. 2009 Mar. 4;360(10):961–972.

[5] Duissaillant GRG, Mintz GSG, Pichard ADA, Kent KMK, Satler LFL, Popma JJJ, et al. Intravascular ultrasound identification of calcified intraluminal lesions misdiagnosed as thrombi by coronary angiography. Am. Heart J. 1996 Aug. 31;132(3):687–689.

[6] Pijls NHJ, Sels JWEM. Functional Measurement of Coronary Stenosis. JAC. Elsevier Inc.; 2012 Mar. 20;59(12):1045–1057.

[7] De Bruyne B, Bartunek J, Sys SU, Pijls NH, Heyndrickx GR, Wijns W. Simultaneous coronary pressure and flow velocity measurements in humans. Feasibility, reproducibility, and hemodynamic dependence of coronary flow velocity reserve, hyperemic flow versus pressure slope index, and fractional flow reserve. Circulation. 1996 Oct. 15;94(8):1842–1849.

[8] Bech GJ, De Bruyne B, Pijls NH, de Muinck ED, Hoorntje JC, Escaned J, et al. Fractional flow reserve to determine the appropriateness of angioplasty in moderate coronary stenosis: a randomized trial. Circulation. 2001 Jun. 19;103(24):2928–2934.

[9] Pijls NH, Van Gelder B, Van der Voort P, Peels K, Bracke FA, Bonnier HJ, et al. Fractional flow reserve. A useful index to evaluate the influence of an epicardial coronary stenosis on myocardial blood flow. Circulation. 1995 Dec. 1;92(11):3183–3193.

[10] Iqbal MB, Shah N, Khan M, Wallis W. Reduction in myocardial perfusion territory and its effect on the physiological severity of a coronary stenosis. Circ Cardiovasc Interv. 2010 Feb. 1;3(1):89–90.

[11] Pijls NH, De Bruyne B. Coronary Pressure (Developments in Cardiovascular Medicine). 2nd ed. Springer; 2010.

[12] McGeoch RJ, Oldroyd KG. Pharmacological options for inducing maximal hyperaemia during studies of coronary physiology. Catheter Cardiovasc Interv. 2008 Jan. 31;71(2):198–204.

[13] Gussenhoven WJ, Bom N, Roelandt J. Intravascular Ultrasound 1991. Kluwer Academic Pub; 1991.

[14] Tardif JCJ, Pandian NGN. Intravascular ultrasound imaging in peripheral arterial and coronary artery disease. Curr Opin Cardiol. 1994 Aug. 31;9(5):627–633.

[15] Hodgson JM, Sheehan HE. Atlas of intravascular ultrasound. Raven Pr; 1994.

[16] Nissen SES, De Franco ACA, Tuzcu EME, Moliterno DJD. Coronary intravascular ultrasound: diagnostic and interventional applications. Coron Artery Dis. 1995 Apr. 30;6(5):355–367.

[17] Mintz GS, Nissen SE, Anderson WD, Bailey SR, Erbel R, Fitzgerald PJ, Pinto FJ, Rosenfield K, Siegel RJ, Tuzcu EM, Yock PG. ACC Clinical Expert Consensus Document on Standards for the acquisition, measurement and reporting of intravascular ultrasound studies: a report of the American College of Cardiology Task Force on Clinical Expert Consensus Documents (Committee to Develop a Clinical Expert Consensus Document on Standards for Acquisition, Measurement and Reporting of Intravascular Ultrasound Studies [IVUS]). J Am Coll Cardiol 2001;37:1478–92.33

[18] Puri R, Kapadia SR, Nicholls SJ, Harvey JE, Kataoka Y, Tuzcu EM. Optimizing outcomes during left main percutaneous coronary intervention with intravascular ultrasound and fractional flow reserve: the current state of evidence. JACC Cardiovasc Interv. 2012 Jul.;5(7):697–707.

[19] Albiero R, Rau T, Schlüter M, Di Mario C, Reimers B, Mathey DG, et al. Comparison of immediate and intermediate-term results of intravascular ultrasound versus angiography-guided Palmaz-Schatz stent implantation in matched lesions. Circulation. 1997 Nov. 3;96(9):2997–3005.

[20] Blasini RR, Neumann FJF, Schmitt CC, Walter HH, Schömig AA. Restenosis rate after intravascular ultrasound-guided coronary stent implantation. Cathet Cardiovasc Diagn. 1998 Jul. 31;44(4):380–386.

[21] Choi JW, Goodreau LM, Davidson CJ. Resource utilization and clinical outcomes of coronary stenting: A comparison of intravascular ultrasound and angiographical guided stent implantation. Am. Heart J. 2001 Jun. 30;142(1):112–118.

[22] Gaster AL, Skjoldborg US, Larsen J, Korsholm L, Birgelen von C, Jensen S, et al. Continued improvement of clinical outcome and cost effectiveness following intravascular ultrasound guided PCI: insights from a prospective, randomised study. Heart. 2003 Aug. 31;89(9):1043–1049.

[23] Russo RJ, Silva PD, Teirstein PS, Attubato MJ, Davidson CJ, Defranco AC, et al. A Randomized Controlled Trial of Angiography Versus Intravascular Ultrasound-Di-

rected Bare-Metal Coronary Stent Placement (The AVID Trial). Circ Cardiovasc Interv. 2009 Mar. 31;2(2):113–123.

[24] Fitzgerald PJ, Oshima A, Hayase M, Metz JA, Bailey SR, Baim DS, et al. Final results of the Can Routine Ultrasound Influence Stent Expansion (CRUISE) study. Circulation. 2000 Jul. 31;102(5):523–530.

[25] Mudra HH, di Mario CC, de Jaegere PP, Figulla HRH, Macaya CC, Zahn RR, et al. Randomized comparison of coronary stent implantation under ultrasound or angiographic guidance to reduce stent restenosis (OPTICUS Study). Circulation. 2001; 104: 1343-1349.

[26] Orford JL, Denktas AE, Williams BA, Fasseas P, Willerson JT, Berger PB, et al. Routine intravascular ultrasound scanning guidance of coronary stenting is not associated with improved clinical outcomes. Am. Heart J. 2004 Aug. 31;148(3):501–506.

[27] Schiele F, Meneveau N, Vuillemenot A, Zhang DD, Gupta S, Mercier M, et al. Impact of intravascular ultrasound guidance in stent deployment on 6-month restenosis rate: a multicenter, randomized study comparing two strategies--with and without intravascular ultrasound guidance. RESIST Study Group. REStenosis after Ivus guided STenting. JAC. 1998 Jul. 31;32(2):320–328.

[28] Frey AWA, Hodgson JMJ, Müller CC, Bestehorn HPH, Roskamm HH. Ultrasound-guided strategy for provisional stenting with focal balloon combination catheter: results from the randomized Strategy for Intracoronary Ultrasound-guided PTCA and Stenting (SIPS) trial. Circulation. 2000; 102: 2497-2502.

[29] Oemrawsingh PV, Mintz GS, Schalij MJ, Zwinderman AH, Jukema JW, van der Wall EE, et al. Intravascular ultrasound guidance improves angiographic and clinical outcome of stent implantation for long coronary artery stenoses: final results of a randomized comparison with angiographic guidance (TULIP Study). Circulation. 2003 Jan. 6;107(1):62–67.

[30] Walters D, Harding S, Walsh C, Wong P. Acute coronary syndrome is a common clinical presentation of in-stent restenosis. The American Journal of Cardiology 2002. Mar 1; 89(5) 491-494

[31] Takarada S, Imanishi T, Liu Y, Ikejima H, Tsujioka H, Kuroi A, et al. Advantage of next-generation frequency-domain optical coherence tomography compared with conventional time-domain system in the assessment of coronary lesion. Catheter Cardiovasc Interv. 2010 Sep. 23;75(2):202–202.

[32] Imola F, Mallus MT, Ramazzotti V, Manzoli A, Pappalardo A, Di Giorgio A, et al. Safety and feasibility of frequency domain optical coherence tomography to guide decision making in percutaneous coronary intervention. EuroIntervention. 2010 Oct. 31;6(5):575–581.

[33] Prati FF, Cera MM, Ramazzotti VV, Imola FF, Giudice RR, Albertucci MM. Safety and feasibility of a new non-occlusive technique for facilitated intracoronary optical

coherence tomography (OCT) acquisition in various clinical and anatomical scenarios. EuroIntervention. 2007 Oct. 31;3(3):365–370.

[34] Yoon JHJ, Di Vito LL, Moses JWJ, Fearon WFW, Yeung ACA, Zhang SS, et al. Feasibility and safety of the second-generation, frequency domain optical coherence tomography (FD-OCT): a multicenter study. J Invasive Cardiol. 2012 Apr. 30;24(5):206–209.

[35] Raffel OC, Akasaka T, Jang I-K. Cardiac optical coherence tomography. Heart. 2008 Aug. 31;94(9):1200–1210.

[36] Shaw LJ, Iskandrian AE. Prognostic value of gated myocardial perfusion SPECT. J Nucl Cardiol. 2004 Feb.;11(2):171–185.

[37] Beller GA, Zaret BL. Contributions of nuclear cardiology to diagnosis and prognosis of patients with coronary artery disease. Circulation. 2000 Mar. 28;101(12):1465–1478.

[38] Davies RF, Goldberg AD, Forman S, Pepine CJ, Knatterud GL, Geller N, et al. Asymptomatic Cardiac Ischemia Pilot (ACIP) study two-year follow-up: outcomes of patients randomized to initial strategies of medical therapy versus revascularization. Circulation. 1997 Apr. 15;95(8):2037–2043.

[39] Shaw LJ, Berman DS, Maron DJ, Mancini GBJ, Hayes SW, Hartigan PM, et al. Optimal medical therapy with or without percutaneous coronary intervention to reduce ischemic burden: results from the Clinical Outcomes Utilizing Revascularization and Aggressive Drug Evaluation (COURAGE) trial nuclear substudy. Circulation. 2008 Mar. 11;117(10):1283–1291.

[40] Tonino PAL, De Bruyne B, Pijls NHJ, Siebert U, Ikeno F, van' t Veer M, et al. Fractional flow reserve versus angiography for guiding percutaneous coronary intervention. N. Engl. J. Med. 2009 Jan. 15;360(3):213–224.

[41] Lima RSL, Watson DD, Goode AR, Siadaty MS, Ragosta M, Beller GA, et al. Incremental value of combined perfusion and function over perfusion alone by gated SPECT myocardial perfusion imaging for detection of severe three-vessel coronary artery disease. JAC. 2003 Jul. 2;42(1):64–70.

[42] Topol EJ, Nissen SE. Our preoccupation with coronary luminology. The dissociation between clinical and angiographic findings in ischemic heart disease. Circulation. 1995 Oct. 15;92(8):2333–2342.

[43] Meijboom WB, Van Mieghem CAG, van Pelt N, Weustink A, Pugliese F, Mollet NR, et al. Comprehensive assessment of coronary artery stenoses: computed tomography coronary angiography versus conventional coronary angiography and correlation with fractional flow reserve in patients with stable angina. J Am Coll Cardiol. 2008 Aug. 19;52(8):636–643.

[44] Tobis J, Azarbal B, Slavin L. Assessment of intermediate severity coronary lesions in the catheterization laboratory. J Am Coll Cardiol. 2007 Feb. 26;49(8):839–848.

[45] Kern MJ, Samady H. Current Concepts of Integrated Coronary Physiology in the Catheterization Laboratory. JAC. Elsevier Inc.; 2010 Jan. 19;55(3):173–185.

[46] Pijls NHJ, De Bruyne B, Peels K, van der Voort PH, Bonnier HJRM, Bartunek J, et al. Measurement of fractional flow reserve to assess the functional severity of coronary-artery stenoses. N Engl J Med. Mass Medical Soc; 1996;334(26):1703–1708.

[47] De Bruyne B, Pijls NH, Kalesan B, Barbato E, Tonino PA, Piroth Z, et al. Fractional Flow Reserve–Guided PCI versus Medical Therapy in Stable Coronary Disease. N Engl J Med. 2012 Aug. 26;:120827230013003–120827230013003.

[48] Pijls NH, van Son JA, Kirkeeide RL, De Bruyne B, Gould KL. Experimental basis of determining maximum coronary, myocardial, and collateral blood flow by pressure measurements for assessing functional stenosis severity before and after percutaneous transluminal coronary angioplasty. Circulation. 1993 Apr.;87(4):1354–1367.

[49] Pijls N, Van Gelder B, Van der Voort P, Peels K. Fractional flow reserve: a useful index to evaluate the influence of an epicardial coronary stenosis on myocardial blood flow. Circulation. 1995 Dec 1;92(11):3183-93.

[50] De Bruyne B, Baudhuin T, Melin JA, Pijls NH, Sys SU, Bol A, et al. Coronary flow reserve calculated from pressure measurements in humans. Validation with positron emission tomography. Circulation. 1994 Mar.;89(3):1013–1022.

[51] Jiménez-Navarro M, Alonso-Briales JH, Hernández García MJ, Rodríguez Bailón I, Gómez-Doblas JJ, de Teresa Galván E. Measurement of fractional flow reserve to assess moderately severe coronary lesions: correlation with dobutamine stress echocardiography. J Interv Cardiol. 2001 Oct.;14(5):499–504.

[52] Bartunek J, Van Schuerbeeck E, De Bruyne B. Comparison of exercise electrocardiography and dobutamine echocardiography with invasively assessed myocardial fractional flow reserve in evaluation of severity of coronary arterial narrowing. Am. J. Cardiol. 1997 Feb. 15;79(4):478–481.

[53] Abe M, Tomiyama H, Yoshida H, Doba N. Diastolic fractional flow reserve to assess the functional severity of moderate coronary artery stenoses: comparison with fractional flow reserve and coronary flow velocity reserve. Circulation. 2000 Nov. 7;102(19):2365–2370.

[54] Layland J, Wilson AM, Whitbourn RJ, Burns AT, Somaratne J, Leitl G, et al. Impact of right atrial pressure on decision-making using fractional flow reserve (FFR) in elective percutaneous intervention. International Journal of Cardiology. Elsevier B.V.; 2012 Apr. 1;:1–3.

[55] Hausmann D, Erbel R, Alibelli-Chemarin M. The safety of intracoronary ultrasound: a multicenter survey of 2207 examinations. Circulation. 1995.

[56] Nishioka TT, Amanullah AMA, Luo HH, Berglund HH, Kim CJC, Nagai TT, et al. Clinical validation of intravascular ultrasound imaging for assessment of coronary

stenosis severity: comparison with stress myocardial perfusion imaging. JAC. 1999 May 31;33(7):1870–1878.

[57] Takagi A, Tsurumi Y, Ishii Y, Suzuki K, Kawana M, Kasanuki H. Clinical Potential of Intravascular Ultrasound for Physiological Assessment of Coronary Stenosis : Relationship Between Quantitative Ultrasound Tomography and Pressure-Derived Fractional Flow Reserve. Circulation. 1999 Jan. 20;100(3):250–255.

[58] Briguori C, Anzuini A, Airoldi F, Gimelli G, Nishida T, Adamian M, et al. Intravascular ultrasound criteria for the assessment of the functional significance of intermediate coronary artery stenoses and comparison with fractional flow reserve. Am. J. Cardiol. 2001 Jan. 15;87(2):136–141.

[59] Gonzalo N, Escaned J, Alfonso F, Nolte C, Rodriguez V, Jimenez-Quevedo P, et al. Morphometric Assessment of Coronary Stenosis Relevance With Optical Coherence Tomography. JAC.; 2012 Mar. 20;59(12):1080–1089.

[60] Magni V, Chieffo A, Colombo A. Evaluation of intermediate coronary stenosis with intravascular ultrasound and fractional flow reserve: Its use and abuse. Catheter Cardiovasc Interv. 2009 Feb. 28;73(4):441–448.

[61] Barlis P, Gonzalo N, Di Mario C, Prati F, Buellesfeld L, Rieber J, et al. A multicentre evaluation of the safety of intracoronary optical coherence tomography. EuroIntervention. 2009 Apr. 30;5(1):90–95.

[62] Yamaguchi T, Terashima M, Akasaka T, Hayashi T, Mizuno K, Muramatsu T, et al. Safety and feasibility of an intravascular optical coherence tomography image wire system in the clinical setting. Am. J. Cardiol. 2008 Mar. 1;101(5):562–567.

[63] Tahara S, Bezerra HG, Baibars M, Kyono H, Wang W, Pokras S, et al. In vitro validation of new Fourier-domain optical coherence tomography. EuroIntervention. 2011 Feb.;6(7):875–882.

[64] Gonzalo N, Serruys PW, a HCMGA-G, van Soest G, Okamura T, Ligthart J, et al. Quantitative ex vivo and in vivo comparison of lumen dimensions measured by optical coherence tomography and intravascular ultrasound in human coronary arteries. Rev Esp Cardiol. 2009 May 31;62(6):615–624.

[65] Fearon WFW, Luna JJ, Samady HH, Powers ERE, Feldman TT, Dib NN, et al. Fractional flow reserve compared with intravascular ultrasound guidance for optimizing stent deployment. Circulation. 2001 Oct 16;104(16):1917-22.

[66] Koo B-K, Kang H-J, Youn T-J, Chae I-H, Choi D-J, Kim H-S, et al. Physiologic assessment of jailed side branch lesions using fractional flow reserve. JAC. 2005 Aug. 15;46(4):633–637.

[67] Niemelä MM, Kervinen KK, Erglis AA, Holm NRN, Maeng MM, Christiansen EHE, et al. Randomized comparison of final kissing balloon dilatation versus no final kissing balloon dilatation in patients with coronary bifurcation lesions treated with main

vessel stenting: the Nordic-Baltic Bifurcation Study III. Circulation. 2011 Jan 4;123(1): 79-86. Epub 2010 Dec 20.

[68] Aarnoudse WW, van den Berg PP, van de Vosse FF, Geven MM, Rutten MM, Van Turnhout MM, et al. Myocardial resistance assessed by guidewire-based pressure-temperature measurement: in vitro validation. Catheter Cardiovasc Interv. 2004 Apr. 30;62(1):56–63.

[69] Fearon W, Shah M, Ng M, Brinton T, Wilson A. Predictive value of the index of microcirculatory resistance in patients with ST-segment elevation myocardial infarction. JACC 2008 51(5):560-565. doi:10.1016/j.jacc.2007.08.062.

[70] Yusuf S, Zucker D, Peduzzi P, Fisher LD, Takaro T, Kennedy JW, et al. Effect of coronary artery bypass graft surgery on survival: overview of 10-year results from randomised trials by the Coronary Artery Bypass Graft Surgery Trialists Collaboration. Lancet. 1994 Aug. 27;344(8922):563–570.

[71] Caracciolo E, Davis K, Sopko G. Comparison of Surgical and Medical Group Survival in Patients With Left Main Coronary Artery Disease: Long-Term CASS Experience. Circulation. 1995 May 1;91(9):2325-34.

[72] Conley MJ, Ely RL, Kisslo J, Lee KL, McNeer JF, Rosati RA. The prognostic spectrum of left main stenosis. Circulation. 1978 May;57(5):947–952.

[73] Moharram MA, Yeoh T, Lowe HC. Swings and roundabouts: Intravascular Optical Coherence Tomography (OCT) in the evaluation of the left main stem coronary artery. International Journal of Cardiology. 2011 Apr. 14;148(2):243–244.

[74] Bech GJ, Droste H, Pijls NH, De Bruyne B, Bonnier JJ, Michels HR, et al. Value of fractional flow reserve in making decisions about bypass surgery for equivocal left main coronary artery disease. Heart. 2001 Nov.;86(5):547–552.

[75] Lindstaedt M, Yazar A, Germing A, Fritz M. Clinical outcome in patients with intermediate or equivocal left main coronary artery disease after deferral of surgical revascularization on the basis of fractional flow measurements. Am Heart J. 2006 Jul; 152(1):156.e1-9

[76] Courtis J, Rodés-Cabau J, Larose E, Potvin J. Usefulness of coronary fractional flow reserve measurements in guiding clinical decisions in intermediate or equivocal left main coronary stenoses. Am J Cardiol. 2009 Apr 1;103(7):943-9. Epub 2009 Feb 7.

[77] Jiménez-Navarro M, Hernández-García JM, Alonso-Briales JH, Kühlmorgen B, Gómez-Doblas JJ, García-Pinilla JM, et al. Should we treat patients with moderately severe stenosis of the left main coronary artery and negative FFR results? J Invasive Cardiol. 2004 Aug.;16(8):398–400.

[78] Hamilos M, Muller O, Cuisset T, Ntalianis A, Chlouverakis G, Sarno G, et al. Long-term clinical outcome after fractional flow reserve-guided treatment in patients with angiographically equivocal left main coronary artery stenosis. Circulation. 2009 Oct. 13;120(15):1505–1512.

[79] Legutko J, Dudek D, Rzeszutko L, Wizimirski M, Dubiel JS. Fractional flow reserve assessment to determine the indications for myocardial revascularisation in patients with borderline stenosis of the left main coronary artery. Kardiol Pol. 2005 Nov.; 63(5):499–506; discussion 507–8.

[80] Suemaru S, Iwasaki K, Yamamoto K, Kusachi S, Hina K, Hirohata S, et al. Coronary pressure measurement to determine treatment strategy for equivocal left main coronary artery lesions. Heart Vessels. 2005 Nov.;20(6):271–277.

[81] Jasti V, Ivan E, Yalamanchili V, Wongpraparut N, Leesar MA. Correlations between fractional flow reserve and intravascular ultrasound in patients with an ambiguous left main coronary artery stenosis. Circulation. 2004 Nov. 2;110(18):2831–2836.

[82] Jeremias A, Whitbourn RJ, Filardo SD, Fitzgerald PJ, Cohen DJ, Tuzcu EM, et al. Adequacy of intracoronary versus intravenous adenosine-induced maximal coronary hyperemia for fractional flow reserve measurements. Am. Heart J. 2000 Oct.;140(4):651–657.

[83] Seo M-K, Koo B-K, Kim J-H, Shin D-H, Yang H-M, Park K-W, et al. Comparison of hyperemic efficacy between central and peripheral venous adenosine infusion for fractional flow reserve measurement. Circ Cardiovasc Interv. 2012 Jun.;5(3):401–405.

[84] De Luca G, Venegoni L, Iorio S, Giuliani L, Marino P. Effects of increasing doses of intracoronary adenosine on the assessment of fractional flow reserve. JACC Cardiovasc Interv. 2011 Oct.;4(10):1079–1084.

[85] Leone A, Porto I, De Caterina A, Basile E. Maximal hyperemia in the assessment of fractional flow reserve: intracoronary adenosine versus intracoronary sodium nitroprusside versus intravenous adenosine: the NASCI (Nitroprussiato versus Adenosina nelle Stenosi Coronariche Intermedie) study. JACC Cardiovasc Interv. 2012 Apr; 5(4):402-8

[86] Abizaid AS, Mintz GS, Abizaid A, Mehran R, Lansky AJ, Pichard AD, et al. One-year follow-up after intravascular ultrasound assessment of moderate left main coronary artery disease in patients with ambiguous angiograms. JAC. 1999 Sep.;34(3):707–715.

[87] Ricciardi MJ, Meyers S, Choi K, Pang JL, Goodreau L, Davidson CJ. Angiographically silent left main disease detected by intravascular ultrasound: a marker for future adverse cardiac events. Am. Heart J. 2003 Sep.;146(3):507–512.

[88] Fassa A-A, Wagatsuma K, Higano ST, Mathew V, Barsness GW, Lennon RJ, et al. Intravascular ultrasound-guided treatment for angiographically indeterminate left main coronary artery disease: a long-term follow-up study. JAC. 2005 Jan. 18;45(2): 204–211.

[89] la Torre Hernandez de JM, Hernández Hernandez F, Alfonso F, Rumoroso JR, Lopez-Palop R, Sadaba M, et al. Prospective application of pre-defined intravascular ultrasound criteria for assessment of intermediate left main coronary artery lesions

results from the multicenter LITRO study. J Am Coll Cardiol. 2011 Jul. 19;58(4):351–358.

[90] Jasti V, Ivan E, Yalamanchili V, Wongpraparut N. Correlations between fractional flow reserve and intravascular ultrasound in patients with an ambiguous left main coronary artery stenosis. Circulation. 2004 Nov 2;110(18):2831-6. Epub 2004 Oct 18

Chapter 14

Coronary Angiography – Technical Recommendations and Radiation Protection

Maria Anna Staniszewska

Additional information is available at the end of the chapter

http://dx.doi.org/10.5772/54034

1. Introduction

According to recent World Health Organization statistics for 2007, cardiovascular deaths account for 33.7% of all deaths worldwide, whereas cancer represents 29.5%, other chronic diseases 26.5%, injury and communicable diseases 4.3%. [1]. Coronary artery disease (CAD) is the leading cause of cardiovascular death throughout the world. In the light of this, special attention has to be paid to CAD.

Imaging is an integral part of diagnostics and treatment of the disease, especially of surgical and transcatheter cardiological interventions. Pre-procedural imaging provides detailed understanding of the operative field prior to the procedure.

Traditional two-dimensional (2D) imaging, i.e. standard echocardiography and conventional angiography, relies on acquisition of a limited number of planes/projections, which cannot be changed during the review, while three-dimentional (3D) imaging allows fast acquisition of volumetric data sets and subsequent off-line reconstructions along unlimited 2D planes and 3D volumes. 3D imaging of the cardiovascular structures is pursued with computed tomography, magnetic resonance and also echocardiography.

Cardiovascular surgery is a dynamically developing field and many procedures are performed under control of dedicated imaging systems but most of these procedures start from coronary angiography.

Quantitative coronary angiography is the method for visualization of coronary vessels during exposure to x-rays, after their filling up with contrast agents. This allows to assess coronary artery stenoses for hybrid revascularization or quantifying stenoses in bypass grafts.

Depending on a further proceeding expected for a patient two versions of the procedure are possible: CCA – conventional coronary angiography and CTA- CT angiography.

CCA is performed under the control of x-ray unit with C-arm and is preferred if further cardiovascular surgery is planned for the patient.

CTA is performed under the control of computerized tomography (CT scanner) and has only diagnostic meaning.

This chapter is divided into three parts concerning both: the techniques of coronary angiography (CCA and CTA) and the new technical solutions in this field. Some details concerning the standards of CCA and CTA performance have already been published [2] and are used here with addition of new information.

2. CCA

2.1. Description of the procedure

A patient lies in supine position on the table being a part of C-arm unit. X-ray tube moves rotationally in two perpendicular planes (horizontal and vertical) which makes any required type of projection possible. (The most common projections are: LAO, LAO/Cranial, LAO/Caudal, RAO). The principal current-voltage parameters are chosen automatically.

Good practice rules require that the x-ray tube is kept under the table. This allows to avoid unnecessary irradiation of the staff and makes the doses to patient lower.

In order to visualize coronary vessels a contrast agent is administered intravenously: a thin catheter is previously introduced to the brachial artery or the femoral artery (there are two alternative access routes) and its movement is traced by fluoroscopy and observed on monitor by the operator.

(The physiological parameters of a patient are permanently monitored during the procedure.)

The operating team consists of 3 to 4 persons: usually they are an operator (with an assistant if necessary), a scrub nurse and an anaesthetic nurse. All the persons stay around the patient table and thus may be exposed to even high doses of radiation. (There are scattered x-rays mainly.) An especially exposed member of the team is the operator: the doses registered for such persons may achieve the highest level measured for occupational exposures [3,4].

Patient exposure results mainly from primary x-ray beam which covers a part of back surface (the area of left shoulder) by most time of the procedure. The remaining body of a patient is exposed to rather scattered radiation.

Three types of images can be created during the procedure:

a. Real-time images (fluoroscopic images) observed by the operator (visible also on the technical console),

b. Radiographic images for saving some chosen moments of the procedure (so-called acquisition),

http://dx.doi.org/10.5772/54034

c. The long periods of exposure can be recorded in so-called "cine-mode" (if x-ray system is technically predicted to this mode of work).

The results of CCA procedure are analyzed by cardiologists during its performance and also retrospectively after that.

2.2. Technical requirements for x-ray systems with C-arm

Cardiovascular surgery covers a wide array of procedures and methods, each with specific imaging requirements. Consequently, x-ray systems are offered by the vendors in many versions.

Two types of construction are proposed generally: a fixed C-arm system and mobile C-arm.

A fixed C-arm system can be floor-mounted or ceiling-mounted. The solution is chosen by the user in dependence on the space condition of operating room. Fixed C-arm systems are required for CCA and further surgery procedures such as: percutaneous coronary interventions (PCI) and endovascular aortic repair (EVAR).

A powerful mobile C-arm can be used for pacemakers or defibrillator implants and carotid artery stenting. However, fixed C-arm systems can offer added security and are preferred for complex cases and lengthier procedures.

Diagnostic procedures and a structural heart disease treatment in children using imaging system require a high temporal resolution, which is provided by dedicated fixed C-arm systems with very high frame rates.

Any x-ray system used for CCA procedures should be equipped as follows:

- high frequency converter generator of minimum 80 kW (in possibly rectangular pulses),
- x-ray tube focuses not larger than 1.2/0.5mm,
- minimum two dose-rate modes (Low-Medium-High or Low- Standard),
- x-ray tube – image detector distance tracking (minimum focus skin distance 30 cm),
- patient table made from low-attenuating materials,
- display of fluoroscopy time, total dose-area product (fluoroscopy and radiographic) and estimated skin entrance dose,
- image hold system (for example default storage of the last 20 sec. of fluoroscopy for reference or archiving).

Despite of the general features, the system should fulfil the following requirements:

- generator should be controlled by microprocessor, power switch accurately controlled, with short switching time (about 1 ms); voltage should cover the range of (40-120) kV,
- a high power tube with high heat dissipation,
- dose-area product meter with display visible for operator,

- should be equipped with additional filtration (Cu preferred), enabling to select a proper filtration in dependence on x-ray spectrum,
- overcouch image detector,
- collimators incorporating circular shutters,
- flexibility of pulsed fluoroscopy mode (grid- switched and individually programmed with a different composition of x-ray dose rate, digital processing and filter settings),
- staff protective shielding,
- a possibility of AEC mode choice by the user (IMAGE or DOSE weighted).

Additionally in some x-ray systems are also available partially absorbent contoured filters (so-called wedge filters) to absorb radiation in the low density areas surrounding the heart.

Another proposal for coronary angiography appears in 2009 [5], i.e. biplane system in which simultaneous accurate images of the heart are provided from two different points of view. This allows to reduced contrast volume and radiation exposure. Biplane angiography helps to visualize complex coronary or structural cardiac anatomy. The clinical settings in which biplane system is the most critical occur in the paediatric population and in those patients with renal failure. The value of biplane angiography must be balanced against cost and difficulty of use: such system requires the patient's heart to be in the exact centre of the two planes (the isocentre) and then AP and lateral planes were properly angled in orthogonal protections.

2.2.1. Image recording

Most of x-ray units used in cardiology nowadays are equipped with the digital image recording system. There are two types of it: (1) an image intensifier based system and (2) a flat-panel fluoroscopy system. The first one utilizes conventional technology: the output screen of image intensifier is projected in a video camera or a CCD camera to produce an electronic information. Such systems are still used in many interventional labs. The older systems have got image intensifiers, which cause a significant loss of signal intensity because of the construction principle.

The digital Flat Detectors (FD) are smaller and easier to operate. Image quality may be better, but the modern x-ray systems have much higher output capacity and thus higher doses are probable.

Maximum field of view FD has to be large enough: 30x36 cm (11.8x14.4 inch), but the used area may be part of the maximum in dependence on current medical needs.

Image matrix size should be also large – especially for the acquisitions recording, and can be smaller for fluoroscopic observations (the signals are then summarized).

Nyquist frequency of FD fluoroscopy systems are better than 3 lp/mm.

Quite important are the monitors in the system: they can be monochrome or colour LCD of 18-19 inch.

http://dx.doi.org/10.5772/54034

2.3. Dosimetric quantities

Presently used fluoroscopic equipment measures air kerma with the use of an ionization chamber incorporated into the x-ray tube envelope and reports the dose-area product (DAP), equal to air kerma (dose) multiplied by x-ray beam cross-sectional area. (This is legal requirement.) X-ray systems used for fluoroscopic procedures are obligatory equipped in DAP-meter to summarize emission in all the modes of work (i.e. fluoroscopy, radiography, cine). (Dose Area Product= DAP [$Gy.m^2$]). Measurements are performed by the transmission chamber placed on the x-ray tube output.

DAP is independent on the distance from x-ray source (according to the inverse-square law). Some systems show also peak skin dose (in grays) treated as the highest dose received by any location on the patient's skin, including both incident and back-scattered radiation. Although thought to be the best predictor of skin injury, peak skin dose is difficult to measure in practice and the values displayed by the x-ray system can be treated as an approximation of real value.

DAP (and entrance air kerma) values have to be displayed on the monitors of x-ray system and should be registered in the patient record. (Especially when entrance air kerma is over 1Gy and exceeds the threshold of deterministic skin effects.)

For a given projection mean entrance skin dose (or entrance air kerma) can be calculated as the ratio of DAP and the area of the incident x-ray beam (at the level of patient's skin). The relationship is not valid for DAP summarized for the whole procedure because of the incidence angle variation.

The actual dose received by a patient from a given x-ray procedure can be evaluated by the following approaches:

- **a.** with calculation based on dosimetric measurements made in physical phantoms,
- **b.** with Monte Carlo simulations using mathematical phantoms,
- **c.** with DLP values provided by the x-ray system and a body region-specific conversion coefficient averaged for multiple scanners.

Dosimetric measurements are commonly made with termoluminescent dosimeters (lithium fluoride or calcium fluoride) or solid state detectors. The detectors are distributed inside the phantom which is exposed as a patient. The most popular are Rando Man or Rando Woman phantoms (representing adult humans) and the family of CIRS phantoms (representing children as well as adults).

Monte Carlo simulation assumes a mathematical phantom representing a patient from a given age group and model photon transitions through this phantom. The older solutions used the "family" of Cristy' phantoms for simulation, modelling organs as geometrical solids. The newer studies use voxel phantoms which are more anatomical being created on the basis of CT human images.

The last approach, i.e. taking some conversion coefficients from literature and multiplying by DAP is the simplest but on the condition that the values are really adequate for the given procedure and type of x-ray system. The range of conversion factor reported for CCA varies from 0.12 to 0.26 mSv/(Gy.cm^2) [6].

Regardless of the way, the effective dose estimates the radiation charge for some "typical" (standard) patient, without taking into consideration the anatomy of a given human, and thus should be referred to the category of patients undergoing the given x-ray procedure.

2.4. Doses to patients

The doses obtained by the patients undergoing CCA procedures depend on:

- patient architecture (BMI-body mass index),
- emission effectiveness of the x-ray system,
- applied dose-rate mode,
- total exposure time,
- mode of work (number of acquisitions -radiographic or cine).

Doses received by patients in CCA are evaluated both for the whole body and to the skin.

The entrance surface dose to patient dramatically increases when the focus-to-skin distance becomes too short.

The patient doses are significantly higher when the high dose-rate mode is activated or if pulsed fluoroscopy of high number of pulses per second is chosen. These doses are also inversely proportional to the size of image detector.

During coronarography an entrance dose for a small area of patient's back can be very high while a dose to the remaining part of the trunk can be very low. In consequence, the effective dose may be low and the deterministic effects can appear. (Skin injuries for patients undergoing interventional procedures are reported [7].)

Number of patients	DAP [Gy.cm^2]	Time of fluoroscopy [min]	Number of frames
130	72 +/-55	0.35+/-0.25	1550+/-775
78	73	9.9	1079
100	60.6	-	412
117	1.1 – 11.3	0.3 - 22	-
106	35 - 160	4.8+/-3.5	39+/-11
62	37-190	4.2+/-3.0	30+/-10
90	3.1-57.2	1.5-5.1	639
194	64 - 281	0.4 - 33	200-1911

Table 1. The doses to patients in CCA procedures (according to [8])

http://dx.doi.org/10.5772/54034

Paediatric patients also undergone CCA procedures. The doses for 50 children examined using Allura Xper F20 system are given in Table 2 (the own data from the paediatric clinic).

Number of patients	The range of PSD [mGy] (*)
6	0-20
7	20-40
2	40-60
7	60-80
5	80-100
11	100-200
4	200-300
4	300-400
3	400-500
1	"/>500

(*) the value of Peak Skin Dose is displayed by x-ray system

Table 2. The values of PSD [mGy] for paediatric patients during CCA

The values of effective doses in non-paediatric population undergoing CCA is presented and discussed in [6]. The values were published during ten years (from 1997 to 2007). The mean value is 7.4 mSv but standard deviation is very high (5.4 mSv) because of a wide range of reported doses (from 2.3 to 22.7 mSv). Similar value of ≈7mSv as typical effective dose for adult patients in CCA is also cited by the UNSCEAR [6].

2.5. Doses to staff

Radiation risk to staff in CCA procedures is caused by necessity to work in the radiation filed, standing near patient during exposure. Staff is exposed mainly to scattered radiation although accidentally can be irradiated by primary x-rays.

The factors affecting staff dose are as follows:

- relative position with respect to patient,
- patient architecture (BMI),
- irradiated patient volume,
- x-ray tube position,
- time of exposure,
- effective use of protection shielding.

Thus, staff and patient doses are partially linked: higher exposure for a patient means higher irradiation to staff. This is especially true for the operator and the person standing nearby him (an assistant or scrub nurse). Additional factor determining the doses to staff is professional experience and good training in the procedure performance: good manual skills cause the exposure time shorter.

The problem of radiation risk to staff in interventional cardiology had been widely discussed many times.The essential conclusions resulted from that are the recommendations concerning performance of the interventional procedures and elaboration of the methodology for evaluation radiation risk for the staff [4, 9].

According results of the survey performed by European research group SENTINEL in a sample of European cardiac centres [10] doses for the first operator are as follows:

a. annual effective dose: median 1.3mSv, third quartile 1.4mSv,

b. equivalent dose over the apron: median 11.1mSv, third quartile 14mSv.

Although the above values are rather low it should be underlined that these values may be higher many times (even up the annual limits), especially for inexperienced staff or in a case of clinically difficult patient.

Currently Philips as the only global healthcare company offered a real-time dosimetric system Dose Aware. The system does not replace the thermoluminescence dosimeter (TLD) as a legal dose meter. TLD reports accumulated x-ray dose from the exposure for a period of time but does not include any time stamp or awareness where and when the x-ray dose was acquired.

Dose Aware is a system that gives real-time feedback of scattered x-ray dose reception and instant access to time-stamped dose history. The system is completed from:

- Base Station : an LCD touchscreen displays real time dose data from all PDMs within range. The Base Station stores PDM data as well. Multiple Base Stations can be network linked to a computer running Dose Manager software for analysis.
- Personal Dose Meter (PDM) –worn by the staff; smart badge measures scatter radiation and transmit this information to the Base Station where is displayed.
- Cradle: for placement of the PDM (outside of the exposure time)
- Dose View: PC software package is included together with the Base Station.

Staff working in an x-ray environment wears a PDM. This PDM measures x-ray dose reception and is wirelessly connected to the Base Station. The Base Station is mounted in the examination room where all staff can directly see whether received dose is in red, yellow or green area. The "yellow" or "red" status means a necessity of immediate action to reduce x-ray exposure. X-ray dose history information can be automatically retrieved from any Base Station or from any PDM by using a Cradle with Dose View software or Dose Manager software.

http://dx.doi.org/10.5772/54034

3. CTA

Cardiac CT procedures were an engine for development of new technical solutions in CT: visualization of quickly moving anatomical structures needs extremely short time for acquisition and reconstruction of images. This is available in the new multislice CT scanners, with rotation time not longer than 0.4s and slice collimation 8 cm or more (up to 16 cm). Improvements in spatial and temporal resolution, scan time, scan range and advanced image postprocessing (very important in clinical practice) have made CT angiography (CTA) an excellent tool for identifying patients in need of invasive therapy and for mapping out the best percutaneous or surgical approach. In some cases CTA provides complementary information to that of conventional angiography (CCA).

Although history of cardiac CT began with the four-slice scanners, the real development started with 64-slice scanners with appropriate combination of spatial and temporal resolution. However, the intensity of x-rays emitted in the multislice CT scanners has to be higher and then a number of dose-reduction mechanisms is implemented for patients' safety.

According the American College of Cardiology Foundation (ACCF) the principal indications to cardiac CT are as follows [11]:

- low and intermediate pretest probability of obstructive coronary artery disease (CAD),
- noncontrast CT calcium scoring for patients at intermediate risk of coronary heart disease and for low-risk patients with a family history of disease,
- coronary CT is especially recommended for patients with reduced left ventricular ejection fraction at low or intermediate pretest probability of disease,
- preoperative CT angiography for both heart surgery and noncoronary indications in the setting of risk of CAD.

The current role of coronary CT angiography in the assessment of coronary artery disease is based on its high negative predictive value in ruling out significant stenosis in intermediate risk populations. [12]. A precise preprocedural visualization of complex coronary lesions with CT angiography would be complementary to conventional angiography and allow optimization of the interventional approach during subsequent PCI [13].

The main benefit from CTA is evaluation of cardiac structure and function and also evaluation of anatomical structures surrounding the heart.

3.1. Description of the procedure

From technological reasons the possibilities of CT are limited to diagnostics, without further therapeutic activity (means angioplasty).

The main stages of CT study protocol are as follows:

1. the heart rate control and regulation,
2. calcium scoring,

3. i.v. injection of contrast agent,

4. CT angiography.

As coronary disease is jointed with calcification of coronary arteries, evaluation of this process is a good indicator of pathology. CTA gives possibility to display calcifications (3D) and to assess them quantitatively: it is so-called "calcium scoring".

Generally, the heart can be imaged well if its structures do not move significantly during the scanning time. This condition is fulfilled during the diastolic phase of cardiac cycle. For selection of the proper phase for CT images recording ECG gating (triggering) is applied.

General rules for exposure parameters:

Slice thickness <1mm, pitch<1, $t_{rot} \leq 0.5$sec, kilovoltage U≥100kV, mAs and physical filtration are dependent on the CT scanner, ECG-gating.

Set of parameters for a given CT scanner is determined by the model of a scanner and the version of software dedicated to coronary procedures and offered by the vendor on a user's requirement.

The parameters have also be optimal for the patient's clinical status. The heart rate has here special importance: at the high cardiac rate the registered imaging data have also to be reconstructed very quickly (practically immediately). This is available only for the newest scanners and is applied for paediatric procedures. As usual, it does not exceed 65 bpm but the required value depends on the scanner software. Lowering of the heart rate is achieved pharmacologically.

After completing acquisition of primary data elaboration on them begins, i.e. post-processing.

The possibilities of CT scanner are determined by the installed version of software which may be changed.

The principal algorithms for image post-processing are [14]:

- curved and multiplanar reformats (MPR),
- shaded-surface display (SSD),
- maximum intensity projection (MIP),
- volume rendering (VR).

The axial images produced by hardware (so-called row data) are essential and should be used but reformed images may improve lesion detection and classification (particularly coronal and oblique views). The axial images and MPRs are used for diagnosis and the SSD and MIPs are for display purposes.

The results of CTA are evaluated or consulted by a cardiologist.

3.2. Dosimetric quantites

Practical dosimetric quantities used for CT are a dose-length-product (DLP) and computed-tomography-dose- index (CTDI).

http://dx.doi.org/10.5772/54034

A dose-length-product (DLP) is directly measured by a dosemeter with a pencil chamber. Measured in units of mGy.cm, DLP reflects the integrated radiation dose (in a given position) for the total length of scanning.

The first estimation of a dose received by a patient during the CT procedure is the value of the $CTDI_{vol}$ displayed on the console monitor of the scanner. The $CTDI_{vol}$ represents an average dose over the scanned volume. The quantity is computed on the basis of exposure parameters (voltage, mAs per scan, pitch) according to the calibration stored in the computer memory of the scanner. The calibration is performed for the standard dosimetric cylindrical phantom from PMMA. By convention, a phantom 16 cm in diameter is used to model the head, and a 32 cm phantom is used to model the body (for adult patient). The displayed $CTDI_{vol}$ is used as a measure of radiation charge in the procedure.

$CTDI_{vol}$ can be computed on the basis of DLP measurements using a practical formula given below:

$CTDI_{vol} = (DLP_{ave}/L)$ [mGy]

where $DLP_{ave} = (1/3)DLP_c + (2/3)DLP_p$, L- the accurate length of scan., i.e. the difference between start and end positions of the table.

DLP_c and DLP_p are measured in the centrum and at periphery of the adequate PMMA phantom (i.e. "HEAD" Ø=16cm or "BODY" Ø=32cm).

The absorbed organ doses and then the effective dose received by a patient from a given CT procedure may be evaluated by the following approaches:

a. with calculation based on dosimetric measurements made in physical phantoms,

b. with Monte Carlo simulations using mathematical phantoms,

c. with $CTDI_{vol}$ values provided on the scanner console and a body region-specific conversion coefficient averaged for multiple scanners.

Dosimetric measurements are commonly made with termoluminescent dosimeters (lithium fluoride or calcium fluoride) or solid state detectors. The detectors are distributed inside the phantom which is exposed as a patient. The most popular are Rando Man or Rando Woman phantoms (representing adult humans) and the family of CIRS phantoms (representing children as well as adults).

Monte Carlo simulation assumes a mathematical phantom representing a patient from a given age group and model photon transitions through this phantom. The older solutions used the "family" of Cristy' phantoms for simulation, modelling organs as geometrical solids. The newer studies use voxel phantoms which are more anatomical being created on the basis of CT human images.

The last approach, i.e. taking some conversions coefficient from literature and multiplying by $CTDI_{vol}$ is the simplest, but under condition, that the both values are really adequate for the given scanner.

Regardless of the way, the effective dose estimates the radiation charge for some "typical" (standard) patient, without taking into consideration the anatomy of a given human, and thus should be referred to the category of patients undergoing the given x-ray procedure.

3.3. Doses to patients and radiation protection in CTA

Computerized tomography is treated as a high-dose imaging technique although in the currently produced scanners a lot of mechanisms for dose reduction is implemented and the high doses can be avoided.

Because of exposure conditions in CTA (thin slices and low pitch) the doses to patients are relatively high, especially at 64-slice scanners. It was an inspiration to implement the methods of dose reduction without loss of image quality. (According to Sun et.al [1] 64-slice CT scanners are the most commonly used for coronary CT angiography, although 16-slice are still in use. The next place have dual-source CT scanners as dedicated to angiographic procedures.)

The mean effective doses in CTA for adult patients undergoing the procedure using 64-slice scanners are from 8 mSv to 21.4 mSv [6].

The doses can be reduced through lowering current-voltage parameters, implementation of x-rays intensity modulation (for three axis), shortening of scanned body length and ECG gating (specially for cardiac procedures). ECG-controlled tube current modulation is very common approach utilized in CTA [1].

An example of the impact of different scan protocols on radiation dose and image quality is taken from [15]. The data concern the randomly selected adult patients examined for the evaluation of coronary artery disease. Two CT scanners were used: 16-slice and 64-slice.

	16 –slice CT			64-slice CT		
	120 kV without EGC	120 kV with EGC	100 kV with EGC	120 kV without EGC	120 kV with EGC	100 kV with EGC
No. of patients	30	50	50	50	50	30
Heart rate [bpm]	61.3±11.3	60.7±9.5	57.8±5.3	61.1±10.4	57.5±7.2	57.0±8.2
Tube current [mA]	510.0±40.3	304.5±42.3	387.6±18.9	870.0±55.6	551.0±58.2	537.8±50.7
$CTDI_{vol}$ [Gy]	42.1±3.6	25.2±2.9	19.4±1.0	58.8±6.5	38.3±3.11	22.0±1.8
Signal-to-noise ratio	11.1±3.9	11.9±4.3	11.9±3.7	8.9±2.5	9.2±2.8	9.2±2.5
Effective dose [mSv]	10.6±1.2	6.4±0.9	5.0±0.3	14.8±1.8	9.4±1.0	5.4±1.1

Table 3. Data for different protocols of CTA (from [15])

The special solution for dose reduction being dedicated to cardiac CT examinations is the change of image acquisition technique from RGH to PGA [8].

RGH = Retrospectively Gated Helical: the patient and table move through the gantry at a steady speed. A low pitch (0.2 to 0.4) is needed to cover the entire cardiac volume, especially to compensate for any ectopic beats, which can result in misregistration and gaps in coverage. Thus, the same anatomy can be exposed to the x-ray beam many times (up to five) to ensure enough coverage, causing high absorbed doses.

PGA= Prospectively Gated Axial: the table is stationary during PGA image acquisition, then moves to the next location for another scan that is initiated by the next normal cardiac cycle.

The x-rays emission is then dynamically predicted on the basis of ECG signal.

Diagnostic value of images obtained for PGA protocol was found not lower than for RGH while the doses where substantially lower [8]. In the same study including 203 CTA exams (82 with routine RGH and 121 with the PGA) the doses were evaluated for protocol including scout images, low-dose calcium scoring scans, test-bolus scan and CT coronary angiogram. The exams were performed using 64-slice CT scanner (LightSpeed VCT XT, GE). The effective doses were as follows:

RGH: (8.7-23.2) mSv, mean: 18.4 mSv;

PGA: (0.75-6.67) mSv; mean: 2.84 mSv.

The similar dose values (16.3 mSv and 3.5 mSv for RGH and PGA, respectively) are drawn as a conclusion from the papers published from 2007 to 2011 [1] and prospective ECG-triggering is recommended as the most commonly applied technique for dose reduction [16, 17].

Lowering of tube voltage is another technique frequently proposed for dose reduction. The results of multicenter, multivendor randomized trial using 80 kVp was published by LaBounty et. al. [18]. The authors concluded that CTA using 80 kVp instead of 100 kVp was associated with a nearly 50% reduction in radiation dose with no significant difference in interpretability and noniferior image quality despite lower signal-to-noise and contrast-to-noise ratios.

4. C-arm CT

The newest technique for cardiac imaging is so-called C-arm CT (also Rotational Angio, dyna-CT). This is a special option of the new models of C-arm units introduced as a potential modality for intra-operative 3D imaging. This is possible for C-arm systems equipped with flat panel detectors and appropriate software for image reconstructions.

The C-arm is rotated over a wide range (>180°) with or without continuous contrast injection, acquiring multiple views of the cardiovascular structure with subsequent 3D reconstruction. This is advanced post processing giving images like 3D reconstructions from CT. For ECG-referenced cardiac imaging, identical alternating forward and backward rotations are triggered by the ECG signal to acquire projections covering the entire acquisition range at a similar cardiac phase [19, 20, 21].

Because of the relatively slow rotation of the C-arm, the temporal resolution of these systems is significantly inferior to the new multislice CT scanners [19].

The acquisition of 3D data directly from the angiography system may facilitate co-registration of angiographic data with pre-procedurally acquired 3D CT images, with subsequent automatic registration to the 2D-fluoroscopy images obtained using the same system. The availability of real-time 3D anatomical information from the patient may offer advantages beyond those of pre-procedural images.

C-arm CT as a technical solution joins some benefits of CT with C-arm techniques, giving possibility to continue the diagnostic procedure (angiography) as a therapeutic one, and subsequently to provide CT-like images during an interventional procedure without moving the patient to a CT or MRI scanner.

The results of comparison of both CA modes (CCA and rotational angiography) performed for the same patients (over 200) revealed a hih degree of diagnostic agreement for 3 independent cardiologist and for each coronary segment [22]. Contrast medium volume during rotational CA and conventional CA amounted to 31.9± 4.5 mL versus 52.2±8.0 mL, and patient radiation exposure amounted to 5.0±2.6 Gy.cm^2 versus 11.5±5.5 Gy.cm^2, respectively.

Author details

Maria Anna Staniszewska

Dept. of Medical Imaging Techniques, Medical University, Lodz, Poland

References

[1] Sun Z, Ng K-H. *Coronary CT angiography in coronary artery disease*. WJC, 2011 September 26; 3(9): 303-310

[2] Advances in the Diagnosis of Coronary Atherosclerosis, Edited by Suna F.Kirac. InTech, 2011. Chapter 5: Coronary Angiography- Physical and Technical Aspects, by M.A.Staniszewska

[3] Vano E, Gonzales L, Guibelalde E, et al:Radiation exposure to medical staff in interventional and cardiac radiology. Br.J.Radio., 71,954-960,1998.

[4] International Commission on Radiological Protection, Publication 85, Avoidance of Radiation Injuries from Medical Interventional Procedures, 2001.

[5] http://www.cathlabdigest.com/articles/Biplane-Coronary-Angiography, by M.Kern

[6] Einstein AJ, Moser KW, Thompson RC, Cerqueira MD, Hezlova MJ. *Contemporary Reviews in Cardiovascular Medicine*. Circulation, 2007; 116: 1290-1305

[7] Vano E, Arranz L, Sastre JM, et al: *Dosimetric and radiation protection considerations based on some cases of patient skin injuries in interventional cardiology*. Br.J.Radiol., 71, 510-516, 1998.

[8] Bor D, Olgar T, Toklu T, et al.: *Patient doses and dosimetric evaluations in interventional cardiology*. Physica Medica, 25,31-42, 2009.

[9] International Commission on Radiological Protection, Publication 75, General Principles of Monitoring for Radiation Protection of Workers, 1997.

[10] Padovani R: Optimisation of patient and staff exposure in interventional radiology. In: Radiation Protection in Medical Physics, edited by Y.Lemoigne and A.Caner, Springer in Cooperation with NATO Public Diplomacy Division, The Netherlands, 2011.

[11] Taylor A, Cerquiera M in Journal of the American College of Cardiology, October 2010: according to AuntMinnie.com (November 1,2010): *New cardiac CT guidelines expand use for low-risk patients*.

[12] Hamon M, Biondi-Zoccai GG, Malagutti P, Agostoni P, Morello R, Valgimigli M, Hamon M. *Diagnostic performance of multi slice spiral computed tomography of coronary arteries as compared with conventional invasive coronary angiography. A meta-analysis*. J Am Coll Cardiol 2006; 48: 1896-1910

[13] Wink O. Hecht HS, Ruijters D. *Coronary computed tomographic angiography in the cardiac catheterization laboratory: current applications and future developments*. Cardiol Clin 2009; 27: 513-529

[14] W.A.Kalender: Computed Tomography. Publicis MCD Verlag, Munich 2000

[15] Hausleiter J, Meyer T, Hademitzky M, Huber E, Zankl M, Martinoff S, Kastrati A, Schomig A. *Radiation Dose Estimates From Cardiac Multislice Computed Tomography in Daily Practice*. Circulation, 2006, March; 113:1305-1310

[16] Sabarudin A, Sun Z, Ng K-H. *Radiation dose associated with coronary CT angiography and invasive coronary angiography: an experimental study of the effect of dose-saving strategies*. Radiat Prot Dosimetry, 2012; 150(2): 180-187

[17] Hong YJ, Kim SJ, Lee SM, Min PK, Yoon YW, Lee BK, Kim TH. *Low-dose coronary computed tomography angiography using prospective ECG-triggering compared to invasive coronary angiography*. Int J Cardiovasc Imaging, 2011 Mar; 27(3): 425-431

[18] LaBounty TM, Leipsic J, Poulter R, Wood D, Johnson M, Srichai MB, Cury RC, Heibron B, Hague C, Lin FY, et al. *Coronary CT angiography of patients with a normal body mass index using 80 kVp versus 100 kVp: a prospective, multicenter, multivendor randomized trial*. Am J Radiol, 2011, Nov,; 197(5): W860-867

[19] Schoenhagen P, Numburi U, Halliburton SS, Aulbach P, von Roden M, Desai MY, Rodriguez LL, Kapadia SR, Tuzcu EM, Lytle BW. *Three-dimensional imaging in the context of minimally invasive and tanscatheter cardiovascular interventions using multi-detector computed tomography: from pre-operative planning to intra-operative guidance*. European Heart Journal, 2010; 31: 2727-2741

[20] Neubauer AM, Garcia JA, Messenger JC, Hansis E, Kim MS, Klein AJ, Schoonenberg GA, Grass M, Carroll JD. *Clinical feasibility of a fully automated 3D reconstructions of rotational coronary X-ray angiograms*. Circ Cardiovasc Interv, 2010; 3: 71-79

[21] Tommassini G, Camerini A, Gatti A, Derelli G, Bruzzone A, Veccio G. *Panoramic coronary angiography*. J Am Coll Cardiol, 1998; 31: 871-877

[22] Empen K, Kuon E, Hummel A, Gebauer C, Dorr M, Konemann R, Hoffmann W, Staudt A, Weitmann K, Reffelmann T, Felix SB. *Comparison of rotational with conventional coronary angiography*. Am Heart J, 2010, Sept.; 160(3): 552-563

Chapter 15

Transradial Versus Transfemoral Coronary Angiography

Amir Farhang Zand Parsa

Additional information is available at the end of the chapter

http://dx.doi.org/10.5772/54077

1. Introduction

Although trans-brachial approach via brachial cut done, that has been introduced by Sones in 1959, was the prefer method for coronary angiography in the 1950s and 1960s, because of the complexity of the procedure, it lost its popularity during last decades. Meanwhile trans-femoral (TF) approach became popular and dominant method for catheterization and angiography, because of the simplicity of the technique and operator-friendly. Whereas trans-radial (TR) approach in aortography for the first time was reported by Radner S, in 1948 [1], due to small vessel size, this technique has been abandoned until 1989, that Campeau did relive this technique and introduced it as an ideal approach for coronary angiography [2]. Although TF approach still is dominant approach worldwide, during the last decade TR approach has emerged as a new method for coronary angiography and angioplasty, mostly in European countries and Japan. Because of its advantages, less vascular complication and early mobilization of patients, TR approach is going to be the method of choice for cardiac catheterization and angiography. TR technique encompasses vast majority of procedures, including diagnostic and interventional procedures, and suitable for most patients.

There is no doubt that all three above mentioned approaches are applicable in invasive and interventional cardiology but we are looking for the most feasible and safest approach for vascular access for coronary angiography and intervention.

The purpose of this chapter is to compare the different approaches in coronary angiography and intervention regarding their applicability, feasibility and safety.

2. Anatomical considerations

Operators should be prepared for these approaches theoretically. The knowledge of anatomy of the femoral, brachial and radial arteries is necessary and helpful for doing these techniques successfully.

Femoral Access: Common femoral artery is the continuation of external iliac artery. It begins just below the inguinal ligament outside the femoral vein and inside to the femoral nerve. Common femoral artery and vein enclosed in a fibrous sheath that has been called, femoral sheath. It lies anterior and adjacent to the one third of internal aspect of the head of femur and crosses to the median side of the body of the femur (figure 1, A). One of the reasons that TF approach is prone to more complication is its proximity to the femoral nerve, femoral vein and pelvic cavity. Because puncturing of superficial femoral artery is more susceptible to pseudo-aneurysm, common femoral artery (first 3 centimeter) must be chosen for arterial puncture.

Radial access: The radial artery is the continuation of the brachial artery. It begins at the bifurcation of the brachial artery in the cubital fossa, and passes along the radial side of the forearm to the wrist toward the styloid process of the radius [3]. Then it passes between the two heads of the first Interosseous dorsalis into the palm of the hand (figure 1, B). At the wrist where arterial puncture should be done there is no nerve, vein or cavity at the vicinity of the radial artery, i.e. they are not enclosed in the same fibrous sheath. Deep palmar arch is a connection between the radial and the ulnar artery that protect hand from ischemia due to the occlusion of each branches. The radial artery serves mainly as an arterial conduit to the hand [4]. These are the reasons that radial approach is less prone to complication. The radial artery diameter is about 3.1mm±0.2mm [5]. However, its size is variable and depends on patients' race, gender and size.

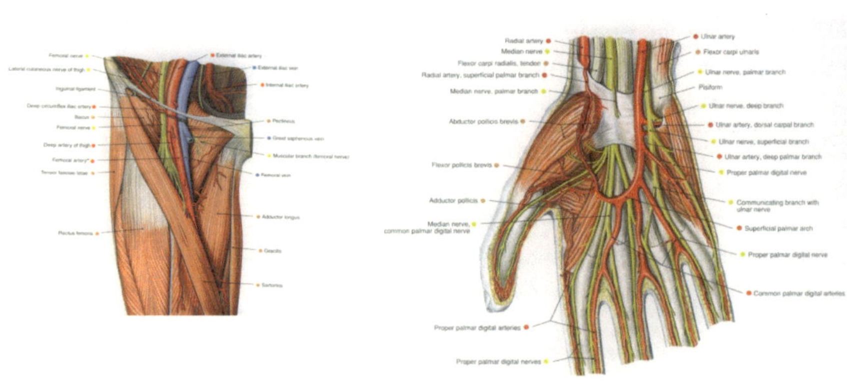

A B

Figure 1. A; The femoral artery, femoral vein and femoral nerve at the groin, B; The radial and the ulnar arteries at the wrist (adapted from: R. Putzand, R. pubast, Sobotta Atlas of Human Anatomy, Urban & Fisher, 14th edition, 2008, p. 245, 614) [6]

http://dx.doi.org/10.5772/54077

3. Technical aspects

Awareness of operators of instruments and devices (catheters, wires and etc....) compatible with each approach and method is crucial for doing these procedures successfully.

Arterial puncture: For doing catheterization and angiography the most important job is to find an accesses route. All cardiologists and interventionists are familiar with the transfemoral access. It is a large caliber artery and easy to be punctured and it is the advantage of this rout over the transbrachial or transradial approach. The only point that should be mentioned regarding TF approach is that the arterial puncture must be done in the groin not farther than 3 centimeter (cm) from the inguinal ligament.

The most difficulty in the transradial technique that operators confront with is the arterial puncture and almost always it is responsible for the failure of the procedure. This is the main reason that this technique needs more experience. Learning curve in this technique dose has profound impact on the procedural success rate and procedural time [7, 8]. Access to the radial artery is a challenging job and needs learning curve for getting skill and to be expert.

Before trying to do radial puncture, it is necessary to do Allen's test for making sure that ulnar artery is patent and collateral supply of the hand is sufficient. The Allen's test for the first time was described by Dr.Allen in 1929 to evaluate collateral circulation of patients suffering from thromboangitis obliterans [9]. For this purpose the patient will be asked to clench his/her hand. Meanwhile operator compresses both the radial and the ulnar arteries by thumb fingers and again the patient will be asked to open his/her hand. After a few second compression on the ulnar artery will be released. In normal situation red color of finger tips will be restored within 10 seconds (positive Allen's test). Pulse Oxymetery of fingers is an alternative method. The test considered positive if the pulse waveform reappeared after releasing compression on the ulnar artery while compressing the radial artery (figure 2) [10, 11]. However the necessity of the evaluation of collateral blood flow to the hand before TR approach is controversial [12].

Before doing radial puncture, the wrist should be prepared by hyperextending it over an arm board or positioned the arm beside the body with the wrist expanded. Sterilization with betadine must be done from elbow to the tips of fingers. Then the skin of the area is anaesthetized with 2-3 ml lidocain 1%-2%. The puncture site is approximately 1-2 centimeter proximal to the radial styloid.

After identifying the radial artery a small incision of the skin of the prepared puncture site is done, and then the radial artery is punctured with a 20- 21- gauge (G) needle through the incision. Appearances of pulsatile flow from the end of the needle confirmed that the needle is inside the lumen of the artery. It can be occurred when the needle is pushing inside the radial artery or when the needle that deeply seated in the posterior wall of the artery is pulling back until pulsatile flow from the needle reappears. Then a 0.018 – 0.035- inch hydrophilic guide wire is introduced through the needle for inserting 5 to 6- French (Fr), 11-25- cm long sheath in the radial artery (figure 3). Just after the insertion of a sheath, a cocktail consisted of 2mg verapamil, 100 microgram (μgr) nitroglycerin and 2500 unit unfractionated heparin (UFH) or 200 μgr nitroglycerin and 2500 unit UFH should be administered through the side arm of the sheath, for preventing vasospasm and thrombus formation. Right radial artery was preferred rout by the majority of operators so far but recently left radial artery has been introduced by some operators as a preferred method.

Although conventional catheters (pigtail, judkin's (left and right), XB, EB and etc....) can be used for catheterization and coronary angiography via radial access, usually new catheters such as Tiger (terumo) are used for coronary angiography (figure 3). The advantage of new catheters is that both left and right coronary arteries can be opacified by one catheter.

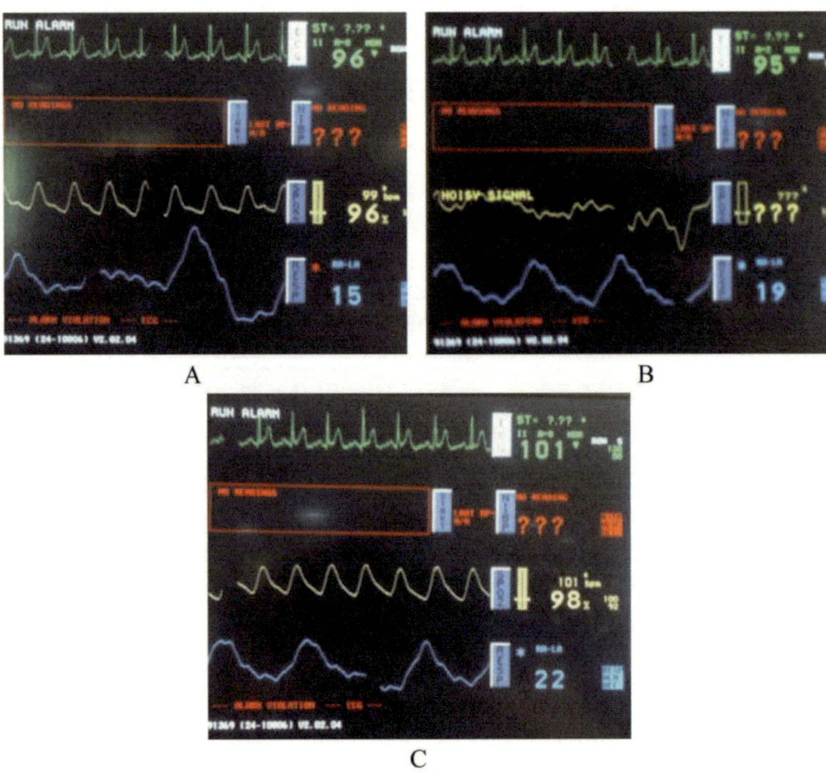

Figure 2. Pulse waveform and oxygen saturation before (A), during (B) and after (C) Allen's test. (Adapted from: Natarajan D. Coronary Angiography – The Need for Improvement in Medical and Interventional Therapy. *Edited by Branislav Baškot, Publisher: InTech, 2011; p=55*) [13]

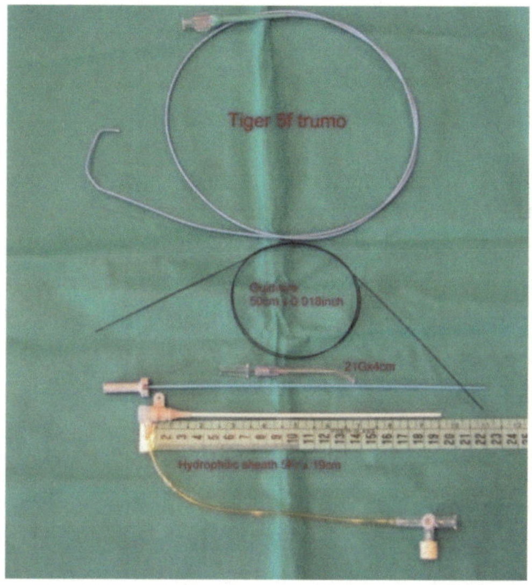

Figure 3. 5-Fr □Tiger catheter, 50-Cm □0.018-inch□Nitinol hydrophilic guide wire, 21-G □needle and 5-Fr □19-Cm sheath, from top to below respectively.

4. Limitations of each approach

Transbrachial approach: The transbrachial approach that for the first time was introduced by F Mason Sones in 1958 has been done via arteriotomy (cut done) technique [14, 15]. Due to the complexity of the procedure this approach lost its popularity and no longer has been used as a routine approach for coronary angiography and intervention. However in recent years this approach is used for selected cases (in the presence of severe peripheral vascular disease and ect…) percutaneously. But the dominant approaches are either radial or femoral approach.

Transfemoral approach: Transfemoral approach that was introduced by Sven Ivar Seldinger in 1953 has been done percutaneously, figure 4 [16]. Because Seldinger's method was feasible and easy to do, very soon did get popularity among invasive and /interventional cardiologists and radiologists. For more than 50 years it has been the method of choice for angiography and/ angioplasty worldwide.

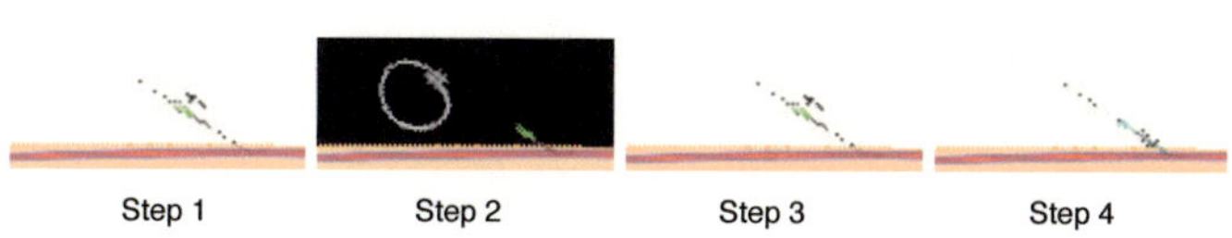

Figure 4. Steps of percutaneous technique for coronary angiography, Seldinger's method. (from Seldinger SI. Catheter replacement of the needle in percutaneous arteriography. A new technique. Acta Radiologica 1953; 39: 368-76) [16].

Limitations for TF approach are: 1) severe peripheral vascular disease, 2) obese patients, 3) presence of severe musculoskeletal abnormalities such as spine or hip malformation, 4) coagulopathies or patients who received high doses of anticoagulation. Not only these limitations decrease the success rate of procedures but also increase the complication rates that will be discussed later.

Transradial approach: Since the first time in1989 that Campeau L reported 100 cases of coronary angiography via getting access through the radial artery without major complication [2] and in 1993 that Ferdinand Keimeneij and colleagues did percutaneous coronary angioplasty (PTCA) by TR approach, that was comparable with TF approach, TR approach emerged as a new technique for coronary angiography and angioplasty. In 1997 Ferdinant Keimeneij et al,reported comparison between transradial, transbrachial and transfemoral PTCA in 900 patients. Although in their study access failure in TR approach was more common than transbracial and TF approaches, major access site complication were more frequent in the two latters [17]. However, with getting more experience the rate of failure in the TR approach has declined significantly [18]. Indeed transradial success rate depends to the operator learning curve.

TR approach is suitable for most patients and limitation of this approach is very low; however, there is some limitations for this approach that are as below: 1) inadequate ulnar artery collateral circulation (abnormal Allen's test), 2) needs for using large sheath, catheter and / devices, 3) the other limitation of this approach is need for repeating the procedure; however, it has been reported by Sakai and colleagues that transradial approach can be repeated for three to five times in the same access site, especially in men [19]. 4) The other limitation is the need for right heart catheterization and / endomyocardial biopsy simultaneously. However, some studies proposed forearm vein for right heart catheterization in the same time [20, 21].

5. Complications

Usually complications are vascular and mostly dependent to the access site. Although access site complication is more common in the TF approach compared to TR approach, it can occur in both approaches.These complications are:

1. Bleeding and hematomas; the most common complications in these approaches are bleeding and hematomas and their occurrence increase in the setting of anticoagulant and antiplatelet therapy that is usual in these patients. Bleeding complication in the femoral approach in the era of intervention is about 3% that 1% of them need blood transfusion; however, in the radial approach it is nearly 0% [22, 17]. Keimeneij et al in a randomized study involving 900 patients did compare TF, transbrchial and TR approaches in patients undergoing percutaneous coronary intervention. In their study access site complications were significantly lower in the TR approach (Major access site bleeding occurred in seven patients (2.3%) in the transbrachial group, six (2.0%) in the transfemoral group and none in the transradial group, $p = 0.035$ [17]. A systematic review of randomized trials has shown reduction of access site complications by 73% when TR approach was employed instead of TF approach. In this met-analysis major

http://dx.doi.org/10.5772/54077

bleeding occurred in 13 (0.05%) of 2,390 patients in the radial access group compared to 48 (2.3%) of 2,068 patients in the femoral access group (OR 0.27, 95% CI 0.16-0.45; P <0.001), figure 5 [23]. Also according to this meta-analysis of trials occurrence of haematomas was significantly lower in the radial access group compared with femoral access group (HR 0 40, 95% CI 0 28-0 57; p<0 0001) [23].

2. Pseudoaneurysm; pseudoaneurysmcan is a potentially life threatening complication that particularly occurred in the TF approach. Its incidence in the TF approach was about 0.03% to 0.2% [24]. But it seems to be more prevalent in the era of intervention. Although in the above mentioned meta-analysis, that included all trials of percutaneous coronary intervention, few cases [7 0f 3507 patients) in the radial group has been reported [23], its incidence in the TR approach in coronary angiography is near zero.

Anticoagulation is the main risk factor for occurring pseudoaneurysm that followed by; receiving thrombolytic agents or potent antiplatelet (Gp IIb/IIa), obesity, female gender, large sheath size, interventional procedures and multipuncture of the left groin. Although the size of the pseudoaneurysm is not an absolute predictor of the need for surgical repair, pseudoaneurysm smaller than 18 mm in diameter is safe and will be closed spontaneously. Ultrasound-guided compression is the first choice treatment of this complication.

Major bleeding

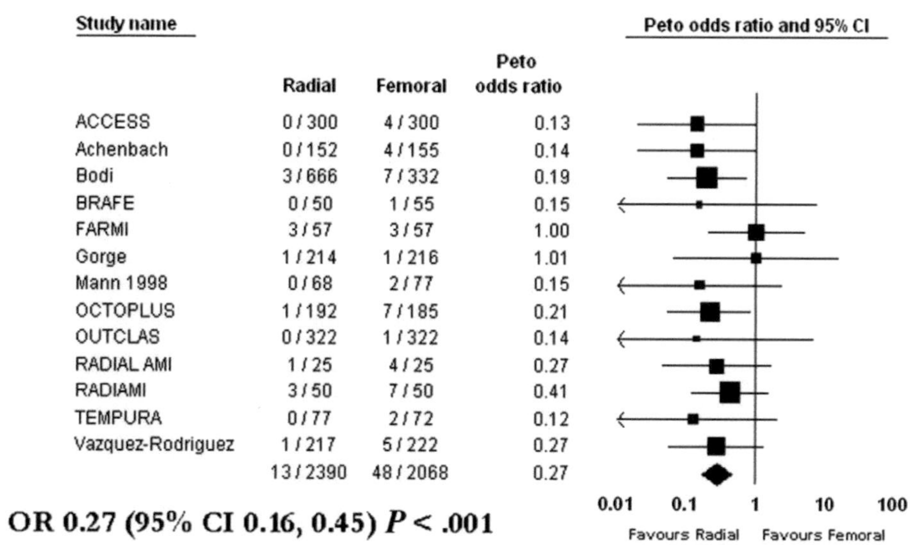

Figure 5. Forest plot for major bleeding of radial versus femoral access. (from; Jolly SS, Amlani S, Haman M, Yusuf S, Mehta SR. Radial versus femoral access for coronary angiography or intervention and the impact on major bleeding and ischemic events: A systematic review and meta-analysis of randomized trials. Am Heart J 2009;157:132-40) [23]

3. Arteriovenous fistula; Occurrence of arteiovenous fistula (AVF) after catheterization is more infrequent than pseudoaneurysm and such as other vascular access complications

is more common in the TF approach. Its incidence in the femoral access site particularly in the era of interventional procedures according to some studies is about 0.3% to 0.8% [25, 26]. Although occurrence of AVF is very rare in the TR approach, there is sporadic case report of its occurrence after using radial access for coronary angioplasty but not in diagnostic coronary angiography. In my best knowledge four cases of AVF after TR approach for intervention have been reported, table 4 [27]. Interestingly majority of catheter induced AVFs, either in the femoral access site or in the radial access site are asymptomatic.

4. Arterial occlusion is the most important but rare access site complication that more frequently occur in the TR approach. Radial artery occlusion has been reported 2%-60% in the studies using absence of pulse as a criterion for arterial occlusion [28], and 3%-6% in the studies using Doppler ultrasound findings [29]. Also Keimeneij et al reported 5% radial artery occlusion at discharge and 3% at one month follow up in their cases without any femoral artery occlusion [17]. Usually radial artery occlusion does not associate with ischemic complication. Duel arterial supply of the hand increases the safety of this procedure regarding thrombotic or traumatic occlusion of the radial artery. Generally speaking, the incidence of ischemic damage to the hand following TR approach is much lower and more infrequent compare to TF approach.

	Authers	Year	Age/Sex	Lession & site	Symptom or sign	Diagnostic tool	Surgical repair
Case 1	Pulikal et al	2005	64/male	AVF of Rt radial artery	1-Venous dilation & palpable thrill at puncture site	Doppler ultrasound imaging	yes
Case 2	Spence et al	2007	59/male	Radial artery pseudoaneurysm	Painless pulsatile mass at puncture site	Doppler ultrasound imaging	yes
Case 3	Spence et al	2007	61/male	AVF of radial artery	Painless pulsatile mass at puncture site	Doppler ultrasound imaging	yes
Case 4	Kwac et al	2010	67/male	AVF of radial artery	Pulsatile mass & thrill at puncture site	Doppler ultrasound imaging	yes

Table 1. Some cases which developed radial arteriovenous fistula after cardiac catheterization (adapted from: Kwac MS, Yoon SJ, Oh SJ, Jeon DW, Kim DH, and Yang JY. A rare case of radial arteriovenous fistula after coronary angiography. Korean Circ J 2010;40:677-79) [23]

AVF: arteriovenous fistula, Rt: right

5. Nerve injury; because of superficial course of radial artery and being far from nerve, in contrast to femoral artery (figure 1), nerve injury is more infrequent in TR approach compare to TF approach.

Although as randomized trials did reveal significant reduction of access site complication by using TR approach [23], many invasive and/ interventional cardiologist do perceive that the decrease in vascular complications with TR approach are balanced by technical difficulties and increased radiation exposure with TR approach.

6. Procedural duration and success rate

As a whole TR approach was associated with a little bit longer procedural duration compare to TF approach, but in the hand of expert operators there was no significant difference (12.4±5.8min versus 11.2±3.3min), CARAFE study [7]. In the recent study that has been done by Bruek et al that was larger than CARAFE study and involved operators who were in their early learning curves of TR approach [8]. The median procedural duration for TR and TF approaches were 40.2min and 37min respectively, that difference was statistically significant (p=0.046). Also in a meta-analysis of randomized trials that has been done by Jolly et al, TR approach was associated with longer procedural duration, when weighted mean difference, 3.1 minutes (95% CI 2.4-3.8 p<0.001). When comparing non-radial expert (4.8min, 95% CI 3.7-5.8min) to radial expert (1.7min, 95% CI 07-2.6min), there is significant heterogeneity [23]. It means that operator experience plays a major role in the procedural duration for TR approach.

Usually procedural success rate in the TR approach is less than TF approach that generally is due to failed radial puncture. The success rate (successful angiography without occurrence of significant hematomas) for TR approach compare to TF approach in the Bruek et al, study [8] was 96.5% versus 99.8% respectively (p<0.0001]. However, recent studies revealed no significant difference in procedural success rate between two techniques [30].

Age didn't have any impact on procedural success rate on the TR approach. Procedural success in patient older than and younger than 70 years old was the same [95.1% versus 94.8% respectively, p=NS) [31]. Also there was no significant difference in the procedural success rate in patients who had prior brachial arteriotomy (cut-down) and those who didn't [93.6% versus 95.3% respectively, p=NS) [18].

7. Advantages and disadvantages of two techniques

As mentioned above both techniques have advantages and disadvantages over each other.

Advantages of TF approach over TR approach are: i) because of large caliber vessel it provides easier access site canulation for inserting different sheath size, particularly, large lumen sheaths, that is necessary in the era of interventional cardiology for using large lumen catheters and/large caliber devices. ii) The other advantageous of this technique is that it made simultaneous venoul canulation possible. iii) It takes X ray tube far from operator, and iv) repeatable for unlimited and/several times. iiv) As a whole this technique was associated with higher procedural success rate particularly in the era of interventional cardiology.

However; disadvantages of TF approach are: i) bleeding that is common in the setting of antiplatelet and anticoagulation therapy, that is usual in these patients, is the most important and prevalent complication of TF approach. Major bleeding results >3 fold increases in-hospital and one year mortality (odds ratio= 3.5) and re-infarction [32]. ii) Pseudoaneurysm, atriovenous fistula and retroperitoneal hemorrhage are serious and life-threatening complication of this procedure. iii) Another disadvantageous of TF approach, albeit rare, is thromboembolic or ischemic events of lower extremities, that more often occurred in the presence of peripheral vascular disease or as a result of traumatization and/ dissection of iliac or illeofemoral arteries.

TR approach has gained popularity in recent years and is going to be the technique of choice in coronary angiography and even coronary intervention due to its advantages over TF approach.

The advantages of TR approach over TF approach are; i) reduction of vascular complications in terms of hematomas, bleeding and etc…, even in the setting of acute coronary syndrome (ACS) and/ in patients receiving antithrombotic and antiplatelet therapies. Due to achieving easy hemostasis the bleeding complication and need for transfusion have decreased dramatically by this technique compare to TF approach. In the MORTAL (Mortality Benefit of Reduced Transfusion after PCI via the Arm or Leg) TR approach was associated with 50% reduction in blood transfusion rate, and 29% and 17% reduction in 30-day and one year mortality respectively (p<0.001) [33]. Although in the RIVAL study TR approach was superior to TF approach regarding access site complications (bleeding, hematoma, pseudoaneurysm, etc...), and the incidence of access site complications even in the presence of aggressive anticoagulant regimen were negligible, they concluded that both techniques are safe and effective [34]. ii) Early ambulation and hospital discharge of patients, decreasing hospital cost and increasing patient comfort and satisfaction are other advantages of TR approach over TF approach. In a meta- analysis of more than 20 randomized trials [23], TR approach reduced hospital stay by 0.4 day (95% CI 0.2-0.5, p=0.0001).

The most important disadvantages of TR approach are; the increasing radiation exposure of the operator, access failure and procedural failure, which is higher in comparison with the TF approach and absolutely depend to the operator's learning curve and skill.

7.1. Post procedural hemostasis

Because of the small size and superficiality of the radial artery, hemostasis can be achieved by manual compression. Usually the arterial sheath is removed at the catheterization laboratory at the end of procedure. Hemostasis is obtained by manual compression of the puncture site, and then compression is applied with a cotton pillow tourniquet or by using pressure bandage with elastic sticky straps. In any way the bandage is removed after 6 hours.

In the TF approach also the sheath is removed in the catheterization laboratory and hemostasis is obtained by manual compression, then a bandage and sandbag is applied proximal to the puncture site. The patient should be restricted to bed rest for at least 6 hours. In the case of extensive anticoagulation, vascular closure device can be used for hemostasis. However, in the presence of severe atherosclerosis and small diameter of the femoral artery closure device shouldn't be used.

8. Summary

Both transfemoral and transradial techniques are safe, feasible and comparable techniques for cardiac catheterization, angiography and intervention. However, each of these two techniques has own applications and limitations. Although TF approach is dominant approach worldwide, TR approach is going to be the technique of choice for coronary angiography and percutaneous coronary intervention in the near future. TR approach reduces hospital stay, procedural cost and vascular complications and also increases patients comfort and satisfaction. However, this approach needs more experience and greater learning curve compare to TF approach. In another word, TF approach is the easier and more operator-friendly technique for catheterization and angiography; but with substantial access site complications. On the other hand, TR approach is safer and more patient-friendly technique for catheterization and angiography but it needs more experience and higher learning curve.

Case selection is mater in this regard. For example obese patients, patients with severe peripheral vascular disease and / severe musculoskeletal abnormalities and patients with coagulopathies or under aggressive anticoagulation are not good candidate for TF approach. The prefer approach for these patients is TR approach. On the other hand patients with abnormal Allen's test, patients who need simultaneous right and left heart catheterization and when insertion of a large sheath is needed are not good candidate for TR approach. The prefer approach for these patients is TF approach. Indeed these two vascular access techniques can be reconciled.

Author details

Amir Farhang Zand Parsa

Imam Khomeini Hospital Complex, Tehran University of Medical Sciences, Tehran, Iran

References

[1] Rander S. Thoracal aortography by catheterization from radial artery; preliminary report of a new technique. Acta Radiol 1948; 29: 178-80

[2] Campeau L. Percutaneous radial artery approach for coronary angiography. Cathet Cardiovasc Diagn 1989; 16: 3-7

[3] Karlsson S, Neichajev IA. Arterial anatomy of the upper extremity. Acta Radiol Diagn 1982; 23: 115-21

[4] Haerle M, Hafner HM, Dietz K, Schaller HE, Brunelli F. Vascular dominance in the forearm. Plast Reconstr Surg 2003;111: 1891-8

[5] Fazan VP, Borges CT, Dasilva JH, Caetano AG, Filho OA. Superficial palmar arch: an arterial diameter study. J Anat 2004; 204: 307-11

[6] Putzand R, pubast R. Sobotta ; Atlas of Human Anatomy, Urban & Fisher, 14th edition, 2008; p.245, 614

[7] Louvard Y, Lefevre T, Allain A, Morice M. Coronary angiography through the radial or the femoral approach: the CARAFE study. Cathet Cardiovasc Interv 2001; 52: 181-7

[8] Brueck M, Bandorski D, Kramer W, Wieczorek M, Holtgen R, Tillmans H. A randomized comparison trasradial versus transfemoral approach for coronary angiography and angioplasty. J Am Coll Cardiol 2009; 2: 1047-54

[9] Allen E. Thromboangitis obliterans: methods of chronic occlusive arterial lesions distal to the wrist with illustrative cases. Am J Med Sci 1929; 178: 237-44

[10] Benit E, Vranckx P, Jaspers L, Jackmaer TR, Poelmans C, Coninx R. Frequency of a positive modified Allen's test in 1000 consecutive patients undergoing cardiac catheterization. Cathet Cardiovasc Diagn 1996; 38: 352-4

[11] Barbeau G, Arcenault F, Dugas L, Lariviere M. A new and objective method for transradial approach screening. J Am Coll Cardiol 2001; 37: 34A-36A

[12] Slogoff S, Keats AS, Arlund C. On the safety of radial artery cannulation. Annesthesiology 1983; 59: 42-7

[13] Natarajan D. Coronary Angiography – The Need for Improvement in Medical and Interventional Therapy; Edited by Branislav Baškot, Publisher: InTech, Published: 2011; p=51-74

[14] Sones FM Jr, Shirely EK. Cine coronary angiography. Mod Concepts Cardiovasc Dis 1962; 31: 735-8

[15] Proudfit WL, Shirely EK, Sones FM Jr. Selective coronary angiography. Correlation with clinical findings in 1000 patients. Circulation 1966; 33: 901-10

[16] Seldinger SI. Catheter replacement of the needle in percutaneous arteriography: a new thechnique. Acta Radiologica 1953;39: 368-76

[17] Kiemeniej F, Laarman GJ, Odekerken D, Slagboom T, Vanderwieken R. A randomized comparison of percutaneous transluminal coronary angiography by the radial, brachial and femoral approaches: the access study. J Am Coll Cardiol 1997; 29: 1269-75

[18] Caputo RP, Simons A, Giambartolomei A, Grant W, Fedele K, Esente P. Transradial cardiac catheterization in patients with prior brachial artery cut down. Cathet Cardiovasc Interv 1999; 48: 271-4

[19] Sakai H, Ikeda S, Harada T, Yonashiro S, Ozumi K, Ohe H, et al. Limitations of successive transluminal approach in the same arm: the Japanese experience. Cathet Cardiovasc Interv 2001; 54: 204-8

[20] Moyer CD, Gilchrist IC. Transradial bilateral cardiac catheterization and endomyocardial biopsy: a feasibility study. Cathet Cardivasc Interv 2005; 64: 134-7

[21] Gilchrist IC, Moyer CD, Gascho JA. Transradial right and left heart catheterization: a comparison to traditional femoral approach. Cathet Cardiovasc Interv 2006; 67: 585-88

[22] Rao SV, Eikelboom JA, Granger CB, Harrington RA, Callif RM, Bassand JP. Bleeding and blood transfusion issues in patients with non-ST- segment elevation acute coronary syndromes. Eur Heart J 2007; 28: 1193-204

[23] Jolly SS, Amlani S, Haman M, Yusuf S, Mehta SR. Radial versus femoral access for coronary angiography or intervention and the impact on bleeding and ischemic events: a systematic review and meta-analysis of randomized trials. Am Heart J 2009; 157: 132-40

[24] Souka H, Burkenham T. Management plan of post-angiography false aneurysm of the groin. Ann Saudi Med 1999;19:101-5

[25] Kent KC, Mc Ardel CR, Kennedy B, Baim DS, Anninos E, Skillman JJ. A prospective study of the clinical outcome of femoral pseudoaneurysms and arteriovenous fistulas induced by arterial puncture. J Vasc Surg 1993;17:125:33

[26] Perings SM, Kelm M, Jax T, Strauer BE. A prospective study on incidence and risk factors of arteriovenous fistula following transfemoral cardiac catheterization. Int J Cardiol 2003; 88: 223-8

[27] Kwac MS, Yoon SJ, Oh SJ, Jeon DW, Kim DH, Yang JY. A rare case of radial arteriovenous fistula after coronary angiography. Korean Circ J 2010; 40: 677-79

[28] Stella PR, Keimeneij F, Laarman GJ, Odekerken D, Stagboom T, Vanderwieken R. Incidence and outcome of radial artery occlusion following transradial artery coronary angiography. Cathet Cardiovasc Diagn 1977; 40: 156-8

[29] Chen JY, Lo PH, Hung JS. Color doppler ultrasound evaluation of radial artery occlusion in transradial catheterization. Acta Cardiol Sin 2001; 17: 193-200

[30] Rao SV, Ou FS, Wang TY, Roe MT, Brindis R, Rumsfeld JS, Peterson ED. Trends in the prevalence and outcomes of radial and femoral approaches to percutaneous coronary intervention: a report from the national cardiovascular data registry. J Am Coll Cardiol 2008; 1: 379-86

[31] Caputo RR, Simons A, Giambartolomei A, Grant W, Fedele K, Abraham S, Rejer MJ, Walford GD, Esente P. Transradial cardiac catheterization in elderly patients. Cathet Cardivasc Interv 2000; 51: 287-90

[32] Fei T, Voeltz MD, Attubato MI, Lincoff AM, Chew DP, Bittl JA, Topol EJ, Manoukian SV. Predictors and impact of major hemorrhage on mortality following percutaneous coronary intervention from Replace-2 trial. Am J Cardiol 2007; 100: 1364-69

[33] Chase AJ, Fretz EB, Warburton WP, Klinke WP, Carere RG, Pi D, Berry B, Hilton JD. Association of the arterial access sites at angioplasty with transfusion and mortality study (mortality benefit of reduced transfusion after percutaneous coronary intervention via the arm or leg). Heart 2008, 91: 1019-25

[34] Jolly SS, Yusuf S, Cairns J, Neimelä K, Xarier D, Widimsky p, Budaj A, Neimelä M, Valentin V, Lewis BS, Avezum A, Step PG, Rao SV, Gao P, Afzal R, Joyner CD, Chrolacius S, Mehta SR; RIVAL trial group. Radial versus femoral access for coronary angiography and intervention in patients with acute coronary syndrome (RIVAL): a randomized parallel group multicenter trial. Lancet 2011; 377:1409-20

Chapter 16

Contrast-Induced Nephropathy

Omer Toprak

Additional information is available at the end of the chapter

http://dx.doi.org/10.5772/54032

1. Introduction

Diagnostic and therapeutic angiographic procedures are increasingly performed. Many complex interventions are lengthy and require large dosages of contrast medium (CM). Radiological procedures such as coronary angiography require intravascular administration of iodinated CM is becoming a great source of an iatrogenic disease known as contrast-induced nephropathy (CIN). The pathogenesis of CIN is unclear. The proposed mechanisms are outer-medullary hypoxia due to decreased renal blood flow secondary to renal artery vasoconstriction. Tubular obstruction, apoptosis and oxidative damage, endothelial dysfunction, defective prostaglandin synthesis, and autonomic dysfunction are other proposed mechanisms.

Patients who develop CIN have higher complication rates, longer hospital stays, and higher mortality than patients who not develop CIN. Nearly one-third of the patients who require in-hospital dialysis because of CIN die prior to discharge. No current treatment can reverse or ameliorate CIN once it occurs. The occurrence of CIN is directly related to the number of pre-existing patient risk markers. After the high-risk patient population has been identified and risk markers addressed, the next step in preventing CIN is the use of different prophylactic therapies. The strongly associated risk markers for CIN are pre-existing renal failure, diabetes mellitus, age greater than 70 years, concurrent use of nephrotoxic drugs, hypovolemia, use of a large amount of CM or an ionic hyperosmolar CM, and congestive heart failure.

Aim of the present chapter is to summarize the knowledge about the risk factors and prophylactic treatments of CIN according to the ultimate clinical research and developments.

2. Definition of CIN

A universally accepted definition of CIN does not exist. The most commonly used definition for CIN is the elevation of serum creatinine by ≥0.5mg/dl or ≥25% occurring within 48 hours after administration of CM, and the absence of an alternative etiology. Using the Cockcroft-Gault and the Modification of Diet in Renal Disease equations are useful in estimation of the GFR. Serum cystatin C has been proposed as an alternative endogenous marker of GFR showing higher correlation to standard clearance methods such as inulin or iohexol clearance. Serum cystatin C may detect CIN one to two days earlier than creatinine. Recent studies documented that serum and urine neutrophil gelatinase-associated lipocalin is an early predictive biomarker of CIN (Shaker et al., 2010). Urinary interleukin 18 and urinary liver-type fatty acid-binding protein are new potential biomarkers of CIN (Perrin et al., 2012). Cholesterol atheroemboli, volume depletion, and interstitial nephritis should consider in differential diagnosis of CIN. The incidence of CIN is reported to be 0.6-2.3% in general population who do not have any risk factor for CIN, but the incidence can be increased to 90% in patients at high risk for CIN (Toprak, 2007).

2.1. Pathophysiology of CIN

The potential pathophysiologic mechanisms of CIN were summarized in Figure 1. Medullary hypoxia due to decreased renal blood flow secondary to renal artery vasoconstriction, tubular obstruction, direct tubular toxicity of the CM due to apoptosis, oxidative damage, endothelial dysfunction, and renal microcirculatory alterations may play a role in the pathogenesis of CIN.

2.2. Clinical course and outcomes

CIN may range in severity from asymptomatic, nonoliguric transient renal dysfunction to oliguric severe renal failure that necessitates permanent dialysis. CIN is reported to be the third leading cause of in-hospital acute renal failure after hypotension and surgery. Approximately $180 million is spent annually to manage CIN in the US. Dangas et al. showed that in-hospital outcomes such as death (6.3% vs 0.8%), cardiac death (4.0% vs 0.5%), coronary artery bypass grafting (5.8% vs 0.5%), major adverse cardiac event (9.3% vs 1.1%), packed red cell transfusion (28% vs 6%), vascular surgery of access site (5.6% vs 2.6%), post-procedure length of stay (6.8±7.1 vs 2.3±2.5) were significantly higher in CIN developed patients compare with control ($p<0.0001$). In cumulative one-year outcome death, out-of-hospital death and major adverse cardiac events were significantly higher in CIN developed patients ($p<0.0001$) (Dangas et al., 2005). In a study of acute myocardial infarction patients undergoing primary angioplasty, it was found that CIN developed patients have significantly higher incidence of high-rate atrial fibrillation ($p=0.01$), high-degree conduction disturbances requiring permanent pacemaker ($p=0.04$), acute pulmonary edema ($p=0.008$), respiratory failure requiring mechanical ventilation ($p<0.0001$), cardiogenic shock requiring intra-aortic balloon ($p<0.0001$), and acute renal failure requiring renal replacement therapy ($p<0.0001$) (Marenzi et al., 2004).

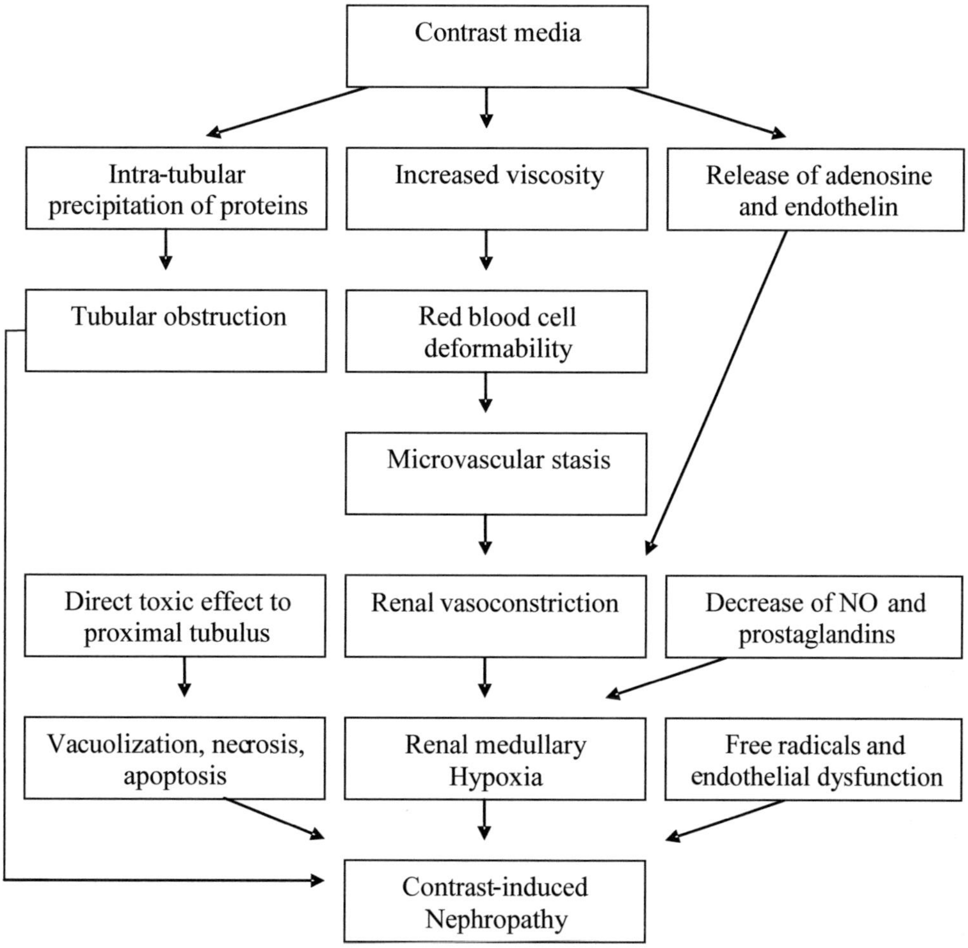

Figure 1. Pathogenesis of contrast-induced nephropathy. NO: nitric oxide.

2.3. Risk Factors for CIN

Specific factors that increase the risks for development of CIN are related to the patient, the contrast media, and the procedure (Table 1).

Risk Factors	Odds Ratio (95%CI)	p Value
Kidney Related Risk Factors		
Pre-existing renal failure		
Preprocedural creatinine 2.0-2.9 mg/dl	7.37 (4.78-11.39)	<0.0001
Preprocedural creatinine ≥ 3mg/d	12.82 (8.01-20.54)	<0.0001
Diabetes mellitus-Diabetic nephropathy		

Risk Factors	**Odds Ratio (95%CI)**	**p Value**
Preprocedural creatinine≤ 1.1mg/dl	1.86 (1.20-2.89)	0.005
Preprocedural creatinine 1.2-1.9 mg/dl	2.42 (1.54-3.79)	<0.001
Use of nephrotoxic drugs		
Low effective circulatory volume	1.19 (0.72-1.95)	0.05
Cardiovascular System Related Risk Factors		
Class III-IV congestive heart failure	2.20 (1.60-2.90)	<0.0001
Left ventricle ejection fraction<40%	1.57 (1.14-2.16)	0.005
Acute myocardial infarction ≤ 24 h	1.85 (1.31-2.63)	0.0006
Hypertension	2.00 (1.40-2.80)	0.0001
Periprocedural hypotension	2.50 (1.70-3.69)	<0.00001
Multi-vessel coronary involvement	3.24 (1.07-9.82)	0.038
Peripheral vascular disease	1.90 (1.40-2.70)	<0.0001
Preprocedure shock	1.19 (0.72-1.96)	0.05
Using intra-aortic balloon pump	15.51 (4.65-51.64)	<0.0001
Bypass graft intervention	4.94 (1.16-20.9)	0.03
Time-to-reperfusion ≥6 h	2.51 (1.01-6.16)	0.04
Pulmonary edema	2.56 (1.42-4.52)	0.001
Demographic Risk Factors		
Age "/>75 years	5.28 (1.98-14.05)	0.0009
Female gender	1.4 (1.25-1.60)	0.0001
Contrast Media Related Risk Factors		
High total dose of contrast agent ("/>300 ml)	2.8 (1.17-6.68)	0.02
Osmolality (Low- vs. high-osmolality)	0.50 (0.36-0.68)	
Short duration of two contrast administration	4.4 (2.9-6.5)	<0.0001
Other Possible Risk Factors		
Procedural success	0.27 (0.19-0.38)	<0.0001
Baseline hematocrit	0.95 (0.92-0.97)	<0.00001
Hyperuricemia	4.71 (1.29-17.21)	0.019
ACE inhibitors	3.37 (1.14-9.94)	0.028
Angiotensin Receptor Blockers	2.70 (1.25-5.81)	0.011
Metabolic Syndrome	426 (1.19-15.25)	0.026
Hypoalbuminemia	5.79 (1.71-19.64)	0.005
Hypercholesterolemia		
Renal transplant		
Multiple myeloma		
Diuretics		
Intra-arterial contrast administration		
Sepsis, cirrhosis		

Table 1. Risk factors for the development of contrast-induced nephropathy

http://dx.doi.org/10.5772/54032

2.3.1. Patient-related risk factors

2.3.1.1. Pre-existing renal disease

The major risk factor for CIN is a GFR<60 ml/min/1.73 m^2. Chronic kidney disease is associated with decreased vasodilatory response, which is important in developing CIN, and in patients with renal insufficiency, the clearance of CM is slower than in normal subjects. In a study of 7586 patients who underwent coronary intervention, CIN developed in 22.4% of the patients who had serum creatinine levels of 2.0 to 2.9 mg/dl and in 30.6% of those with serum creatinine levels of 3.0 mg/dl or higher, compared with 2.4% of patients with serum creatinine levels <1.1 mg/dl (Rihal et al., 2002). Two other studies (Moore et al., 1992; Barrett et al., 1992) reported that the incidence of CIN increased from 4% to 20% as the baseline serum creatinine increased from 1.2 to 2.9 mg/dl. In another study, the incidence of CIN increased from 8% to 92% as the serum creatinine increased from 1.5 to 6.8 mg/dl. Furthermore, the probability of CIN requiring dialysis increases from 0.04% to 48% as the baseline GFR decreases from 50 to 10 ml/min (McCullough et al., 1997).

2.3.1.2. Diabetes mellitus

Nitric oxide-dependent renal vasodilatation is characteristically altered and renal outer medullary pO_2 is significantly reduced in diabetes mellitus. Chronic kidney disease and DM are associated with endothelial dysfunction and decreased vasodilatory responses. Diabetic nephropathy has been identified as a powerful and independent risk factor for CIN. Patients with diabetic nephropathy and a mean serum creatinine of 6.8 mg/dl had a 92% incidence of CIN after coronary angiography (Weinrauch et al., 1977). Patients with diabetes who have advanced chronic renal failure because of causes other than diabetic nephropathy are at significantly higher risk of developing CIN like diabetic nephropathy. On the other hand, studies have shown that when pre-existing renal disease is present, patients with and without diabetes are similarly at risk of CIN, which correlates with the degree of renal disease. Some authors have suggested that DM in the absence of nephropathy, particularly in insulin-dependent patients with diabetes, is associated with an increased risk of CIN (McCullough et al., 1997; Toprak 2007). In a study, it was found that the incidence of CIN was rather low (2%) in patients with neither diabetes nor azotemia, significantly higher (16%) in individuals with diabetes but preserved renal function, and much higher (38%) in patients who had both diabetes and azotemia (Lautin et al., 1991). In another study, the incidence of CIN was found to be 2% in patients without diabetes and 3.7% in patients with diabetes with a baseline creatinine of 1.1 mg/dl or less (OR=1.86, p=0.005). When renal function is mildly impaired (serum creatinine level 1.2 to 1.9 mg/dl), the risk of CIN in patients with diabetes mellitus increases to 4.5% (OR=2.42, p<0.001) (Rihal et al., 2002). Other studies have failed to corroborate this connection (Parfrey et al., 1989). However, given that, those with diabetes alone were found to be at slightly higher risk of CIN than the general population.

2.3.1.3. Pre-diabetes

In a study of 421 patients who underwent coronary angiography with renal insufficiency, we presented that pre-DM increase the incidence of CIN 2.1-fold in comparison to patients with normal fasting glucose (NFG) but pre-DM is not as strong as DM as a risk of developing CIN. CIN occurred in 20% of the DM (RR=3.6, p=0.001), 11.4% of the pre-DM (RR 2.1, p=0.314) and 5.5% of the NFG group. The decrease of GFR was higher in DM and pre-DM (p=0.001 and p=0.002, respectively). Length of hospital stay was 2.45 ± 1.45 day in DM, 2.27 ± 0.68 day in pre-DM, and 1.97 ± 0.45 day in NFG (p<0.001, DM vs. NFG and p=0.032, pre-DM vs. NFG). The rate of major adverse cardiac events was 8.7% in DM, 5% in pre-DM, and 2.1% in NFG (*P*=0.042, DM vs. NFG). Hemodialysis was required in 3.6% of DM, and 0.7% in pre-DM (*P*=0.036, DM vs. NFG), and the total number of hemodialysis sessions during 3 months was higher in DM and pre-DM (*P*<0.001). Serum glucose ≥124 mg/dl was the best cut-off point for prediction of CIN (Toprak et al., 2007).

2.3.1.4. Metabolic syndrome, impaired fasting glucose and hypertriglyceridemia

In a prospective cohort study of 219 non-diabetic elderly patients with reduced kidney function who underwent elective coronary angiography, we reported that metabolic syndrome was a risk indicator of CIN (OR=4.26, p=0.026). CIN occurred in 14% of the metabolic syndrome group and 3.6% of the non-metabolic syndrome group (relative risk 3.93, p=0.007). Impaired fasting glucose (OR=4.72, p=0.007), high triglyceride (OR=4.06, p=0.022); and multivessel involvement (OR=3.24, p=0.038) in the metabolic syndrome group were predictors of CIN (Toprak et al., 2006).

2.3.1.5. Hyperuricemia

Contrast agents have a uricosuric effect, which appears to be caused by enhanced renal tubular secretion of uric acid. Furthermore, hyperuricemia is accompanied by enhanced synthesis of reactive oxygen species, tubular obstruction by uric acid, an activated renin–angiotensin–aldosterone system, increased endothelin-1, and an inhibited nitric oxide system which plays a role in the pathogenesis of CIN. In a prospective cohort study we evaluated 266 patients who undergoing elective coronary angiography and we found that patients with hyperuricemia are at risk of developing CIN (OR=4.71, p=0.019). CIN occurred in 15.1% of the hyperuricemic group and 2.9% of the normouricemic group (p<0.001). Length of hospital stay (p<0.001) and CIN requiring renal replacement therapy (p=0.017) were significantly higher in hyperuricemic group. Serum uric acid ≥7 mg/dl in males and ≥5.9 mg/dl in females were found the best cut-off value for prediction of CIN (Toprak et al., 2006).

2.3.1.6. Hypercholesterolemia

Altered nitric oxide-dependent renal vasodilatation is prevalent in hypercholesterolemia. Hypercholesterolemia aggravates CIN through the reduced production of nitric oxide (Yang et al., 2004).

http://dx.doi.org/10.5772/54032

2.3.1.7. Multivessel Coronary involvement, peripheral vascular disease, and renal artery stenosis

If a patient has multivessel coronary involvement, the other vessels in the body, such as the renal artery, can be involved. If the renal artery is involved, the renal blood supply may decrease and the kidneys may be more susceptible to CIN. Factors related to accelerated or diffuse atherosclerosis are linked to the development of CIN. The treatment of multivessel disease, challenging chronic total occlusions and extensively diseased coronary segments, may require high doses of CM for providing an optimal image quality, thus enhancing the potential toxic effects on the renal function. In a study of 177 patients who underwent cardiac catheterization, subjects were also evaluated for renal artery stenosis. Coronary artery disease was detected in 110 patients (62%), and significant renal artery stenosis was detected in 19 patients (11%). Using multivariate analysis, it was found that the extent of coronary artery disease was an independent predictor of renal artery stenosis (Weber-Mzell et al., 2002). In a study a total of 5571 patients who underwent PCI were evaluated for CIN risk factors, and it was found that multivessel coronary involvement was only a univariate predictor of CIN ($p=0.003$) (Mehran et al., 2004). In two other cohort studies it was found that peripheral vascular disease is a risk for CIN in patients who underwent PCI ($OR=1.9$, $p<0.0001$ and $OR=1.71$, $p=0.001$, respectively) (Bartholomew et al., 2004; Rihal et al., 2002). In a study a total of 219 non-diabetic patients who underwent coronary angiography we have found that multivessel coronary involvement is a risk for CIN ($OR=3.24$, $p=0.038$) (Toprak et al., 2006).

2.3.1.8. Older age

In a prospective study in which elderly patients (≥70 years) were subjected to cardiac catheterization, 11% developed CIN (Rich & Crecelius, 1990). In another study, CIN incidence was 17% in elderly patients (>60 years) as compared with 4% in younger patients (Kohli et al., 2000). In 208 patients with acute myocardial infarction who underwent coronary intervention, it was found that an age of ≥75 years was an independent risk for CIN ($OR=5.28$, $p=0.0009$) (Marenzi et al., 2004). The possible reasons of the high incidence of CIN in elderly were age-related changes in renal function, more difficult vascular access following tortuosity, calcification of the vessels requiring greater amount of CM, defective prostaglandin synthesis, and the presence of renovascular disease. Furthermore, hypovolemia is very common in elderly patients.

2.3.1.9. Gender

Ovarian hormones can affect the renin–angiotensin system and renal blood flow. In a retrospective study of 8628 patients who underwent PCI, female sex was an independent predictor of CIN ($OR=1.4$, $p<0.0001$). One-year outcome analyses by gender showed a higher mortality among females than among males in a cohort of CIN patients (14% vs 10%, $p=0.05$) (Iakovou et al., 2003). The findings of this study contradict those of a previous randomized controlled trial of ionic vs nonionic CM, in which a multivariate analysis identified male gender as an independent risk factor for CIN (Rudnick et al., 1995).

2.3.1.10. Hypovolemia

Hypovolemia leads to active sodium reabsorbtion, which is an oxygen-demanding process, and increases neurohumoral vasoconstrictive stimuli that might compromise medullary oxygenation. The toxic effects of CM on the renal tubular lumen may be exacerbated in hypovolemia. Decreased effective circulating volume and reduced renal perfusion potentiate renal vasoconstriction after administration of intravascular CM. Volume expansion reduces the activity of the renin–angiotensin system, minimizes increases in blood viscosity and osmolality, and increases medullary perfusion. At present the most convincing preventive procedure of CIN is adequate hydration with isotonic saline or sodium bicarbonate. Before coronary angiography, the volume status of patients can be assessed through the inferior vena cava index, mean atrial pressure, noninvasive pulmonary-capillary wedge pressure or bioimpedance spectroscopy (Toprak & Cirit, 2005).

2.3.1.11. Congestive heart failure and reduced left ventricular ejection fraction

Advanced heart failure and reduced LVEF are characterized by effective volume depletion caused by low cardiac output and increased neurohumoral vasoconstrictive stimuli and impaired nitric oxide-dependent renal vasodilatation that might compromise medullary oxygenation. Studies have shown that reduced left ventricular ejection fraction (LVEF) (≤49%) and advanced congestive heart failure (New York Heart Association class III or IV) are independent risk factors for CIN. In a study, Dangas et al. showed that LVEF below 40% is an independent predictor of CIN (Dangas et al., 2005). We have previously reported that if the LVEF is greater than 30%, this condition does not show any significant effect on the development of CIN (Toprak et al., 2003). In a study it was shown that congestive heart failure was an independent risk for CIN (OR=1.53, p=0.007) (Rihal et al., 2002). In a cohort study it was found that congestive heart failure is a risk for CIN in patients who underwent PCI (OR=2.2, p<0.0001) (Bartholomew et al., 2004).

2.3.1.12. Hypertension

An explanation for hypertension as a risk factor for CIN is: alterations in the intrarenal expression of vasoactive mediators, such as the renin-angiotensin system or nitric oxide, may be contributing factors. Impaired nitric oxide-dependent renal vasodilatation is prevalent in individuals who are hypertensive. Finally, a reduced number of nephrons could predispose hypertensive patients to CIN. In a study of 8628 patients who underwent percutaneous interventions, hypertension was found to be an independent predictor of CIN (OR=1.2, p=0.0035). In a cohort study Bartholomew et al. found that hypertension is a risk for CIN in patients who underwent PCI (OR=2.0, p=0.0001) (Bartholomew et al., 2004).

2.3.1.13. Nephrotoxic drugs

Directly, nephrotoxic drugs and those that inhibit the vasodilatory effects of prostaglandins have been reported to render the kidney more vulnerable to CM. Sulfonamides, aminoglycosides, and their combinations with furosemide are particularly potent. Cyclosporin A may

http://dx.doi.org/10.5772/54032

intensify medullary hypoxia, and cisplatin can attach to sulfhydryl groups. Mannitol can increase the metabolic workload in the kidney, and amphotericin B can cause the effect of a combination of mannitol and cyclosporine A. Nonselective NSAIDs and selective COX-2 inhibitors decrease the vasodilatory prostaglandins in the kidney and potentiate the vasoconstrictive effect of CM.

2.3.1.14. Metformin

Patients who are receiving metformin may develop lactic acidosis as a result of CIN. A decline in renal function after contrast exposure could adversely affect the clearance of metformin. The complication was almost always observed in diabetic patients with decreased renal function before injection of CM. A meta-analysis by the Cochrane Library with pooled data from 176 comparative trials and cohort studies revealed no cases of fatal or nonfatal lactic acidosis in 35,619 patient-years of metformin use or in 30,002 patients-years in the non-metformin group. It seems safer to instruct patients especially at high risk for CIN not to take this drug for 48 h or so after CM administration and resume taking the drug only if there are no signs of nephrotoxicity.

2.3.1.15. ACE inhibitors and angiotensin receptor blockers

ACE inhibitors have been identified as a risk factor for CIN because of their potential to reduce renal function. On the other hand, some small studies have shown that the nephrotoxicity of CM may be reduced because of decreased renal vasoconstriction by inhibition of angiotensin II. Renal vasoconstriction occurs after the CM administration and the renin–angiotensin system is responsible for this vasoconstriction. In a randomized controlled study with 71 patients with diabetes who underwent coronary angiography randomized to captopril or control, 25-mg captopril was given three times daily. There was a significant decrease in CIN in the patients who received captopril compared with the control group (6% vs 29%, respectively, $p<0.02$) (Gupta et al., 1999). We have performed a randomized controlled study in 80 patients with serum creatinine below 2 mg/dl who underwent coronary angiography. Captopril was administered in 48 patients before coronary angiography. Five patients (10.4%) in the captopril group developed CIN, compared with only one patient (3.1%) in the control group ($p=0.02$) (Toprak et al., 2003). In a study of 230 patients with renal insufficiency and age ≥65 years we found that chronic ACE inhibitor administration was a risk for developing CIN. CIN occurred in 17 patients (15.6%) in the ACE inhibitor group and 7 patients (5.8%) in the control group ($p=0.015$). Serum creatinine level increased from 1.34 ± 0.20 to 1.53 ± 0.27 mg/dl in the ACE inhibitor group and from 1.33 ± 0.18 to 1.45 ± 0.19 mg/dl in the control group ($p<0.001$). Chronic ACE inhibitor administration was a risk indicator of CIN (OR=3.37, $p=0.028$) (Cirit et al., 2006). In another study, 421 patients with renal insufficiency who underwent coronary angiography, use of ACE inhibitors or ARB was a risk for CIN in multivariate analysis (OR=2.7, $p=0.011$) (Toprak et al., 2007). In a recent study, the impact of renin-angiotensin and aldosterone system blockade on the frequency of CIN was assessed retrospectively. Patients treated with ACE inhibitors or ARB (n=269) and were not treated with them (n=143) underwent coronary angiography included to the study. CIN developed

11.9% in ACE-inhibitor using group and 4.2% in control group (p=0.006). Use of ARB or ACE inhibitors was found as a risk for CIN (OR=3.08, p=0.016) (Kiski et al., 2010). Checking the use of ACE inhibitors or ARB before coronary angiography seems to be a useful guide in tracking risk assessment for CIN. It is reasonable to suggest that there is a need to hold ACE inhibitor or ARB use before coronary angiography.

2.3.1.16. *Multiple myeloma*

Multiple myeloma has been suggested as a potential risk factor for CIN. The pathomechanism of this process has been explained by the precipitation of CM molecules together with Tamm–Horsfall proteins and other abnormal proteins, tubular epithelial cells damaged and desquamated as a result of ischemia, direct contrast toxicity, or disturbed function of integrins. Intratubular light chains, particularly in the setting of intravascular volume depletion, have been found to augment the nephrotoxic potential of CM (Holland et al., 1985). Studies with a broader scope have since shown that the observed risk is linked to coexisting risk factors, such as pre-existing renal insufficiency, low circulating volume, proteinuria, amyloidosis, hyperuricemia, and hypercalcemia rather than to myeloma itself. Studies showed an incidence of CIN of only 0.6–1.25% in patients with myeloma if dehydration is avoided (McCarthy & Becker, 1992).

2.3.1.17. *Renal transplantation*

Patients with renal transplantation may be at a higher risk of CIN due to concomitant use of cyclosporine and higher prevalence of diabetes and renal insufficiency. In a study, 33 patients with a functioning renal allograft who underwent different contrast studies, the incidence of CIN was 21.2% (Ahuja et al., 2000).

2.3.1.18. *Acute myocardial infarction*

A study by Rihal et al. showed that acute myocardial infarction within 24 h before administration of the CM is a risk factor for CIN (OR=1.85, p=0.0006). This study demonstrates that CIN is a frequent complication in acute myocardial infarction, even in patients with a normal baseline renal function. (Rihal et al., 2002). In a study of 208 acute myocardial infarction patients who underwent primary PCI, anterior acute myocardial infarction was significantly higher in patients who developed CIN (p=0.0015). However, in multivariate analysis, anterior acute myocardial infarction (OR=2.17, p=0.09) was not a risk for CIN (Marenzi et al., 2004). In 2082 percutaneous interventions for acute myocardial infarction, it was reported a more than seven-fold (3.2% vs 23.3%) increase in 1-year mortality in patients who developed CIN (Sadeghi et al., 2003).

2.3.1.19. *Anemia*

Anemia-induced deterioration of renal ischemia may be one plausible explanation for the higher incidence of CIN in patients with a low hematocrit level. A baseline hematocrit value of less than 39% for men and less than 36% for women is a risk for CIN. The relationship between low hematocrit levels and CIN has been investigated in a prospective study of 6773 patients who underwent PCI (Nikolsky et al., 2005). A lower baseline hematocrit was an independent predictor of CIN; and each 3% decrease in baseline hematocrit resulted in a significant increase in the odds of CIN in patients with and without chronic kidney disease (11% and 23%, respectively). Dangas et al. showed that the baseline hematocrit level is an independent predictor of CIN in patients with chronic kidney disease (OR=0.95, p<0.00001) (Dangas et al., 2005).

2.3.1.20. Low serum albumin

Hypoalbuminemia impairs endothelial function, enhances renal vasoconstriction, impairs the synthesis and release of nitric oxide, and decreases antioxidant enzyme activity. In a study, low serum albumin (<3.5 g/dl) was identified as a risk factor for CIN in patients 70 years of age or older who underwent cardiac catheterization (Rich, et al., 1990). Also we have found that in 230 patients who underwent coronary angiography with renal insufficiency, serum albumin level ≤3.5 g/dl was a risk factor for CIN (OR=5.79, p=0.005) (Cirit et al., 2006).

2.3.1.21. Hypotension, sepsis, cirrhosis, and pulmonary edema

A systolic blood pressure of less than 80 mm Hg for at least 1 h that requires inotropic support with medications is a risk factor for CIN. A study by Dangas et al showed that periprocedural hypotension and pulmonary edema are independent predictors of CIN in patients with chronic kidney disease (OR=2.50, p<0.00001 and OR=2.56, p=0.001, respectively) (Dangas et al., 2005) Sepsis, through direct damage by bacterial toxins to renal tubules and impairment of circulation, has also been reported as a risk factor. Reduction of effective intravascular volume caused by liver cirrhosis has been reported as contributing to pre-renal reduction in renal perfusion, thus enhancing the ischemic insult of CM (Toprak, 2007).

2.3.2. Procedure-related risk factors

2.3.2.1. Short duration of the two contrast administration and urgent/emergency procedure

In those who have no risk factors for CIN, angiography should be delayed more than 48 hours after a previous exposure to intravascular contrast media. In patients with diabetes or preexisting renal disease, this time interval should be increased to more than 72 hours. In a cohort study, urgent/emergency procedure was found as a predictor of CIN (OR=4, p<0.0001) (Bartholomew et al., 2004). The higher risk of developing CIN in patients with urgent status was irrespective of baseline renal function.

2.3.2.2. Use of intra-aortic balloon pump

Using intra-aortic balloon pump may signify a very high-risk population due to very severe coronary atherosclerosis and/or indicate a role of atheroembolism. In 208 consecutive acute myocardial infarction patients undergoing percutaneous coronary intervention, use of intra-aortic balloon pump was a risk predictor of CIN (OR=15.51, p<0.0001) (Marenzi et al., 2004). In a study, it has demonstrated that, intra-aortic balloon pump use is an independent predictor of CIN in patients with chronic kidney disease (OR=2.27, p=0.004) (Dangas et al., 2005). In another study, it was found that the use of intra-aortic balloon pump was a risk factor for CIN requiring dialysis after PCI (OR=1.94) (Gruberg et al., 2001). In another derivation and validation cohort study, intra-aortic balloon pump use was a risk for CIN in patients undergoing coronary intervention (OR=5.1, p<0.0001) (Bartholomew et al., 2004).

2.3.2.3. Bypass graft intervention and delayed reperfusion

Procedures with bypass angiography and intervention may be associated with higher complexity, longer duration, and limited success, thus indicating an unstable post-procedural period with impaired cardiac output. Gruberg et al. showed that the risk of CIN requiring dialysis after PCI was increased with bypass graft intervention (OR=4.94) (Gruberg et al., 2001). In a study of 208 acute myocardial infarction patients undergoing primary PCI, the risk of CIN was increased if the time-to-reperfusion is ≥6 h (OR=2.51, p=0.04) (Marenzi et al., 2004)

2.3.3. Contrast medium-related risk factors

2.3.3.1. Increased dose of contrast medium

According to different sources, the relatively safe cutoff point of contrast amount varies from 70 ml up to 220ml. However, doses as low as 20 to 30 ml are capable of inducing CIN. In a study that patients undergoing coronary angiography, each 100 ml of contrast medium administered was associated with a significant increase of 12% in the risk of CIN (OR=1.12, p=0.02) (Rihal et al., 2002). Marenzi et al. showed that contrast volume >300 ml is an independent risk for CIN (OR=2.80, p=0.02) (Marenzi et al., 2004). In another study patients with preexisting renal failure revealed a 10-fold risk of CIN when more than 125 ml of contrast media was administered (Taliercio et al., 1986).

2.3.3.2. High-osmolar and ionic CM

Most side effects attributable to contrast medias are related to hypertonicity. Currently, four main types of contrast media are used in routine practice today, including nonionic low-osmolar, ionic low-osmolar, nonionic iso-osmolar, and ionic high-osmolar contrast media. In a large study which comparing the non-ionic low-osmolality agent iohexol to the ionic high-osmolality agent meglumine/sodium diatrizoate in patients with pre-existing renal dysfunction undergoing angiography, patients with renal insufficiency receiving diatrizoate were 3.3 times as likely to develop CIN compared to those receiving iohexol (Rudnick et al., 1995). NEPHRIC trial is a randomized, prospective study comparing the nonionic iso-osmolar CM iodixanol with the nonionic low-osmolar CM iohexol in 129 renal impairment patients with diabetes undergoing coronary or aorto-femoral angiography. The incidence of CIN was 3% in the iodixanol group and 26% in the iohexol group (p=0.002) (Aspelin et al., 2003). In another randomized study, the renal tolerance of iodixanol and iohexol was compared in 124 patients with creatinine >1.7 mg/dl. The incidence of CIN was 3.7% in iodixanol group and 10% in iohexol group (p>0.05) (Chalmers et al., 1999). The available data do not provide clear evidence that the whole iso-osmolar CM class offers an improvement over the low-osmolar CM class. Other studies with iodixanol in renal failure patients have shown a higher incidence of CIN than that observed in the NEPHRIC study (21% in the RAPPID trial, 30% in the CONTRAST trial) (Baker et al., 2003: Stone et al., 2003). In addition to their osmolarity, contrast medias are characterized as ionic versus non-ionic. Small clinical trials of low-risk patients undergoing coronary angiography have shown little difference in the risk of CIN between the 2 types of CM. However, a randomized trial of 1196 patients undergoing coronary angiography showed that non-ionic CM reduced the incidence of CIN in patients with preexisting renal disease with or without diabetes (Rudnick et al., 1995). In addition, symptomatic or hemodynamic adverse drug events have been shown to occur less often with non-ionic, low-osmolality CM compared with ionic, high-osmolality CM. In high-risk patients, it is reasonable to don't use the high-osmolar and ionic CM to minimize the risk of CIN.

2.3.3.3. Intra-arterial administration of the contrast media

Intra-arterial contrast administration is a risk for CIN. This effect is thought to be due to the fact that the acute intra renal concentration of CM is much higher after intra arterial rather than intravenous injection.

2.3.4. Scoring method to predict high risk patients for CIN

Mehran et al. developed a simple scoring method that integrates eight baseline clinical variables to assess the risk of CIN after percutaneous coronary intervention (PCI). These are hypotension (score 5), use of intra-aortic balloon pump (score 5), congestive heart failure (score 5), serum creatinine>1.5 mg/dl (score 4), age>75 years (score 4), anemia (score 3), diabetes mellitus (score 3), and volume of CM (score 1 per 100 ml). If the total score is 5 or less, the risk category is low; if the total score is 16 or higher, the risk category is very high (Mehran et al., 2004).

2.4. Prevention Strategies for CIN

Extracellular volume expansion with intravenous saline or sodium bicarbonate, minimizing the dose of CM, using low-osmolar non-ionic CM instead of high osmolar ionic CM, stopping the intake of nephrotoxic drugs and avoiding short intervals between procedures requiring CM have all been shown to be effective in reducing CIN. Alternatives to ordinary CM, such as carbon dioxide or gadolinium chelates, can be used in patients at high risk of CIN (Table 2).

Clinical evidence advocating their use	Don't use	With conflicting or limited evidence
Extracellular volume expansion	Nonsteroidal anti-inflammatory drugs, COX-2 inhibitors, aminoglycoside, cisplatin	Acetylcystein
Saline or sodium bicarbonate	Loop diuretics	Theophylline
Low or iso-osmolar contrast	Mannitol	Calcium channel blockers
Minimizing the dose of contrast	Multiple use of contrast within 72 h	Fenoldopam
Alternative imaging techniques	Large doses of contrast	Captopril
Monitoring serum creatinine	High-osmolar contrast	Ascorbic acid
Delaying contrast procedures until hemodynamic status is corrected	Metformin usage especially in patients with renal failure	Atrial natriuretic peptide
≥48 h between contrast procedures		Endothelin antagonist
		PGE1
		Hemofiltration
		Nebivolol
		Statins
		B-type natriuretic peptide
		Pentoxifylline

Table 2. Prevention strategies for contrast-induced nephropathy in high-risk patients

2.4.1. Volume expansion

Volume expansion is the single most important measure that has been documented to be beneficial in preventing CIN. A standardized saline hydration protocol has been proven effective in reducing the risk of CIN and should be used routinely. The most widely accepted protocol is administering isotonic saline at 1 to 1.5 ml/kg/h beginning 6 to 12 hours prior to the procedure and continuing for up to 12 hours following contrast administration. In a randomized trial, two different hydration regimens were compared in 1620 patients undergoing coronary interventions. They showed that the incidence of CIN was significantly lower among patients given an isotonic saline solution than among those given a hypotonic saline solution (0.7% vs. 2.0% respectively, p=0.04) (Mueller et al., 2002). In another trial, a total of 119 patients with serum creatinine exceeding 1.1 mg/dl were randomized to receive isotonic solution of sodium bicarbonate (n=59) or isotonic saline (n=60) at a rate of 3 ml/kg/h for 1 hour before and 1 ml/kg/h for 6 hours after contrast administration. CIN developed in only 1 patient (1.7%) compared with 8 patients (13.6%) in the saline group (p=0.02) (Merten et al., 2004). The authors postulated that a reduction in oxidative injury may have conferred protection against CIN. However, further studies are required to clarify the role of hydration with sodium bicarbonate in preventing CIN. In a prospective study, the effect of combination intravenous and oral volume supplementation on the development of CIN was studied in 425 patients undergoing percutaneous coronary intervention. Patients were randomly assigned to receive hydration with either isotonic or half-isotonic. In addition patients were encouraged to drink plenty of fluids (at least 1500 ml). They found that applying the combination of intravenous and oral volume supplementation results in a very low incidence of CIN (1.4%) (Mueller et al., 2005). Most studies have found that hydration alone is better than hydration combined with a diuretic. In a study, 78 patients with serum creatinine >1.6 mg/dl were randomized to three groups: hydration alone, hydration with mannitol and hydration with furosemide. Half-isotonic saline was used for hydration. CIN occurred in 11%, 28% and 40% of patients in the three groups, respectively (p=0.02), thus showing that forced diuresis is of no benefit in preventing CIN. In a meta-analysis it was found that the administration of sodium bicarbonate is superior to the administration of saline alone in the prevention of CIN (Solomon et al., 1994). The effectiveness of sodium bicarbonate treatment to prevent CIN in high-risk patients remains uncertain.

2.4.2. N-acetylcysteine

Antioxidant N-acetylcysteine (NAC) might scavenge oxygen free radicals, thus attenuate the cytotoxic effects of CM. NAC may also have direct vasodilating effects on the kidneys through an increase in the biologic effects of nitric oxide. Tepel et al. were evaluated the effects of NAC (600 mg orally twice daily), at first time, in 83 patients undergoing computed tomography. Two percent of the patients in the NAC group had CIN versus 21% in the placebo group (p=0.01) (Tepel et al., 2000). Since then, a number of trials have been published. Results from these trials have been inconsistent. In a randomized, placebo-controlled study it was found that NAC is protective against CIN Fifty-four patients were randomized to receive either 600 mg of NAC twice daily for 4 doses or placebo. The incidence of CIN was 8% in the NAC group versus 45% in the placebo group (p=0.005) (Diaz-Sandoval et al., 2002). In addition to oral administration, intravenous administration of NAC to protect against CIN has also been evaluated. In a study, Baker et al. randomly assigned 80 patients to receive either NAC infusion (n=41) versus saline infusion (n=39). CIN developed in only 2 (5%) of patients in the NAC group compared with 8 (21%) in the saline group (p=0.04) (Baker et al., 2003). The authors concluded that NAC infusion protects against CIN. In a meta-analysis, evaluating more than 800 patients at high risk of developing CIN also documented a positive impact of NAC prophylaxis on CIN (Birck et al., 2003). In another meta-analysis, nine randomized controlled trials were included and the difference in mean change in creatinine between the NAC treated group and controls was -0.27 mg/dl. The relative risk of developing CIN was 0.43 in subjects randomized to NAC. They suggest that NAC helps prevent declining renal function and CIN (Liu et al., 2005). In contrast to these reports, some studies failed to find a significant effect of NAC on the occurrence of CINA total of 183 patients with preexisting renal insufficiency undergoing contrast study were randomly assigned to receive NAC at a dose of 600 mg twice daily on the day before and the day of the contrast study plus saline infusion or saline alone. The incidence of CIN was 6.5% in the NAC group versus 11% in the control group (p=0.22) (Briguori et al., 2002). In a multi centric double blind clinical trial 156 patients undergoing coronary angiography or percutaneous coronary intervention with creatinine clearance <50 ml/min were randomly assigned to receive N-acetylcysteine 600 mg orally twice daily for two days or placebo. Sixteen patients developed CIN. Eight of 77 patients (10.4%) in the NAC group and eight of 79 patients (10.1%) in the placebo group ($p=1.00$). No difference was observed in the change in endogenous creatinine clearance, $p=0.28$). They concluded that oral NAC did not prevent CIN in patients at low to moderate risk undergoing cardiac catheterisation with ionic low osmolality CM (Gomes et al., 2005). In another study, 50 patients undergoing elective diagnostic coronary angiography with serum creatinine values above 1.3 mg/dl were included and CIN was detected in 3 of 25 patients (12%) in the NAC group and 2 of 25 patients (8%) in the control group ($p>0.05$). It was detected that in patients planned to undergo elective diagnostic coronary angiography with renal dysfunction, oral NAC and hydration before the procedure was not more effective than hydration alone in the prevention of CIN (Gulel et al., 2005). A direct renoprotective effect of NAC remains questionable. To date, only a few trials described the effects of NAC not only on serum creatinine but also on clinical end points. The serum creatinine can be decrease in administration of NAC without renoprotective effect. In a prospective study, NAC was given at a dose of 600 mg every 12 h for a total of four doses to the volunteers with a normal renal function who did not receive contrast agent. There was a significant decrease of the mean serum creatinine ($p<0.05$) and a significant increase of the GFR ($p<0.02$), whereas the cystatin C concentration did not change significantly (Hoffmann et al., 2004). In patients undergoing emergency diagnostic procedures, in which a full hydration protocol is not possible, an abbreviated hydration regimen plus oral or intravenous administration of NAC can be recommended. NAC may be of benefit mostly in high-risk patients. If NAC is to be used as a preventative measure, it should be given at a dose of 600 mg orally twice daily on the day before and day of the procedure.

2.4.3. Ascorbic acid

Prophylactic oral administration of ascorbic acid may protect against CIN. In a randomized, placebo-controlled trial in 231 patients with serum creatinine ≥1.2 mg/dl who undergoing coronary angiography showed that the use of ascorbic acid was associated with a significant reduction in the rate of CIN. CIN occurred in 11 of the 118 patients (9%) in the ascorbic acid group and in 23 of the 113 patients (20%) in the placebo group ($OR=0.38$; $p=0.02$) (Spargias et al., 2004). Further prospective studies are needed to validate these preliminary results.

2.4.4. Fenoldopam

Fenoldopam mesylate is a selective dopamine-1 receptor agonist that produces systemic, peripheral and renal arterial vasodilatation. Several investigators have reported a positive impact of fenoldopam against CIN in small studies. In a placebo-controlled, double-blind, multicenter trial, 315 patients with creatinine clearance of less than 60 ml/min were randomized to receive fenoldopam infusion [0.05 μg/kg/min titrated to 0.1 μg/kg/min ($n=157$)] or matching placebo ($n=158$). CIN occurred in 33.6% of patients in the fenoldo-

http://dx.doi.org/10.5772/54032

pam group compared with 30.1% of patients in the placebo group (p=0.61) (Stone et al., 2003). The authors concluded that fenoldopam did not protect against CIN. In 2 other large studies comparing fenoldopam with NAC treatment with fenoldopam either had a similar, non significant effect as that of NAC or was inferior to it (Allaqaband et al., 2002; Briguori et al., 2004). The routine use of fenoldopam cannot be recommended at the present time.

2.4.5. Adenosine antagonists

CM stimulate the intrarenal secretion of adenosine, which binds to the renal adenosine receptor and acts as a potent vasoconstrictor, reducing renal blood flow and increasing the generation of oxygen free radicals as it is metabolized to xanthine and hypoxanthine. Theophylline and aminophylline, adenosine antagonists, have also been studied in the prevention of CIN in a number of trials. Studies with these agents have used varying doses and dosage forms and yielded conflicting results (Erley et al., 1999; Kapoor et al., 2001). Based on the conflicting information found in clinical studies, adenosine antagonists should not be routinely used in patients as a preventative measure at this time.

2.4.6. Calcium channel blockers

The calcium channel antagonists verapamil and diltiazem have been found to attenuate the renal vasoconstrictor response after exposure to CM. However, when the efficacy of the felodipine, nitrendipine and nifedipine was evaluated, results were inconsistent. Two small studies performed the use of sublingual nifedipine given prior to contrast administration. Patients (n=20) who received sublingual nifedipine did not have a significant increase in serum creatinine, while those in the placebo group did (Rodicio et al., 1990). In another study, patients (n=30) who received nifedipine had an increase in renal plasma flow following administration of contrast, while patients in the placebo group had a decrease in renal flow (Russo et al., 1990). One other study showed that nitrendipine use cause a significant reduction in the GFR in the placebo group compared to little or no change in GFR in the nitrendipine group (Neumayer et al., 1989). In another study, 27 patients with normal to moderately reduced renal function underwent femoral angiography randomized to receive either oral felodipine or placebo. Patients in the felodipine group had a significant increase in serum creatinine from baseline, while patients in the placebo group did not demonstrate a similar increase (Spangberg-Viklund et al., 1996). More large-scale trials are needed before calcium channel blockers can be routinely recommended in patients prior to CM administration.

2.4.7. Prostaglandin E_1

PGE_1 has vasodilatory effects that may be beneficial in preventing CIN. In one study, 130 patients were randomly assigned to receive either placebo or one of three doses of PGE_1. The increase in serum creatinine level was smaller in all of the three PGE_1 groups than in the placebo group, but the difference was significant only in the medium-dose (20 ng/kg/min) of

PGE_1 group (Koch et al., 2000). More studies need to be done to better understand the role of prostaglandin E1, but results from this pilot study appear promising.

2.4.8. *Atrial Natriuretic Peptide (ANP)*

ANP may prevent CIN by increasing renal blood flow. In a study, ANP was included in one of the four arms. In which dopamine, mannitol, and ANP caused an increase in CIN in diabetic patients as compared to saline alone (Weisberg et al., 1994). In another trial patients were randomized to one of four treatment arms: fluid alone or one of three doses of ANP. Results showed no statistically significant differences in the incidence of CIN between any of the four treatment arms (Kurnik et al., 1998) Based on these results and the limited clinical data, ANP cannot be advocated in the prevention of CIN.

2.4.9. *Endothelin antagonists*

Endothelin-1 is a potent endogenous vasoconstrictor, is thought to play a role in the development of CIN. Endothelin-1 has two primary receptors. In animal studies, endothelin-A antagonists were shown to reduce the incidence of CIN (Liss et al., 2003). However, in a randomized study of 158 patients, the use of a mixed endothelin-A and B antagonist was associated with a significantly higher incidence of CIN than was placebo (56% vs. 29%, p=0.002) (Wang et al., 2000). Endothelin antagonists currently have no role in prevention of CIN.

2.4.10. *Low-dose of dopamine*

At low doses (1-3 mcg/kg/min), dopamine activates two types of dopamine (DA) receptors, DA-1 and DA-2. Activation of the DA-1 receptor results in an increase in natriuresis and renal blood flow. Since dopamine, at low doses, is believed to be more selective for the DA-1 receptors, it has been investigated in the prevention of CIN. Kapoor et al. randomized 40 patients with diabetes scheduled to undergo a coronary angiography to either dopamine or placebo control. None of the patients in the dopamine group developed CIN compared to 50% of patients receiving placebo (Kapoor et al., 2002). In another prospective, randomized trial, Hans et al. evaluated 55 patients (40% had diabetes) with chronic renal insufficiency. Patients were randomized to receive dopamine or an equal volume of saline. The group receiving dopamine had a significantly lower incidence of CIN as compared to the control group (Hans et al., 1998). In contrast to the trials showing a potential benefit of dopamine, other studies have failed to demonstrate this benefit. Abizaid et al. performed a randomized, prospective study involving patients with renal insufficiency who underwent coronary angioplasty. Patients were randomized to continue with the saline, receive aminophylline in addition to the saline, or receive dopamine plus saline. In the dopamine plus saline group, 50% of patients developed CIN, while only 30% of the patients in the saline-alone group developed CIN. This difference did not reach statistical significance, but it appeared that use of dopamine might worsen outcomes (Abizaid et al., 1999). Low-dose dopamine use cannot be supported at this time.

2.4.11. Statins

Whether additional benefits can be achieved with the use of statin in decreasing the risk of CIN remains undetermined. In a recent meta analysis of randomised controlled trials comparing statin pretreatment with non-statin pretreatment for the prevention of CIN, it was found that, the incidence of CIN was not significantly lower in statin pretreatment group as compared with control group (RR=0.76, p=0.30) (Zhang et al., 2011). The current cumulative evidence suggests that statin pretreatment may neither prevent CIN nor reduce the need for renal replacement therapy.

2.4.12. Nebivolol

In an experimental study we demonstrated that nebivolol have a protective role against CIN. Nebivolol leads to a decrease in the systemic and renal oxidative stres (p=0.001) and an increase in renal nitrite production (p=0.027). In addition, contrast-induced proteinuria, proteinaceous cast ($p< 0.001$), and tubular necrosis (p=0.001) are restored by nebivolol (Toprak et al., 2008). Two recent human studies demonstrated the protective effect of nebivolol on CIN. One of the study showed that the use of oral nebivolol for one week at a dose of 5 mg per day decrease the incidence of CIN in patients who underwent coronary angiography with renal dysfunction (p=0.03) (Avci et al., 2011). Another more recent study showed that the use of oral nebivolol for 4 days at a dose of 5 mg per day is protective against nephrotoxic effects of CM in patients who underwent coronary angiography or ventriculography (Gunebakmaz et al., 2012). More large-scale trials are needed before nebivolol can be routinely recommended in prevention of CIN.

2.4.13. Hemofiltration and hemodialysis

Currently available data do not support use of prophylactic hemodialysis for prevention of CIN. In a trial of 113 patients, reported that CIN occurred in 24% of the hemodialysis group as compared with 16% of non-hemodialysis group (Vogt et al., 2001). Clinically relevant events also were not different in two groups. Only continuous venovenous hemofiltration has been shown to protect against CIN. In a study, 114 patients with chronic renal failure undergoing percutaneous coronary intervention were divided in two groups: 56 patients received normal saline and 58 patients underwent hemofiltration at a rate of 1000 ml/h (Marenzi et al., 2003). Hemofiltration seems to have a protective effect, including significant reduction in in-hospital and 1-year mortality compared with routine hydration. The mechanisms of this benefit are not clear. Further studies are needed to confirm the results of this trial.

2.4.14. New types of contrast medias

Gadolinium-enhanced magnetic resonance coronary angiography is a non-invasive method for evaluation of coronary arteries. It has been suggested that gadolinum-based CM could be used in stead of iodinated CM for radiological examinations in patients with significant renal impairment. However, its use has been questioned on the basis of reports of nephrotoxicity and its association with nephrogenic systemic fibrosis, a rare and serious syndrome that involves fibrosis of skin, joints, eyes, and internal organs. In a study by Hoffmann et al. the effect of gadopentetate dimeglumine (iodine-based CM) was studied in 181 patients with normal renal function and the effect of gadolinium was studied in 198 patients with pre-excisting renal failure. There was no statistically significant change in serum creatinine concentration after gadopentetate dimeglumine. In contrary, serum creatinine levels decreased significantly after the administration of gadolinium ($p<0.01$) (Hoffmann et al., 2005). In a retrospective study, the safety of gadolinium was evaluated in 91 patients with stage 3 and 4 renal failure who underwent angiographic MRI procedures. Eleven of 91 patients developed CIN (12.1%) (Ergun et al., 2006). In another randomized study gadobutrol, a gadolinium-based CM, was compared with standard iohexol, an iodinated CM, in 21 patients with renal dysfunction. The incidence of CIN was 50% in gadobutrol group and 45% in iohexol group ($p=0.70$). In this study, gadolinium showed no benefit over iohexol in patients with severely impaired renal function (Erley et al., 2004). More studies need to be done to better understand the role of gadolinum on CIN. Ultrasound contrast agents are micro-bubbles which produce acoustic enhancement. They are pharmacologically almost inert and safe.

3. Conclusion

The development of CIN is associated with adverse outcomes including prolonged hospitalization, the potential need for renal replacement therapy, and most important, increased mortality. The treatment of established CIN is limited to supportive measures and dialysis. For this reason, screening for high-risk patients before CM including -cardiac procedures and taking the appropriate prophylactic regimens is important in reducing CIN. Pre-existing renal dysfunction, especially when secondary to diabetic nephropathy, is the most important risk factor. Extra cellular volume expansion and use of low osmolar CM are the two most effective measures to prevent CIN. Acetylcysteine may use in high-risk patients, and nebivolol may use as a new prophylactic agent for CIN, but this finding has not been uniform or always demonstrated by currently available trials.

Author details

Omer Toprak

Department of Medicine, Division of Nephrology, Balikesir University School of Medicine, Balikesir, Turkey

References

[1] Abizaid, AS., Clark, CE., Mintz, GS., Dosa, S., Popma, JJ., Pichard, AD., Satler, LF., Harvey, M., Kent, KM., & Leon, MB. (1999). Effects of Dopamine and Aminophylline

on Contrast-Induced Acute Renal Failure after Coronary Angioplasty in Patients with Preexisting Renal Insufficiency. *The American Journal of Cardiology*, Vol.83, No.2, (January 1999), pp.260-263, ISSN 0002-9149

[2] Ahuja, TS., Niaz, N., & Agraharkar, M. (2000). Contrast-Induced Nephrotoxicity in Renal Allograft Recipients. *Clinical Nephrology*, Vol.54, No.1, (July 2000), pp.11-14, ISSN 0301-0430

[3] Allaqaband, S., Tumuluri, R., Malik, AM., Gupta, A., Volkert, P., Shalev, Y., & Bajwa, TK. (2002). Prospective Randomized Study of N-Acetylcysteine, Fenoldopam, and Saline for Prevention of Radiocontrast-Induced Nephropathy. *Catheterization and Cardiovascular Interventions*, Vol.57, No.3, (November 2002), pp.279-283, ISSN 1522-1946

[4] Aspelin, P., Aubry, P., Fransson, SG., Strasser, R., Willenbrock, R., & Berg, KJ. (2003). Nephrotoxic Effects in High-Risk Patients Undergoing Angiography. *The New England Journal of Medicine*, Vol.348, No.6, (February 2003), pp.491-499, ISSN 0028-4793

[5] Avci, E., Yeşil, M., Bayata, S., Postaci, N., Arikan, E., & Cirit, M. (2011). The Role of Nebivolol in The Prevention of Contrast-Induced Nephropathy in Patients with Renal Dysfunction. The Anatolian Journal of Cardiology, Vol.11, No.7, (November 2011), pp.613-617, ISSN 1302-8723

[6] Baker, CS., Wragg, A., Kumar, S., De Palma, R., Baker, LR., & Knight, CJ. (2003). A Rapid Protocol for the Prevention of Contrast-Inducted Renal Dysfunction: The RAPPID Study. *Journal of the American College of the Cardiology*, Vol. 41, No. 12, (June 2003), pp.2114-2118, ISSN 0735-1097

[7] Bartholomew, BA., Harjai, KJ., Dukkipati, S., Boura, JA., Yerkey, MW., Glazier, S., Grines, CL., & O'Neill, WW. (2004). Impact of Nephropathy after Percutaneous Coronary Intervention and a Method for Risk Stratification, *The American Journal of Cardiology*, Vol.93, No.12, (June 2004), pp.1515-1519, ISSN 0002-9149

[8] Barrett, BJ., Parfrey, PS., Vavasour HM., McDonald, J., Kent, G., Hefferton, D., O'Dea, F., Stone, E., Reddy, R., & McManamon, PJ. (1992). Contrast Nephropathy in Patients with Impaired Renal Function: High Versus Low Osmolar Media. *Kidney International*, Vol.41, No.5, (May 1992), pp. 1274–1279, ISSN 0085-2538

[9] Birck, R., Krzossok, S., Markowetz, F., Schnulle, P., van der Woude, FJ., & Braun, C. (2003). Acetylcysteine for Prevention of Contrast Nephropathy: Meta-Analysis. *Lancet*, Vol.362, No.9384, (August 2003), pp.598-603, ISSN 0140-6736

[10] Briguori, C., Manganelli, F., Scarpato, P., Elia, PP., Golia, B., Riviezzo, G., Lepore, S., Librera, M., Villari, B., Colombo, A., & Ricciardelli, B. (2002). Acetylcysteine and Contrast Agent-Associated Nephrotoxicity. *Journal of the American College of the Cardiology*, Vol.40, No.2, (July 2002), pp. 298-303, ISSN 0735-1097

[11] Briguori, C., Colombo, A., Airoldi, F., Violante, A., Castelli, A., Balestrieri, P., Paolo Elia, P., Golia, B., Lepore, S., Riviezzo, G., Scarpato, P., Librera, M., Focaccio, A., & Ricciardelli, B. (2004). N-Acetylcysteine Versus Fenoldopam Mesylate to Prevent

Contrast Agent-Associated Nephrotoxicity. *Journal of the American College of the Cardiology*, Vol.44, No.4, (August 2004), pp.762-765, ISSN 0735-1097

[12] Chalmers, N., & Jackson, RW. (1999). Comparison of Iodixanol and Iohexol in Renal Impairment. *The British Journal of Radiology*, Vol.72, No.859, (July 1999), pp.701-703, ISSN 0007-1285

[13] Cirit, M., Toprak, O., Yesil, M., Bayata, S., Postaci, N., Pupim, L., & Esi, E. (2006). Angiotensin-Converting Enzyme Inhibitors as a Risk Factor for Contrast-Induced Nephropathy. *Nephron Clinical Practice*, Vol.104, No.1, (August 2006), pp. c20-c27, ISSN 1660-2110

[14] Dangas, G., Iakovou, I., Nikolsky, E., Aymong, ED., Mintz, GS., Kipshidze, NN., Lansky, AJ., Moussa, I., Stone, GW., Moses, JW., Leon, MB., & Mehran, R. (2005). Contrast-Induced Nephropathy After Percutaneous Coronary Interventions in Relation to Chronic Kidney Disease and Hemodynamic Variables. *The American Journal of Cardiology*, Vol.95, No.1, (January 2005), pp. 13-19, ISSN 0002-9149

[15] Diaz-Sandoval, LJ., Kosowsky, BD., & Losordo, DW. (2002). Acetylcysteine to Prevent Angiography-Related Renal Tissue Injury (The APART Trial). *American Journal of Cardiology*, Vol.89, No.3, (February 2002), pp.356-358, ISSN 0002-9149

[16] Ergun, I., Keven, K., Uruc, I., Ekmekci, Y., Canbakan, B., Erden, I., & Karatan, O. (2006). The Safety of Gadolinium in Patients with Stage 3 and 4 Renal Failure. *Nephrology Dialysis Transplantation*, Vol.21, No.3, (March 2006), pp. 697-700, ISSN 0931-0509

[17] Erley, CM., Bader, BD., Berger, ED., Tuncel, N., Winkler, S., Tepe, G., Risler, T., & Duda, S. Gadolinium-Based Contrast Media Compared with Iodinated Media for Digital Subtraction Angiography in Azotaemic Patients. *Nephrology Dialysis Transplantation*, Vol.19, No.10, (October 2004), pp.2526-2531, ISSN 0931-0509

[18] Erley, CM., Duda, SH., Rehfuss, D., Scholtes, B., Bock, J., Muller, C., Osswald, H., & Risler, T. (1999). Prevention of Radiocontrast Media-Induced Nephropathy in Patients with Pre-Existing Renal Insufficiency by Hydration in Combination with the Adenosine Antagonist Theophylline. *Nephrology Dialysis Transplantation*, Vol.14, No. 5, (May 1999), pp.1146–1149, ISSN 0931-0509

[19] Gomes, VO., Poli de Figueredo, CE., Caramori, P., Lasevitch, R., Bodanese, LC., Araujo, A., Roedel, AP., Caramori, AP., Brito, FS Jr., Bezerra, HG., Nery, P., & Brizolara, A. (2005). N-Acetylcysteine Does Not Prevent Contrast Induced Nephropathy after Cardiac Catheterisation with an Ionic Low Osmolality Contrast Medium: A Multicentre Clinical Trial. *Heart*, Vol.91, No.6, (June 2005), pp.774-778, ISSN 1355-6037

[20] Gruberg, L., Mehran, R., Dangas, G., Mintz, GS., Waksman, R., Kent, KM., Pichard, AD., Satler, LF., Wu, H., & Leon, MB. (2001). Acute Renal Failure Requiring Dialysis after Percutaneous Coronary Interventions. *Catheterization and Cardiovascular Interventions*, Vol.52, No.4, (April 2001), pp.409-416, ISSN 1522-1946

[21] Gulel, O., Keles, T., Eraslan, H., Aydogdu, S., Diker, E., & Ulusoy, V. (2005). Prophylactic Acetylcysteine Usage for Prevention of Contrast Nephropathy after Coronary Angiography. *Journal of Cardiovascular Pharmacology*, Vol.46, No.4, (October 2005), pp. 464-467, ISSN 0160-2446

[22] Gunebakmaz, O., Kaya, MG., Koc, F., Akpek, M., Kasapkara, A., Inanc, MT., Yarlioglues, M., Calapkorur, B., Karadag, Z., & Oguzhan, A. (2012). Does nebivolol prevent contrast-induced nephropathy in humans? Clinical Cardiology, Vol.35, No.4, (April 2012), pp.250-254, ISSN 1932-8737

[23] Gupta, RK., Kapoor, A., Tewari, S., Sinha, N., & Sharma, RK. (1999). Captopril for Preventing of Contrast-Induced Nephropathy in Diabetic Patients: A Randomized Study. *Indian Heart Jouurnal,* Vol.51, No.5, (September 1999), pp.521–526, ISSN 0019-4832

[24] Hans, SS., Hans, BA., Dhillon, R., Dmuchowski, C., & Glover, J. (1998). Effect of Dopamine on Renal Function after Arteriography in Patients With Preexisting Renal Insufficiency. *The American Surgeon,* Vol.34, No.5, (May 1998), pp.1682-1688, ISSN 0003-1348

[25] Hoffmann, U., Fischereder, M., Reil, A., Fischer, M., Link, J., & Kramer, BK. (2005). Renal Effects of Gadopentetate Dimeglumine in Patients with Normal and Impaired Renal Function. *European Journal of Medical Research,* Vol. 10, No.4, (April 2005), pp. 149-154, ISSN 0949-2321

[26] Hoffmann, U., Fischereder, M., Kruger, B., Drobnik, W.; & Kramer, BK. (2004). The Value of N-Acetylcysteine in the Prevention of Radiocontrast Agent-Induced Nephropathy Seems Questionable. *Journal of the American Society of Nephrology,* Vol.15, No.2, (February 2004), pp.407–410, ISSN 1046-6673

[27] Holland, MD., Galla, JH., Sanders, PW., & Luke, RG. (1985). Effect of Urinary pH and Diatrizoate on Bence Jones Protein Nephrotoxicity in the Rat. *Kidney International,* Vol.27, No.1, (January 1985), pp. 46-50, ISSN 0085-2538

[28] Iakovou, I., Dangas, G., Mehran, R., Lansky, AJ., Ashby, DT., Fahy, M., Mintz, GS., Kent, KM., Pichard, AD., Satler, LF., Stone, GW., & Leon, MB. (2003). Impact of Gender on the Incidence and Outcome of Contrast-Induced Nephropathy after Percutaneous Coronary Intervention. *The Journal of Invasive Cardiology,* Vol.15, No.1, (January 2003), pp. 18–22, ISSN 1042-3931

[29] Kapoor, A., Kumar, S., Gulati, S., Gambhir, S., Sethi, RS., & Sinha, N. The Role of Theophylline in Contrast-Induced Nephropathy: A Case-Control Study. *Nephrology Dialysis Transplantation,* Vol. 17, No.11, (November 2002), pp.1936–1941, ISSN 0931-0509

[30] Kapoor, A., Sinha, N., Sharma, RK., Shrivastava, S., Radhakrishnan, S., Goel, PK., & Bajaj R. (1996). Use of Dopamine in Prevention of Contrast Induced Acute Renal Failure: A Randomized Study. *International Journal of Cardiology,*Vol.53, No.3, (March 1996), pp.233-236, ISSN 0167-5273

[31] Kiski, D., Stepper, W., Brand, E., Breithardt, G., & Reinecke, H. (2010). Impact of Renin-Angiotensin-Aldosterone Blockade by Angiotensin-Converting Enzyme Inhibitors or AT-1 Blockers on Frequency of Contrast Medium-Induced Nephropathy: A Post-Hoc Analysis from the Dialysis-Versus-Diuresis (DVD) Trial. . *Nephrology Dialysis Transplantation*, Vol.25, No.3, (May 2010), pp.759-64, ISSN 0931-0509

[32] Koch, JA., Plum, J., Grabensee, B., & Modder, U. (2000). Prostaglandin E1: A New Agent for the Prevention of Renal Dysfunction in High Risk Patients Caused by Radiocontrast Media? *Nephrology Dialysis Transplantation*, Vol. 15, No.1, (January 2000), pp.43-49, ISSN 0931-0509

[33] Kohli, HS., Bhaskaran, MC., Muthukumar, T., Thennarasu, K., Sud, K., Jha, V., Gupta, KL., & Sakhuja, V. (2000). Treatment-Related Acute Renal Failure in the Elderly: A Hospital-Based Prospective Study. . *Nephrology Dialysis Transplantation*, Vol.15, No.2, (February 2000), pp. 212-217, ISSN 0931-0509

[34] Kurnik, BR., Allgren, RL., Genter, FC., Solomon, RJ., Bates, ER., & Weisberg, LS. (1998). Prospective Study of Atrial Natriuretic Peptide for the Prevention of Radiocontrast-Induced Nephropathy. *American Journal of the Kidney Diseases*, Vol.31, No.4, (April 1998), pp.674-680, ISSN 0272-6386

[35] Lautin, EM., Freeman, NJ., Schoenfeld, AH., Bakal, CW., Haramati, N., Friedman, AC., Lautin, JL., Braha, S., Kadish, EG., & Sprayregen, S. (1991). Radiocontrast-Associated Renal Dysfunction: Incidence and Risk Factors. *AJR American Journal of Roentgenology*, Vol.157, No.1, (July 1991), pp. 49–58, ISSN 0033-8419

[36] Liss, P., Carlsson, PO., Nygren, A., Palm, F., & Hansell, P. (2003). ET-A Receptor Antagonist BQ123 Prevents Radiocontrast Media-Induced Renal Medullary Hypoxia. *Acta Radiologica*, Vol.44, No.1, (January 2003), pp.111-117, ISSN 0284-1851

[37] Liu, R., Nair, D., Ix, J., Moore, DH., & Bent, S. (2005). N-Acetylcysteine for the Prevention of Contrast-Induced Nephropathy. A Systematic Review and Meta-Analysis. *Journal of General Internal Medicine*, Vol.20, No.2, (Febrary 2005), pp.193-200, ISSN 0884-8734

[38] McCarthy, CS., & Becker, JA. (1992). Multiple Myeloma and Contrast Media. *Radiology*, Vol.183, No.2, (May 1992), pp.519–521, ISSN 0033-8419

[39] McCullough, PA., Wolyn, R., Rocher, LL., Levin, RN., & O'Neill, WW. (1997). Acute Renal Failure after Coronary Intervention: Incidence, Risk Factors, and Relationships to Mortality. *The American Journal of Medicine*, Vol.103, No.5, (November 1997), pp. 368–375, ISSN 0002-9243

[40] Marenzi, G., Lauri, G., Assanelli, E., Campodonico, J., De Metrio, M., Marana, I., Grazi, M., Veglia, F., & Bartorelli, AL. (2004). Contrast-Induced Nephropathy in Patients Undergoing Primary Angioplasty for Acute Myocardial Infarction. *Journal of the American College of the Cardiology*, Vol.44, No.9, (November 2004), pp. 1780-1785, ISSN 0735-1097

[41] Marenzi, G., Marana, I., Lauri, G., Assanelli, E., Grazi, M., Campodonico, J., Trabattoni, D., Fabbiocchi, F., Montorsi, P., & Bartorelli, AL. (2003). The Prevention of Radiocontrast-Agent-Induced Nephropathy by Hemofiltration. *The New England Journal of Medicine*, Vol.349, No.14, (October 2003), pp.1333-1340, ISSN 0028-4793

[42] Mehran, R., Aymong, ED., Nikolsky, E., Lasic, Z., Iakovou, I., Fahy, M., Mintz, GS., Lansky, AJ., Moses, JW., Stone, GW., Leon, MB., & Dangas, G. (2004). A Simple Risk Score for Prediction of Contrast-Induced Nephropathy after Percutaneous Coronary Intervention: Development and Initial Validation. *Journal of the American College of Cardiology*. Vol.44, No.7, (October 2004), pp.1393-1399, ISSN 0735-1097

[43] Merten, GJ., Burgess, WP., Gray, LV., Holleman, JH., Roush, TS., Kowalchuk, GJ., Bersin, RM., Van Moore, A., Simonton, CA 3rd., Rittase, RA., Norton, HJ., & Kennedy, TP. (2004). Prevention of contrast-induced nephropathy with sodium bicarbonate: a randomized controlled trial. *Journal of the American Medical Association*, Vol.291, No.19, (May 2004), pp.2328-2334, ISSN 0098-7484

[44] Moore, RD., Steinberg, EP., Powe, NR., Brinker, JA., Fishman, EK., Graziano, S., & Gopalan, R. (1992). Nephrotoxicity of High-Osmolarity vs Low-Osmolarity Contrast Media: Randomized Clinical Trial. *Radiology*, Vol.182, No.3, *(March* 1992), pp. 649–655, ISSN 0033-8419

[45] Mueller, C., Seidensticker, P., Buettner, HJ., Perruchoud, AP., Staub, D., Christ, A., & Buerkle, G. (2005). Incidence of Contrast Nephropathy in Patients Receiving Comprehensive Intravenous and Oral Hydration. Swiss Medical Weekly, Vol.135, No.19, (May 2005), pp.286-290, ISSN 1424-7860

[46] Mueller, C., Buerkle, G., Buettner, HJ., Petersen, J., Perruchoud, AP., Eriksson, U., Marsch, S., & Roskamm, H. (2002). Prevention of Contrast Media-Associated Nephropathy: Randomized Comparison of 2 Hydration Regimens In 1620 Patients Undergoing Coronary Angioplasty. *Archives of Internal Medicine*, Vol.162, No.3, (February 2002), pp.329-336, ISSN 0003-9926

[47] Neumayer, HH., Junge, W., Kufner, A., & Wening, A. (1989). Prevention of Radiocontrast-Media-Induced Nephrotoxicity by the Calcium Channel Blocker Nitrendipine: A Prospective Randomized Clinical Trial. *Nephrology Dialysis Transplantation*, Vol.4, No.12, (April 1989), pp.1030-1036, ISSN 0931-0509

[48] Nikolsky, E., Mehran, R., Lasic, Z., Mintz, GS., Lansky, AJ., Na, Y., Pocock, S., Negoita, M., Moussa, I., Stone, GW., Moses, JW., Leon, MB., & Dangas, G. Low Hematocrit Predicts Contrast-Induced Nephropathy After Percutaneous Coronary Interventions. *Kidney International*, Vol.67, No.2, (February 2005), pp.706-713, ISSN 0085-2538

[49] Parfrey, PS., Griffiths, SM., Barrett, BJ., Paul, MD., Genge, M., Withers, J. Farid, N., & McManamon, PJ. (1989). Contrast Material-Induced Renal Failure in Patients with Diabetes Mellitus, Renal Insufficiency, or Both. A Prospective Controlled Study. *The New England Journal of Medicine*, Vol.320, No.3, (January 1989), pp.143-149, ISSN 0028-4793

[50] Perrin, T., Descombes, E., & Cook S. (2012). Contrast-Induced Nephropathy in Invasive Cardiology. Swiss Medical Weekly, Vol.142, No.13608, (June 2012), ISSN1424-7860

[51] Rich, MW., & Crecelius, CA. (1990). Incidence, Risk Factors, and Clinical Course of Acute Renal Insufficiency after Cardiac Catheterization in Patients 70 Years of Age or Older. A Prospective Study. *Archives of Internal Medicine*, Vol.150, No.6, (June1990), pp. 1237-1242), ISSN 0003-9926

[52] Rihal, CS., Textor, SC., Grill, DE., Berger, PB., Ting, HH., Best, PJ., Singh, M., Bell, MR., Barsness, GW., Mathew, V., Garratt, KN., & Holmes, DR Jr. (2002). Incidence and Prognostic Importance of Acute Renal Failure after Percutaneous Coronary Intervention. *Circulation,* Vol.105, No.105, (May 2002), pp. 2259-2264, ISSN 0009-7322

[53] Rodicio, JL., Morales, JM., & Ruilope, LM. (1990). Calcium Antagonists and the Kidney. *Nephrology Dialysis Transplantation*, Vol.5, No.2, (1990), pp.81-86, ISSN 0931-0509

[54] Rudnick, MR., Goldfarb, S., Wexler, L., Ludbrook, PA., Murphy, MJ., Halpern, EF., Hill, JA., Winniford, M., Cohen, MB., & Van Fossen, DB. (1995). Nephrotoxicity of Ionic and Nonionic Contrast Media in 1196 Patients: A Randomized Trial. The Iohexol Cooperative Study. *Kidney International*, Vol.47, No.1, (January 1995), pp. 254-261, ISSN 0085-2538

[55] Russo, D., Testa, A., Della Volpe, L., & Sansone, G. (1990). Randomised Prospective Study on Renal Effects of Two Different Contrast Media in Humans: Protective Role of a Calcium Channel Blocker. *Nephron,* Vo.55, No.3, (1990), pp.254-257, ISSN 0028-2766

[56] Sadeghi, HM., Stone, GW., Grines, CL., Mehran, R., Dixon, SR., Lansky, AJ., Fahy, M., Cox, DA., Garcia, E., Tcheng, JE., Griffin, JJ., Stuckey, TD., Turco, M., & Carroll, JD. (2003). Impact of Renal Insufficiency in Patients Undergoing Primary Angioplasty for Acute Myocardial Infarction. *Circulation,* Vol.108, No.22, (December 2003), pp. 2769-2775, ISSN 0009-7322

[57] Shaker, OG., El-Shehaby, A., & El-Khatib, M. (2010). Early Diagnostic Markers for Contrast Nephropathy in Patients Undergoing Coronary Angiography. *Angiology,* Vol.61, No.8, (November 2010), pp. 731-736, ISSN 0003-3197

[58] Solomon, R., Werner, C., Mann, D., D'Elia, J., & Silva, P. (1994). Effects of Saline, Mannitol and Furosemide to Prevent Acute Decreases in Renal Function Induced by Radiocontrast Agents. *The New England Journal of Medicine*, Vol. 331, No.21, (November 1994), pp.1416–1420, ISSN 0028-4793

[59] Spangberg-Viklund, B., Berglund, J., Nikonoff, T., Nyberg, P., Skau, T., & Larsson, R. (1996). Does Prophylactic Treatment with Felodopine, a Calcium Antagonist, Prevent Low-Osmolar Contrast Induced Renal Dysfunction in Hydrated Diabetic and Nondiabetic Patients with Normal or Moderately Reduced Renal Function? *Scandinavian Journal of Urology and Nephrology,* Vol.30, No.1, (February 1996), pp.63-68, ISSN 0036-5599

[60] Spargias, K., Alexopoulos, E., Kyrzopoulos, S., Iokovis, P., Greenwood, DC., Manginas, A., Voudris, V., Pavlides, G., Buller, CE., Kremastinos, D., & Cokkinos, DV. (2004). Ascorbic Acid Prevents Contrast-Mediated Nephropathy in Patients with Renal Dysfunction Undergoing Coronary Angiography or Intervention. *Circulation,* Vol.110, No.18, (November 2004), pp.2837-2842, ISSN 0009-7322

[61] Stone, GW., McCullough, PA., Tumlin, JA., Lepor, NE., Madyoon, H., Murray, P., Wang, A., Chu, AA., Schaer, GL., Stevens, M., Wilensky, RL., & O'Neill, WW., CONTRAST Investigators. (2003). Fenoldopam Mesylate for the Prevention of Contrast-Induced Nephropathy: A Randomized Controlled Trial. *The Journal of the American Medical Association,* Vol.290, No.17, (November 2003), pp.2284-2291, ISSN 0098-7484

[62] Taliercio, CP., Vlietstra, RE., Fisher, LD., & Burnett, JC. (1986). Risks for Renal Dysfunction with Cardiac Angiography. *Annals of Internal Medicine,* Vol.104, No.4, (April 1986), pp.501-504, ISSN 0003-4819

[63] Tepel, M., van Der Giet, M., Schwarzfeld, C., Laufer, U., Liermann, D., & Zidek, W. (2000). Prevention of Radiographic-Contrast-Agent-Induced Reductions in Renal Function by Acetylcysteine. *The New England Journal of Medicine,* Vol.343, No.3, (July2000), pp.,180-184, ISSN 0028-4793

[64] Toprak, O., Cirit, M., Tanrisev, M., Yazici, C., Canoz, O., Sipahioglu, M., Uzum, A., Ersoy, R., & Sozmen, EY. (2008). Preventive Effect of Nebivolol on Contrast-Induced Nephropathy in Rats. *Nephrology Dialysis Transplantation,* Vol.23, No.3, (March 2008), pp. 853-859, ISSN 0931-0509

[65] Toprak, O. (2007). Conflicting and New Risk Factors for Contrast-Induced Nephropathy. *The Journal of Urology,* Vol. 178, No.6, (December 2007), pp. 2277-2283, ISSN 0022-5347

[66] Toprak, O., Cirit, M., Yesil, M., Bayata, S., Tanrisev, M., Varol, U., Ersoy, R., & Esi, E. (2007). Impact of Diabetic and Pre-Diabetic State on Development of Contrast-Induced Nephropathy in Patients with Chronic Kidney Disease. *Nephrology Dialysis Transplantation,* Vol.22, No.3, (March 2007), pp. 819-826, ISSN 0931-0509

[67] Toprak, O., Cirit, M., Yesil, M., Byrne DW, Postaci, N., Bayata, S., Majchrzak, KM., & Esi, E. (2006). Metabolic Syndrome as a Risk Factor for Contrast-Induced Nephropathy in Non-Diabetic Elderly Patients with Renal Impairment. *Kidney and Blood Pressure Research,* Vol.29, No.1, (June 2006), pp. 2-9, ISSN 1420-4096

[68] Toprak, O., Cirit, M., Esi, E., Postaci, N., Yesil, M., & Bayata, S. (2007). Hyperuricemia as a Risk Factor for Contrast-Induced Nephropathy in Patients with Chronic Kidney Disease. *Catheterization and Cardiovascular Interventions,* Vol.67, No.2, (February 2006), pp. 227-235, ISSN 1522-1946

[69] Toprak, O., & Cirit, M. (2006). Risk Factors and Therapy Strategies for Contrast-Induced Nephropathy. *Renal Failure,* Vol. 28, No. 5, (January 2006), pp. 365-381, ISSN 0886-022X

[70] Toprak, O., & Cirit, M. (2005). Investigating the Volume Status Before Contrast Nephropathy Studies. *Nephrology Dialysis Transplantation,* Vol.20, No.2, (February 2005), pp. 464, ISSN 0931-0509

[71] Toprak, O., Cirit, M., Bayata, S., Yesil, M., & Aslan, SL. (2003). The Effect of Pre-procedural Captopril on Contrast-Induced Nephropathy in Patients who Underwent Coronary Angiography. *Anadolu Kardiyoloji Dergisi,* Vol. 3, No.2, (June 2003), pp. 98-103, ISSN 1302-8723

[72] Toprak, O., Cirit, M., Bayata, S., Aslan, SL., Sarioglu, F., & Cetinkaya, GS. (2003). Is There Any Relationship Between Left Ventricul Ejection Fraction and Contrast Induced Nephropathy? *Türkiye Klinikleri Journal of Medical Sciences,* Vol 23, No. 2, (March 2003), pp. 104-107 , ISSN 1300-0292

[73] Vogt, B., Ferrari, P., Schonholzer, C., Marti, HP., Mohaupt, M., Wiederkehr, M., Cereghetti, C., Serra, A., Huynh-Do, U., Uehlinger, D., & Frey, FJ. (2001). Prophylactic Hemodialysis after Radiocontrast Media in Patients with Renal Insufficiency is Potentially Harmful. *The American Journal of Medicine,* Vol.111, No.9, (December 2001), pp.692-698, ISSN 0002-9243

[74] Wang, A., Holcslaw, T., Bashore, TM., Freed, MI., Miller, D., Rudnick, MR., Szerlip, H., Thames, MD., Davidson, CJ., Shusterman, N., & Schwab, SJ. (2000). Exacerbation of Radiocontrast Nephrotoxicity by Endothelin Receptor Antagonism. *Kidney International,* Vol.57, No.4, (April 2000), pp.1675-1680, ISSN 0085-2538

[75] Weber-Mzell, D., Kotanko, P., Schumacher, M., Klein, W., & Skrabal, F. (2002). Coronary Anatomy Predicts Presence or Absence of Renal Artery Stenosis. A Prospective Study in Patients Undergoing Cardiac Catheterization for Suspected Coronary Artery Disease. *European Heart Journal,* Vol.23, No.21, (November 2002), pp.1684–1691, ISSN 0195-668x

[76] Weinrauch, LA., Healy, RW., Leland, OS Jr., Goldstein, HH., Kassissieh, SD., Libertino, JA., Takacs, FJ., & D'Elia, JA. (1977). Coronary Angiography and Acute Renal Failure in Diabetic Azotemic Nephropathy. *Annals of Internal Medicine,* Vol.86, No.1, (January 1977), pp.56-59, ISSN 0003-4819

[77] Weisberg, LS., Kurnik, PB., & Kurnik, BR. (1994). Risk of Radiocontrast Nephropathy in Patients with and without Diabetes Mellitus. Kidney International, Vol.45, No.1, (January 1994), pp.259-265,ISSN 0085-2538

[78] Yang, DW., Jia, RH., Yang, DP., Ding, GH., & Huang, CX. (2004). Dietary Hypercholesterolemia Aggravates Contrast Media-Induced Nephropathy. *Chinese Medical Journal,* Vol. 117, No.4 (April 2004), pp.542–546, ISSN 0366-6999.

[79] Zhang, L., Zhang, L., Lu, Y., Wu, B., Zhang, S., Jiang, H., Ge, J., & Chen, H. (2011). Efficacy of Statin Pretreatment for the Prevention of Contrast-Induced Nephropathy: A Meta-Analysis of Randomised Controlled Trials. *International Journal of Clinical Practice,*Vol.65, No.5, (May 2011), pp.624-30, ISSN 1368-5031

Chapter 17

Contrast-Induced Nephropathy in Coronary Angiography and Intervention

Chia-Ter Chao, Vin-Cent Wu and Yen-Hung Lin

Additional information is available at the end of the chapter

http://dx.doi.org/10.5772/54081

1. Introduction

Since the advent of coronary angioplasty more than 3 decades ago, the volume of percutaneous coronary interventions (PCI) has been rising progressively, with relative decrease in amount of coronary artery bypass graft (CABG) surgery. Roughly 1.4 million of catheterization procedures are performed in U.S. each year.[1] Contrast medium is widely used in both diagnositc coronary angiography and PCI, and intravenous use of iodinated contrast medium is a common precipitator of contrast-induced nephropathy (or contrast-induced acute kidney injury [AKI]). [2, 3] With the trend of increasing PCI use in the modern era, expectedly more patients will develop contrast-induced AKI in the future. Currently contrast-induced nephropathy has been the third most common cause of hospital-acquired AKI in the large registry studies. [4] This phenomenon is worthy of our attention, since past researchers have identified that contrast-induced AKI can be associated with increased late incidence of acute myocardial infarction (AMI) and target vessel revascularization [5], longer in-hospital stay [6], a more complicated hospitalization course (bleeding episodes requiring transfusion, vascular complications) [7], and higher in-hospital mortality and morbidity [8-10]. More importantly, contrast induced AKI correlates with higher healthcare resource utilization including hospitalization cost [11]. The economical spending increases even further if the episodes of contrast-induced AKI are dialysis-requring.

We have witnessed significant advancement in the development of contrast medium within the past 7 decades. [8] The structure, osmolality and its inherent chemotoxicity have also changed tremendously, and are the focuses of experiments involving various animal models, cell culture systems, and human subjects. [12] In addition, knowledge of the pathogenesis and the relevant risk factors of contrast-induced AKI is also expandng, and this progress contributes significantly to our planning of strategies to prevent this adverse event after contrast medium injection. In this sense, a thorough understanding of the epidemiology, pathophysiology, clinical manifestations, diagnosis, prevention strategy and management of contrast-induced AKI is of critical importance for both primary care physicians and intervention cardiologists.

2. Epidemiology of contrast induced acute kidney injury (AKI)

The reported incidence of contrast-induced AKI varies widely among the existing literature, ranging from 2% to 25% after contrast medium injection [2, 13-15]. The estimations differ according to the cohort being studied, the definition used to identify patients with contrast-induced AKI, the distinction of the baseline risk factors of the population studied, and the intervention administered for prevention. [2] Maioli and coworkers, in a randomized controlled trial (RCT) to evaluate the effectiveness of various preventive strategies, identified a 2~2.5 fold difference in the incidence of contrast-induced AKI (control group, 12%; intervention group, 27.3%). [16] Weisbord and colleagues, in another study, demonstrated the importance of the AKI definition to the estimated incidence (ranging from 0.3% if stringently defined by serum creatinine [sCr] change of 1.0 mg/dL, to 13.7% if loosely defined by sCr change of 0.25 mg/dL). [3] Consequently, a consistent definition of contrast-induced AKI is vital for both clinical and research interest in this field.

2.1. Definition of contrast-induced acute kidney injury (AKI)

The definition of contrast-induced AKI can be divided into 2 main components, the predefined time frame and the change of renal function markers (Table 1). Typically contrast-induced AKI is defined by the current literature as an increase in sCr within the first 24 or 48 hours after contrast injection. [2, 14] There are arguments, however, that a period of 24 hours best captures the group of patients who develop contrast-induced AKI and carry the most favorable outcome; others claim that the elevation of sCr for clinical dignosis of contrast-induced AKI takes at least 48 hours. [17] The European Society of Urogenital Radiology (ESUR) has produced guidelines on contrast-induced AKI in 1999, and updated the content in 2011. [18, 19] Contrast-induced AKI (then termed contrast-induced nephropathy [CIN]) is defined as "a condition in which an impairment in renal function (an increase in sCr by more than 25% or 0.5 mg/dL) occurs within 3 days following intravascular administration of a contrast medium, in the absence of an alternative etiology". [18] Recently, the threshold of sCr change for diagnosis of AKI has been challenged, since minor sCr change has been shown to correlate with outcome measures. [20] In 2007, Acute Kidney Injury Network (AKIN) group has proposed a further fine-tuned classification scheme for staging AKI. [21] Milder AKI was staged as an elevation of sCre of 0.3 mg/dL within 48 hours. This concept further enhances the diagnostic probability of contrast-induced nephropathy, but there concerns that this criteria might be over-sensitive and leads to false positive diagnosis. [22] The researchers are now gradully adopting this scheme in categorzing contrast-induced AKI.

Potential Serum markers	Time frame		
	Within 2-4 hours after procedure	**Within 24 hours after procedure**	**Within 48 hours after procedure**
Serum creatinine		0.5 mg/dL↑	0.5 mg/dL↑
Serum creatinine		1.0 mg/dL↑	
Serum creatinine		25%↑from baseline	25%↑from baseline
Serum creatinine		50%↑from baseline	
Serum cystatin C#	? 25%↑from baseline		
Urinary NGAL#	↑>100-150 ng/mL		

Abbreviations: NGAL, Neutrophil gelatinase-associated lipocalin

Still under investigation

Table 1. The currently available definition of contrast-induced nephropathy

Other rapidly-responsive serum markers aiming at earlier detection of renal function change also are under investigation. Cystatin C is a cationic low molecular weight cysteine protease, produced at a constant rate by all nucleated cells.[23] It is not metabolized in the serum, and is freely filtered by glomeruli, thus serving as a good marker for assessing glomerular filtration rate (GFR).[24] A japanese study utilizing cystatin C and sCr in evaluating post-computed tomographic coronary angiography AKI concluded that serum cystatin C at day one after examination significantly correlates with change of sCr, indicating AKI. [25] Cystatin C is particularly useful in patients with diabetic history. On the other hand, Ribichini et al, in another study comparing sCr and cystatin C for detecting AKI after PCI within 12 hours, found that serum cystatin C performed significantly worse than sCr, with an area under curve (AUC) value of 0.48 only. [26] Neutrophil gelatinase-associated lipocalin (NGAL) is a small stress protein released from injured tubular cells after various stimuli. [27] A multitude of studies have documented its role in earlier detection of AKI, with excellent sensitivity and fair specificity.[28-30] Hirsch and coworkers first demonstrated in pediatric population that, with a cut-off value of 100 ng/mL and timeframe of 2 hours, urinary NGAL predicts contrast-induced AKI well, with 73% sensitivity and 100% specificity. [31] Another study from Austria reached similar findings, with additional benefit of improving renal outcome, possibly due to earlier detection. [32] Besides, there are other potential candidate biomarkers implicated as possessing a role in contrast-induced AKI, including kidney-injury molecules -1 (KIM-1), urinary L type fatty acid-binding protein (L-FABP), but few human studies are available currently.[33] Finally, the exact diagnostic modality of choice for contrast-induced nephropathy remains uncertain. A recent study by Erselcan and colleagues discovered that sCr-based diagnosis can in fact differ substantially from radionuclide-based GFR estimation method. [34] Consequently, the reported incidence of contrast-induced nephropathy in the literature might contain certain degree of deviation. Nonetheless, a close monitoring of sCr change and other markers of renal function change after contrast exposure is still crucial and necessary to detect any evidence of contrast-induced nephropathy after PCI.

3. Risk factors for contrast induced acute kidney injury (AKI)

Identification of patients potentially susceptible of developing contrast-induced AKI before their exposure is important, since modification of the ways we administer contrast medium can lead to a decrease in AKI. [4] Risk factors for developing such injury can be divided into 2 parts: patient-related factors and procedure-related factors. We will give a brief overview of these factors in the following sections.

3.1. Patient-related risk factors

There are several factors identified in the literature that enhances the susceptibility of developing contrast-induced AKI (Table 2).

Patient-related risk factors	Procedure-related risk factors
Advanced age	Higher contrast medium volumes
Diabetes (especially with nephropathy)	Higher contrast medium osmolality
Pre-existing CKD	Intra-arterial (vs. intravenous) route
Arterial hypotension	
Absolute intravascular volume depletion status	
Relative intravascular volume depletion status	
Diuretic use	
NSAID use (?)	
ACE inhibitor/ARB use (?)	

Abbreviations: ACE, angiotensin-converting enzyme; ARB, angiotensin-receptor blocker; CKD, chronic kidney disease; NSAID, non-steroidal anti-inflammatory agent

Table 2. Factors associated with increased risk of contrast-induced acute kidney injury

3.1.1. Diabetes mellitus (DM)

DM has been established as an independent factor for patients developing contrast-induced AKI. Presence of DM is associated with a 1.5 ~ 3 fold higher risk of renal injury after contrast exposure, and it potentially amplifies the risk incurred by pre-existing chronic kidney disease (CKD) alone (see below). [13, 15, 35] DM putatively predisposes host kidneys to ischemic injury (from macro- or micro-vascular stenosis), increases oxidatice stress and free radical damage, as well as endothelial dysfunction.[36] The accompanying comorbidities such as coronary artery diseases also contribute to the increased susceptibility. [37] Fluid retention in DM patients also increases the use of diuretics, which is also reportedly a risk factor for contrast-induced AKI. [38] In addition to the impact of a baseline DM, pre-procedural glucose level higher than 200 mg/dL s is also a risk factor for contrast-induced AKI (2-fold risk). [39]

3.1.2. Advanced age

Advanced age is another risk factor that enhances the probability of developing contrast-induced AKI. The definition of advanced age differs between the reported studies, but generally a range of 65-75 year-old is adopted. [15] Age higher than 75 can associate with a 1.5-5 fold elevated risk, while every one-year increment carries a 2% increased risk. [7, 15, 35] Aging *per se* denotes the physiologic degeneration of the kidney, both structurally and functionally, and the ability of recovery after various nephrotoxic insults also dampens in this population. [40] Most experts agree that a baseline renal function should be measured in older patients before their exposure to contrast medium. [2, 19]

3.1.3. Pre-existing chronic kidney disease (CKD)

Probably the most important risk factor for contrast-induced AKI is a baseline comorbidity of CKD. Almost all clinical trials and scoring models for predicting and stratifying risk of contrast-induced AKI have shown that CKD independently leads to more contrast-induced AKI episodes. [6, 7, 9, 13, 15, 35] The risk of renal dysfunction is directly proportional to the baseline sCr value, and further amplified by the presence of DM. [7, 15] Rihal et al, in a large PCI cohort, identified that patients with pre-procedural sCr 1.2-1.9, 2.0-2.9, >3 mg/dL, had a graded increment in risk of developing contrast-induced AKI (odds ratio [OR] 2.4, 7.4 and 12.8, respectively).[35] One-third of patients with sCr level higher than 2.0 mg/dL receiving contrast medium for radiographic studies will develop contrast-induced AKI. [41, 42]

The definition of CKD seems to vary somewhat between studies. It is generally agreed that patients with CKD should be classified by the stages proposed by the Kidney Disease Outcome Quality Initiative (KDOQI) according to their GFR values. [19] (Table 3) CKD is usually defined as renal function within stage 3 or higher level based on the KDOQI scheme, but there are some controversy about this. [43] GFR can be estimated by the Modification of Diet in Renal Disease (MDRD) formula, which takes account of each patient's sCr, age, ethnicity and gender. [44] However, this equation might be flawed when applied in patients with unstable or changing renal function. Patients with special dietary preference such as vegetarians and high protein diets, and ones with extreme body stature (very obese or lean) may be unsuitable by MDRD formula, too. [44] Recently, Chronic Kidney Disease – Epidemiology Collaboration (CKD-EPI) creatinine equation is found to outperform MDRD formula in these situations, but this equation, too, does not apply during changing renal function. [45] Nonetheless, sCr-based estimation of GFR is currently still the most valuable and timely method of grading patients' baseline renal function. Patients with estimated GFR (eGFR) higher than 60 ml/min/1.73m^2 should be treated as normal unless they have other renal diseases. [46]

3.1.4. Arterial hypotension

Hemodynamic instability has been quoted as a risk factor for contrast-induced AKI. [6, 13, 15] This can be demonstrated in certain parameters like hypotension and placement of intra-aortic balloon pump (IABP). [47] Gruberg and coworkers identified that use of IABP is linked to a 2 fold increase of developing contrast-induced AKI in patients receiving PCI. [48] In addition, anemia *per se* can also be treated in this regard as a factor that reduces tissue oxygenation and predisposes to CIN. [49]

3.1.5. Absolute intravascular volume depletion (dehydration)

Dehydration is commonly cited as a risk factor for contrast-induced nephropathy. [35, 50, 51] However, few clinical trials actually prove this risk, possibly owing to the fact that dehydration status is difficult to demonstrate and quantify.

3.1.6. Relative intravascular volume depletion

Statuses such as congestive heart failure (CHF) also potentiate the development of contrast-induced AKI, through mechanisms similar to dehydration and absolute intravascular volume depletion. [2, 15] CHF is also a risk factor for AKI in critically ill patients. [2] Most clinical trials have shown than CHF (with a New York Heart Association [NYHA] grade 3-4) is associated with elevated risk of contrast-induced AKI (OR around 1.5-2.0). [13, 15, 35] There are also studies showing that AMI within 24 hours of PCI with a low left ventricular ejection fraction (LVEF) independently predicts occurrence of CIN, with a 80% higher risk. [6, 35]

3.1.7. Drugs (Angiotensin-converting enzyme inhibitors [ACEI], angiotensin-receptor blockers [ARB], Non-steroidal anti-inflammatory agents [NSAID])

ACEI and ARB, by virtue of their glomerular hemodynamic effect, have been implicated in predisposing patients to contrast-induced AKI. [42] However, minimal data exists regarding their actual role in the development of such renal injury. Currently, most available results are retrospective in nature, and case numbers are low. Umruddin and colleagues, in a small case control study, demonstrated that use of ACEI or ARB is associated with 2.5-3.0 fold higher risk of developing CIN after coronary angiography. [52] On the contrary, withdrawal of ACEI or ARB before coronary procedures does not seem to reduce the risk of contrast-induced AKI. [53]

NSAIDs are commonly prescribed for analgesic and anti-pyretic purposes, and are notorious for their adverse impact on cardiovascular outcomes after AMI. [54] Through the interruption of intrarenal prostaglandin production, these drugs impede the hemodynamic regulation of kidney during nephrotoxic insults. Intuitively, they should contribute significantly to contrast-induced nephropathy, but there are very few clinical data currently. A Brazilian group identified no obvious increase in risk of CIN in patients taking NSAIDs before they receive coronary procedures, but the case number was low. [55] Further study is warranted before we can conclude that NSAID is neutral or potentially promoting contrast-induced AKI at this time.

Other nephrotoxic agents such as cyclosporin, tacrolimus, platinum-based chemotherapeutic regimen can theoretically enhance the susceptibility of the kidney to the insult of contrast medium. [56] Likewise, few clinical data exists concerning this issue, but physicians and cardiologists are still advised to refrain from these drugs in patients preparing for coronary procedures.

3.1.8. Miscellaneous

Elevated high sensitivity CRP has recently been reported as a risk factor for contrast-induced AKI. [57] The mechanism is putatively related to higher inflammatory status and the cytokine effect, but this remains speculative. Some researchers also claimed that multiple myeloma elevates the risk of CIN, but this association is inconsistent among recent studies. [56, 58, 59] Multiple myeloma by itself might not increase the inherent risk, but patients with myeloma is frequently dehydrated, and such dehydration could underlie the basis of the heightened risk. [19]

3.2. Procedure-related risk factors

Procedure-related risk factors include the volume, the osmolality, and the route of contrast medium administration.

3.2.1. Osmolality of contrast medium

Iodinated contrast media are structurally composed of carbon-based skeletons and iodide atoms, which render the molecules radiopaque. Contrast media are classified according to their osmolality into 3 types: high-osmolal (HOCM) (ex. diatrizoate), with an osmolality of ~2000 mOsm/kg; low-osmolal (LOCM)(ex. Iohexol, iopamidol, ioxaglate), with an osmolality of 600~800 mOsm/kg; and isosmolal (IOCM) (iodixanol), with an osmolality similar to serum. [2] When the contrast media were first introduced decades ago, only HOCM are available for imaging purposes. LOCM/IOCM were later developed in 1980s and 1990s, in order to reduce the accompanied toxicity incurred by high osmolality. [8] Earlier meta-analysis before 1990 demonstrated that the pooled OR for developing CIN decreased substantially after the introduction of LOCM. [60] High osmolality contrast medium is now an established risk factor for contrast-induced AKI. [2, 8, 14, 19] IOCM has been shown to possess the lowest risk for contrast -induced AKI in patients with CKD, but different IOCM agents do not seem to display clinically different effect. [61-64] A systemic review performed several years ago found that IOCM possess the lowest risk of contrast-induced AKI. [64] However, several clinical trials done in recent years yielded conflict results, with similar CIN rates between IOCM and LOCM agents. [65, 66] Despite these controversies, the American College of Cardiology (ACC) /American Heart Association (AHA) guidelines for the management of patients with acute coronary syndrome (ACS) list IOCM as a class I recommendation. [67]

3.2.2. Volume of contrast medium

The volume of administered contrast medium can be another important factor regarding the risk of contrast-induced AKI. Multiple studies have identified that the mean contrast volume is an independent predictor of CIN. [5, 9, 15] Even small volumes of contrast medium (~30ml) might trigger renal injury in high-risk patients. [68] For every 100ml increase in the amount of contrast medium used, there is a concomitant 12% increase of the risk. [35] Several groups proposed that the volume of contrast administered should not exceed twice the number of a given patient's baseline eGFR value (in mililiter), while others found that adjustment of the contrast volume to one's body weight and sCr level could minimize the risk. [2, 69]

3.2.3. Route of contrast medium administration

Circumstantial evidence has pointed out that intra-arterial injection of contrast medium carries a higher risk of contrast-induced AKI than intravenous use. [15, 70] However, no mechanisms have been provided to explain this phenomenon. [2] Some speculative reasons are as follows: the dose used in intravenous enhancement for computed tomography (CT) is usually lower than that for arteriography; patients who received contrast-enhanced CT are usually less hemodynamically unstable than ones receiving intra-arterial studies; intra-arterial angiography may incidentally incur atheroembolism, which would not be expected to happen in intravenous studies. [2, 19] There are also reports suggesting that patients who were at-risk for intra-arterial procedures might not be at-risk for intravenous studies. [3] Nonetheless, based upon the available evidence, it is prudent to evaluate patients regarding the exact necessity, risk and benefit for intra-arterial or intravenous procedures. If both indications exist with equal risk-benefit ratio, a choice of intravenous administration of contrast medium might be better.

4. Clinical course and pathophysiology of contrast-induced AKI

The norm of contrast-induced nephropathy is that sCr begins to rise within 24 hours after contrast medium administration, peaks at 3-5 days, and returns to baseline level or near baseline within 1-3 weeks. [71] It has been shown that even transient rise of sCr can associate with longer hospital stay. [42] Most patients developing contrast-induced AKI do not require dialysis; however, they do have poorer short-term and long-term survival. [9, 48] Gruberg et al, in a large cohort of patients with CIN after coronary angiography, reported that only 0.4% require hemodialysis after AKI occurs, but those necessitating dialytic support have particularly higher mortality (12-35%). [42, 48]

The pathophysiologic sequence of contrast-induced AKI includes a pre-existing impaired renal function, and the superimposed acute events consisting of vasoactive mediator-related vasoconstriction, triggered by iodinated contrast medium. [2] Besides, experimental studies also suggest that contrast-induced nephropathy can be a combination of both: renal ischemia and the direct tubulotoxicity exerted by contrast medium. [42]

4.1. Renal ischemia

Animal studies showed that contrast medium intravascular injection can increase the activity of a variety of vasoactive substances, including vasopressin, angiotensin II, dopamine-1, endothelin and adenosine, while decrease the activity of renal vasodilators such as nitric oxide and prostaglandins. [72, 73] Other mechanisms include high osmolality-related renal blood flow decrease, and the enhanced erythrocyte aggregation induced by contrast medium. [74, 75] This decrease in renal blood flow and GFR after exposure to contrast medium is frequently severer in dehydrated animals than euvolemic ones. [76] In particular, renal medulla is more susceptible to ischemic insult than renal cortex, and contrast medium has been reported to cause shunting of blood flow to the cortex. [77]

4.2. Direct tubulotoxicity

The tubulotoxicity of contrast medium can be demonstrated in the pathological changes it induces, including epithelial vacuolization, cellular necrosis or apoptosis and interstitial inflammation. [78] Contrast medium can additionally reduce antioxidant enzyme activity within the kidney of experimental animals, and free radical mediated cytotoxicity of the renal tubular cells has been detected in these models. [78] The higher osmolality of contrast medium can also contribute to its epithelial cell toxicity. The osmolar-driven solute diuresis with subsequent tubuloglomerular feedback activation can theoretically reduce GFR, and increased tubular hydrostatic pressures might cause compression of surrounding microvasculatures, leading to a decrease in GFR. [42] In an in vitro cell model, apoptosis (presenting as DNA fragmentation) was found to increase in cells exposed to hyperosmolar contrast media, with the degree of fragmentation proportional to the osmolality of contrast media. [79] Consequently, contrast medium possesses direct tubulotoxicity not only through the induction of oxidative stress and cellular injury, but also through the hyperosmolality it carries. It would be interesting to speculate whether the available isosmotic contrast media can reduce the renal abnormality displayed by exposure to their high osmolar and low osmolar counterparts, but there seems to be no difference. [80] A plausible reason is that isosmolar contrast medium still has increased viscosity and might cause more tubular cell vacuolization and cessation of renal microcirculation. [81]

5. Risk prediction and modeling

Many research groups have strived to devise predictive models for patients with high risk of developing contrast-induced AKI. Mehran and colleagues developed a simple scoring method that integrates 8 baseline clinical variables to evaluate the risk of CIN after PCI. These variables include advanced age (defined as age > 75), hypotension, CHF, anemia, DM, CKD (defined as sCr > 1.5 mg/dL), use of IABP and procedural factors (volume of contrast medium), each with different score. [15] Risk categories are divided into low, moderate, high, and very high. They found that the incidence of contrast-induced AKI ranges from 7.5% in the low risk category, to 57.3% in the very high risk category. Bartholomew and coworkers, in another large cohort of post-PCI CIN patients, derived a risk scoring scheme composed of DM, CHF, hypertension, peripheral vascular disease, IABP uses, CKD (defined as creatinine clearance < 60 ml/min), and procedural factors (urgent or emergency procedures, contrast volume ≧260ml). [13] Incidence of CIN ranged from 0.5% in the lowest risk category, to 43% in the highest risk category. These studies did prove that the risk factors identified previously are mutually additive, and the risk of contrast-induced AKI increases prominently as risk factors accumulate. However, none of the reported studies have been prospectively applied to different populations, and the utility in real-world is still in question. It is currently inappropriate to recommend the routine use of these models in risk stratification of specific population [2], but we should bear in mind that the more risk factors our patients possess, the higher risk he/she might develop AKI after receiving PCI.

6. Strategies of prevention for contrast-induced AKI

6.1. Modification of risk factors

Some of the patients' baseline comorbidities cannot be changed (eg. DM, CHF, etc.), but others are potentially modifiable to reduce the risk of developing CIN. First, the selection of the patients for PCI can be important. Patients with unstable hemodynamic status or circulatory collapse are at high-risk of developing contrast-induced AKI, and and the risk/benefit ratio needs to be carefully weighed for these patients. [42] The clinical need for PCI should be scrutinized, and the in-charge cardiologist or hospitalist should consider whether another procedure without the use of iodinated contrast media can act as a substitute. [59] Nonetheless, in the setting of emergency procedures (like primary PCI), where the benefit of very early intervention outweighs the risk of waiting for the results of the blood test, it is still necessary to proceed without available sCr. [2] When possible, it is still desirable to obtain a pre-procedural blood sample for sCr, since the likelihood of impaired renal function pre-procedurally can increase the subsequent risk of developing CIN and other adverse events. Second, patients with DM, HTN, CHF or potentially changing renal function should receive a pre-procedural baseline renal function testing (if they have not received one before), and if possible, a nephrology/radiology specialist consultation could be obtained. [2] Hyperglycemic status should be properly managed before procedure. Agents such as NSAIDs, diuretics (if feasible), and possibly ACEIs should be discontinued 1-2 days before administration of contrast media. [42] Finally, if PCI or diagnostic coronary angiography is warranted, the amount of contrast medium volume should be as little as possible, and the choice of contrast medium should be iso-osmolar or low osmolar agents, especially in patients with high risk. [2, 8, 14, 42] Repeated exposure should be delayed for 48 hours in patients at-risk of developing contrast-induced AKI, and an even longer delay if patients are diabetic or have pre-existing CKD. [42] Ideally, the interval between procedures should be 2 weeks, the expected recovery time for kidney after an acute insult, but frequently this is not possible, especially in patients with AMI and complicating courses. [19] In this situation, the interval should still be as long as clinically acceptable.

6.2. Volume expansion

There is broad consensus that volume expansion (through isotonic saline hydration) is capable of reducing the risk of contrast-induced nephropathy. The putative benefit of adequate volume expansion includes improving renal blood flow, inducing diuresis with dilution of contrast medium within renal tubules, suppression of the renin-angiotensin-aldosterone system, lowering the secretion of arginine vasopressin, and less reductions in the renal production of endogenous vasodilators (nitric oxide, prostaglandin). [82] However, firm evidence regarding the benefit of volume expansion is not available and not expected to exist, since randomized, double-blinded trials comparing hydration and a control group without hydration cannot be perfomed for lack of ethical acceptability.

6.2.1. Route of volume expansion

The route of volume expansion has been debated. Earlier expert group consensus suggested that intravenous hydration is more favorable than oral hydration [18], but clinical evidence seemed conflicting. Trivedi and coworkers prospectively evaluated the efficacy of unrestricted oral fluids or intravenous normal saline for 24 hours (at a rate of 1ml/kg/hr, 12 hours before and 12 hours after procedures) in a small group of elective PCI patients. [83] Contrast-induced AKI occurred significantly less frequently in the intravenous hydration group than the oral fluid group (3.7% vs. 34.6%). Dussol et al perfomed another study comparing intravenous normal saline (at a rate of 15 ml/kg for 6 hours before procedure) to oral salt tablet (1g/10kg body weight for 2 days before procedure) in a moderately-sized cohort receiving various radiologic studies. [84] Oral salt supplement was found to be as effective as intravenous saline hydration for the prevention of contrast-induced AKI. However, the pre-procedural fasting policy routinely instituted in some groups might make oral salt tabley not feasible. Nonetheless, most groups currently use intravenous hydration for volume expansion purposes in clinical practice.

6.2.2. Formula of hydration

Currently the most popular and effective solution for preventing CIN is isotonic saline (0.9%). Earlier studies comparing saline and other solutions including mannitol or mannitol with furosemide have demonstrated the superiority of saline infusion. [85, 86] The strategy of forced diuresis is also not favored by existing evidence. In the PRINCE study (Prevention of Radiocontrast Induced Nephropathy Clinical Evaluation), Stevens and coworkers found no benefit from forced diuresis with intravenous crystalloid, furosemide, mannitol or low-dose dopamine therapy, compared with hydration alone in at-risk patients. [86] The lack of benefit of mannitol and furosemide might come from their renal untoward effects, including osmotic diuresis-related increase of renal oxygen consumption, vasoconstrictor effect of mannitol and diuretic-induced hypovolemia. [42] In addition, Mueller et al, in a large group of patients receiving PCI, compared the strategy of siotonic saline (0.9%) infusion to half-isotonic saline infusion (0.45%, + plus 5% glucose) starting one day before procedures. [87] Isotonic hydration is superior to half-isotonic hydration in the efficacy for prevention of contrast-induced AKI.

The issue of sodium bicarbonate for preventing contrast-induced AKI is also controversial. It is suggested that sodium bicarbonate might result in urine alkalinization and reduce the generation of free radical through scavenging reactive oxygen species. [19] Bicarbonate can also increase urine flow, while on the contrary, the large amount of chloride from isotonic saline infusion may lead to constriction of the renal vasculature. [88] Merten and colleagues first performed a pilot study comparing sodium bicarbonate (154 mEq/L in dextrose 5% water at a rate of 3ml/kg/hour) started one hour before procedure and continued for six hours after (at a rate of 1ml/kg/hour), to infusion of sodium chloride at a similar rate. [89] The more favorable effect of sodium bicarbonate prophylaxis inspired multiple follow-up studies focusing on similar issues, with more-or-less similar results. Several metanalysis concluded that sodium bicarbonate is more effective than sodium chloride in protecting against CIN, but the heterogeneity of included studies exist, with even publication bias in some studies. [88, 90] Besides, the lower risk of contrast-induced AKI does not seem to translate into lower mortality or less need for dialytic support. [91] The potential risk of al kalemia induced by sodium bicarbonate infusion in patients with CHF and electrolyte disturbance (hypocalcemia, hypokalemia) is another concern. Nonetheless, based upon existing evidence, sodium bicarbonate serves as an equal or even better choice for prevention of contrast-induced AKI, compared with sodium chloride. [19]

6.2.3. *Amount and rate of volume expansion*

There is currently no clear evidence for the optimal rate and duration of volume expansion. Correlation with patients' body weight seems reasonable, and expert consensus agrees that 1.0-1.5 ml/kg/hour of infusion is appropriate. [19] However, there are clinical trials comparing overnight hydration before elective procedures to bolus hydration immediately before the procedures, and continuous hydration seems to provide better protection. [92] It is recommended now that intravenous hydration should start 12 hours before PCI or coronary angiography and continue for 12 hours after, at a rate provided above. [19]

6.3. Pharmacological prophylaxis

Other than intravenous hydration, pharmacologic prophylaxis for at-risk patients against CIN has been tested with multiple drugs, but currently no single agent is approved specifically for this purpose. [19] Several candidate drugs have been attempted, with conflicting results. We will briefly review these drugs in the following section.

6.3.1. *N-acetylcysteine (NAC)*

NAC has been the center of investigation during the last decade. It possesses antioxidant and potentially vasodilatory properties. [8] Usually NAC is given orally but intravenous formula is also available, and owing to its low price, the availability is also high. NAC has minimal side effects and is generally considered safe. The most common protocol of NAC is to give this agent orally 600mg twice a day for 24 hours on the day before and the day of procedure. [19]

More than 30 randomized controlled trials have been performed regarding the efficacy of NAC for preventing contrast-induced AKI, and most studies involve patients receiving PCI or diagnostic coronary angiography. The results are conflicting, with some displaying lower incidence of CIN, while others demonstrating no significant benefit. [93-95] Some researchers proposed that higher dose NAC might be more effective than standard dose NAC [96], but we should remind ourselves that intravenous NAC at higher doses might be associated with significant side effects (hypotension, bronchospasm, etc.) Meta-analysis of existing studies also display conflicting results, depending on the studies included. [97-99] However, most studies are under-powered, and the beneficial effect of NAC is mostly deducted by earlier studies, with small size and lower quality. [19] Furthermore, there have been observations that NAC might lower sCr without affecting GFR, devoid of benefit to renal function. [100] In conclusion, the benefit of NAC in preventing contrast-induced AKI remains unproven, and the use of NAC should be carefully weighed against the potential side effects listed above.

6.3.2. Fenoldopam

Fenoldopam mesylate is a selective dopamine-1 receptor agonist that produces systemic and renal artery vasodilatation. [42] It is found to exhibit desirable renal effects including decrease in renal vascular resistance and increase in renal blood flow, GFR, with natriuresis. Small-group studies have identified potential benefit of fenoldopam with normal saline in the amelioration of renal blood flow reduction caused by contrast media, but this is not validated in a subsequent large, multicenter, double-blind randomized placebo-controlled trial. [101] It is also found to perform inferiorly to NAC in several controlled trials. [102] Currently, the routine use of fenoldopam to protect against contrast-induced AKI could not be recommended.

6.3.3. Theophylline

Theophylline, through cyclic AMP generation, is found to relieve the renal vasoconstrictive reponse to contrast media injection potentially mediated by adenosine in animal models. [103] Multiple investigators have evaluated the competitive adenosine antagonists, theophylline and aminophylline as candidate agents for reducing the risk of CIN. A meta-analysis concluded that prophylactive theophylline use appears to protect against contrast-induced AKI, but the included trials are few, and publication bias is likely. [103] There are also studies suggesting the superiority of theophylline over NAC. [104] Further evaluation is needed in this regrad. Significant side effect resulting from use of theophylline is rarely observed during short-term use and if serum concentration being kept low.

6.3.4. Ascorbic acid

Ascorbic acid is a potent, water-soluble antioxidant capable of scavening reactive oxygen species that potentially introduces damage to vital macromolecules. Ascorbic acid has been shown to attenuate renal damage from various types of insult, including post-ischemic stress, cisplatin-related and aminoglycoside-related injury in animal models. [105] It also possesses extensive safety record as a harmless dietary supplement. Randomized controlled trials utilizing oral ascorbic acid as a prophylactive strategy for reducing CIN have been performed, and the results appear to be positive. [106] Boscheri et al, in a small cohort, failed to display benefit of ascorbid acid. [107] In this sense, definite conclusion also can not be made at this time, owing similarly to low case numbers and somewhat flawed study design.

6.3.5. *Statin*

Statin, also hydroxymethylglutaryl coenzymeA reductase (HMG-CoA) inhibitor, improves the lipid profiles of patients, and has reportedly pleiotropic effects on vasculature, including decreasing low-density lipoprotein (LDL), lipid peroxidation, improving inflammation, lowering risk of cellular necrosis and elevated collagen content in human plaques. [108] Statin therapy significantly reduces cardiovascular mortality and morbidity in patients with hyperlipidemia, and post-procedural statin also is shown to reduce cardiovascular events in patients receiving PCI. [109] Although the exact mechanism by which statin reduces iodinated contrast media-induced AKI is still unclear, it is likely that one of the anti-oxidation, anti-inflammatory, and anti-thrombotic effects can be the principle reason. [110] In a large group of PCI patients, statin use was found to reduce incidence of CIN (OR 0.87). [110] Patti et al further demonstrated that pre-procedural statin use not only prevents against contrast-induced AKI but also leads to a better long-term survival after 4 years of follow-up. [111] Several recent meta-analyses yielded conflicting results, and some researchers proposed that statin might be helpful mostly in patients with more advanced CKD. [112, 113] Thus, it remains unknown whether statins is beneficial for preventing contrast-induced AKI at present, and further clinical trials are awaited to determine the specific group of patients that acquire the most benefit from statin use.

6.3.6. *Iloprost*

Iloprost is a stable prostaglandin I2 (prostacyclin) analogue, which exerts renal vasodilatory effect and has been shown to protect animal kidneys against ischemic and toxic insults. [114] Development of contrast-induced AKI might partially originate from attenuation of the renal prostacylin response, and thus iloprost is theoretically beneficial for the prevention of CIN. Spargias and coworkers first conducted a pilot study on iloprost, with a regimen of 1-2 ng/kg/min infusion from 30-90 minutes before procedures and continuing until 4 hours after procedures, for prevention of CIN. [115] The result was promising. Subsequent larger confirmatory trials yielded similarly positive findings. [116] However, these results were all produced by a single group, and other researchers have not been able to replicate their findings. The other drawbacks of iloprost are its tolerability issues. [116] Further studies are needed to affirm the role of iloprost in our armamentarium against contrast-induced AKI.

6.3.7. *Miscellaneous*

There is limited evidence regarding low-dose dopamine, calcium channel blockers, atrial natriuretic peptides, L-arginine, endothelin antagonists in their roles in the prevention of contrast-induced nephropathy. [19]

http://dx.doi.org/10.5772/54081

7. Conclusion

Contrast-induced AKI, or contrast-induced nephropathy, is a growing issue in the contemporary field of intervention cardiology and also in fields like diagnostic radiology. Although the definitions of contrast-induced AKI are still changing with the advancement of new biomarkers reflecting renal function and injury, the most popular and cost-effective method is still serum creatinine. As the understanding of the pathogenesis of CIN also progresses, more and more strategies for prevention of contrast-induced AKI are being developed and tested clinically. It will be vital for primary care physicians and cardiologists to carefully select their patients as candidates of contrast medium containing procedures, knowledgeably stratify the risk, and implicate evidence-based prophylactic means to reduce the incidence of contrast-induced AKI.

Author details

Chia-Ter Chao, Vin-Cent Wu and Yen-Hung Lin*

*Address all correspondence to: austinr3@yahoo.com.tw

Division of Cardiology, Departments of Internal Medicine, National Taiwan University Hospital and National Taiwan University College of Medicine, Taipei, Taiwan

References

[1] Riley RF, Don CW, Powell W, Maynard C, Dean LS. Trends in Coronary Revascularization in the United States From 2001 to 2009. Circulation: Cardiovascular Quality and Outcomes 2011; 4:193-197.

[2] McCullough PA. Contrast-Induced Acute Kidney Injury. Journal of the American College of Cardiology 2008; 51:1419-1428.

[3] Weisbord SD, Mor MK, Resnick AL, Hartwig KC, Palevsky PM, Fine MJ. Incidence and Outcomes of Contrast-Induced AKI Following Computed Tomography. Clinical Journal of the American Society of Nephrology 2008; 3:1274-1281.

[4] Nash K, Hafeez A, Hou S. Hospital-acquired renal insufficiency. American Journal of Kidney Diseases 2002; 39:930-936.

[5] Lindsay J, Apple S, Pinnow EE, et al. Percutaneous coronary intervention-associated nephropathy foreshadows increased risk of late adverse events in patients with normal baseline serum creatinine. Catheterization and Cardiovascular Interventions 2003; 59:338-343.

[6] Dangas G, Iakovou I, Nikolsky E, et al. Contrast-Induced nephropathy after percutaneous coronary interventions in relation to chronic kidney disease and hemodynamic variables. The American Journal of Cardiology 2005; 95:13-19.

[7] Marenzi G, Lauri G, Assanelli E, et al. Contrast-induced nephropathy in patients undergoing primary angioplasty for acute myocardial infarction. Journal of the American College of Cardiology 2004; 44:1780-1785.

[8] Barrett BJ. Contrast nephrotoxicity. Journal of the American Society of Nephrology 1994; 5:125-137.

[9] McCullough Md MPHPA, Wolyn Md R, Rocher Md LL, Levin Md RN, O'Neill Md WW. Acute Renal Failure After Coronary Intervention: Incidence, Risk Factors, and Relationship to Mortality. The American Journal of Medicine 1997; 103:368-375.

[10] Weisbord SD, Chen H, Stone RA, et al. Associations of Increases in Serum Creatinine with Mortality and Length of Hospital Stay after Coronary Angiography. Journal of the American Society of Nephrology 2006; 17:2871-2877.

[11] Subramanian S, Tumlin J, Bapat B, Zyczynski T. Economic burden of contrast-induced nephropathy: implications for prevention strategies. Journal of Medical Economics 2007; 10:119-134.

[12] VanZEE BE, Hoy WE, Talley TE, Jaenike JR. Renal Injury Associated with Intravenous Pyelography in Nondiabetic and Diabetic Patients. Annals of Internal Medicine 1978; 89:51-54.

[13] Bartholomew BA, Harjai KJ, Dukkipati S, et al. Impact of nephropathy after percutaneous coronary intervention and a method for risk stratification. The American Journal of Cardiology 2004; 93:1515-1519.

[14] Solomon R, Dauerman HL. Contrast-Induced Acute Kidney Injury. Circulation 2010; 122:2451-2455.

[15] Mehran R, Aymong ED, Nikolsky E, et al. A simple risk score for prediction of contrast-induced nephropathy after percutaneous coronary intervention: Development and initial validation. Journal of the American College of Cardiology 2004; 44:1393-1399.

[16] Maioli M, Toso A, Leoncini M, Micheletti C, Bellandi F. Effects of Hydration in Contrast-Induced Acute Kidney Injury After Primary Angioplasty. Circulation: Cardiovascular Interventions 2011; 4:456-462.

[17] Guttterez NV, Diaz A, Timmis GC, et al. Determinants of Serum Creatinine Trajectory in Acute Contrast Nephropathy. Journal of Interventional Cardiology 2002; 15:349-354.

[18] Morcos SK, Thomsen HS, Webb JAW, members of the Contrast Media Safety Committee of the European Society of Urogenital R. Contrast-media-induced nephrotoxicity: a consensus report. European Radiology 1999; 9:1602-1613.

[19] Stacul F, van der Molen A, Reimer P, et al. Contrast induced nephropathy: updated ESUR Contrast Media Safety Committee guidelines. European Radiology 2011; 21:2527-2541.

[20] Kwon SH, Hyun J, Jeon JS, Noh H, Han DC. Subtle change of cystatin C, with or without acute kidney injury, associated with increased mortality in the intensive care unit. Journal of Critical Care 2011; 26:566-571.

[21] Cruz D, Ricci Z, Ronco C. Clinical review: RIFLE and AKIN - time for reappraisal. Critical Care 2009; 13:211.

[22] Molitoris BA, Levin A, Warnock DG, et al. Improving outcomes of acute kidney injury: report of an initiative. Nat Clin Pract Neph 2007; 3:439-442.

[23] Jacobsson B, Lignelid H, Bergerheim USR. Transthyretin and cystatin C are catabolized in proximal tubular epithelial cells and the proteins are not useful as markers for renal cell carcinomas. Histopathology 1995; 26:559-564.

[24] Inker LA, Okparavero A. Cystatin C as a marker of glomerular filtration rate: prospects and limitations. Current Opinion in Nephrology and Hypertension 2011; 20:631-639 610.1097/MNH.1090b1013e32834b38850.

[25] Takeuchi T, Isobe S, Sato K, et al. Cystatin C: A Possible Sensitive Marker for Detecting Potential Kidney Injury After Computed Tomography Coronary Angiography. Journal of Computer Assisted Tomography 2011; 35:240-245 210.1097/RCT.1090b1013e31820a39465.

[26] Ribichini F, Gambaro G, Graziani MS, et al. Comparison of Serum Creatinine and Cystatin C for Early Diagnosis of Contrast-Induced Nephropathy after Coronary Angiography and Interventions. Clinical Chemistry 2012; 58:458-464.

[27] Bolignano D, Coppolino G, Lacquaniti A, Buemi M. From kidney to cardiovascular diseases: NGAL as a biomarker beyond the confines of nephrology. European Journal of Clinical Investigation 2010; 40:273-276.

[28] Chen T-H, Chang C-H, Lin C-Y, et al. Acute Kidney Injury Biomarkers for Patients in a Coronary Care Unit: A Prospective Cohort Study. PLoS ONE 2012; 7:e32328.

[29] Haase M, Bellomo R, Devarajan P, Schlattmann P, Haase-Fielitz A. Accuracy of Neutrophil Gelatinase-Associated Lipocalin (NGAL) in Diagnosis and Prognosis in Acute Kidney Injury: A Systematic Review and Meta-analysis. American Journal of Kidney Diseases 2009; 54:1012-1024.

[30] Mishra J, Dent C, Tarabishi R, et al. Neutrophil gelatinase-associated lipocalin (NGAL) as a biomarker for acute renal injury after cardiac surgery. The Lancet 2005; 365:1231-1238.

[31] Hirsch R, Dent C, Pfriem H, et al. NGAL is an early predictive biomarker of contrast-induced nephropathy in children. Pediatric Nephrology 2007; 22:2089-2095.

[32] Schilcher G, Ribitsch W, Otto R, et al. Early detection and intervention using neutrophil gelatinase-associated lipocalin (NGAL) may improve renal outcome of acute contrast media induced nephropathy: A randomized controlled trial in patients undergoing intra-arterial angiography (ANTI-CIN Study). BMC Nephrology 2011; 12:39.

[33] Malyszko J. Biomarkers of Acute Kidney Injury in Different Clinical Settings: A Time to Change the Paradigm? Kidney and Blood Pressure Research 2010; 33:368-382.

[34] Erselcan T, Egilmez H, Hasbek Z, Tandogan I. Contrast-induced nephropathy: controlled study by differential GFR measurement in hospitalized patients. Acta Radiologica 2012; 53:228-232.

[35] Rihal CS, Textor SC, Grill DE, et al. Incidence and Prognostic Importance of Acute Renal Failure After Percutaneous Coronary Intervention. Circulation 2002; 105:2259-2264.

[36] Deedwania P, Kosiborod M, Barrett E, et al. Hyperglycemia and Acute Coronary Syndrome. Circulation 2008; 117:1610-1619.

[37] Zaytseva NV, Shamkhalova MS, Shestakova MV, et al. Contrast-induced nephropathy in patients with type 2 diabetes during coronary angiography: Risk-factors and prognostic value. Diabetes Research and Clinical Practice 2009; 86, Supplement 1:S63-S69.

[38] Hoste E, Doom S, De Waele J, et al. Epidemiology of contrast-associated acute kidney injury in ICU patients: a retrospective cohort analysis. Intensive Care Medicine 2011; 37:1921-1931.

[39] Stolker JM, McCullough PA, Rao S, et al. Pre-Procedural Glucose Levels and the Risk for Contrast-Induced Acute Kidney Injury in Patients Undergoing Coronary Angiography. Journal of the American College of Cardiology 2010; 55:1433-1440.

[40] Anderson S, Eldadah B, Halter JB, et al. Acute Kidney Injury in Older Adults. Journal of the American Society of Nephrology 2011; 22:28-38.

[41] Parfrey PS, Griffiths SM, Barrett BJ, et al. Contrast Material-Induced Renal Failure in Patients with Diabetes Mellitus, Renal Insufficiency, or Both. New England Journal of Medicine 1989; 320:143-149.

[42] Goldenberg I, Matetzky S. Nephropathy induced by contrast media: pathogenesis, risk factors and preventive strategies. Canadian Medical Association Journal 2005; 172:1461-1471.

[43] Glassock RJ, Winearls C. The Global Burden of Chronic Kidney Disease: How Valid Are the Estimates? Nephron Clinical Practice 2008; 110:c39-c47.

[44] Hudson JQ, Nyman HA. Use of estimated glomerular filtration rate for drug dosing in the chronic kidney disease patient. Current Opinion in Nephrology and Hypertension 2011; 20:482-491 410.1097/MNH.1090b1013e328348c328311f.

[45] Levey AS, Stevens LA, Schmid CH, et al. A New Equation to Estimate Glomerular Filtration Rate. Annals of Internal Medicine 2009; 150:604-612.

[46] Delanaye P, Cohen EP. Formula-Based Estimates of the GFR: Equations Variable and Uncertain. Nephron Clinical Practice 2008; 110:c48-c54.

[47] McCullough PA, Soman SS. Contrast-Induced Nephropathy. Critical care clinics 2005; 21:261-280.

[48] Gruberg L, Mehran R, Dangas G, et al. Acute renal failure requiring dialysis after percutaneous coronary interventions. Catheterization and Cardiovascular Interventions 2001; 52:409-416.

[49] Nikolsky E, Mehran R, Lasic Z, et al. Low hematocrit predicts contrast-induced nephropathy after percutaneous coronary interventions. Kidney Int 2005; 67:706-713.

[50] Krumlovsky FA, Simon N, Santhanam S, del Greco F, Roxe D, Pomaranc MM. Acute Renal Failure: Association with administration of radiographic contrast material. JAMA: The Journal of the American Medical Association 1978; 239:125-127.

[51] McCullough PA, Adam A, Becker CR, et al. Risk Prediction of Contrast-Induced Nephropathy. The American Journal of Cardiology 2006; 98:27-36.

[52] Umruddin Z, Moe K, Superdock K. ACE inhibitor or angiotensin II blocker use is a risk factor for contrast-induced nephropathy. Journal of Nephrology 2012:DOI 10.5301/jn.5000059.

[53] Thomsen H, Morcos S. Risk of contrast-medium-induced nephropathy in high-risk patients undergoing MDCT – A pooled analysis of two randomized trials. European Radiology 2009; 19:891-897.

[54] Gislason GH, Jacobsen S, Rasmussen JN, et al. Risk of Death or Reinfarction Associated With the Use of Selective Cyclooxygenase-2 Inhibitors and Nonselective Nonsteroidal Antiinflammatory Drugs After Acute Myocardial Infarction. Circulation 2006; 113:2906-2913.

[55] Diogo LP, Saitovitch D, Biehl M, et al. Há uma associação entre anti-inflamatórios não-esteroides e nefropatia induzida por contraste? Arquivos Brasileiros de Cardiologia 2010; 95:726-731.

[56] Kitajima K, Maeda T, Watanabe S, Sugimura K. Recent issues in contrast-induced nephropathy. International Journal of Urology 2011; 18:686-690.

[57] Liu Y, Tan N, Zhou Y-L, Chen Y-Y, Chen J, Luo J-F. High-sensitivity C-reactive protein predicts contrast-induced nephropathy after primary percutaneous coronary intervention. J Nephrol 2011:DOI 10.5301/jn.5000007.

[58] McCarthy CS, Becker JA. Multiple myeloma and contrast media. Radiology 1992; 183:519-521.

[59] Preda L, Agazzi A, Raimondi S, et al. Effect on renal function of an iso-osmolar contrast agent in patients with monoclonal gammopathies. European Radiology 2011; 21:63-69.

[60] Barrett BJ, Carlisle EJ. Metaanalysis of the relative nephrotoxicity of high- and low-osmolality iodinated contrast media. Radiology 1993; 188:171-178.

[61] Aspelin P, Aubry P, Fransson S-G, Strasser R, Willenbrock R, Berg KJ. Nephrotoxic Effects in High-Risk Patients Undergoing Angiography. New England Journal of Medicine 2003; 348:491-499.

[62] Chalmers N, Jackson RW. Comparison of iodixanol and iohexol in renal impairment. British Journal of Radiology 1999; 72:701-703.

[63] McCullough PA, Bertrand ME, Brinker JA, Stacul F. A Meta-Analysis of the Renal Safety of Isosmolar Iodixanol Compared With Low-Osmolar Contrast Media. Journal of the American College of Cardiology 2006; 48:692-699.

[64] Solomon R. The role of osmolality in the incidence of contrast-induced nephropathy: A systematic review of angiographic contrast media in high risk patients. Kidney Int 2005; 68:2256-2263.

[65] Barrett BJ, Katzberg RW, Thomsen HS, et al. Contrast-Induced Nephropathy in Patients With Chronic Kidney Disease Undergoing Computed Tomography: A Double-Blind Comparison of Iodixanol and Iopamidol. Investigative Radiology 2006; 41:815-821 810.1097/1001.rli.0000242807.0000201818.0000242824.

[66] Solomon RJ, Natarajan MK, Doucet S, et al. Cardiac Angiography in Renally Impaired Patients (CARE) Study. Circulation 2007; 115:3189-3196.

[67] Anderson JL, Adams CD, Antman EM, et al. ACC/AHA 2007 Guidelines for the Management of Patients With Unstable Angina/Non–ST-Elevation Myocardial Infarction: A Report of the American College of Cardiology/American Heart Association Task Force on Practice Guidelines (Writing Committee to Revise the 2002 Guidelines for the Management of Patients With Unstable Angina/Non–ST-Elevation Myocardial Infarction) Developed in Collaboration with the American College of Emergency Physicians, the Society for Cardiovascular Angiography and Interventions, and the Society of Thoracic Surgeons Endorsed by the American Association of Cardiovascular and Pulmonary Rehabilitation and the Society for Academic Emergency Medicine. Journal of the American College of Cardiology 2007; 50:e1-e157.

[68] Manske CL, Sprafka JM, Strony JT, Wang Y. Contrast nephropathy in azotemic diabetic patients undergoing coronary angiography. The American Journal of Medicine 1990; 89:615-620.

[69] Cigarroa RG, Lange RA, Williams RH, Hillis D. Dosing of contrast material to prevent contrast nephropathy in patients with renal disease. The American Journal of Medicine 1989; 86:649-652.

[70] Moore RD, Steinberg EP, Powe NR, et al. Nephrotoxicity of high-osmolality versus low-osmolality contrast media: randomized clinical trial. Radiology 1992; 182:649-655.

[71] McCullough PA, Sandberg KR. Epidemiology of contrast-induced nephropathy. Reviews in Cardiovascular Medicine 2003; 4:S3-S9.

[72] Bakris GL, Lass NA, Glock D. Renal hemodynamics in radiocontrast medium-induced renal dysfunction: A role for dopamine-1 receptors. Kidney Int 1999; 56:206-210.

[73] Russo D, Minutolo R, Cianciaruso B, Memoli B, Conte G, De Nicola L. Early effects of contrast media on renal hemodynamics and tubular function in chronic renal failure. Journal of the American Society of Nephrology 1995; 6:1451-1458.

[74] Nygren A, Ulfendahl HR. Effects of high- and low-osmolar contrast media on renal plasma flow and glomerular filtration rate in euvolaemic and dehydrated rats. A comparison between ioxithalamate, iopamidol, iohexol and ioxaglate. Acta Radiologica 1989; 30:383-389.

[75] Liss P, Nygren A, Olsson U, Ulfendahl HR, Erikson U. Effects of contrast media and mannitol on renal medullary blood flow and red cell aggregation in the rat kidney. Kidney Int 1996; 49:1268-1275.

[76] MOREAU J-F, DROZ D, NOEL L-H, LEIBOWITCH J, JUNGERS P, MICHEL J-R. Tubular Nephrotoxicity of Water-soluble Iodinated Contrast Media. Investigative Radiology 1980; 15:S54-S60.

[77] Heyman SN, Brezis M, Epstein FH, Spokes K, Silva P, Rosen S. Early renal medullary hypoxic injury from radiocontrast and indomethacin. Kidney Int 1991; 40:632-642.

[78] Ueda J, Nygren A, Hansell P, Ulfendahl HR. Effect of intravenous contrast media on proximal and distal tubular hydrostatic pressure in the rat kidney. Acta Radiologica 1993; 34:83-87.

[79] Hizóh I, Sträter J, Schick CS, Kübler W, Haller C. Radiocontrast-induced DNA fragmentation of renal tubular cells in vitro: role of hypertonicity. Nephrology Dialysis Transplantation 1998; 13:911-918.

[80] Liss P, Nygren A, Erikson U, Ulfendahl HR. Injection of low and iso-osmolar contrast medium decreases oxygen tension in the renal medulla. Kidney Int 1998; 53:698-702.

[81] Lancelot E, Idée J-M, Laclédère C, Santus R, Corot C. Effects of Two Dimeric Iodinated Contrast Media on Renal Medullary Blood Perfusion and Oxygenation in Dogs. Investigative Radiology 2002; 37:368-375.

[82] Stacul F, Adam A, Becker CR, et al. Strategies to Reduce the Risk of Contrast-Induced Nephropathy. The American Journal of Cardiology 2006; 98:59-77.

[83] Trivedi HS, Moore H, Nasr S, et al. A Randomized Prospective Trial to Assess the Role of Saline Hydration on the Development of Contrast Nephrotoxicity. Nephron Clinical Practice 2003; 93:c29-c34.

[84] Dussol B, Morange S, Loundoun A, Auquier P, Berland Y. A randomized trial of saline hydration to prevent contrast nephropathy in chronic renal failure patients. Nephrology Dialysis Transplantation 2006; 21:2120-2126.

[85] Solomon R, Werner C, Mann D, D'Elia J, Silva P. Effects of Saline, Mannitol, and Furosemide on Acute Decreases in Renal Function Induced by Radiocontrast Agents. New England Journal of Medicine 1994; 331:1416-1420.

[86] Stevens MA, McCullough PA, Tobin KJ, et al. A prospective randomized trial of prevention measures in patients at high risk for contrast nephropathy: Results of the P.R.I.N.C.E. study. Journal of the American College of Cardiology 1999; 33:403-411.

[87] Mueller C, Buerkle G, Buettner HJ, et al. Prevention of Contrast Media-Associated Nephropathy: Randomized Comparison of 2 Hydration Regimens in 1620 Patients Undergoing Coronary Angioplasty. Arch Intern Med 2002; 162:329-336.

[88] Joannidis M, Schmid M, Wiedermann CJ. Prevention of contrast media-induced nephropathy by isotonic sodium bicarbonate: a meta-analysis. Wiener Klinische Wochenschrift 2008; 120:742-748.

[89] Merten GJ, Burgess WP, Gray LV, et al. Prevention of Contrast-Induced Nephropathy With Sodium Bicarbonate. JAMA: The Journal of the American Medical Association 2004; 291:2328-2334.

[90] Brar SS, Hiremath S, Dangas G, Mehran R, Brar SK, Leon MB. Sodium Bicarbonate for the Prevention of Contrast Induced-Acute Kidney Injury: A Systematic Review and Meta-analysis. Clinical Journal of the American Society of Nephrology 2009; 4:1584-1592.

[91] Meier P, Ko D, Tamura A, Tamhane U, Gurm H. Sodium bicarbonate-based hydration prevents contrast-induced nephropathy: a meta-analysis. BMC Medicine 2009; 7:23.

[92] Krasuski RA, Beard BM, Geoghagan JD, Thompson CM, Guidera SA. Optimal timing of hydration to erase contrast-associated nephropathy: the OTHER-CAN study. J Invasive Cardiol 2003; 15:699-702.

[93] Briguori C, Manganelli F, Scarpato P, et al. Acetylcysteine and contrast agent-associated nephrotoxicity. Journal of the American College of Cardiology 2002; 40:298-303.

[94] Marenzi G, Assanelli E, Marana I, et al. N-Acetylcysteine and Contrast-Induced Nephropathy in Primary Angioplasty. New England Journal of Medicine 2006; 354:2773-2782.

[95] Kay J, Chow WH, Chan TM, et al. Acetylcysteine for Prevention of Acute Deterioration of Renal Function Following Elective Coronary Angiography and Intervention. JAMA: The Journal of the American Medical Association 2003; 289:553-558.

[96] Briguori C, Colombo A, Violante A, et al. Standard vs double dose of N-acetylcysteine to prevent contrast agent associated nephrotoxicity. European Heart Journal 2004; 25:206-211.

[97] Kelly AM, Dwamena B, Cronin P, Bernstein SJ, Carlos RC. Meta-analysis: Effectiveness of Drugs for Preventing Contrast-Induced Nephropathy. Annals of Internal Medicine 2008; 148:284-294.

[98] Fishbane S. N-Acetylcysteine in the Prevention of Contrast-Induced Nephropathy. Clinical Journal of the American Society of Nephrology 2008; 3:281-287.

[99] Pannu N, Wiebe N, Tonelli M, Network ftAKD. Prophylaxis Strategies for Contrast-Induced Nephropathy. JAMA: The Journal of the American Medical Association 2006; 295:2765-2779.

[100] Hoffmann U, Fischereder M, Krüger B, Drobnik W, Krämer BK. The Value of N-Acetylcysteine in the Prevention of Radiocontrast Agent-Induced Nephropathy Seems Questionable. Journal of the American Society of Nephrology 2004; 15:407-410.

[101] Stone GW, McCullough PA, Tumlin JA, et al. Fenoldopam Mesylate for the Prevention of Contrast-Induced Nephropathy. JAMA: The Journal of the American Medical Association 2003; 290:2284-2291.

[102] Briguori C, Colombo A, Airoldi F, et al. N-acetylcysteine versus fenoldopam mesylate to prevent contrast agent-associated nephrotoxicity. Journal of the American College of Cardiology 2004; 44:762-765.

[103] Ix JH, McCulloch CE, Chertow GM. Theophylline for the prevention of radiocontrast nephropathy: a meta-analysis. Nephrology Dialysis Transplantation 2004; 19:2747-2753.

[104] Huber W, Eckel F, Hennig M, et al. Prophylaxis of Contrast Material–induced Nephropathy in Patients in Intensive Care: Acetylcysteine, Theophylline, or Both? A Randomized Study1. Radiology 2006; 239:793-804.

[105] Lloberas N, Torras J, Herrero-Fresneda I, et al. Postischemic renal oxidative stress induces inflammatory response through PAF and oxidized phospholipids. Prevention by antioxidant treatment. The FASEB Journal 2002; 16:908-910.

[106] Spargias K, Alexopoulos E, Kyrzopoulos S, et al. Ascorbic Acid Prevents Contrast-Mediated Nephropathy in Patients With Renal Dysfunction Undergoing Coronary Angiography or Intervention. Circulation 2004; 110:2837-2842.

[107] Boscheri A, Weinbrenner C, Botzek B, Reynen K, Kuhlisch E, Strasser RH. Failure of ascorbid acid to prevent contrast-media induced nephropathy in patients with renal dysfunction. Clin Nephrol 2007; 68:279-286.

[108] Crisby M, Nordin-Fredriksson G, Shah PK, Yano J, Zhu J, Nilsson J. Pravastatin Treatment Increases Collagen Content and Decreases Lipid Content, Inflammation, Metalloproteinases, and Cell Death in Human Carotid Plaques : Implications for Plaque Stabilization. Circulation 2001; 103:926-933.

[109] Serruys PWJC, de Feyter P, Macaya C, et al. Fluvastatin for Prevention of Cardiac Events Following Successful First Percutaneous Coronary Intervention. JAMA: The Journal of the American Medical Association 2002; 287:3215-3222.

[110] Khanal S, Attallah N, Smith DE, et al. Statin therapy reduces contrast-induced nephropathy: An analysis of contemporary percutaneous interventions. The American Journal of Medicine 2005; 118:843-849.

[111] Patti G, Nusca A, Chello M, et al. Usefulness of Statin Pretreatment to Prevent Contrast-Induced Nephropathy and to Improve Long-Term Outcome in Patients Undergoing Percutaneous Coronary Intervention. The American Journal of Cardiology 2008; 101:279-285.

[112] Zhou Y, Yuan WJ, Zhu N, Wang L. Short-term, high-dose statins in the prevention of contrast-induced nephropathy: a systematic review and meta-analysis. Clin Nephrol 2011; 76:475-483.

[113] Zhang L, Lu Y, Wu B, et al. Efficacy of statin pretreatment for the prevention of contrast-induced nephropathy: a meta-analysis of randomised controlled trials. International Journal of Clinical Practice 2011; 65:624-630.

[114] Krause W, Muschick P, Krüger U. Use of Near-Infrared Reflection Spectroscopy to Study the Effects of X-Ray Contrast Media on Renal Tolerance in Rats: Effects of a Prostacyclin Analogue and of Phosphodiesterase Inhibitors. Investigative Radiology 2002; 37:698-705.

[115] Spargias K, Adreanides E, Giamouzis G, et al. Iloprost for prevention of contrast-mediated nephropathy in high-risk patients undergoing a coronary procedure. Re-

http://dx.doi.org/10.5772/54081

sults of a randomized pilot study. European Journal of Clinical Pharmacology 2006; 62:589-595.

[116] Spargias K, Adreanides E, Demerouti E, et al. Iloprost Prevents Contrast-Induced Nephropathy in Patients With Renal Dysfunction Undergoing Coronary Angiography or Intervention. Circulation 2009; 120:1793-1799.

Chapter 18

Contrast-Induced Nephropathy: Risk Factors, Clinical Implication, Diagnostics Approach, Prevention

Frantisek Kovar, Milos Knazeje and Marian Mokan

Additional information is available at the end of the chapter

http://dx.doi.org/10.5772/54036

1. Introduction

Contrast induced nephropathy (CIN) is an important and well-known complication in patients with chronic renal insufficiency undergoing both coronary angiography and coronary interventions. The estimated incidence of CN after coronary angiography was around 15%. In fact, CIN is the third leading cause of acute renal failure in hospitalized patients [1]. CIN is usually transient disorder, but in some cases may result in residual permanent renal damage, prolong hospital stay and increase medical cost [2]. Renal failure increases the risk of developing severe nonrenal complications that can lead to death. The mortality rate in subjects without renal failure was 7%, compared with 34% in patients with renal failure [3]. With the increasing number of patients undergoing percutaneous coronary intervention, it is expected that the burden of such iatrogenic complications will exponentially increase and effective preventive measures are necessary.

2. Definition of CIN

Contrast induced nephropathy is an important cause of nosocomial renal impairment. This deleterious effect of contrast agents on renal function is defined as an impairment of renal function with increase in serum creatinine level by more than 25% or 44umol/l occurring within 3 days after intravascular administration of contrast agents and in the absence of alternative cause [4].

3. Incidence and clinical significance of CIN:

The incidence of CIN in the general population has been estimated to be less than 2% [5]. However in high risk patients the incidence can increase to more than 50%. Pre-existing renal impairment and diabetes mellitus have been identified as the main conditions predisposing to the development of CIN. Other risk factors include decreased effective blood volume, age > 75 years, heart failure, use of non-steroid anti-inflammatory drugs, diuretics, previous parenteral contrast medium administration within 72 hours and large volume of contrast medium [6].

During the last two decades the number of computed tomographies has increased by 800% and between 1979 and 2002 the number of percutaneous cardiac interventions in the USA has risen by 390% [7]. As the number of susceptible patients exposed to parenteral iodinated contrast media expands, contrast-induced nephropathy represents an ever-growing clinical problem. Meanwhile, the main predisposing factors for CIN, namely diabetes mellitus and previous renal impairment are currently augmented. CIN represents the third most frequent cause of hospital acquired acute renal failure.

The first reported case of CIN was an acute renal failure following intravenous pyelography with 20 ml of Diodrast in patient with myelomatosis in 1954 year [8].

Renal failure following exposure to radiocontrast agents is usually nonoliguric. Creatinine rises within 48 hours, peaks 4 to 5 days after exposure and returns to baseline in 7 to 10 days. Complete recovery is expected in more than 75% of patients, who develop this complication, but approximately 10% requires dialysis [9]. Introduction of low- and iso-osmolar contrast media has resulted in decreased frequency of contrast-induced nephropathy [10].

Effect and safety of iodixanol, a new generation iso-osmolar contrast medium, even when administered to high-risk patients was assessed in the Nephrotoxicity in High-Risk Patients Study of Iso-Osmolar and Low-Osmolar Non-Ionic Contrast Media (NEPHRIC) study [11]. In this multicenter randomized study were enrolled patients with diabetes mellitus (type 1 or 2) and either a stable serum creatinine concentration (133 to 308 μmol per liter for men and 115 to 308 μmol per liter for women) as measured within three months before enrollment referred for coronary or aortofemoral angiography, had or a calculated creatinine clearance of no more than 60 ml per minute, according to the formula of Cockcroft and Gault. Study was designed to compare the renal effects of a nonionic, iso-osmolar, dimeric contrast medium, iodixanol (320 mg of iodine per milliliter; 290 mOsm per kilogram of water), with nonionic, low-osmolar, monomeric contrast medium iohexol (350 mg of iodine per milliliter; 780 mOsm per kilogram of water). Iodixanol induced a significantly smaller mean increase in the serum creatinine level than did iohexol. The peak increase in the serum creatinine concentration within three days after the administration of contrast medium was 11.2 μmol per liter in the iodixanol group, as compared with 48.2 μmol per liter in the iohexol group (P=0.001). The effect of the base-line serum creatinine concentration was different in the two groups. Among patients who received iohexol, but not among those who received iodixanol, a higher base-line serum creatinine concentration was associated with a higher peak increase between day 0 and day 3 (P for interaction <0.001). Peak increase of serum creatinine level was higher in iohexanol group (Figure 1).

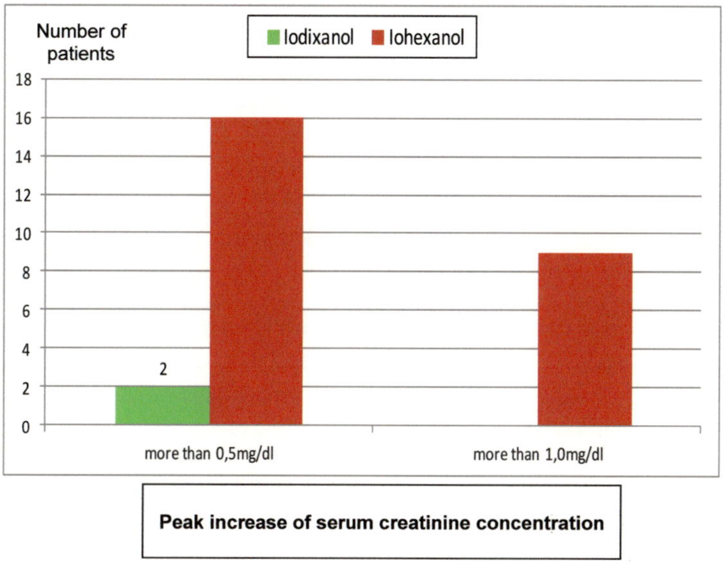

Figure 1. Nephrotoxicity in iodixanol and iohexanol

All seven serious events deemed to be related to contrast medium occurred in the iohexol group; five patients in this group had acute renal failure related to the use of iohexol, and one patient had both acute renal failure and arrhythmia related to the use of iohexol. Three of these six patients recovered, two died, and one had persistent renal failure. [11].

CIN is a significant cause of morbidity and mortality.

Renal failure increases the risk of developing severe nonrenal complications that can lead to death. In analysis of 16 248 patients undergoing radiocontrast procedures, were identified 183 subjects who developed contrast media associated renal failure. These cases were matched for age and baseline serum creatinine level, with 174 paired subjects, who underwent similar contrast procedures but without developing renal failure. The mortality rate in subjects without renal failure was 7%, compared with 34% in patients with renal failure (odds ratio, 6,5; P<0,001). After adjusting for differences in co morbidity, renal failure was associated with an odds ratio of dying of 5,5. Subjects who died after developing renal failure had complicated clinical courses characterized by sepsis, bleeding, delirium, and respiratory failure; most of these complications developed after the onset of renal failure [3].

Likelihood of death increases approximately 8.5-13.5 times in patients with CIN and need for hemodialysis comparing with CIN patients but without hemodialysis [12, 13].

Observation made by Gruber and coworkers confirmed that acute renal failure that requires dialysis after percutaneous coronary interventions is associated with very high in-hospital and 1-year mortality rates and a dramatic increase in hospital resource utilization. They compared clinical course in 51 consecutive patients who were not on dialysis on admission and developed acute renal failure that required in-hospital dialysis after coronary intervention and 7 690 patients who did not require dialysis after PCI. Patients who required dialysis were older, with a higher incidence of hypertension, diabetes, prior bypass surgery, chronic renal failure, and a significantly lower left ventricular ejection fraction. Despite similar angiographic success, these patients had a higher incidence of in-hospital mortality (27.5% vs. 1.0%, $P < 0.0001$), non–Q-wave myocardial infarction (45.7% vs. 14.6%, $P < 0.0001$), vascular and bleeding complications, and longer hospitalization. At 1-year follow-up, mortality (54.5% vs. 6.4%, $P < 0.0001$), myocardial infarction (4.5% vs. 1.6%, $P = 0.006$), and event-free survival (38.6% vs. 72.0%, $P < 0.0001$) were significantly worse in patients who required dialysis compared to patients who did not [12].

Similarly, analysis of 1 826 consecutive patients undergoing coronary intervention from aspect of the incidence, predictors, and mortality related to acute renal failure (ARF) and acute renal failure requiring dialysis (ARFD) after coronary intervention has shown that occurrence of ARFD after coronary intervention is rare (<1%) but is associated with high in-hospital lethality and poor long-term survival. Individual patient risk can be estimated from calculated CrCl, diabetic status, and expected contrast dose prior to a proposed coronary intervention [13]. The incidence of ARF and ARFD was 144,6/1,000 and 7,7/1,000 cases respectively. The cutoff dose of contrast below which there was no ARFD was 100 ml. No patient with a CrCl > 47 ml/min developed ARFD. These thresholds were confirmed in the validation set. Multivariate analysis found CrCl [odds ratio

Variable (%)	CIN (n=254)	**No CIN (n=7332)**	**P-value**
Procedural success	72,8	94,0	< 0,0001
Death	22,0	1,4	< 0,0001
Q-wave myocardial infarction	3,9	0,9	< 0,0001
Creatinine kinase elevation	16,9	6,1	< 0,0001
Shock	13,0	3,1	< 0,0001
Cardiac arrest	11,4	1,5	< 0,0001
Intraaortic balloon pump use	11,4	3,1	< 0,0001
Femoral bleeding	3,1	1,4	0,03
Stroke	1,2	0,03	0,05
Adult respiratory distress syndrome	9,4	0,7	< 0,0001
Gastrointestinal bleeding	4,3	1,2	< 0,0001

CIN = contrast induced nephropathy

Table 1. Procedural complications in patients both with and without CIN after coronary intervention

(OR) = 0.83, 95% confidence interval (CI) 0.77 to 0.89, P <0.00001], diabetes (OR = 5.47, 95% CI 1.40 to 21.32, P = 0.01), and contrast dose (OR = 1.008, 95% CI 1.002 to 1.013, P = 0.01) to be independent predictors of ARFD. The in-hospital mortality for those who developed ARFD was 35,7% and the 2-year survival was 18,8% [13].

Moreover, development of CIN significantly prolongs hospitalization among survive patients and is often associated with increased procedural complications rate (table 1) [2].

4. Contrast agents

All modern contrast agents are based on iodine, because of its high atomic number and chemical versatility has proved to be an excellent agent for intravascular opacification. First reported parenteral application of an iodinated contrast agents was during an intravenous pyelography in 1919. Inorganic sodium iodide cause often toxic reactions. In 1929 was explored an organic iodide preparation with one iodine atom per benzoic acid ring and in 1950s, more substituted tri-iodobenzoic acid derivates were developed (with three iodine atoms per ring). Specific side chains in position 1, 3 and 5 influence both solubility and toxicity.

First generation contrast agents were ionic monomers containing a benzene ring with three iodine atoms, exhibiting high osmolarity in the range of 1500 to 1800 mOsm/kg (high osmolar contrast agents), roughly six times that of blood. This ratio-1,5 ionic compounds are substituted ionic triiodobenzoic acid derivatives that contain three atoms of iodine for every two ions (substituted benzoic acid ring and accompanying cation). To have an iodine concentration of 320 do 370 mg I/ml, as is required for coronary artery angiography, solution of these agents are extremely hypertonic with osmolarity more than 1500 mOsm/kg (Figure 2).

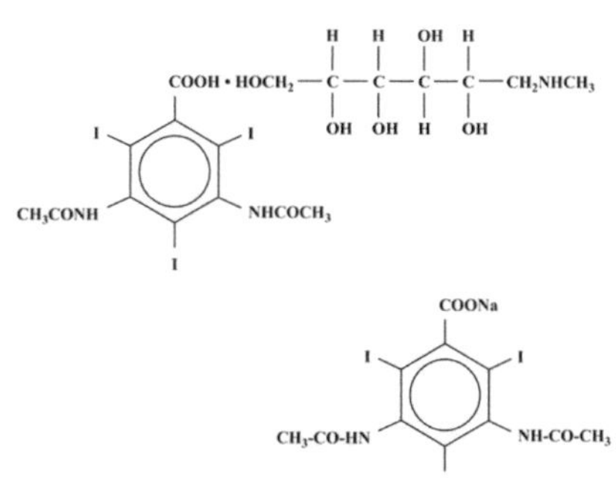

Figure 2. Ionic monomer contrast agent (Diatrizoat)

Ratio-3 lower-osmolarity contrast agents were introduced in 1980s. This contrast ages (ioxaglate) was still ionic with dimeric structure that include six molecules iodine on the dimeric ring (three atoms of iodine per one ion) (Figure 3).

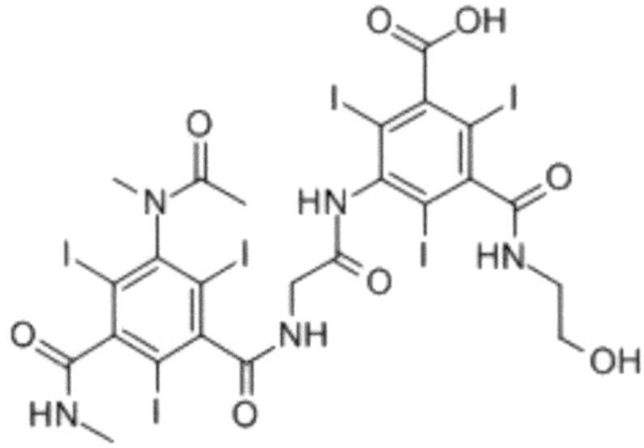

Figure 3. Ionic dimeric contrast agent (Ioxaglate)

The introduction of nonionic ratio-3 contrast agents was very important step in late 1980s. An iodine content of 320 to 370 mg I/ml can be achieved with an osmolarity of 600 to 700 mOsm/kg (between two and three times that of blood) (low osmolar contrast agents). Their viscosity is approximately 6 to 10 times that of water (Figure 4).

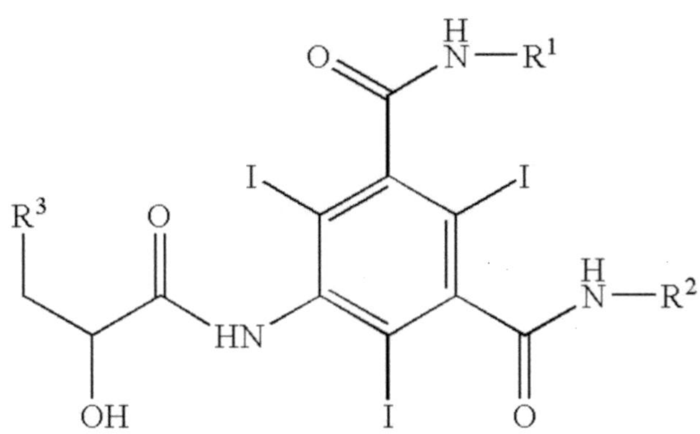

Figure 4. Nonionic monomer contrast agent (iopamidol)

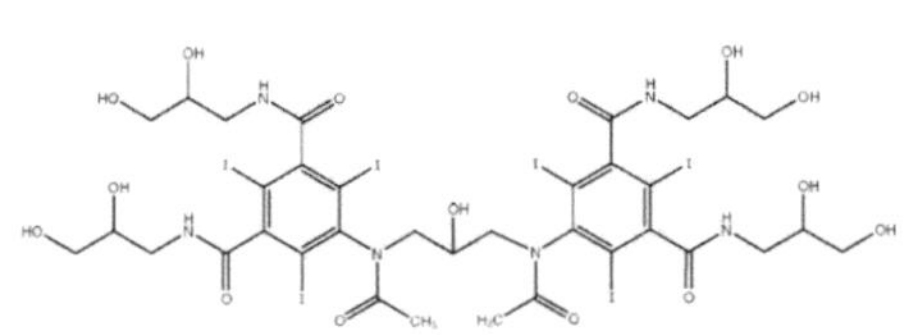

Figure 5. Nonionic dimeric contrast agent (Iodixanol)

Third generation agents are dimmers almost iso-osmolar to plasma (iso-osmolar contrast agents) but with increased viscosity, which results in complicated injection through small vascular catheters. This iso-osmolar contrast agent is a ratio-6 nonionic dimeric compound (iodixanol). There are data suggesting a reduction of nephrotoxicity with this agent [11]. Nevertheless even third generation contrast agents have been implicated by some authors for potential nephrotoxicity [14] (Figure 5).

The osmolarity of a solution is proportional to the number of dissolved particles (ions, molecules). Thus, the osmolarity of contrast agent solution can be decreased by increasing the number of iodine atoms per dissolved particle (Table 2).

COMPOUND	Iodine atoms	Particles	Ratio
Ionic monomers	3	2	1,5
Nonionic monomers	3	1	3,0
Ionic dimmers	6	2	3,0
Nonionic dimmers	6	1	6,0

Table 2. Osmolarity in the four categories of contrast media

In table 3 are summarized properties of current available contrast agents.

CLASS	EXAMPLES	IODINE (mg I/ml)	Osmolarity (mOsm/kg)	Viscosity (at 37°C)
High-osmolar ionic Ratio 1,5 (3:2)	Diatrizoate	370	2076	8,4
	iothalmate	325	1797	2,8
Low-osmolar nonionic Ratio 3 (3:1)	Iopamidol	370	796	9,4
	Iohexol	350	844	10,4
	Ioversol	350	792	9,0
	Ioxilan	350	695	8,1
Low-osmolar ionic dimmer Ratio 3 (6:2)	Ioxaglate	320	600	7,5
Iso-osmolar nonionic dimmer Ratio 6 (6:1)	Iodixanol	320	290	11,8

Table 3. Properties of available contrast agents

5. Patothophysiology of CIN:

The exact pathogenesis of CIN is still unclear. Several injury pathways have been proposed. Important possible pathogenetic mechanisms of CIN involve:

a. a medullar hypoxia due to altered hemodynamics, which in the presence of impaired adaptive responses leads to tubular damage and

b. a direct cytotoxic effect of the contrast agents on tubular cells.

Probably, a combination of various pathophysiologic mechanisms is involved. The contrast agent may have direct cytotoxic effects due to relatively high tissue osmolarity. The contrast medium induces renal vasoconstriction, leading to tubular injury or even necrosis.

It has been shown in experimental animal model that after parenteral administration of contrast media they exhibit short-term renal vasodilatation, which is followed by prolonged vasoconstriction, resulting in a decrease in total renal blood flow and a reduction of glomerular filtration rate [15].

Elevated endothelia levels and other vasoconstrictor levels were detected in patients with CIN. Administration of radiocontrast agents in normal rats induces endothelia release [16]. Subsequent reperfusion injury may increase free radical formation and create oxidative stress. The contrast medium may precipitate with Tamm- Horsfall glycoprotein in distal tubule lumen and form casts [17].

Increased adenosine-induced renal vasoconstriction in combination with attenuated renal NO-dependent vasodilatation, may account for the predisposition of diabetic patients to CIN [18].

There is a relationship between osmolarity and viscosity in monomeric contrast media (Figure 6) [19].

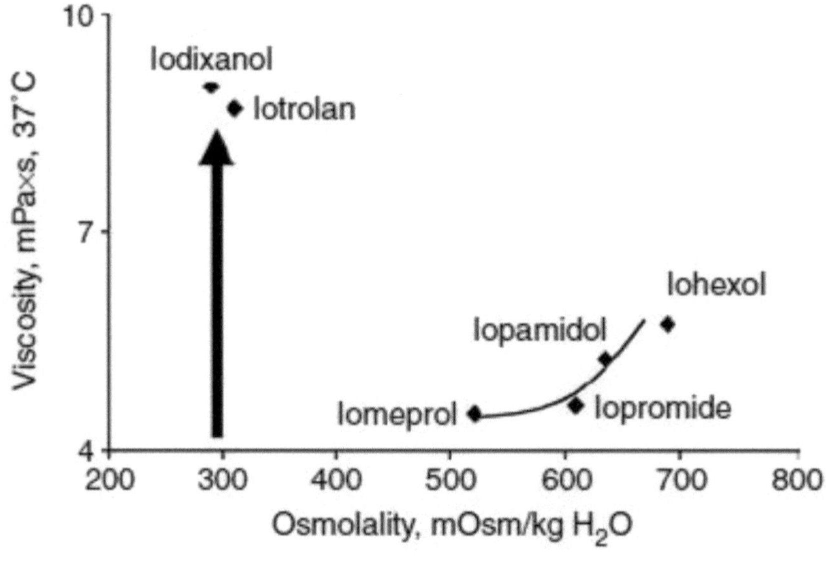

Figure 6. Osmolarity and viscosity for I-concentration of 300 mg/ml

http://dx.doi.org/10.5772/54036

Available izo-osmolar contrast agents exhibit considerably higher viscosity and should impair renal medullar blood flow to a greater extent than low osmolar agents. This situation is indicated by a particularly reduced pO2 levels caused by iso osmolar contrast media in experimental model (Figure 7) [20].

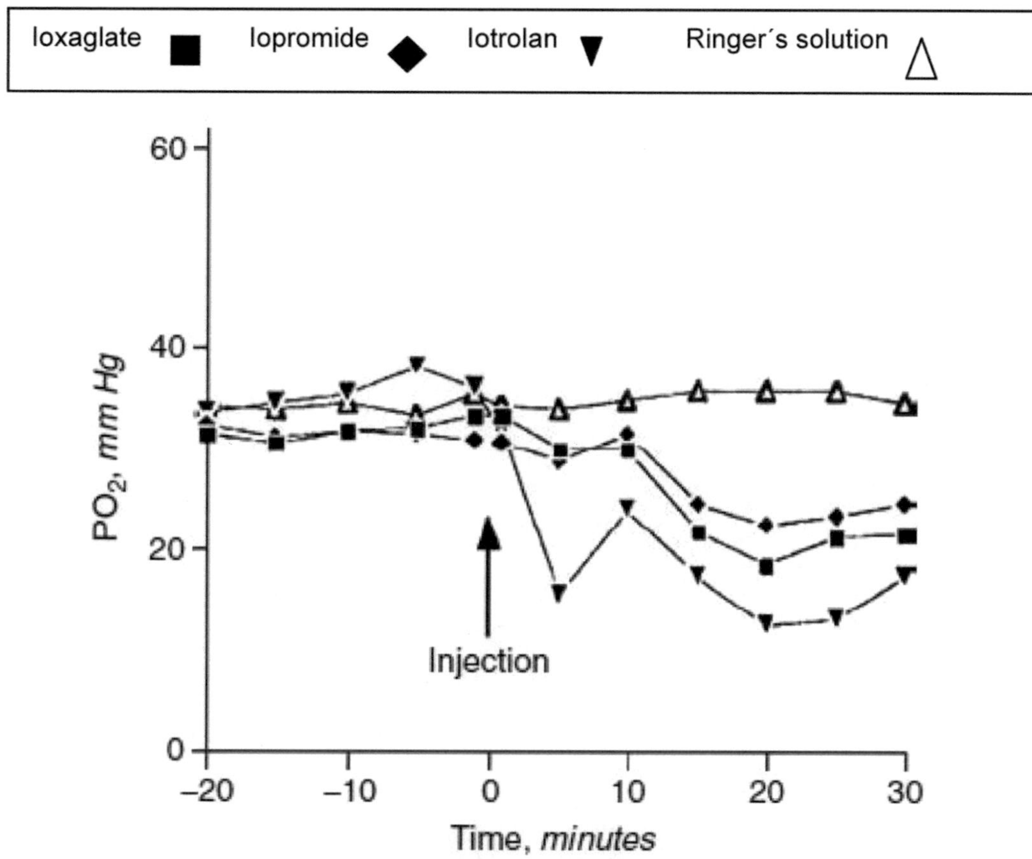

Figure 7. Medullar hypoxia induced by contrast media (ioxaglate, iopromide, and iotrolan in comparison to Ringer's solution).

Reduction of pO2 is greater for iotrolan (iso-osmolar nonionic dimer) followed by ioxaglate (low-osmolar ionic dimer). Iopromide (low-osmolar monomer) had the least effect of the contrast media.

Tubular viscosity will increase markedly toward distal sections of the kidney due to fluid reabsorbtion. When urine becomes very concentrated, tubular fluid viscosity will increase and tubular plugging may occur. Hydration attenuates fluid reabsorbtion in the collecting ducts and is therefore very beneficial [19].

Adverse effects of pronounced increases of viscosity on the kidney are schematically shown in figure 8 [19].

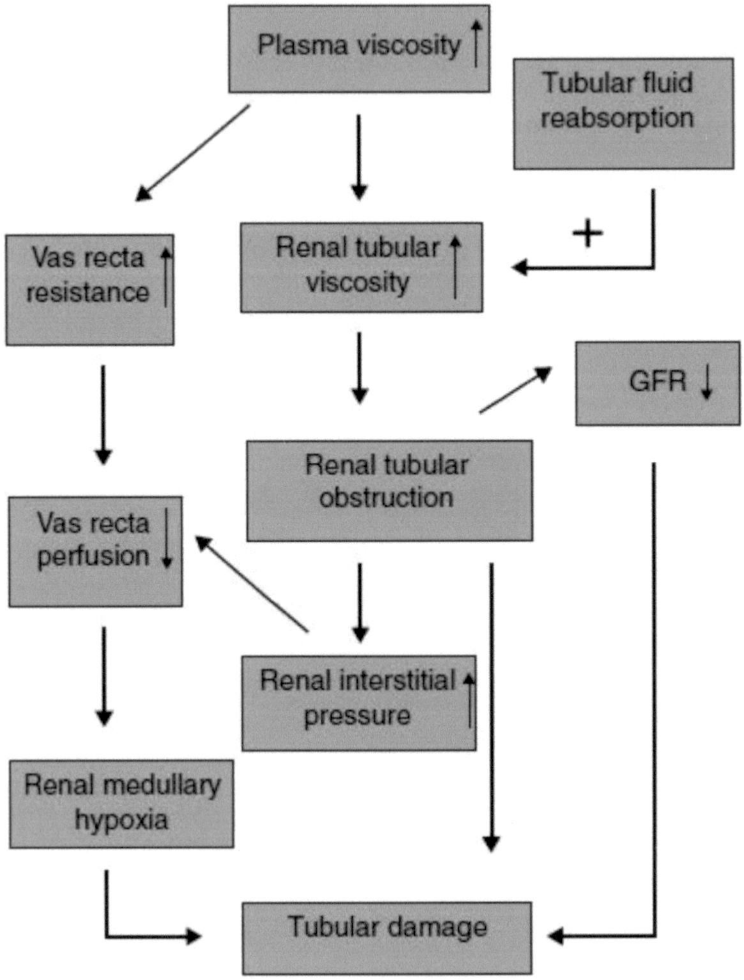

Figure 8. Flow chart of mechanisms linking fluid osmolarity to renal damage, GFR = glomerular filtration rate

As a consequence of contrast media administration, tubular cell damage can occur. Except for vacuolization, there was described pertubation of mitochondrial enzyme activity and mitochondrial membrane potential as a cause of alteration of proximal tubular functions (Figure 9) [21].

Extend of mitochondrial enzyme activity impairment relies primarily on two features of the contrast media: ionicity and the molecular structure. Remarkably, low-osmolar (monomeric) contrast media had the least effect, followed by the iso-osmolar (dimeric, nonionic) agents. Ionic compounds revealed the most profound effects [21].

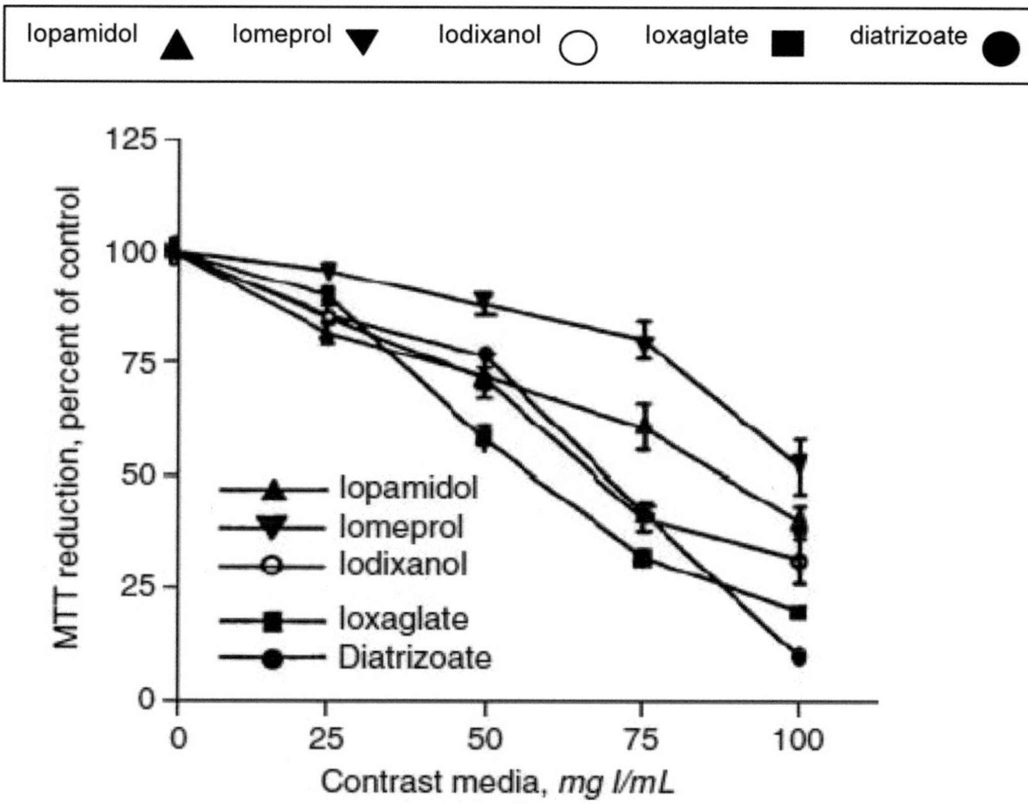

Figure 9. Altered mitochondrial function in a proximal tubular cell line as determined by 3- (4,5-dimethylthiasol-2-yl)-2,5-diphenyltetrazolium bromide (MTT) reduction (24-hour treatment)

The least influence was found by the low-osmolar agents, followed by theiso-osmolar contrast media (Iodixanol). The ionic substances showed the greatest effect.

6. Risks factors

Numerous studies have identified predisposing risk factors such as preexisting chronic kidney disease, particularly diabetic kidney disease, degree of renal dysfunction, volume depletion, co administration of nephrotoxic agents, high doses of radiocontrast, particularly ionic and high osmolar, repeated examinations at short intervals, as well as advanced cardiac failure [22, 23], perhaps also age, smoking, and hypercholesterolemia [23].

Multiple CIN risk factors, including both patient's factors and procedural factors are summarized in table 4 and 5.

Baseline creatinine level or creatinine clearance
Diabetes mellitus
Female gender
Advanced age ("/> 70 year)
Nephrotoxic medication
Anemia
Acute coronary syndrome
Volume depletion, hypotension, hypovolemia
Low cardiac output
Intra aortic balloon pump use
Congestive heart failure
Renal transplantant patient
Hypoalbuminemia
Multiple myeloma

Table 4. Patients factors associated with CIN

Contrast agents amount
Osmolarity of contrast agents
Multiple contras media application within 72 hours

Table 5. Procedural factors associated with CIN

Risk factor	Score
Hypotension (syst. BP < 80mmHg for 1 h requiring inotropic support	5
Intra aortic balloon pump (within 24h periprocedurally)	6
Congestive heart failure. NYHA class III/IV	5
Age "/> 75 years	4
Anemia (hematocrit < 39% for mean and <36% for women)	3
Diabetes mellitus	3
Contrast media volume	1 for each 100 ml
Serum creatinine "/> 1,5 mg/ml	4
Estimated glomerular filtration rate < 60 ml/min/1,73m2	2 for 40-60ml/min/1,73m2 4 for 20-40ml/min/1,73m2 6 for < 20ml/min/1,73m2

Table 6. Risk factor scores for a predictive score for CIN

Most important predictor of CIN is baseline renal function (creatinine clearance < 60 ml/s). Presence of diabetes mellitus and the type and amount of contrast agents are strong risk factors as well ([24, 25].

Using these risk factors, there have been simple and reliable predictive scores for CIN developed (Table 6 and 7) [6, 26].

Risk score	Risk of CIN	Risk of dialysis
≤ 5	7,5%	0,04%
6-10	14,0%	0,12%
11-16	26,1%	1,09%
≥ 16	57,3%	12,6%

Table 7. Risk scores for CIN and outcomes

7. Prevention of CIN

At present there is no specific therapy, which could reduce or reverse development of the CIN, once it is occurs. However, there is possibility of CIN prophylaxis. There are available published data on many different methods of prevention, but many of them failed in efficiency and quality of study design. The most important step in preventing CIN is to determine whether a patient belongs to a risk group. If it is not so, there are not specific measures required. In the case of risk, it should be consider using another method of investigation without need for contrast agent.

7.1. Hydration

Hydration is the most important preventing tool consistently resulting in a decrease of CIN incidence.

In long-term study of 537 consecutive patients undergoing angiography (average dose of contrast agent 2ml/kg) there was not observed either clinical nor biochemical instance of acute renal failure, despite high risk profile of population. Prevalence of underlying clinical abnormalities was: prior stroke or myocardial infarction (58%), diabetes mellitus (33%), hypertension (46%), renal insufficiency (27%), liver disease (14%), proteinuria (14%), elevated uric acid level (13%). In 53% of patients two or more clinical abnormalities was detected. In 24%, there were two or more of the risk factors witch increased likelihood of renal failure. There was not restriction of fluids prior to angiography, infusing about 500 ml/hr during the procedure and encouraging fluids following the examination [27].

An important aspect is to ensure optimal volume repletion prior the procedure. It is recommended to parenterally administer of at least total 1 l of isotonic saline. Infusion usually begins at least 3 hours before and continues 6-8 hours after procedure. Initial infusion rate of

100-150ml/hr are recommended with adjustment post procedure as clinically indicated [28].Caution should be applied in the patient with reduced left ventricular ejection fraction or congestive heart failure.

Prospective, randomized, controlled, open-label study was organized to compare the incidence of CIN with isotonic or half-isotonic hydration [29]. Patient scheduled for elective or emergency coronary angioplasty were randomly assigned to receive isotonic (0,9% saline) or half-isotonic (0,45% sodium chloride plus 5% glucose) hydration beginning the morning of the procedure for elective intervention or immediately before emergency intervention. CIN was defined as increase of serum creatinine at least 44umol/l within 48 hours. There were 15,7% diabetics, 25,6% women and 20,7% patients had chronic renal insufficiency, in this study population (Table 8),

Characteristic	Isotonic (n=685)	Half-isotonic (n=698)	P value
Age, year	64 (63-65)	64 (63-65)	0,71
Female sex	178 (26%)	176 (25%)	0,74
Chronic renal insufficiency	138 (20%)	148 (21%)	0,92
Diabetes mellitus	107 (16%)	110 (16%)	0,94
Arterial hypertension	445 (65%)	425 (61%)	0,12
Previous MI	327 (48%)	353 (51%)	0,29
Acute MI	54 (8%)	60 (9%)	0,63
Single vessel disease	244 (36%)	251 (36%)	0,90
3-vessel disease	252 (37%)	236 (34%)	0,25
LVEF ≥ 60%	287 (42%)	285 (41%)	0,70
LVEF 45-60%	292 (43%)	313 (45%)	0,39
LVEF 30-45%	88 (13%)	82 (12%)	0,54
LVEF < 30%	18 (3%)	17 (2%)	0,82

LVEF= left ventricular ejection fraction, MI=myocardial infarction

Table 8. Baseline clinical characteristics

CIN developed in 5 patients with isotonic infusion vs. 14 patients with half-isotonic infusion. Therefore, incidence of CIN was significantly reduced with isotonic (0,7%, 95% confidence interval, 0,1%-1,4%) vs. half-isotonic (2%, 95% CI, 1,0%-3,1%) hydration (p=0,04) (Figure 10).

http://dx.doi.org/10.5772/54036

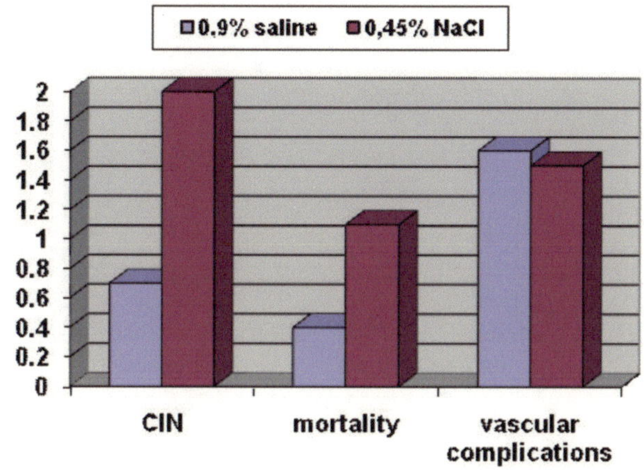

Figure 10. Incidence of CIN, mortality and peripheral vascular complications

Length of hospital stay was significantly increased in patients developing CIN in comparison without nephropathy (8,1 vs. 4,7 days, p<0,001). However, it was similar in both treatment regimens.

In multivariate risk factors analysis, female sex and baseline creatinine level were revealed as independent risk factors for CIN (Table 9).

Risk factor	P value	Odds ratio (95% confident interval)
Female sex	0,005	3,9 (1,5-10,1)
Baseline creatinine	<0,001	6,6 (3,2-13,8) *
Isotonic hydration	0,037	0,3 (0,1-0,9)

* for an increase in baseline creatinine of 88 μmol/l

Table 9. Multivariate risk factor analysis for the development of CIN

7.2. Bicarbonate

In single-center, randomized controlled trial was compared infusion of sodium chloride vs. sodium bicarbonate as the hydration fluid to prevent renal failure in patients with stable renal insufficiency undergoing diagnostic or interventional procedures requiring radiographic contrast [30]. Patients received 154 mEq/L of either sodium chloride or sodium bicarbonate, as a bolus of 3 ml/kg per hour for 1 hour before iopamidol contrast, followed by an infusion of 1 ml/kg per hour for 6 hours after the procedure.

The primary outcome (development of contrast-induced nephropathy, defined by an increase in serum creatinine of 25% or more within 2 days after administration of the radiographic contrast) was observed in 1.7% (1 of 60) patients receiving sodium bicarbonate compared with 13.6% (8 of 59) in patients who received sodium chloride (mean difference, 11.9%; 95% confidence interval [CI], 2.6%-21.2%; *P* = 0,02) Figure 11).

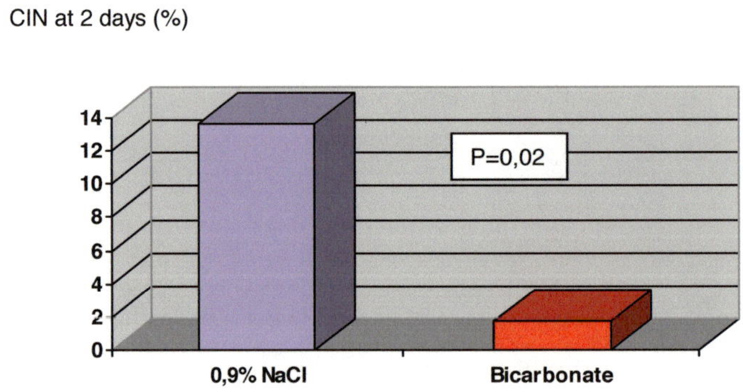

Figure 11. Prevention of CIN by bicarbonate

The absolute risk reduction of CIN, using sodium bicarbonate compared with sodium chloride was 11.9%, resulting in a number needed to treat of 8.4 patients to prevent 1 case of renal failure.

When results were analyzed by another common definition of CIN (at least ≥44.2 μmol/l change in serum creatinine), 7 (11.9%) of 59 patients who were treated with sodium chloride developed contrast nephropathy vs. only 1 (1.7%) of 60 who received sodium bicarbonate (mean difference, 10.2%; 95% CI, 1.3%-19.1%; *P* =0,03).

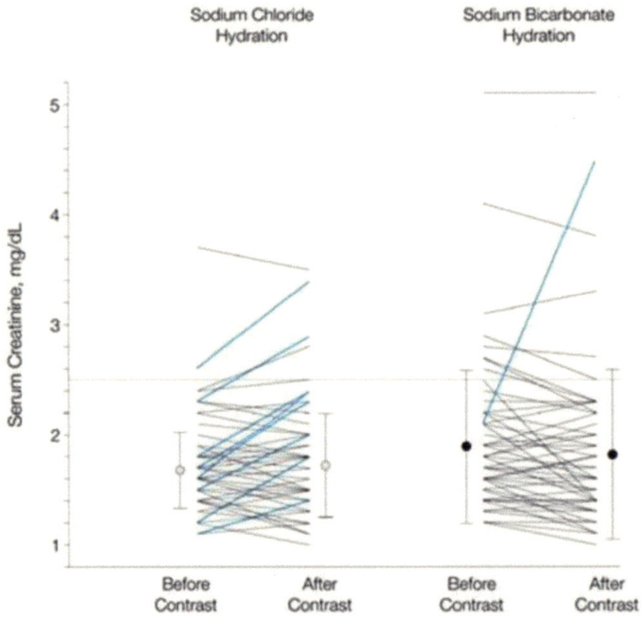

Figure 12. Percentage change in estimated glomerular filtration rate in randomized patients following contrast

Post hoc analysis revealed that the percentage change in glomerular filtration rate after contrast was significantly improved in patients receiving sodium bicarbonate treatment (+8.5%) compared with those receiving sodium chloride (–0.1%) (mean difference, –8.6%; 95% CI, −17.0% to −0.2%; $P = 0{,}02$) (Figure 12) [30].

Blue heavy lines represent cases of contrast-induced renal failure. Dotted line indicates threshold for severe renal insufficiency (serum creatinine ≥221 μmol/L).

Solomon R et al performed randomized comparison saline hydration and different types of diuretic strategies in patients scheduled for cardiac angiography who had serum creatinine concentrations exceeding 140 μmol/l or creatinine clearance rates below <1.0 ml/s [31].

All the patients received 0.45% saline intravenously at a rate of 1 ml /kg of body weight/1 hour beginning 12 hours before the angiography. This saline infusion was continued during the angiography (saline group) or was supplemented with 25 g of manitol, infused intravenously during the 60 minutes immediately before angiography (manitol group), or with 80 mg of furosemide, infused intravenously during the 30 minutes immediately before angiography (furosemide group). All the patients continued to receive 0.45 % saline intravenously at the same rate for 12 hours after angiography. A CIN was defined as an increase in the base-line serum creatinine concentration of at least ≥ 44 μmol per liter within 48 hours after the injection of radiocontrast medium.

Study confirmed that hydration with 0.45 percent saline for 12 hours before and 12 hours after the administration of radiocontrast agents was the most effective means of preventing acute decreases in renal function in patients with chronic renal insufficiency with or without diabetes mellitus. Neither manitol nor furosemide offered any additional benefit when added to this hydration protocol (Figure 13).

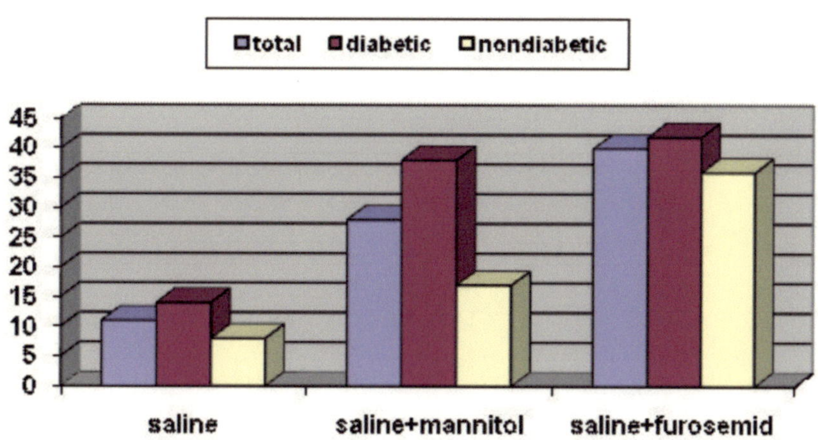

Figure 13. Effect of saline, manitol, and furosemide on the prevention of contrast-induced nephropathy

It is necessary for optimal preprocedural management of patients at risk for CIN, carefully evaluate pharmacotherapy and withdrawn potentially nephrotoxic drugs, as clinically appropriate, (nonsteroidal anti-inflammatory drugs, aminoglycoside antibiotics, antirejection therapy) [2, 29, 31]. Angiotensin converting enzyme inhibitor therapy should continue without neither initiating nor changing dose until the patient safely past the risk period for CIN development [28]. In patient with diabetes mellitus, metformin should be withheld after procedure until it is clear that renal functions are without deterioration because risk of lactate acidosis [32].

7.3. Dopamine

Dopamine in low doses (0.5 to 2.5 μg/kg/min) stimulates dopaminergic receptors in the renal and mesenteric vasculature, resulting in selective vasodilatation. Low dose of dopamine increases renal plasma flow, glomerular filtration rate, and sodium excretion in subjects with normal renal function and with congestive heart failure [27, 33, 34].

Effect of low-dose dopamine in prevention of CIN was studied in prospective randomized trial in patients with chronic renal failure (CRF) (serum Cr <200 μmol/l) and/or diabetes mellitus who underwent coronary angiography. All patients received intravenous hydration for 8 to 12 h before and 36 to 48 h after angiography with 0.45% saline/5% dextrose. In addition, the patients were randomly assigned to receive either 120 ml/day of 0.9% saline plus dopamine 2 μg/kg/min (Dopamine group), or saline alone (Control group) for 48 h [35].

There were 36 Dopamine-treated (30 diabetics and 6 with CRF) and 33 Control (28 diabetics and 5 with CRF) patients compared. Plasma creatinine (Cr) level increased in the Control group from 100,6 ± 5,2 before to 112,3 ± 8,0 μmol/liter within five days after angiography (p = 0,003), and in the Dopamine group from 100,3 ± 5,4 before to 117,5 ± 8,8 μmol/liter after angiography (p = 0,0001), respectively. There was no significant difference in the *change* of Cr level (ΔCr) between the two groups (Figure 14).

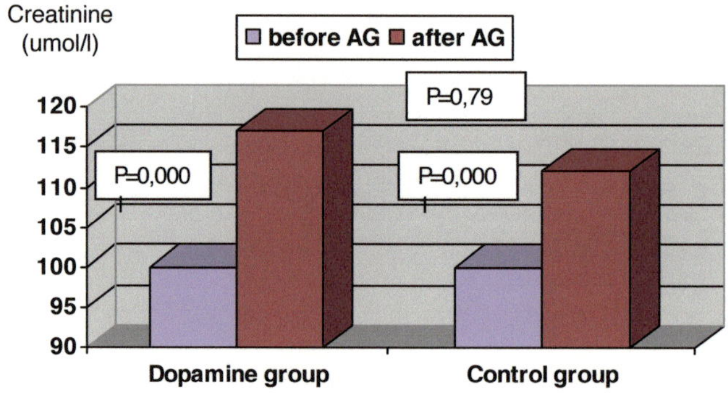

Figure 14. Effect low-dose dopamine on creatinine level in patients after angiography, AG=coronary angiography

http://dx.doi.org/10.5772/54036

However, in a subgroup of patients with peripheral vascular disease (PVD), ΔCr was −2,4 ± 2,3 in the Control group and 30,0 ± 12,0 μmol/l in the Dopamine group (p = 0,01). No significant difference occurred in ΔCr between Control and Dopamine in subgroups of patients with preangiographic CRF or DM.

Administration of contrast agent caused a small but significant increase in Cr blood level in high-risk patients. There is no advantage of dopamine over adequate hydration in patients with mild to moderate renal failure or DM undergoing coronary angiography [35].

7.4. Fenoldopam

Fenoldopam mesylate is a dopamine A1 receptor agonist, augment renal plasma flow and preserves renal blood flow after iodinated contrast administration. It appeared promising in prevention of CIN in a pilot randomized placebo controlled double blind study in 45 patients with chronic renal insufficiency who underwent angiography [36]. Patients were randomized to receive normal saline solution or saline solution with fenoldopan mesylate at 0,1 ug/kg/min at lease 1hr before administration of contrast agent.

Renal plasma flow (primary endpoint) at 1 hour after angiography was 15,8% above baseline in fenoldopan group compared with 33,2% below baseline in the normal saline group (p<0,05). Incidence of CIN at 48 hour (secondary endpoint) was 41,0% in the normal saline group vs. 21% in the fenoldopam group (p=0,148). Renal plasma flow was significantly (p<0,001) reduced in patients with CIN compared with patients without development of CIN [36].

Effect of fenoldopam mesylate was investigated in larger prospective randomized controlled CONTRAST study [37]. There were 315 patients with creatinine clearance less than 1.00 ml/s at 28 centers in the United States randomized to receive fenoldopam mesylate (0.05 μg/kg/min titrated to 0.10 μg/kg/min) (n = 157) or placebo (n = 158), starting 1 hour prior to angiography and continuing for 12 hours. Within 96 hours, the primary end point of contrast-induced nephropathy had been reached in 33.6% of patients in the fenoldopam group vs. 30.1% of patients in the placebo group (relative risk [RR], 1.11; 95% confidence interval [CI], 0.79-1.57; *P* =.61) (Figure 15).

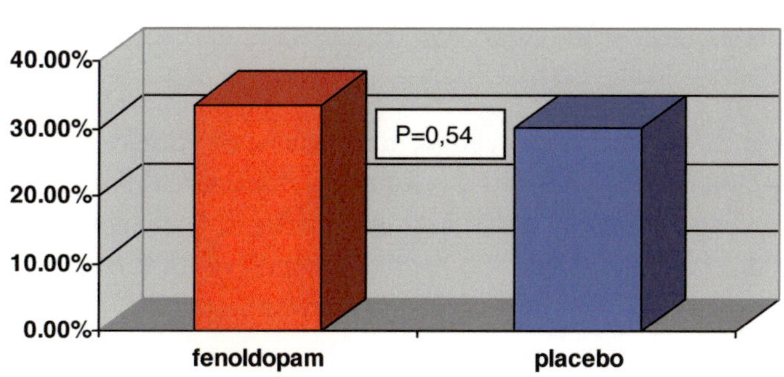

Figure 15. Effect of fenoldopam on CIN prevention

The incidence of contrast-induced nephropathy was also similar in both groups when defined by an absolute increase in serum creatinine level. There were no significant interactions between treatment group and diabetic status, hypertension, baseline renal function, N-acetylcysteine use, or amount of hydration or contrast use.

7.5. Acetylcystein

N-acetylcysteine is a modified form of the amino acid cysteine, which is a nitrogen atom bound via an acetyl group (Figure 16). Molecular weight of N-acetylcysteine is 163,2. The main therapeutic indication is its use as an antidote for paracetamol overdose, as well as a mucolytic therapy.

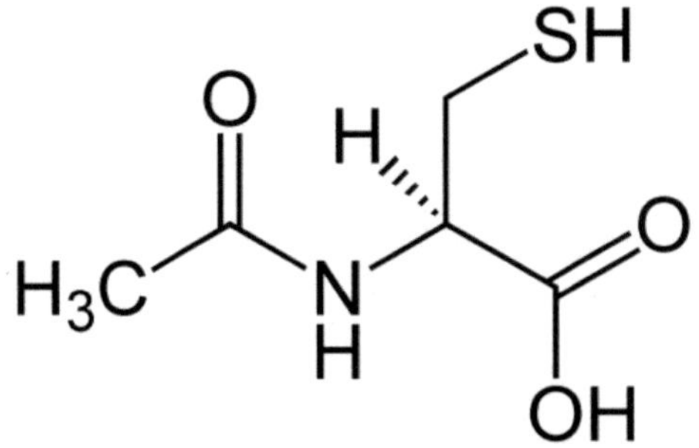

Figure 16. Formula N-acetyl cysteine.

The mechanism by which N-acetylcysteine may reduce the incidence of CIN remains unclear so far. In its most important feature is considered a strong antioxidant effect, which can dispose of a wide range of oxygen radicals. Moreover, N-acetylcysteine is the precursor of the endogenous antioxidant glutathione. Reduce damage from oxygen radicals by N-acetylcysteine have been observed in myocardial infarction [38]. Similarly, N-acetylcysteine can preserve cell death in ischemia-reperfusion renal injury [39]. N-acetylcysteine increases the expression of NO synthase and also enhances the biological effect of nitric oxide itself by creating a compound S-nitrozotiole, which is also a strong and stable vasodilator. In this way, N-acetylcysteine reduces the renal vasoconstriction, and thereby improves blood flow to the kidneys.

N-Acetylcysteine is a free-radical scavenger and has been shown to be renoprotective in some studies [40]. There were performed a lot of randomized trials and meta-analysis with an acetylcysteine in prevention of CIN in high risk patients. Some contradictory results from these studies may be caused by different type or volume of used contrast agents as well as different dosage, timing and route of acetylcystein administration.

Tepel at al. prospectively assessed 83 patients with chronic renal insufficiency (serum creatinine level 216+/-116 μmol/l, mean +/-SD) who were undergoing computed tomography with a nonionic, low-osmolarity contrast agent. Patients were randomly assigned either to receive the antioxidant acetylcysteine (600 mg orally twice daily) and 0.45 percent saline intravenously, before and after administration of the contrast agent, or to receive placebo and saline [40].

Ten of the 83 patients (12 percent) had an increase of creatinine level at least 44 μmol/l at 48 hours after administration of the contrast agent: 1 of the 41 patients in the acetylcysteine group (2 percent) and 9 of the 42 patients in the control group (21 percent; P=0.01; relative risk, 0.1; 95 percent confidence interval, 0.02 to 0.9) (Figure 17).

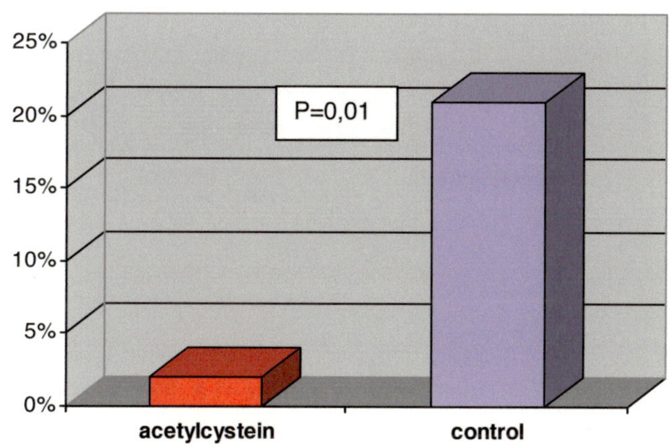

Figure 17. Effect of an acetylcystein on incidence of CIN

In the acetylcysteine group, the mean serum creatinine concentration decreased significantly (P<0.001), from 220+/-118 to 186+/-112 μmol/l at 48 hours after the administration of the contrast medium, whereas in the control group, the mean serum creatinine concentration increased nonsignificantly (P=0.18), from 212+/-114 to 226+/-133 μmol/l (P<0.001 for the comparison between groups).

In prospective randomized RAPPIDE study, 80 patients with stable renal dysfunction undergoing coronary angiography and/or intervention were allocated to an administration of 150mg/kg acetylcystein in 500 ml saline over 30 min immediately before contrast followed by 50mg/kg acetylcystein in 500 ml saline over 4 hours or intravenously hydration (1ml/kg saline for 12hours pre and post-contrast) [41].

Acute CIN occurred in 10 of the 80 patients (12,5%), 2 of the 41 (5%) in acetylcysteine group and in 8 of the 39 fluid-treated patients (21%), p=0,045, relative risk: 0,28; 95% confidence interval: 0,08 to 0,98 (Figure 18).

Prophylactic preventive double dose of N-acetylcystein was investigated in prospective randomized trial in population of 224 patients with chronic renal insufficiency (creatinine level ≥1.5mg/dl or eGFR< 1ml/s) undergoing intravascular administration of non-ionic, low-osmolarity contrast agent [42].

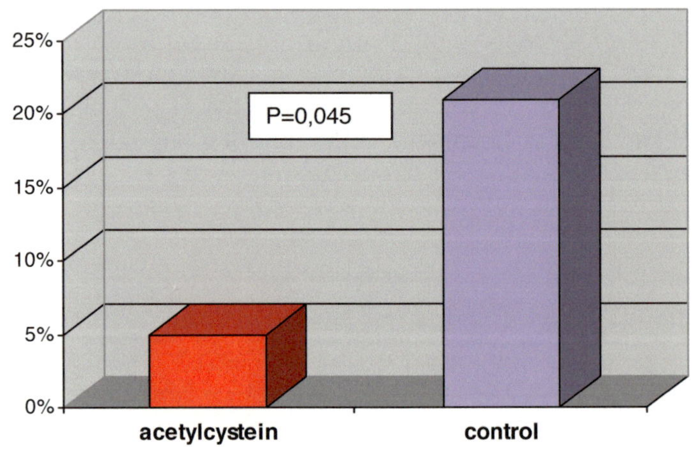

Figure 18. Incidence of CIN, RAPPIDE study results

Patients were randomly assigned to receive 0.45% saline intravenously and acetylcysteine at the standard dose (600mg orally twice daily; *n*=110) or at a double dose (1200mg orally twice daily; *n*=114) before and contrast agent administration.

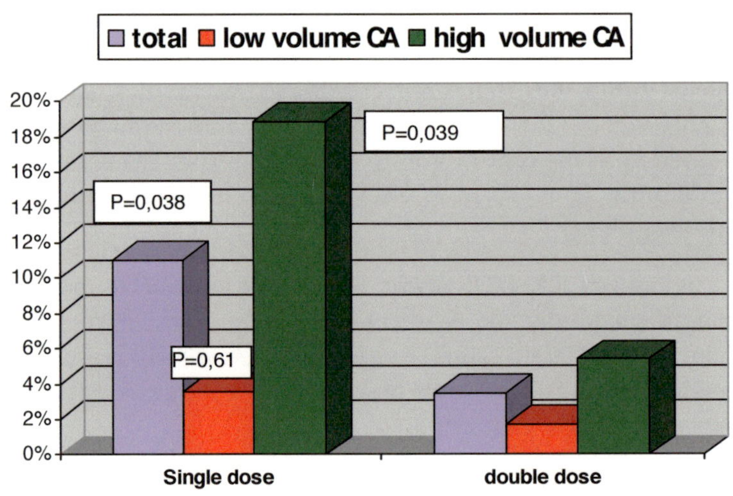

Figure 19. Effect of single and double dose of N-acetylcystein on CIN incidence at 48h, CA=contrast agent

Increase of the creatinine level at least 44umol/l at 48h after the procedure occurred in 12/109 patients (11%) in the standard dose group and 4/114 patients (3.5%) in the double dose group (*P*=0.038; OR=0.29; 95% CI=0.09–0.94). In the subgroup (n=114) with low (<140ml) contrast dose (mean value 101±23ml), no significant difference in renal function deterioration occurred between the 2 groups (3,6% in single dose group vs. 1,7% in double dose group, p=0,61). In the subgroup (n=109) with high (≥140ml) contrast dose (mean value 254±102ml), the event was significantly more frequent in the single dose group vs. double dose group (18,9% vs. 5,4%, p=0,039, OR=0,24; CI=0,06-0,94) (Figure 19).

Effect of N-acetylcysteine was studied in several meta-analyses (Table 10) [43-51].

First author	Year of publication	No of trials included in meta analysis	Relative risk (99% CI)
Birck	2003	7	0,435 (0,215-0,879)
Isenbarger	2003	7	0,370 (0,160-0,840)
Alonso	2004	12	0,550 (0,340-0,910)
Bangshaw	2004	14	0,540 (0,320-0,910)
Pannu	2004	15	0,650 (0,430-1,000)
Kshirsagar	2004	16	ND
Nallamothu	2004	20	0,730 (0,520-1,000)
Liu	2005	9	0,430 (0,240-0,750)
Duong	2005	14	0,570 (0,370-0,840)

Table 10. Meta-analyses of randomized prospective trials on effect of acetylcysteine for prevention of CIN

7.6. Hemodialysis

Although hemodialysis is an appropriate method in rapid elimination of the contrast agent, but in clinical trials it did not showed to be effective in the prevention of CIN [52, 53]. The probably reason is, that the potential kidney damage by contrast media occurs rapidly after its application. Although dialysis starts 1 hour before procedure or concurrently with administration of contrast medium, it did not reduce the incidence of CIN.

7.7. Hemofiltration

Hemofiltration has been shown to be effective in reducing CIN in high-risk patients with advanced stage renal failure undergoing coronary intervention and is associated with improved in-hospital and long-term outcomes.

In a prospective study were 114 consecutive patients with serum creatinine level > 176,8umol/l randomly assigned to groups [54]. One group consisted of patients who undergone hemofiltration 4 to 6 hours before and 18 to 24 hours after coronary intervention, in the second patient group was given isotonic saline in the same time frame. A mean [±SD] serum creatinine level was 265,2±88,4 μmol/l in hemofiltration group and 274,0±88,.4 μmol/l in control group (p=0,63).

Incidence of CIN in patients undergoing hemofiltration was much lower than that of only hydrated patients (5% vs. 50%, p<0,001). The rate of in-hospital events was 9 percent in the hemofiltration group and 52 percent in the control group (P<0.001). In-hospital mortality was 2 percent in the hemofiltration group and 14 percent in the control group (P=0.02), and the cumulative one-year mortality was 10 percent and 30 percent, respectively (P=0.01) (Figure 20) [54].

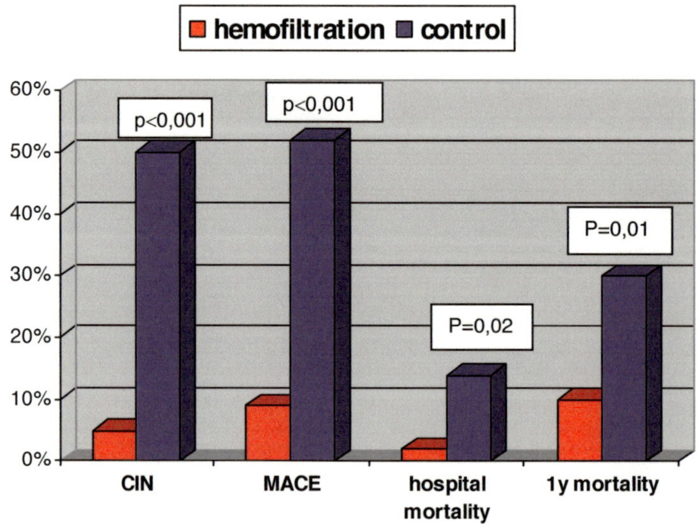

Figure 20. Influence of hemofiltration on incidence of CIN and both hospital and long-term outcome

Important post procedural complications were similar in both groups, except of pulmonary edema, renal replacement therapy (Table 11).

Complication	Hemofiltration group (n=58)	Control group (n=56)	P value
Q MI	0	2(4%)	0,24
nonQ MI	1(2%)	1(2%)	1,00
Emergency CABG	0	0	1,00
Pulmonary edema	0	6(11%)	0,02
Hypotension or shock	1(2%)	3(5%)	0,36
Blood transfusion	1(2%)	3(5%)	0,36
Renal replacement the	2(3%)	14(25%)	<0,001
All clinical events	5(9%)	29(52%)	<0,001

Table 11. Post procedural complications in both hemofiltration and control groups

Interpretation of the study results has some limitations. CIN was defined as more than 25% increase in serum creatinine, but hemofiltration itself remove creatinine from the blood, thus it is impossible to objectively evaluate true creatinine growth. Since the incidence of CIN in the control group far exceed the percentage incidence observed in other studies, it is likely that patients included in this study represent the specific, high risk group that is way the result cannot be simply applied to a wide population. Furthermore, hemofiltration is also an expensive elimination method, and thus cannot be generally recommended as a standard measure for CIN prevention.

Practical recommendations for prevention of CIN are summarized in Table 12 (Schweiger MJ, 2006)

Identify risk
Low risk – eGFR "/> 60ml/min/1,73m2
Optimize hydration status
High risk – eGFR < 60ml/min/1,73m2
Schedule outpatient for early or delay procedure time to allow time to accomplish the hydration
Consider the following recommendation (No 2-No 5)
Manage medications
Withhold, if clinically appropriate, potentially nephrotoxic drugs including aminoglycoside antibiotics, anti-rejection drugs and nonsteroidal anti-inflammatory drugs
Administer N-acetylcysteine
600mg orally q 12hrs "/> 4 doses beginning prior to contrast
Manage intravascular volume (avoid dehydration)
Administer a total of at least 1 l of isotonic saline beginning at least 3hrs before and continuing at least 6-8hr after procedure
Initiation infusion rate 100-150ml/hr adjusted post procedure as clinically indicated
Sodium bicarbonate
154mEq/l @ 3ml/kg/hr starting 1hr before contrast
154mEq/l @ 1ml/kg/hr for 6hrs following contrast
Radiographic contrast media
Minimize volume
Low- or iso-osmolar contrast agents
Postprocedure: discharge/follow-up
Obtain follow-up S-Cr 48 hrs post procedure
Consider holding appropriate medications until renal function returns to normal, i.e. metformin, nonsteroidal anti-inflammatory drugs

eGFR = estimated glomerular filtration rate, S-Cr = serum creatinine level

Table 12. Recommendation for prevention of CIN

8. Contrast induced nephropathy among patients undergoing coronary angiography or percutaneous coronary intervention. Results from 12-months' consecutive cases analysis from University Hospital Martin, Slovakia

8.1. Objective

The primary objective of this work was to evaluate the incidence of contrast-induced nephropathy in patients undergoing coronary angiography examination (KG) or percutaneous coronary intervention (PCI) and was hospitalized at the coronary care unit, I. Internal clinic, University hospital, Martin, Slovakia.

A secondary objective was to identify and assess the impact of major risk factors for developing CIN. At the same time, we assessed the incidence of CIN according to the recommended definition, significance of serum creatinine at 24 hours, and at third to fifth day after administration of contrast medium and the use of scoring systems to estimate the risk of CIN development.

8.2. Methods

In the period from January 2008 to February 2009, we prospectively followed patients admitted to the coronary care unit and department of invasive and interventional cardiology of I. Internal clinic, who underwent coronary angiography or coronary intervention. We studied basal serum creatinine level (SCr0), creatinine value at 16-24 hours after contrast administration (SCr1) and creatinine value at 3rd-5th day after contrast administration (SCr2), which was mostly obtained after hospitalization discharge during ambulatory collection and sent via mail by patients or their GPs. If there was a significant increase in creatinine level at 24 hours after invasive procedures, we recommend extending hospitalization in patients till normalization of values.

Patients without obtained SCr2 values and patients in chronic hemodialysis were excluded from the analysis.

Major risk factors for developing CIN (age, sex, diabetes mellitus, chronic kidney disease, type and amount of contrast medium administration) were monitored at the same time as well.

The invasive procedures contrast agent iopamidol (SCANLUX 370 ®) was used in all patients. Iopamidol represents a non-ionic low-osmolar contrast agent with osmolarity 796 mOsm / kg. It is therefore hypertonic compared with blood plasma osmolarity which is approximately 300 mOsm / kg. Its half-life after intravascular administration is approximately 2 hours with normal renal function. In patients with renal insufficiency there is prolonged elimination, depending on the degree of renal impairment and may takes several days.

In order to determine the risk of CIN, patients were divided into four groups according to the CIN risk score by Mehran. Patients at low and medium risk for the CIN developing were orally hydrated (with the recommendation approximately 2000 ml of fluid on the examination day), High risk patients were hydrated parenteral with saline at a dose of 0,5 to 1 ml / kg body weight per hour.

8.3. Definitions

Contrast-induced nephropathy (CIN) was defined as an increase in baseline creatinine level of ≥ 25% (CIN25) or ≥ 44,2 micromol / l (CIN 0,5) or decrease baseline GFR of ≥ 25% within 24 to 48 hours after administration of contrast medium. Baseline glomerular filtration rate (eGFR) was calculated according to the Cockcroft-Gault formula.

Severe renal dysfunction (SRD) was defined as an acute renal failure requiring dialysis or a rise in baseline creatinine over 50% during 24 hours to 120 hours after the procedure.

Chronic kidney disease was determined according to the history with the presence of kidney disease in nephrologic observation.

8.4. Statistic methods

The incidence of contrast-induced nephropathy was evaluated by Pearson Chi-square test. Quantitative parameters (age, BMI, sex, number of KL, SCr0, GFR0, left ventricular ejection fraction), were evaluated by the Mann-Whitney U - test and qualitative parameters (age over 75 years, DM, chronic renal disease), by the Fisher's exact test.

To assess correlation of the endpoints, we used the Spearmen correlation coefficient. Numerical values are expressed as median and quartile range or as a percentage of the total amount. As statistically significant, we considered the value of $p < 0.05$.

8.5. Results

There were excluded 19,2% patients with incomplete documentation of sampling creatinine values at 24 hours (SCr1) or at third to fifth day after contrast agent administration (SCr2) and patients in the chronic hemodialysis. In the final data analysis was then included 529 patients, whose basic clinical characteristics are listed in Table 13.

Age "/> 75 years	15,1% (80/529)
Diabetes mellitus (DM)	30,3% (160/529)
Preexisting renal disease (CKD)	14,6% (77/529)
DM + CKD	6,6% (35/529)
PCI procedure	62,38% (330/529)

DM = diabetes mellitus, CKD = chronic kidney disease, PCI = percutaneous coronary intervention

Table 13. Clinical characteristics

CIN25 was observed in 3, 97% (21/529) patients and CIN 0,5 in 2,27% (12/529) patients. The decrease of eGFR ≥ 25% occurred in 2, 27% (12/529) patients. SRD occurred in 1, 51% (8/529) patients, dialysis was needed in 0,76% (4/529) patients. Severe hypotension requiring combined inotropic support was observed in 3 patients (0, 57%). There were 4 deaths from529 patients (0, 76%) as a consequence of the contrast induced nephropathy (2 men and 2 women). Mortality rate of patients with CIN was 19% (4/21).Distribution of patients according to Mehranś risk score model is shown in Table 14.

Score	**Number of pts**	**CIN25 incidence**
Low risk	77,5% (410/529)	2,44% (10/410)
Medium risk	17,9% (95/529)	4,21% (4/95)
High risk	3,59% (19/529)	21,05% (4/19)
Very high risk	0,95% (5/529)	60% (3/5)

Table 14. Distribution of patients according risk score model (Mehran)

Patients with the development of CIN, compared with patients in whom CIN was not confirmed, differed statistically significantly in age (p = 0.043), left ventricle systolic function (p <0.001), and the amount of administered contrast medium (p = 0.004). On the contrary statistically significant differences were not found in sex, BMI, the initial value of creatinine (SCr0), or the initial value calculated glomerular filtration rate (eGFR0). Both groups of patients also differed significantly in the presence of chronic kidney disease (p <0.001) and in the combined appearance of diabetes and chronic kidney disease (p = 0.001). In contrast, both groups of patients did not differ significantly according of the risk age (over 75 years), or diabetes mellitus (Table 15, Figure 21).

Parameter	**with CIN**	**without CIN**	**P value**
	(n = 508)	**(n = 21)**	
Age (year)	62	71	0,043
Age > 75y (No of pts)	14,8% (75/508)	23,8% (5)	0,345
Sex (men/women)(No of pts)	63/37%(318/190)	62/38%(13/8)	1,00
BMI (kg/m2)	28,4 (25,8-31,2)	29,8 (27,7-34,0)	0,121
Diabetes mellitus (No of pts)	30% (152/508)	38,1% (8)	0,469
CKD (No of pts)	13,2% (67/508)	47,6% (10)	< 0,001
Both DM and CKD (No of pts)	5,7% (29/508)	28,6% (6)	0,001
LVEF (%)	55 (50-60)	45 (40-50)	< 0,001
Serum creatinine level (μmol/l)	100 (88-112)	105 (91-136)	0,129
eGFR (ml/min)	72,6 (60,6-90,0)	62,4 (45,6-91,2)	0,291

CKD = chronic kidney disease, LVEF = left ventricle ejection fraction, BMI = body mass index, eGFR = estimated glomerular filtration rate, DM = diabetes mellitus

Table 15. Comparison of clinical parameters in patients with and without the occurrence of CIN

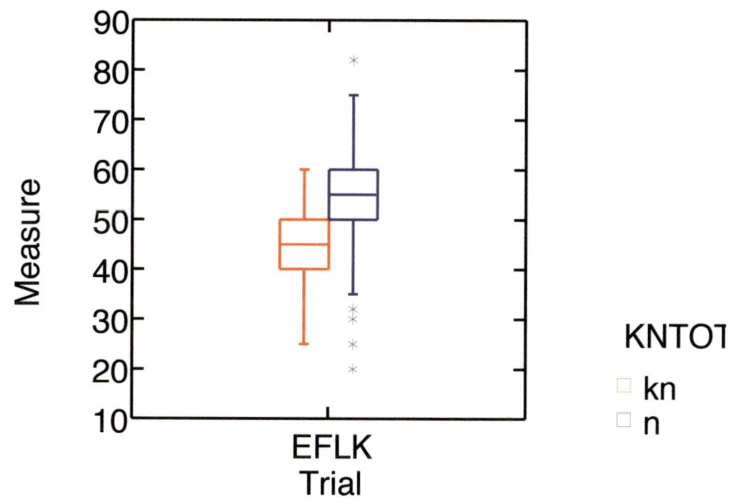

Figure 21. Left ventricle ejection fraction (EFLK) (%) in patients with CIN (kn) and without CIN (n)

There was not observed correlation between the amount administered contrast agent and development of CIN (0.50), although patients with the development of CIN received significantly higher amount of contrast agent (Figure 22).

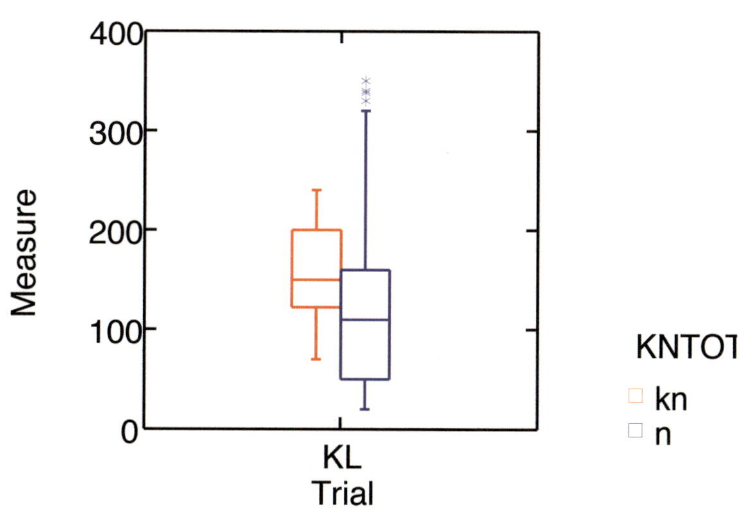

Figure 22. Amount of contrast agent administered in patients with CIN (kn) and without CIN (n)

If the criterion value was chosen CIN25, diagnosis of CIN was determined by the value of delta SCr1 in 1,89% (10/519) and the delta SCr2 in 2,65% (14/515) of cases, together in the 3,97% (21/509) of cases. If the criterion value was determined CIN 0,5, CIN, diagnosis of CIN was established based on the value deltaSCr1 in 0,76% (4/524) and deltaSCr2 in 2,08% (11/517) of cases, together in 2,27% (12/516) of cases.

If the definition of CIN was used decrease in creatinine clearance, than diagnosis of CIN was determined by delta eGFR1 in 0.57% (3/524) of patients and delta eGFR2 in 1, 9% (10/517) of cases, together in 2,28% (12/515) of cases.

In a subset of patients with CIN, according of CIN25 definition, there were based on result of SCr1, diagnosed 47, 62% (10/21) and on SCr2 52,38% (11/21) patients. Using the definition CIN 0,5 there were based on result of SCr1 diagnosed 33,33% (4/12) and on SCr2 66,67% (8/12) patients. According of the reduction in eGFR as a definition of CIN, there were based on result of SCr1 diagnosed 25% (3/12) and on SCr2 75% (9/12) cases.

8.6. Discussion

The incidence of CIN depends on the study population and diagnostic criteria that define it and is reported in the range 4.4% -20%. While in the general population is low and ranges from 0,6 to 2,3% [55], significantly increases in patients with risk factors especially with documented cardiovascular disease and the acute coronary syndromes and may be as high as 57,3% [56]. In 250 patients with creatinine clearance <60 ml/min, the incidence of CIN ranged from 6,0% -21,6%. Similarly, using different definitions of CIN incidence was 4,4% -20% in diabetics and 2,8% -17,3% in 469 patients with elevated cardiac markers before PCI [57]. There are four currently used CIN definitions, but only two (CIN CIN25 and 0,5) allow more consistently predict the clinical course. In comparison to CIN25, the definition of CIN 0,5 provides greater differences between unselected group of patients and patients with high risk of CIN and is a stronger indicator of the unfavorable course.

A large variation in the incidence of CIN emphasizes the need for a uniform definition of CIN, which would allow proper comparison of results from different databases. The CIN25 and CIN 0,5 independently correlated with the clinical course. Patients with a seemingly small increase in creatinine level have adverse cardiovascular variables. The relationship between increases in serum creatinine and glomerular filtration current is nonlinear. A small increase in creatinine level may represent significant deterioration in renal function, particularly at lower values of basal serum creatinine. Moreover, work dealing with a rise in serum creatinine showed that the peak levels are often not achieved until several days after exposure to contrast medium [58-60]. Because most of the patients are discharged after 24-48 hours after PCI, a small increase in creatinine may be a sign of further renal damage in the coming days. Besides of a consistent prognostic value, ideal definition of CIN should distinguish between patients with moderate and high risk. Although the value of CIN25 and CIN 0,5 provide consistent prognostic value, CIN 0,5 clearly distinguishes between a whole population and a subgroup of patients with chronic kidney disease at highest risk. In contrast, CIN25 has only low discriminatory value, but very high in patients with the lowest risk. Combining these two definitions, we can divide the patients into 3 groups: The lowest risk for adverse events - level 0 (deltaCr <25% <44 μmol / l), the highest (deltaCr> 25%> 44 μmol / l) - level 2 and intermediate (deltaCr> 25% <44 μmol / l) - level 1. Trend toward a worse clinical outcome is observed in patients at higher degrees of nephropathy. Multivariate analysis revealed stage 1 and 2 as an independent and significant indicator of 6-month MACE (major adverse cardiovascular events) compared with the degree 0. This scoring system reflects the fact that those patients who experienced an increase in CIN CIN25 or CIN0,5 are in fact two prognostic categories (nephropathy Level 1 and nephropathy Level 2) [57].

In our study, the overall incidence of CIN varied, according to the chosen definition of the baseline increase in serum creatinine, from 2,27% with the definition of CIN 0.5 to 3,97% using the definition of CIN25. Using the definition of impairment eGFR of ≥ 25% compared to baseline, the overall incidence of CIN was 2,28%. Therefore, as the most-sensitive diagnostic tool for CIN, was the determination of the CIN25 value.

In most of the studies was the incidence of CIN based on an increase in creatinine levels at 24 hours after contrast agent administration. Management of patients with complete follow-up serum creatinine at 48 hours after contrast medium administration evaluated only Huber et al., while many others have failed to adequate monitoring of all patients enrolled, which bring potentially serious problem in interpreting their results. While our results suggest that CIN can be diagnosed according to the definition based on SCr1 value only in 25 - 47,6% cases and in 52,4 -75% of cases based on SCr2 value. Moreover, among patients developing severe renal dysfunction in the future (hemodialysis or death), 60% (3/5) had CIN diagnosed until just based on the SCr2 value. This raises the question of the need for routine clinical assessment of SCr2 (in the third to fifth day after contrast administration) in all patients at risk [61, 62].

The overall low incidence of CIN in our study can be attributed to several factors. There was present very high proportion of patients with low and moderate risk of developing CIN (77,5%, respectively. 17,96%). Moreover, before invasive procedure were patients hydrated both oral and parenteral way with saline. Hydration is widely recognized as the simplest and most effective preventive measure of CIN. In our series we noted paradoxical decrease in serum creatinine level after 16-24 hours following invasive procedure compared to baseline in 35,16% (186/529) patients, despite of administration of contrast agent. This finding demonstrates importance of standard saline hydration for patients prior to invasive procedures, as patients are admitted for coronary angiography or percutaneous coronary intervention often dehydrated. Another factor that can be attributed to a low incidence of CIN is the type and amount of contrast medium. In our study, non-ionic low-osmolar contrast medium iopamidol was used. This contrast agent has safety renal profile that is comparable with the safety profile of iso-osmolar contrast agent iodixanol.

In our study was not confirmed a significant relationship between amount of used contrast agent and the incidence of CIN. However, dose of contrast medium was significantly higher in patients with development of CIN25, in comparison with dose used in patients who did not develop CIN25 (150 ml vs. 110 ml, p = 0,004).

This may explain the low prevalence of patients with age above 75 years (15,12%), diabetes mellitus (30,24%), with chronic kidney disease (14,56%) and also low doses of used contrast medium, the maximum dose was 350 ml.

Generally, a safe dose of intravascular administrated iodinated contrast media is considered below 70 ml. The dose more than 5 ml / kg of patient weight is considered high risk [63, 64]. In patients with chronic kidney disease, dose of contrast medium for coronary angiography should be planned below 30 ml and if procedure will be followed by percutaneous coronary intervention than dose should be below 100 ml [64]. Even in our study, we confirmed that the dose of contrast medium into 70 ml can be considered relatively safe, because in this dose no CIN did occur in our study group.

Results of several studies suggested that the prevalence of CIN is more common in women than men in older age groups, mainly in the context of low eGFR in this group. These findings are supported by other studies that found a higher risk for developing of renal complications after angiography in women than in men. However, previous findings were related to influencing factors such as age, which caused that women seemed to be a higher risk for developing CIN than men. In our group of patients had preexisting renal impairment 12,63% women and 16,61% men, which is one possible explanation for higher incidence of CIN in males.

Anemia seems also to be an independent risk factor for CIN. Several studies have shown that women more incline to anemia before angiography than men and have a trend to higher risk of bleeding during periprocedural period [55]. The decrease in hematocrit of more than 6% doubles the risk of developing CIN, especially in women. Such a reduction in hematocrit can cause renal hypoperfusion, which potentiates renal damage caused by exposure to contrast media.

Patients with chronic kidney disease have a reduced vasodilatory response that is important factor in the development of CIN. At the same time, in these patients due to reduced glomerular filtration extends elimination of contrast agent from circulation, thus potentiating its both cytotoxic and hemodynamic effect. Chronic kidney disease as a highly significant predictor of CIN was also confirmed by our study.

In our study, age was a marginally significant predictor of CIN and age over 75 years has not been demonstrated as important.

Advanced congestive heart failure and reduced left ventricle ejection fraction are characterized by reduced cardiac output, increased neurohumoral vasoconstrictor activity and reduced NO-dependent renal vasodilatation, which can lead to hypoperfusion of renal medulla [64]. Left ventricle systolic dysfunction was in our study recognized as highly significant predictor of CIN.

Diabetes mellitus was not an independent predictor, but in combination with chronic kidney disease has become a significant predictor of CIN development.

http://dx.doi.org/10.5772/54036

9. Conclusion

Contrast induced nephropathy is common cause of renal functions impairment. Incidence of CIN in unselected patients undergoing angiographic procedures (coronary angiography, percutaneous coronary intervention) varies approximately 2-30%. Once occurs, CIN is associated with a significant increase in potentially serious morbidity and mortality. If possible, in patients at the highest risk for development of CIN, very useful is avoiding of contrast agent administration (or strongly limiting contrast volume of low or iso-osmolar contrast agents). To this high risk group are usually includes patients with diabetes mellitus, preexisting renal insufficiency, hypotension (or incipient shock), congestive heart failure, anemia or at advanced age. This risky patients population requires appropriate both peri and post-procedural management. Most important measure is adequate hydration in order to avoid hypovolemia. Preferred type of solutions is parenteral isotonic saline or an isotonic sodium bicarbonate. Still limited evidence is for pharmacologic intervention (N-acetylcystein) in CIN prevention.

Since most cases of CIN, including patients with an unfavorable course in the future, were diagnosed on the basis of serum creatinine level at third to fifth day after administration of contrast medium, it is recommended for high-risk patients to assess serum creatinine level at day 3 to 5 after invasive procedures.

Author details

Frantisek Kovar, Milos Knazeje and Marian Mokan

*Address all correspondence to: fkovar8@gmail.com

I. Internal Clinic, University Hospital, Martin, Slovak Republic

References

[1] Hou SH, Bushinsky DA, Wish JB et al.: Hospital-acquired renal insufficiency: a prospective study. Am J Med 1983; 74: 243–248

[2] Rihal CS, Textor SC, Grill DE at al.: Incidence and prognostic importance of acute renal failure after percutaneous coronary intervention. Circulation 2002; 105: 2259-2264

[3] Levy EM, Viscoli CM, Horwitz RI: Effect of acute renal failure on mortality. A cohort analysis. JAMA. 1996; 275: 1489-1494

[4] Morcos SK, Thomsen HS, Web JAW: Contrast media safety committee of the European society of urogenital radiology. Contrast – media induced nephrotoxicity: a consensus report. Eur Radiol 1999; 9: 1602-1613

[5] Gleeson TG, Bulugahapitiya S. Contrast-induced nephropathy. AJR Am J Roentgenol.2004; 183: 1673–1689

[6] Mehran R, Aymong ED, Nikolsky E et al. A simple risk score for prediction of contrast-induced nephropathy after percutaneous coronary intervention: development and initial validation. J Am Coll Cardiol. 2004; 44: 1393–1399

[7] Efstratiadis G, Pateinakis P, Tambakoudis G et al.: Contrast media-induced nephropathy: case report and review of the literature focusing on pathogenesis. Hippokratia 2008; 12: 87–93

[8] Bartels ED, Brun GV, Gammeltoft A et al.: Acute anuria following intravenous pyelography in a patient with myelomatosis. Acta Med Scand. 1954; 150: 297–302

[9] Scanlon PJ, Faxon DP, Audet AM, et al.: ACC/AHA guidelines for coronary angiography. A report of the American College of Cardiology/American Heart Association Task Force on practice guidelines (Committee on Coronary Angiography). J Am Coll Cardiol. 1999; 33: 1756–1824

[10] Solomon R. Radiocontrast-induced nephropathy. Semin nephrol. 1998; 18: 551–557

[11] Aspelin P, Aubry P, Fransson SG et al.: Nephrotoxic effects in high-risk patients undergoing angiography. N Engl J Med 2003; 348: 491-499

[12] Gruberg L, Mehran R, Dangas G et al.: Acute renal failure requiring dialysis after percutaneous coronary interventions. Catheter Cardiovasc Interven 2001; 52: 409–416

[13] McCullough PA, Wolyn R, Rocher LL et al: Am J Med. 1997;103:368-75. Acute renal failure after coronary intervention: incidence, risk factors, and relationship to mortality

[14] Sandler CM: Contrast-agent-induced acute renal dysfunction--is iodixanol the answer? N Engl J Med.2003; 348: 551–553

[15] Solomon R. Contrast-medium-induced acute renal failure. Kidney Int 1998; 53: 230–242

[16] Heyman SN, Clarc BA, Kaiser N et al.: Radiocontrast agents induce endothelin release in vivo and in vitro. J Am Soc Nephrol 1992; 3: 58-65

[17] Fishbane S, Durham J H, Marzo K. et al.: N-acetylcysteine in the prevention of radiocontrast-induced nephropathy. J Am Soc Nephrol 2004; 15: 251–260

[18] Pflueger A, Larson TS, Nath KA et al.: Role of adenosine in contrast media-induced acute renal failure in diabetes mellitus. Mayo Clin Proc. 2000; 75: 1275–1283

[19] Persson PB, Hansell P, Liss P: Pathophysiology of contrast medium induced nephropathy. Kidney Int 2005; 68: 14-22

[20] Liss P, Nygren A, Erikson U et al.: Injection of low and iso-osmolar contrast medium decreases oxygen tension in the renal medulla. Kidney Int 1998; 53: 698-702

[21] Hardiek K, Katholi RE, Ramkumar V et al.: Proximal tubule cell response to radiographic contrast media. Am J Physiol Renal Physiol 2001; 280: F61-F70

[22] Chertow GM: Prevention of radiocontrast nephropathy: Back to basics. JAMA 2004; 291: 2376 –2377

[23] Weisbord SD, Palevsky PM: Radiocontrast-induced acute renal failure. J Intensive Care Med 2005; 20: 63 –75

[24] Berns AS: Nephrotoxicity of contrast media. Kidney Int 1989; 36: 730-740

[25] Davidson CJ, Hlatky M, Morris KG et al.: Cardiovascular and renal toxicity of a nonionic radiographic contrast agent after cardiac catheterization. A prospective trial. Ann Intern Med 1989; 110: 557-560

[26] Bartholomew BA, Harjai KL, Dukkipati S et al.: Impact of nephropathy after percutaneous coronary intervention and a method for risk stratification. Am J Cardiol 2004; 93: 1515-1519

[27] Eisenberg RL, Bank WO, Hedgock MW et al.: Renal failure after major angiography can be avoided with hydration. Am J Roentgenol 1981; 136: 859-861

[28] Schweiger MJ, Chambers CE, Davidson CJ et al.: Prevention of contrast induced nephropathy: Recommendations for the high rist patient undergoing cardiovascular procedures. Cathet Cardiovasc Interv 2007; 69: 135-140

[29] Mueller C, Buerkle G, Heinz J et al.: Prevention of contrast media associated nepropathy. Randomized of two hydration regimen in 1620 patients undergoing coronary angioplasty. Arch Intern Med 2002; 162: 329-336

[30] Merten GJ, Burgess WP, Gray LV, MD et al: Prevention of contrast-induced nephropathy with sodium bicarbonate. A randomized controlled trial. JAMA. 2004; 291: 2328-2334

[31] Solomon R, Werner C, Mann D et a.: Effects of saline, manitol, and furosemide on acute decreases in renal function Idnuced by radiocontrast agents. N Engl J Med 1994; 331:1416-1420

[32] Heupler FA: Guidelines for performing angiography in patients taking metformin. Catheter Cardiovasc Diagn 1998; 43: 121-123

[33] Kolonko A, Wiecek A, Kokot F: The nonselective adenosine antagonist theophylline does prevent renal dysfunction induced by radiographic contrast agents, J Nephrol 1998; 11: 151-156

[34] Szerlip HM: Renal-dose dopamine. fact and fiction, Ann Int Med 1991; 115: 153-154

[35] Gare M, Haviv YS, Ben-Yehuda A et al.: The renal effect of low-dose dopamine in high risk patients undergoing coronary angiography. J Am Coll Cardiol 1999; 34: 1682-1688

[36] Tumlin JA, Wang A, Murray PT: Fenoldopam mesylate blocks reductions in renal plasma flow after radiocontrast dye infusion: a pilot trial in the prevention of contrast nephropathy. Am Heart J 2002; 143: 894-903

[37] Stone GW, McCullough PA, Tumlin JA at al: CONTRAST investigators. Fenoldopam mesylate for the prevention of contrast induced nephropathy: a randomized controled trial. JAMA 2003; 290: 2284-2291

[38] Arstall MA, Yang J: Nacetylcysteine in combination with nitroglycerin and streptokinase for treatment of evolving acute myocardial infarction: safety and biochemical effects. Circulation 1995; 92: 2855-2862

[39] Safirstein R, Andrade L, Vieira, JM: Acetylcysteine and nephrotoxic effects of radiocontrast agents—A new use for an old drug. New Engl J Med 2000; 343: 210-212

[40] Tepel M, van der Giet M, Schwarzfeld C et al.: Prevention of radiographic-contrast-agent-induced reductions in renal function by acetylcysteine. N Engl J Med 2000; 343: 180-184

[41] Baker CSR, Wragg A, Kumar S et al.: A rapid protocol for the prevention of contrast induced denal dysfunction: the RAPPID study. J Am Coll Cardiol 2003; 41: 2114-2118

[42] Briguori C, Colombo A, Violante A at al.: Standard vs double dose of N-acetylcysteine to prevent contrast agent associated nephrotoxicity. Eur Heart J. 2004; 25: 206–211

[43] Tepel M, Aspelin P, Lameire N: Contrast induced nephropathy. A clinical and evidence based approach. Circulation 2006; 113: 1799-1806

[44] Nallamothu BK, Shojania KG, Saint S et al.: Is acetylcysteine effective in preventing contrast-related nephropathy? A meta-analysis. Amer J Med 2004; 117: 938–947

[45] Pannu N, Manns B, Lee H et al.: Systematic review of the impact of acetylcysteine on contrast nephropathy. Kidney Int 2004; 65: 1366–1374

[46] Bangshaw SM, Ghali WA: Acetylcysteine for prevention of contrast induced nephropathy after intravascular angiography: a systematic review and meta-analysis. BMC 2004; 2: 38

[47] Birck R, Krzossok S, Markowetz F et al.: Acetylcysteine for prevention of contrast induced nephropathy: meta-analysis. Lancet 2003; 362: 598-603

[48] Isenbarger DW, Kent SM, O'Malley PG: Meta-analysis of randomized clinical trials on the uselfuness of acetylcysteine for prevention of contrast nephropathy. Am J Cardiol 2003; 92: 1454-1458

[49] Alonso A, Lau J, Jaber BL et al.: Prevention of radiocontrast nepropathy with N-acetylcysteine in patients with chronic kidney disease: a meta-analysis od randomized, controlled trials. Am J Kidney Dis 2004; 43: 1-9

[50] Liu R, Nair D, Ix J et al.: Acetylcysteine for prevention of contrast induced nephropathy after intravascular angiography: a systematic review and meta-analysis. J Gen Intern Med 2005; 20: 193-200

[51] Duong MH, Mackenzie TA, Malenka DJ et al.: N-acetylcysteine prophylaxis significantly reduces the risk of radiocontrast induced nephropathy: comprehensive meta-analysis. Catheter Cardiovasc Interv 2005; 64: 471-479

[52] Frank H, Werner D, Lorusso V et al. Simultaneous hemodialysis during coronary angiography fails to prevent radiocontrast-induced nephropathy in chronic renal failure. In Clinical Nephrology 2003; 60: 176 -182

[53] Schindler R, Stahl C, Venz S et al. Removal of contrast media by different extracorporeal treatments. Nephrol Dialys Transplant 2001; 16: 1471-1474

[54] Marenzi G, Marana I, Lauri G et al. The prevention of radiocontrast-agent-induced nephropathy by hemofiltration. New Engl J Med 2003; 349: 1333-1340

[55] Mehran R, Nikolsky E.: Contrast -induced nephropathy: Definition, epidemiology, and patients at risk. Kidney Int 2006; 69: S11-S15Osten MD, Ivanov J, Eichhofer J et al.: Impact of renal insufficiency on angiographic, procedural, and in-hospital outcomes following percutaneous coronary intervention. Amer J Cardiol 2008; 101: 780–785

[56] McCullough PA: Contrast-induced AKI. J Amer Coll Cardiol 2008; 51: 1419-1428

[57] Guitterez NV, Diaz A, Timmis GC et al. Determinants of serum creatinine trajectory in acute contrast nephropathy. J Interv Cardiol 2002; 15: 349-354Neugarten J, Kasiske B, Silbiger SR et al.: Effects of sex on renal structure. Nephron 2002; 90: 139-144

[58] Iakovou I, Dangas G, Mehran R, et al.: Impact of gender on the incidence and outcome of contrast-induced nephropathy after percutaneous coronary intervention. J Invas Cardiol 2003; 15: 18-22

[59] Sidhu RB, Brown JR, Robb JF et al.: Interaction of gender and age on post cardiac catheterization contrast-induced acute kidney injury. Amer J Cardiol 2008; 102: 1482-1486

[60] Toprak O, Cirit M..: Risk factors for contrast-induced nephropathy. Kidney Blood Pressure Respir 2006; 29: 84-93

[61] Krusová D, Ševela K.: Kontrastní látkou indukovaná nefropatie. Interní Medicína 2007; 3: 118-122

[62] Martínek V.: Poškození ledvin kontrastními látkami. Interv Akut Kardiol 2002; 1: 37-40

Chapter 19

Myocardial Bridges in the ERA of Non-Invasive Angiography

Mohamed Bamoshmoosh and Paolo Marraccini

Additional information is available at the end of the chapter

http://dx.doi.org/10.5772/54083

1. Introduction

Cardiovascular (CV) and cerebrovascular (CBV) diseases are the leading causes of mortality in developed countries. In these countries CV risk factors like smoke, obesity, sedentary life, dyslipidemias, hypertension and diabetes are well recognized and efforts have been efficaciously undertaken so that CV and CBV mortality in the second half of the last century has been significantly reduced. Cardiovascular and CBV diseases are also the leading cause of mortality in the developing world where in the last century we witnessed a rapid epidemiological as well as nutritional transition related mainly to increased urbanization and market globalization. Now the majority of CV and CBV mortality occurs in low and middle-income countries [1].

Indeed the major responsible of CV as well as CBV diseases is the vascular atherosclerotic process. In particular the atherosclerotic calcified and non calcified plaques that cause coronary artery vessel lumen reduction are worldwide the leading cause of myocardial ischemia, which can lead to asymptomatic myocardial dysfunction, life threatening arrhythmias, angina, myocardial infarction and sudden death.

Besides the atherosclerotic coronary artery diseases there are also other non atherosclerotic coronary artery vessel lumen reductions, although their prevalence is less common. The non atherosclerotic coronary artery diseases are related to prolonged coronary artery spasm, hypertrophic cardiomyopathy, vasculitis and congenital coronary anomalies.

Congenital coronary artery anomalies are a heterogeneous group of diseases. In the majority of cases congenital coronary artery anomalies lack clinical significance and are merely epiphenomena found accidentally during necropsies, while performing invasive or non invasive coronarography or during surgical interventions. However in some cases they may be responsible for chest discomfort, malignant arrhythmias, fatal or non fatal acute myocardial infarction, ventricular septum rupture, myocardial stunning, paroxysmal atrio-ventricular block, syncope and sudden death. In particular 19% of sudden deaths in young athletes are due to coronary artery anomalies [2].

In this chapter we will focus our attention on describing the second most common type of coronary congenital anomaly: the myocardial bridges (MBs). We will discuss the nature of MBs and how to diagnose them with particular attention to the use of cardiac computed tomography (CCT).

2. Classifications

In describing coronary anomalies Angelini et al. proposed that a condition should be considered "normal when it is observed in > 1% of an unselected population; normal variant, an alternative, relatively unusual, morphological feature seen in > 1% of the same population; and anomaly, a morphological feature seen in < 1% of that population". These Authors performed their study using cine-angiograms [3]. The procedure used to define a normal from an abnormal coronary may be a bias. In fact coronary angiography is performed in symptomatic patients while necropsies are usually done for medico-legal purposes especially for violent non hospital based deaths whereas necropsy for hospital based deaths is decreasing. This bias explains why coronary anomalies of origination and course are rare during autopsy (0.17% of the cases) while their incidence is higher in the population of patients referred for coronary angiography (0.6-1.3%).

Clinically coronary anomalies are evaluated with the same diagnostic tests used to study the atherosclerotic coronary artery diseases: electrocardiogram, exercise stress test, trans-thoracic and trans-esophageal echocardiography, stress echocardiography, stress single photon emission computed tomography, myocardial perfusion imaging, magnetic resonance, fractional flow reserve, electron beam computed tomography, invasive coronary angiography (ICA) and non-invasive coronary angiography with CCT.

Myocardial bridges in humans are inborn coronary anomalies of intrinsic coronary arterial anatomy with an intramural course. Although it was Reyman in 1737 and then Black in 1805 who first described, as a curiosity during necropsy, the presence of a MB overlaying the left anterior descending coronary artery (LAD), the first detailed postmortem analysis of this anomaly was reported by Geiringer in 1951 [4].

In fact in humans coronary arteries and their main branches have an epicardial course running over the cardiac musculature. In the presence of a MB a portion of one coronary artery or more dips into and underneath the heart muscle to come back out again in the majority of the cases. This condition is also known also as "intramuscular coronary artery", "tunnelled artery", "myocardial loop", "mural coronary artery", "intramural coronary artery", "myocardial bridging" or "coronary artery over bridging".

http://dx.doi.org/10.5772/54083

The real incidence of this entity is unknown and varies according to the procedure used to study it. Myocardial bridges are rare in patients referred for cardiac surgery (0.2-0.3%) or ICA (0.4-4.9%) while they are very frequent during autopsy (5.4-85.7%) [5]. Such disparate autopsy prevalence rates may result from the selection and preparation of the hearts as well as variations in definitions of MBs and probably also to ethnicity [6]. On average MBs are present in about one third of adults [7]. Thus, MB should not be defined as a congenital coronary anomaly, but rather as a normal variant [3]. According to some Authors superficial MBs may not be exclusively congenital in origin, but may result from adulthood disease processes that partially cover the artery with fibro-fatty connective tissue [7].

There are also myocardial loops that are thinner and derive from atrial myocardium, surround the vessel three quarters of the circumference, and return to atrial myocardium. Occasionally, a bridge may involve also a coronary vein. Both, myocardial loops and venous bridges appear to have no clinical relevance [7].

The wide variation in frequency of MBs indicates that many MBs do not produce symptoms. Subjects may become symptomatic after the third decade of life unless MBs are associated with precipitating factors (i.e. high heart rate, myocardial contractility state, hypertrophic cardiomyopathy, decreased peripheral vascular resistance). Myocardial ischemia due to MB could be attributed to a combination of the following factors: increased heart rate compromising the diastolic filling, exercise-induced spasm, and systolic kinking which may cause endothelium damage with platelet activation and thrombus formation [4, 7].

A milestone work in studying MBs is that of Ferreira *et al.* These Authors found a MB in 50 of the 90 hearts studied (55.6%) mainly on LAD. They distinguished MBs into two types. In the superficial type (75% of cases) the myocardial fibres cross the artery transversely towards the apex of the heart at an acute angle or perpendicularly. In the deep type (25% of cases) the myocardial fibres arise from the right ventricular apical trabeculae, surround the LAD with a muscle bundle that crosses the artery transversely, obliquely, or helically before terminating in the interventricular septum. In the deep variant, no direct contact occurs between the MB and the adventitial wall of the tunnelled artery. In addition, adipose, neural, and loose connective tissues are interposed between the MB and the artery. The Authors speculated that the vessel may be more distorted and compressed in the deep type of MB [8].

Some superficial MBs may be not completely covered by myocardial fibres, but by a thin layer of connective tissue, nerves and fatty tissue [7]. Obviously in these cases the systolic compression is light and may not be appreciated during angiographic studies.

Recently the use of multi-detector computed tomography (MDCT) made it possible to visualize in vivo the MBs. Konen *et al.* were moreover able to describe three types of MBs. Beside the superficial type (29% of cases) and deep type (41% of cases) described by Ferreira *et al.* the Authors characterized a third one called "right ventricular type" (29% of cases. In this type the descending coronary artery "disappears" and is visible only in the axial images where it has a course near the right ventricular wall. This type of MB seems to be more potentially pathologic and more difficult to treat surgically [5].

Myocardial bridges can be classified also depending on the thickness, the length and the number (one or more) of MBs. Obviously MBs are also classified according to the coronary artery and the segment of the coronary artery involved. The majority of MBs are in the mid portion of LAD. However MBs have been found also over the proximal and distal parts of the LAD, the diagonal and marginal branches and over the posterior interventricular branch of the LAD. Bridging of the circumflex or the right coronary artery or one of their branches is not so common [9]. In the presence of two parallel LADs one of them frequently takes an intramural course [7].

Although autopsy studies did not demonstrate any difference in the frequency of MBs by age or sex [8, 10] angiographic studies indicate that males have a higher incidence and longer MBs probably owing to a higher musculature of the body in respect to females [9, 11].

A fairly large percentage of subjects with MBs may have concomitant atherosclerotic, muscular, or valvular heart diseases, which may independently affect the clinical outcome as well as the treatment strategy [4]. Typically, the MB patients are 5 to 10 years younger than those with symptomatic coronary disease. Typical angina is present in 55% to 70% of the cases, and atypical angina is often reported in association with rest angina. The co-presence of MBs with atherosclerotic coronary artery disease should be taken into account when it is not possible to detect a culprit lesion in symptomatic patients. Although MBs have excellent prognosis even in patients with ≥ 50% systolic compression, early diagnosis and treatment are important due to their possible complications [5].

Nowadays there is a debate concerning the evaluation of asymptomatic young athletes who have a low probability to have an atherosclerotic coronary artery disease. Some of these athletes however during or just after physical exertion or in circumstances non-associated with sports, during routine daily activities, while sedentary or even asleep may have an unexpected death. In an autopsy-based registry comprising 1866 young athletes (19 ± 6 years) the cause of sudden death was in 56% of the cases due to CV disease. Of these the cause of sudden death was attributable to hypertrophic cardiomyopathy in 36% of the cases and to coronary artery anomalies in 19% of the cases (119 cases of coronary artery anomalies of wrong sinus origin and 24 cases of MBs) [2].

3. Anatomic properties of myocardial bridges

In a necropsy study Morales et al. found that hearts with MBs but with no evidence of other cardiac abnormalities had gross or microscopic alterations (or both), such as interstitial fibrosis, replacement fibrosis, contraction-band necrosis, or increased vascular density, in areas of the myocardium supplied by the bridged LAD. According to the Authors, the histologic heterogeneity of these findings, with closely interspersed patches of normal myocardium, is related to the attenuation of blood flow due to the intramural course of the vessel. These blood flow alteration may induce chronic and/or acute transient myocardial ischemia. The myocardial ischemia may be responsible of life threatening arrhythmias, such as ventricular fibrillation. In fact many of the analyzed hearts with MBs were from subjects who died of sudden death [12].

Recently several histopathologic studies clearly demonstrated that while the arterial intima beneath the MB is significantly spared from atherosclerotic changes, the segments proximal to the MB are not interested by this atherosclerosis suppression. By scanning electron microscopy the endothelial cells in the tunnelled segment had a helical, spindle-shaped orientation along the course of the segment as a sign of laminar flow and high shear. In the segments proximal to the MB the endothelium was flat, polygonal, and polymorph, indicating low shear. Low shear stress facilitates adhesion and aggregation of platelets followed by subsequent thrombosis and is associated with a release of endothelial vasoactive agents such as endothelin-1, nitric oxide synthase and angiotensin-converting enzyme which favour mass transfer of lipids into subentothelial space [13, 14]. Higher shear stress on the other side, results in lower levels of these vasoactive agents and in a suppression of lipid infiltration into subentothelial space. It has also been found that the intima beneath the bridged segment always consisted of contractile-type smooth muscle cells, while the segment proximal to the MB had synthetic-type smooth muscle cells. These types of cells usually proliferate and produce collagen fibrils and elastic fibres in the intima as atherosclerosis progresses. Moreover in the proximal segments to the MB the flow is turbulent accentuated by the retrograde blood flow caused by the "squeezing" of the MB during systole and a "sucking effect" of the proximal segment during the early phases of diastole. The increase of local wall tension and stretch in the segment proximal to MB may induce endothelial injury and plaque fissuring with subsequent thrombus formation. All these complex hemodynamic alterations may explain the atherosclerotic plaque formation, mainly eccentric, at the entrance of the tunnelled segment [4, 7, 9, 10, 14]. However, although the endothelium of MB is spared from atherosclerotic lesions its function seems to be significantly impaired as estimated by the vasoactive response to achetylcoline and increased vasoconstriction [15]. These data suggest that MB itself may have a dysfunctional endothelium, a strong atherogenic factor that can cause myocardial ischemia, chest pain, life threatening arrhythmias, and sudden cardiac death [5].

4. Angiographic findings

The current gold standard technique for diagnosing MBs is coronary angiography. Portman and Iwing in 1960 were the first to report the radiological appearance of transient stenosis in a segment of the LAD during systole in a 19 year old patient. The typical angiographic finding of a MB is a systolic narrowing of an epicardial artery, known also as a "milking effect" phenomenon induced by systolic compression of the tunnelled segment. Another angiographic finding is the presence of the "step down-step up" appearance, namely, a significant tortuosity of the segment beneath MB at the entrance (step-down) and the exit (step-up) sites [4, 10] (Fig 1).

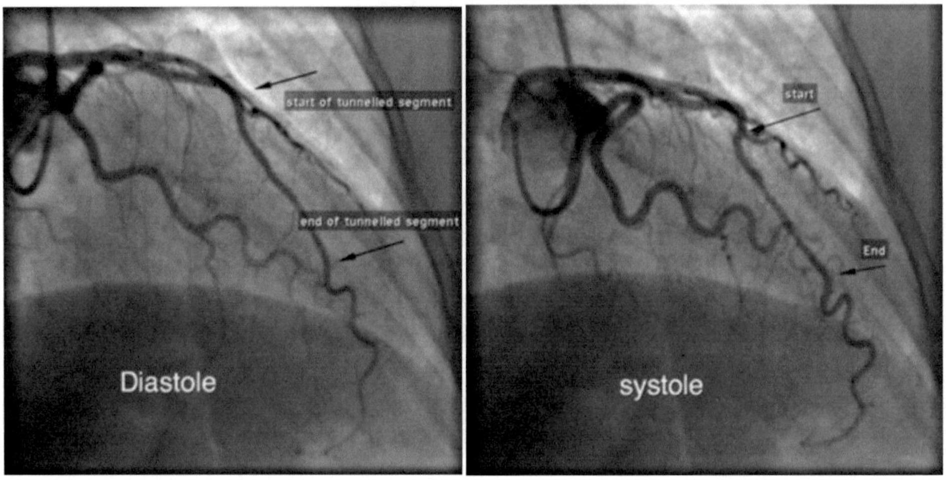

Figure 1. Myocardial bridging on conventional coronary angiography in diastole and systole. Compression at the middle of the left descending coronary artery occurs during systole with a clear step-down and step us phenomenon. Arrows indicate the beginning and the end of the tunnelled segment. The left descending coronary artery and the circumflex artery are free of atherosclerotic lesions.

The systolic compression is usually eccentric rather than concentric [11]. However, also the diastole is compromised. In fact measurements in patients with MB have shown a persistent diastolic diameter reduction enduring mid diastole. In a series of 42 patients a mean maximum systolic diameter reduction of 71% was found with a persistent reduction of 35% during mid diastole, while 12% of patients showed a reduction of more than 50% in mid diastole [16]. Almost the same results were found by Bourassa et al. in a frame-by-frame analysis of cine-angiograms during a complete cardiac cycle. The Authors were able to demonstrate that 17 of 20 patients (85%) with a ≥ 75% milking effect of the LAD had an extension of the obstruction into diastole, which averaged 136 ms or 26% (range 4% to 50%) of diastole [4]. In borderline cases intracoronary nitroglycerine administration may uncover the systolic coronary compression. The milking effect is evaluated as grade I when the narrowing is less than 50%, grade II when it is between 50 and 75%, and grade III when it is greater than 75% [4].

The frequency of MBs reported in angiographic studies varies from 0.5 to 33%. This wide variation at angiography may in part be attributable to technologic advances in cine-angiography; to the orientation of the coronary artery and myocardial fibres; to the state of myocardial contractility; to the fact that small and thin bridges cause little compression badly detectable during angiography specially with no previous percentage of systolic narrowing specified for the designation of MB; if the study was retrospectively reviewed for the specific purpose of assessing the frequency of MBs; to sample size and finally to different population selection and probably also to ethnicity. In patients with MBs chest pain is the common reason for angiography. At angiography the mid portion of the LAD is the most frequently affected vessel.

http://dx.doi.org/10.5772/54083

A limit of ICA is that it estimates coronary artery diameter as a percent by comparing it with the adjacent segment, which arbitrarily is considered normal. This visual procedure to estimate lesions has a high degree of intra and inter-observer variability. These limits have been reduced by improving the software (quantitative coronary angiography) and hardware (flat panel digital detectors) of angiographs.

5. Intravascular ultrasound, intracoronary Doppler and intracoronary pressure

The performance of ICA increased with the introduction of important tools such as intravascular coronary ultrasound (IVUS), that for the first time visualized, in vivo, both vessel lumen and walls, intracoronary Doppler-ultrasound and intracoronary pressure-wire. These tools increased our understanding of the morphological and functional features of MBs.

Although its anatomy and physiology are not fully understood the "half moon phenomenon" is a characteristic and highly specific IVUS observation of MBs as it is only found in the tunnelled segments, but not in the proximal or distal segments of the vessel or in other arteries. The "half moon phenomenon" appears as an echolucent area surrounding the bridge segment. In the presence of a "half-moon phenomenon" the milking effect can be induced by intracoronary provocation tests, such as intracoronary nitroglycerin injection, even if the bridge was previously angiographically undetectable [11]. Ultrasound pullback studies confirmed the histological findings of absence of atherosclerosis within the tunnelled segments, whereas there was a plaque in the segment proximal to the MB in about 90% of subjects. None of these proximal atherosclerotic lesions detected by IVUS has been seen on angiography confirming the known superiority of IVUS on angiography in detecting atherosclerotic plaques [11].

In presence of MB the pullback of the intracoronary Doppler (0.0014 inch wire) reveals a characteristic flow pattern: "fingertip phenomenon" or "spike-and-dome pattern" which is present in most of the patients with MBs. This flow pattern described by Ge et al. [17] can be observed within and just proximal to the tunnelled segment and consists in a sharp acceleration of flow in early diastole followed by immediate marked deceleration and a mid to late diastolic pressure plateau. The Authors explain this flow pattern as an increase in the pressure gradient in the early diastole as a result of reduced distal coronary resistance while there is a delay in the relaxation of the myocardial fibres. The subsequent sharp deceleration in the coronary flow velocity results from the relaxation of the myocardial fibres and an increase in the vascular lumen. After the release of the compression, the lumen of the bridge segment remains unchanged in the second half of diastole and this corresponds to the plateau of the flow pattern at this phase. In deep myocardial bridges, rapid diastolic forward flow may be preceded by end-systolic flow inversion as a result of systolic squeezing of the bridge segment. In the subjects where the "fingertip phenomenon" is not present (13% of cases) this may be related to the fact that the bridging segment was not so severe to induce the hemodynamic disorders that lead to the "fingertip phenomenon" formation [17]. The consequence of these phenomena is that in the segment proximal to the MB the pressure can become even higher than that in the aorta. At the entrance of the MB the high wall stress and disturbance in blood flow promote atherosclerosis [17]. Finally in subjects with MBs the coronary flow reserves, defined as the ratio of mean flow velocity achieved at peak hyperemia obtained after intracoronary injection of papaverine or adenosine to mean resting flow velocity, is frequently reduced (2.0-2.6), values below 3.0, which is regarded as the lower normal limit [4].

6. Cardiac computed tomography

The introduction of multidetector row systems in the field of cardiac computed tomography (CCT) has made imaging of the heart and in particular of epicardial coronary arteries feasible. In the last two decades CCT has been used to study different group of subjects becoming in some cases the new "gold standard technique" instead of invasive coronary angiography (ICA), because of it's ability to visualize correctly coronary arteries and most interestingly to obtain this information non-invasively [18, 19, 20].

In particular CCT is widely used to study coronary artery anomalies. In fact ICA has some limits as it provides a few 2D view images of the coronary arteries and sometimes it fails to clearly visualize the relationship between the coronary vessels and the surrounding structures. With ICA it is not always easy to selectively engage the anomalous coronary vessel, which may lead to the erroneous assumption that the coronary vessel is occluded. In addition with this traditional 2D technique is more difficult to understand the course of the coronary vessels within the heart and discern the anterior versus the posterior direction of the anomalous vessels. On the other side CCT provides an unlimited number of 2D reformatted images as well as 3D images of the single vessel making it possible to have a 3D depiction of the whole heart [19].

The CCT information is very useful to the surgeon as it helps him to plan the surgery by seeing the exact course of the vessel and its relationship within the heart and with the other intra-thoracic organs and chest wall [19]. In addition, in case of extensive and deep MB there may be a technical challenge during coronary arterial bypass. The intramuscular coronary artery may be difficult to localize and may require the use of intraoperative echocardiographic Doppler to explore the coronary artery to avoid, for example, accidental opening of the right ventricle during dissection of intramuscular LAD. It has also been suggested that a preoperative diagnosis of MBs on CCT may help in planning the surgery strategy allowing a key information for selecting the standard midsternotomy with or without cardiopulmonary bypass (coronary artery bypass graft or off-pump coronary bypass graft, respectively) or a minimally invasive approach through the small left anterior thoracotomy [5].

In the recent American Appropriate Use Criteria Task Force for CCT, the use of CCT in the "assessment of anomalies of coronary arterial and other thoracic arteriovenous vessels" was pointed to be most appropriate (i.e. the test is acceptable and considered a reasonable ap-

http://dx.doi.org/10.5772/54083

proach to study the disease and its expected incremental information, combined with clinical judgment exceeds the expected negative consequences by a sufficiently wide margin) with a score of 9 out of 9 [20].

Cardiac computed tomography has however some important limits that must be considered. Invasive coronary angiography is still superior over CCT because it has, for the moment, a higher spatial (<0.16 mm vs approximately 0.4 mm of CCT) as well as temporal resolution (33 msec. vs 140 to 200 msec. of the recent cardiac computed systems or 83 msec. of the dual source system). Another limit of CCT present also with the currently available 64 channel systems is related to patient's heart rate which must be rhythmic and around or less than 60-64 beats per minute. Patients with atrial fibrillation or with a heart rate that can not be reduced to a rate of 60-64 beats per minute, for the moment, are not eligible to undergo this kind of examination. The introduction of new tools like the "ECG-tube current modulation" and the "step and shoot" procedures and the 128, 256, 320 and 640 channel or dual source scanners offers the possibility to study also patients with higher heart rates and with atrial fibrillation, making it possible to image the entire heart not only, as it is now, in a single breath hold, but in a single heartbeat [19]. Moreover less than or equal to 5% of patients have a un-valuable CCT scans due to motion artefacts, because the patient cannot follow breathing commands, involuntary motion of the diaphragm or because the patient is overweigh or has respiratory problems.

Particular attention must be also given to the dose of radiation delivered to patients. In the commonly used CCT systems the amount of radiation, expressed as units of millisieverts (equivalent to millijoules per kilogram of tissue), absorbed by patients during the test is 2-4 folds that of ICA [19]. However the introduction of improvements in CCT technologies decreased significantly the radiation dose to equal almost that of traditional coronary angiography [21]. Finally it is worth noting that both ICA and CCT use non-ionic contrast medium to visualize coronary artery lumen. For this reason particular attention must be given in allergic patients and in patients with a pre-existing renal impairment [19].

While studying MBs it is also important to consider that CCT analysis are mainly performed with images reconstructed during diastole (70-80% of the cardiac cycle) when there is the maximal vasodilatation and minimal motion artifacts. Conversely maximal lumen narrowing of MB is during the systolic phase (30-40% of cardiac cycle) where usually there are more motion artifacts. To better evaluate patient's MB it is therefore important to analyze the whole cardiac cycle, but good quality CCT images in both the diastolic and systolic phases are obtained only with the more recent CCT machines.

7. Myocardial bridges and cardiac computed tomography

For the final interpretation of MBs conventional post-processing tools are used, namely: cross-sectional imaging, multiplanar reconstructions (MPR), curved MPR (cMPR), maximum intensity projections (MIP) and three-dimension volume rendering (Fig 2).

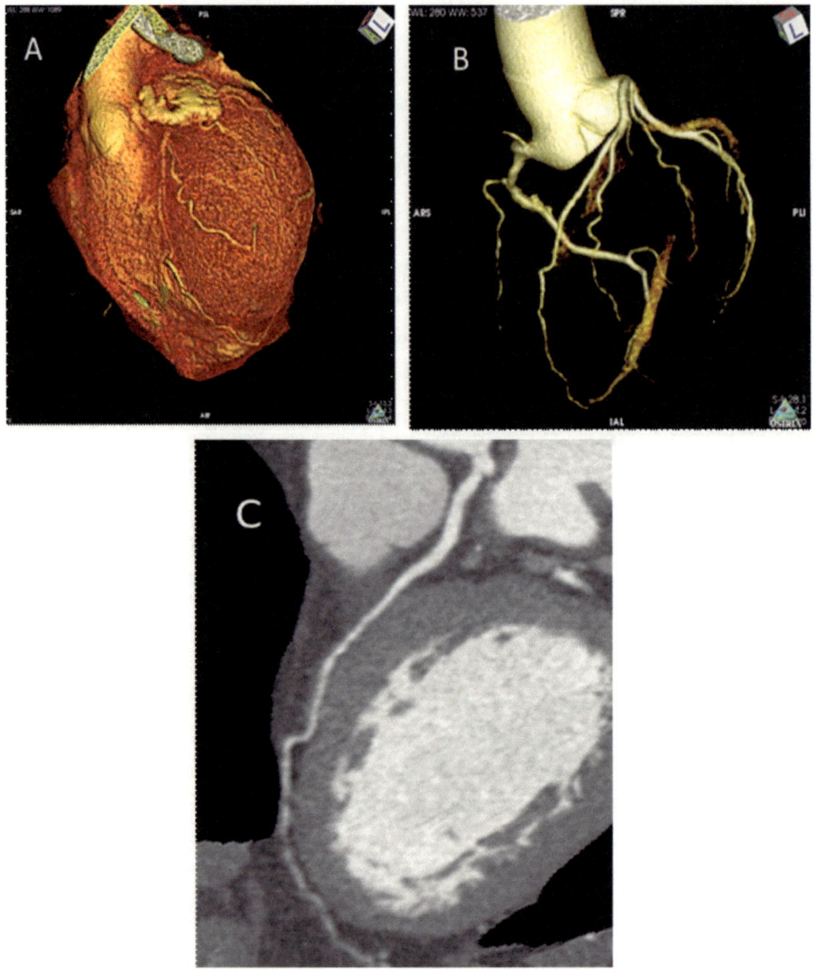

Figure 2. Myocardial bridging at 64 multi-detector computed tomography. Volume rendering image of the heart (A). 3D image of the coronary tree (B). Multiplanar reconstructed image of the left descending coronary artery. The middle segment of the vessel is tunnelled by overlying myocardium (C). It is clearly evident the step up phenomenon.

The high temporal resolution obtained with the most recent scanners or dual source scanners enable the visualization of the vessel lumen during most of the cardiac cycle, and thus permit the observation of the milking effect in the 4-dimensional reconstruction [22]. Cardiac computed tomography helped to better evaluate the anatomical properties of MB. Several Authors using CCT confirmed what was already know from necropsies, CCA and IVUS studies that the tunnelled segments are spared from atherosclerotic changes [23]. However Zeina et al. found that the thickness and length of the bridge correlated with the presence of stenosis in the LAD proximal to the MB suggesting that the MB may predispose to the development of atherosclerosis in the coronary artery segment proximal to the bridge and that MB should be considered an anatomic risk factor in the evaluation of coronary artery disease patients [23]. Also Takamura et al. demonstrated that, in patients with culprit lesions in the LAD segment proximal to MB, the length and thickness of MBs were significantly greater, and the distance from the orifice of the left coronary artery to the entrance of MB was significantly shorter than those in patients with no culprit lesion in the LAD segment proximal to MB [24]. These results are similar to those of the autopsy studies that demonstrated that the anatomical properties of MB muscle were closely associated with a shift of coronary intimal lesion more proximally, an effect that may increase the risk of myocardial infarction [14].

Since the introduction of CCT in the last decade of last century many papers have been published showing the feasibility of CCT in evaluating patients with MB (Fig 3).

In particular many papers compared CCT to ICA. Recently a significant correlation was found between the within-MB diameters obtained with CCT and ICA during the systolic (1.3±0.3 mm vs. 1.2±0.5 mm: r= 0.394, P=0.028) and diastolic phases (1.4±0.4 mm vs. 1.6±0.6 mm: r= 0.524, P=0.001) [25]. However CCT is superior to ICA in diagnosing the presence of MB. Kim et al. found that while dynamic compression was present in 13.3% of the subjects (40/300) who underwent ICA, CCT revealed that 58% of the subjects (178/300) had myocardial bridging (partial encasement in 57 and full encasement in 117 subjects) [26]. Leschka et al. found that MB was revealed with CCT and ICA respectively in 26 and 12 of the 100 subjects studied [27].

When comparing CCT with IVUS, the sensitivity of detecting MB by CCT was found to be 93%, specificity 100%, positive predictive value and negative predictive value 100% and 91% respectively. A significant correlation was also observed between lumen diameters derived from CCT and IVUS (systolic phase: r=0.87, P<0.05; diastolic phase: r=0.92, P<0.05). Although minimal and maximal diameters of MB during systolic and diastolic phases derived from CCT were significantly smaller than those from IVUS (2.4±0.4 mm vs 2.6±0.5 mm, P<0.05) and (2.9±0.3 mm vs 3.3±0.3 mm, P<0.05) the narrowing percent derived from the two methods was similar ((21.4±10.9% vs 17.4±7.6%, P>0.05). The Authors however note that CCT offers a safer, more comfortable and cost-effective examinations (in China the prices of IVUS and MSCT are 1500 US $ and 95 US $ respectively [28].

Usually in the CCT studies where MB is evaluated the coronary arteries are classified according to the American Heart Association classification system: right coronary artery: 1, proximal; 2, mid; 3, distal; 4a, posterior descending; 4b, posterolateral; left main coronary artery: 5, LAD; 6, proximal; 7, mid; 8, distal; 9, first diagonal; 10, second diagonal; circumflex coronary artery: 11, proximal; 12, first marginal; 13, mid; 14, second marginal; 15, distal.

All studied performed the evaluation of MB mainly in the diastolic phase while a few studies performed it in the systolic phase due to technical problems related to the increased motion of the heart due to myocardial contraction in the systolic phase and to the limited temporal resolution of routinely available scanners [5, 22, 27, 29].

In the literature there is not a consensus in the definition of MB. Usually MB is defined as the existence of tissues exhibiting soft tissue density covering a part of the vessel, which had the same contrast enhancement as myocardial tissue [24].

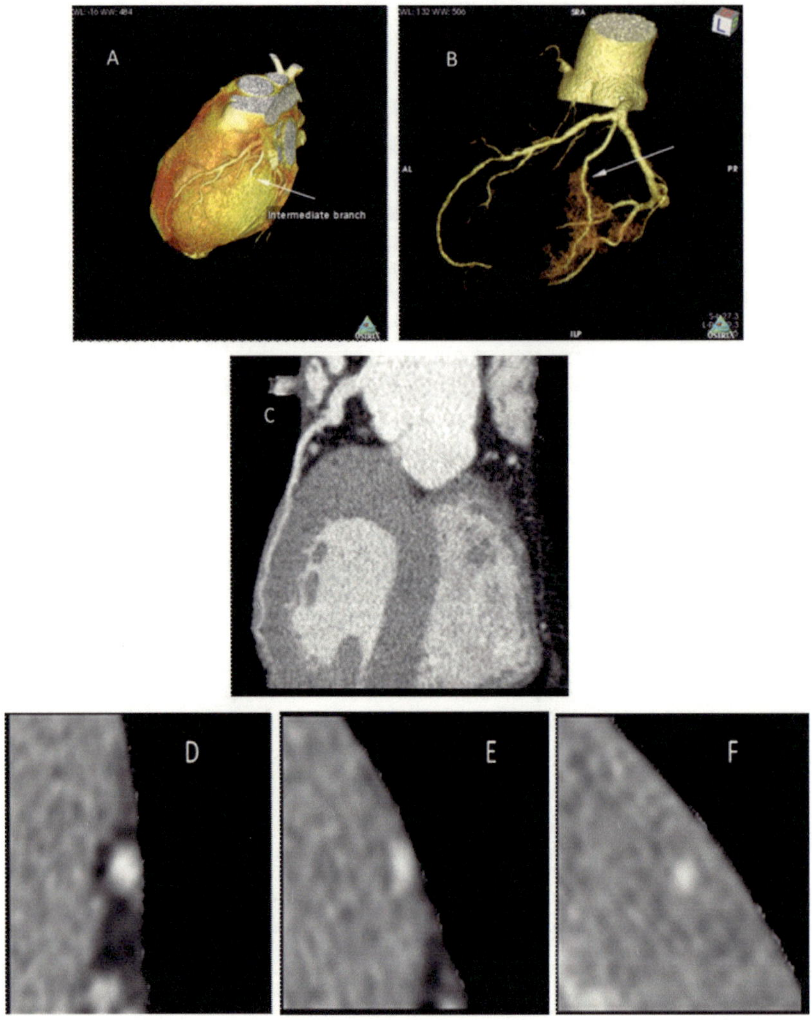

Figure 3. Myocardial bridging at 64 multi-detector computed tomography. Volume rendering image of the heart (A). 3D image of the coronary tree (B). Multiplanar reconstructed image of intermediate branch which is tunnelled by overlying myocardium (C). While in D the vessel has an epicardial course in E and especially F the vessel is completely encompassed by the myocardium.

The length of MB is usually defined as the distance of the covering myocardial tissue from the entrance to the exit of the tunnelled artery, which is measured by curved MPR images (i.e. parallel to the course of the vessel) [24].

There are several definitions to describe the depth of MB. In the majority of the papers the depth is defined as the thickness of the deepest part from the surface of the covering myocardial tissue to the tunnelled artery, which is measured in an axial image (i.e. perpendicular to the course of the vessel) (Fig. 3) [24]. Myocardial bridges were divided into two types: superficial and deep. In the superficial type a myocardial band overlies the vessel with no de-

http://dx.doi.org/10.5772/54083

viation of the vessel into the myocardium. In the deep type the vessel dips as a U-shaped curve into the myocardium [30]. Another classification divided MB in complete or incomplete. The complete types of MB were those where it was possible to demonstrate the continuity of myocardium over the tunnelled segment [31].

Another definition of superficial and deep MB was given by Jodecy et al. These Authors defined the MB as "deep" when the vessel was surrounded entirely by myocardium in depth of a more than 2 mm, whereas it was defined as "superficial" when the vessel appeared either not entirely surrounded (but with a minimum of 75% of the circumference), or entirely surrounded by myocardium in less than 2 mm depth [29].

Author [reference]	type of MDCT	number of pts (% of MB)	% of MB in LAD	length mean (range)	depth mean (range)
Kawaka et al. [34]	16 slices	148 (26)	91	20±8.6 (10.5-50.2)	1.8±0.7 (1.1-3.7)
Kantraci et al. [35]	16 slices	626 (3.5)	100	17 (6-22)	2.5 (1.2-3.3)
Ko et al. [36]	16 slices	401 (5.7)	91	15.7 (5-27)	3.2 (1.0-7.0)
Canyigit et al. [31]	16 slices	280 (38.5)	81.6	15.8 (4-50.9)	1.7 (1-6.4)
Chen et al. [37]	16 slices	276 (8.7)	76.7	24.6±11.8 (5.2-50.6)	3.7±1.9 (0.5-9.1)
Takamura et al. [24]	16 slices	228 (18.8)	100	20.0 (2.4-54.7)	1.7 (0.4-9.7)
Zeina et al. [23]	16/64 slices	300 (15.8)	87.5	19.5±5.7 (8-30)	2±0.6 (1-3.1)
Konen et al. [5]	40/64 slices	118 (30.5)	72	23±9 (13-50)	(0.1-6.2)
Lubarsky et al. [38]	64 slices	245 (44)	100	28.7±16.5	NA
Johansen et al. [32]	64 slices	152 (32)	69.4	NA	NA
Kim PJ et al. [26]	64 slices	300 (58)	100	29.1±15.5	1.4±1.0
Leschka et al. [27]	64 slices	100 (26)	98	24.3±10 (8-53)	2.6±0.8 (1.4-4.8)
Koşar et al. [39]	64 slices	700 (37)	NA	NA	NA
Kim SY et al. [30]	64 slices	607 (6.4)	84.2	16.3±6.3 (6.9-30)	1.8±0.8 (0.5-3.9)
Jeong et al. [25]	64 slices	120 (25)	47.4	20.5±6.8 (8-35)	2.3±1.2 (0.8-6.6)
Jodocy et al. [29]	64 slices	221 (23)	91	14.9±6.5 (2.5-43.8)	2.6±1.6 (0.5-9.4)
La Grutta et al. [40]	64 slices	254 (29)	93	NA	NA
Wrianta et al. [33]	64 slices	934 (16.3)	94	NA	NA
Jacobs et al. [41]	64 slices-DSCT	506 (10.4)	96	23.4 (4.1-53.9)	2.6 (1-7.8)
Lu et al. [22]	DSCT	53 (39.6)	57	23.2±9.5	3.5±1.0
Hwang et al. [42]	DSCT	1275 (42)	100	21.0±11.6	3.0±1.4

MDCT: multidetector computed tomography; pts: patients; MB: myocardial bridges; LAD left anterior descending coronary artery; NA : non available; DSCT: dual source computer tomography.

Table 1. Cardiac computed tomography papers where myocardial bridges were evaluated

Arterial segments located in a deep gorge but covered only by a thin layer of muscle or fibrous-fatty tissue were also considered by some Authors as MB because they also may be compressed during systole by the surrounding muscle [5]. According to other Authors the presence of myocardial bridging was defined as myocardium completely encompassing a section of coronary artery in at least one transverse image [32]. For Wirianta et al. MB was defined when at least half of the coronary artery was imbedded within the myocardium with a normal epicardial course of the proximal and distal portion [33].

The prevalence of MB according to CCT studies increased progressively with the introduction of more modern scanners approaching values found in autopsy studies, which should be considered the ultimate gold standard method, rather than the results obtained in the ICA studies. This wide variation may be related to different reasons: differences between temporal and spatial resolution parameters of the scanners; different post processing techniques; different inclusion or exclusion of borderline cases; retrospective observation of arteries with the specific purpose to analyze MB; different population selection (i.e presence of symptomatic or asymptomatic patients, patients with hypertrophic cardiomyopathy); probably also to ethnicity (Tab 1).

8. Conclusion

Myocardial bridges are normal variants of intrinsic coronary arterial anatomy with an intramural course that till 20 years ago were visualized during necropsies, surgery or conventional coronary angiography. Invasive coronary angiography alone or with the use of important tools such as intravascular coronary ultrasound, intracoronary Doppler-ultrasound and intracoronary pressure-wire, is still considered the gold standard technique to study in vivo MBs. The introduction in the cardiac arena of CCT, that with very good accuracy investigates coronary arteries, gave us a complementary and sometimes an alternative test to ICA and more interestingly provides this information non-invasively. In particular settings such as that of a coronary artery with MB, CCT seems to be even superior to ICA and to have results similar to autopsy which is the real gold standard technique to evaluate MBs. However to better understand the real usefulness of CCT in this particular field, further multi-centric interdisciplinary studies must be performed, to link the morphological with the clinical information especially in those patients who have MB and normal coronary arteries or coronary arteries with no culprit atherosclerotic lesions, but who may be at risk for cardiovascular morbidity or mortality.

Acknowledgements

We gratefully thank the radiology team of Fanfani Clinical Research Institute (Florence, Italy) and in particular Dr. Fabio Fanfani, the Cardiopulmonary Radiological Research group of CNR Institute of Clinical Physiology of Pisa (Italy) and the Fondazione Monasterio of Pisa

http://dx.doi.org/10.5772/54083

(Italy), for their collaboration, Dr. Alessandro Mazzarisi for the technical support and Dr. Haifa Alsakkaf for the assistance with the manuscript.

Author details

Mohamed Bamoshmoosh[1,2*] and Paolo Marraccini[3]

*Address all correspondence to: bamoshmoosh@hotmail.it

1 Fanfani Clinical Research Institute, Florence, Italy

2 University of Science and Technology, Sana'a, Yemen

3 CNR Institute of Clinical Physiology, Pisa, Italy

References

[1] Lopez AD, Mathers CD, Ezzati M, Jamison DT, Murray CJL. Global and regional burden of disease and risk factors, 2001: systematic analysis of population health data. Lancet 2006; 367: 1747-57

[2] Maron BJ, MD, Doerer JJ, Haas TS, Tierney DM, Mueller FO. Sudden deaths in young competitive athletes. Circulation 2009; 119: 1085-1092

[3] Angelini P, Velasco JA, Flamm S. Coronary anomalies: incidence, pathophysiology, and clinical relevance. Circulation 2002; 105: 2449-2454

[4] Bourassa MG, Butnaru A, Lespérance J, Tardif JC. Symptomatic myocardial bridges: overview of ischemic mechanisms and current diagnostic and treatment strategies. J Am Coll Cardiol 2003; 41: 351-9

[5] Konen E, Goitein O, Sternik L, Eshet Y, Shemseh J, Di Segni E. The prevalence and anatomical patterns of intramuscular coronary arteries. J Am Coll Cardiol 2007; 49: 587-93

[6] Saidi H, Ongeti WK, Ogeng.o J. Morphology of human myocardial bridges and association with coronary artery disease. African Health Sciences 2010; 10: 242-247

[7] Möhlenkamp S, Hort W, Ge J, Erbel R. Update on myocardial bridging. Circulation 2002; 106: 2616-2622

[8] Ferreira Jr AG, Trotter SE, Konig Jr B, Decourt LV, Fox K, Olsen EGJ. Myocardial bridges: morphological and functional aspects. Br Heart J 1991; 66: 364-7

[9] Loukas M, Von Kriegenbergh K, Gilkes M, Tubbs RS, Walker C, Malaiyand D, Anderson RH. Myocardial bridges: a review. Clinical Anatomy 2011; 24: 675-683

[10] Alegria JR, Herrmann J, Holmes Jr DR, Lerman A, Rihal CS. Myocardial bridging. European Heart Journal 2005: 26, 1159-1168

[11] Ge J, Jeremias A, Rupp A, Abels M, Baumgart D, Liu F, Haude M, Gorge G, von Birgelen C, Sack S Erbel R. New signs characteristic of myocardial bridging demonstrated by intracoronary ultrasound and Doppler. European Heart Journal 1999; 20: 1707-16

[12] Morales AR, Romanelli R, Tate LG, Boucek RJ, De Marchena E. Intramural left anterior descending coronary artery. Significance of the depth of the muscular tunnel. Human Pathology 1993; 27: 693-700

[13] Masuda T, Ishikawa Y, Akasaka Y, Itoh K, Kiguchi H, Ishii T. The effect of myocardial bridging of the coronary artery on vasoactive agents and atherosclerosis localization. J Pathol 2001; 193: 408-414

[14] Ishikawa Y, Akasaka Y, Ito K, Akishima Y, Kimura M, Kiguchi H, Fujimoto A, Ishii T. Significance of anatomical properties of myocardial bridge on atherosclerosis evolution in the left anterior descending coronary artery. Atherosclerosis 2006; 186: 380-389

[15] Kim JW, Seo HS, Na JO, Suh SY, Choi CU, Kim EJ, Rha S-W, Park CG, Oh DJ. Myocardial bridging is related to endothelial dysfunction but not to plaque as assessed by intracoronary ultrasound. Heart 2008; 94: 765-769.

[16] Schwarz E, Klues HG, Vom Dahl J, Klein I, Krebs W, Hanrath P. Functional, angiographic and intracoronary Doppler flow characteristics in symptomatic patients with myocardial bridging: effect of short-term tntravenous beta-blocker medication. J Am Coll Cardiol 1996; 27; 1637-45

[17] Ge J, Erbel R, G6rge G, Haude M, Meyer J. High wall shear stress proximal to myocardial bridging and atherosclerosis: intracoronary ultrasound and pressure measurements. Br Heart J 1995; 73: 462-465

[18] Bamoshmoosh M. When cardiac computed tomography becomes the gold standard technique to evaluate coronary artery disease patients. In: Baskot B (ed.) Coronary angiography. Advance in non invasive imaging approach for evaluation coronary artery disease Rijeka: InTech; 2011. p199-214.

[19] Mark DB, Berman DS, Budoff MJ, Carr JJ, Gerber TC, Hecht HS, Hlatky MA, Hodgson JM, Lauer MS, Miller JM, Morin RL, Mukherjee D, Poon M. Rubin GD, Schwartz RS. ACCF/ACR/AHA/NASCI/SAIP/SCAI/SCCT 2010 Expert Consensus Document on Coronary Computed Tomographic Angiography. J Am Coll Cardiol 2010; 55: 2663-99

[20] Taylor AJ, Cerqueira M, Hodgson JM, Mark D, Min J, O'Gara P, Rubin GD. ACCF/SCCT/ACR/AHA/ASE/ASNC/NASCI/SCAI/SCMR 2010 appropriate use criteria for cardiac computed tomography. J Am Coll Cardiol 2010; 56: 1864-94

[21] Hausleiter J, Meyer T, Hadamitzky M, Huber E, Zankl M, Martinoff S, Kastrati A, Schömig A. Radiation dose estimates from cardiac multislice computed tomography in daily practice: impact of different scanning protocols on effective dose estimates. Circulation 2006; 113: 1305-10

[22] Lu G-M, Zhan L-J, Guo H, Huang W, Merges RD. Comparison of myocardial bridging by dual-source CT with conventional coronary angiography. Circ J 2008; 72: 1079-1085

[23] Zeina A-R, Odeh M, Blinder J, Rosenschein U, Barmeir E. Myocardial bridge: evaluation on MDCT. American Journal of Radiology 2007; 188: 1069-1073

[24] Takamura K, Fujimoto S, Nanjo S, Nakanishi R, Hisatake S, Namiki A, Ishikawa Y, Ishii T, Yamazaki J. Anatomical characteristics of myocardial bridge in patients with myocardial infarction by multi-detector computed tomography. Circ J 2011; 75: 642-648

[25] Jeong Y-H, Kang M-K, Park S-R, Kang Y-R, Choi H-C, Hwang S-J, Jeon K-N, Kwak CH, Hwang J-Y. A head-to-head comparison between 64-slice multidetector computed tomographic and conventional coronary angiographies in measurement of myocardial bridge. International Journal of Cardiology 2010; 143: 243-248

[26] Kim PJ, Hur G, Kim SY, Namgung J, Hong SW, Kim YH, Lee WR. Frequency of myocardial bridges and dynamic compression of epicardial coronary arteries. Circulation 2009; 119: 1408-1416

[27] Leschka S, Koepfli P, Husmann L, Plass A, Vachenauer R, Gaemperli O, Schepis T, Genoni M, Marincek B, Eberli FR, Kaufmann PA, Alkadhi H. Myocardial bridging: depiction rate and morphology at CT coronary angiography-comparison with conventional coronary angiography. Radiology 2008; 246:754-762

[28] Wang M-H, Sun A-J, Qian J-Y, Ling Q-Z, Zeng M-S, Ge L, Wang K-Q, Fan B, Yan W, Zhang F, Erberl R, Ge J. Myocardial bridging detection by non-invasive multislice spiral computed tomography: comparison with intravascular ultrasound. Chinese Medical Journal 2008; 121: 17-21

[29] Jodocy D, Aglan I, Friedrich G, Mallouhi A, Pachinger O, Jaschke W, Feuchtner GM. Left anterior descending coronary artery myocardial bridging by multislice computed tomography: Correlation with clinical findings. European Journal of Radiology 2010; 73: 89-95

[30] Kim SY, Lee YS, Lee JB, Ryu JK, Choi YI, Chang SG, Kim K-S. Evaluation of myocardial bridge with multidetector computed tomography. Circ J 2010; 74: 137-141

[31] Canyigit M, Hazirolan T, Karcaaltincaba M, Dagoglu MG, Akata D, Aytemir K, Oto A, Balkanci F, Akpinar E, Besim A. Myocardial bridging as evaluated by 16 row MDCT. European Journal of Radiology 2009; 69: 156-164

[32] Johansen C, Kirsch J, Araoz P, Williamson E. Detection of myocardial bridging by 64 row computed tomography angiography of the coronaries. J Comput Assist Tomogr 2008; 32: 448-451

[33] Wirianta J, Mouden M, Ottervanger JP, Timmer JR, Juwana YB, de Boer MJ, Suryapranata H. Prevalence and predictors of bridging of coronary arteries in a large Indonesian population, as detected by 64-slice computed tomography scan. Neth Heart J Published online 06 June 2012. DOI 10.1007/s12471-012-0296-4

[34] Kawawaa Y, Ishikawa Y, Gomia T, Nagamotoa M, Terada H, Ishii T, Kohda E. Detection of myocardial bridge and evaluation of its anatomical properties by coronary multislice spiral computed tomography. European Journal of Radiology 2007; 61: 130-138

[35] Kantarci M, Duran C, Durur I, Alper F, Onbas O, Gulbaran M, Okur A. Detection of myocardial bridging with ECG-Gated MDCT and multiplanar reconstruction. American Journal of Radiology 2006; 186: S391-S394

[36] Ko S-M, Choi J-S, Nam C-W, Hur S-H. Incidence and clinical significance of myocardial bridging with ECG-gated 16-row MDCT coronary angiography. Int J Cardiovasc Imaging 2008; 24: 445-452

[37] Chen Y-D, Wu M-H, Sheu M-H, Chang Y-C. Myocardial bridging in Taiwan: depiction by multidetector computed tomography coronary angiography. J Formos Med Assoc 2009; 108: 469-474

[38] Lubarsky L, Gupta MP, Hecht HS. Evaluation of myocardial bridging of the left anterior descending coronary artery by 64-Slice multidetector computed tomographic angiography. Am J Cardiol 2007; 100: 1081-1082

[39] Koşar P, Ergun E, Öztürk C, Koşar U. Anatomic variations and anomalies of the coronary arteries: 64-slice CT angiographic appearance. Diagn Interv Radiol 2009; 15: 275–283

[40] La Grutta L, Runza G, Galia M, Maffei E, Lo Re G, Grassedonio E, Tedeschi C, Cademartiri F, Midiri M. Atherosclerotic pattern of coronary myocardial bridging assessed with CT coronary angiography. Int J Cardiovasc Imaging 2012; 28: 405-414

[41] Jacobs JE, Bod J, Kim DC, Hecht EM, Srichai MB. Myocardial bridging: evaluation using single and dual-source multidetector cardiac computed tomographic angiography. J Comput Assist Tomogr 2008; 32: 242-246

[42] Hwang JH, Ko SM, Roh HG, Song MG, Shin JK, Chee HK, Kim JS. Myocardial bridging of the left anterior descending coronary artery: depiction rate and morphologic features by dual-source CT coronary angiography. Korean J Radiol 2010; 11: 514-521

Percutaneous. Recanalization of Chronic Total Occlusion (CTO) Coronary Arteries: Looking Back and Moving Forward

Simona Giubilato, Salvatore Davide Tomasello and Alfredo Ruggero Galassi

Additional information is available at the end of the chapter

http://dx.doi.org/10.5772/54079

1. Introduction

Chronic total occlusion (CTO) of coronary arteries is one of the most challenging PCI, usually defined as more than three-month-old obstruction of a native coronary artery. This coronary lesion subset is a frequent finding in patients with coronary artery disease (CAD) as CTOs have been reported in approximately one-third of patients undergoing diagnostic coronary angiography. However only 7-15% of CTOs were treated with percutaneous coronary intervention (PCI) [1] (Figure 1). Perhaps for the fact that procedural success is hampered by the difficulties associated with crossing and/or dilating the occluded segment with guidewires and recanalization devices and by a high incidence of restenosis and reocclusion.

Despite these obstacles, several studies have documented that successful PCI of CTOs leads to an improvement in anginal status, normalization of functional tests, improvement of left ventricular function and avoidance of coronary artery bypass graft surgery (CABG) [2-6]. Patients with untreated CTOs face a threefold increase in cardiac mortality or complications in case of future acute events [7-9].

Historically, a procedural success rate of 60-70% was achieved using anterograde approach [6]. Nowadays, specifically trained operators are able to improve the rate of CTO recanalization thanks to several new techniques and dedicated device developments. In particular, the retrograde CTO PCI approach, that was first mastered by Japanese operators, has evolved rapidly, resulting in higher success rates, shortened procedural time and reduced exposure to radiation.

It should keep in mind that reopening of a CTO needs to be carefully considered in the presence of symptoms or objective evidence of viability/ischaemia in the territory of the occluded artery.

The aim of this chapter will be to provide a systematic overview of the current state-of-the art in percutaneous recanalization of CTO, to enhance the understanding of this complex procedure and, consequently, promote safe and effective PCI for patients who present with this lesion subset. Specifically, after a brief introduction about CTO anatomy and definitions, the chapter will be divided into five paragraphs that address the most important clinical and technical aspects of CTO PCI. In the first paragraph the complex clinical CTO decision-making process will be described. This crucial step consists in the evaluation of clinical indication, patient selection and revascularization strategies. In the second paragraph, specific tools for CTO recanalization will be illustrated focusing on improvements in guidewire and dedicate device technology, responsible for improved procedural success in PCI of CTO. A further paragraph will be dedicated to the stent choice for the treatment of CTO. In fact, there is overwhelming evidence in the literature that drug eluting stent (DES) rather than bare metal stent (BMS) reduce significantly the restenosis and reocclusion rates after recanalization of CTOs. The fourth paragraph, will deal with the description of all techniques to cross CTO by anterograde and retrograde techniques. In this paragraph, the attention will be focused on common pitfalls and difficulties and related tips and tricks. Finally, the last paragraph will be focused on the strategies to prevent and treat the possible procedural complications including complications related to vascular access or to procedure such as coronary dissection, perforation or rupture and coronary thrombosis.

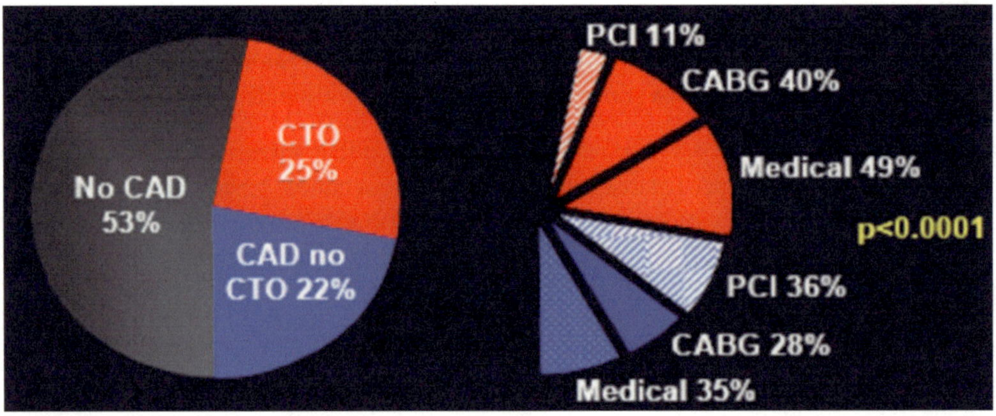

Figure 1. Diagnostic catheterization results stratified by treatment strategy. Adapted from Christofferson et al. [1]

http://dx.doi.org/10.5772/54079

2. CTO anatomy and definitions

A deeper understanding of CTO histopathology might offer insights into the development of new techniques and procedural strategies. The occluded part of the lumen in CTOs consists of two types of tissue: atheromatous plaque and old thrombus (Figure 2). The respective amount of these items are largely dependent on CTO formation which may be grossly classified as the two following phenomena:

1. The late organization and development of an acute occlusion due to a plaque rupture, generally apart from the maximal narrowing area.

2. The progressive occlusion of a long term and high-degree stenosis (with a large amount of plaque and sometimes several layers of additional thrombi).

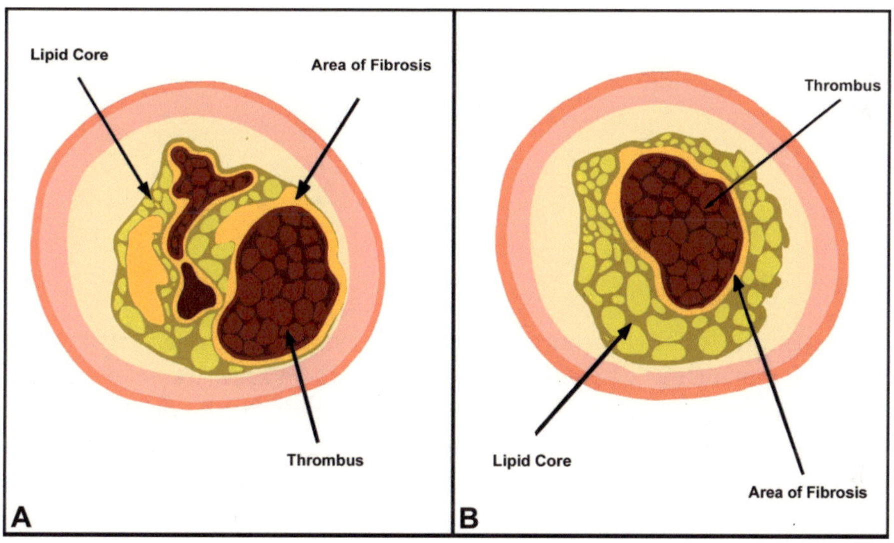

Figure 2. The two mechanisms of CTO formation: A) late evolution of an acute occlusion of an eccentric stenosis B) progressive occlusion of a long standing concentric stenosis.

The histopathology of CTOs was comprehensively described by Srivatsa and coll. in 1997 [10]. These lesions are characterized by a mix of luminal plaque, thrombin, fibrin, inflammatory cells and neovascular channels (Figure 3). The occlusive thrombus is mainly composed of collagen-rich extracellular matrix, intra and extracellular lipids, smooth muscle cells and mixed components, including a small quantity of cholesterol, dense collagen and calcium deposits. The core composition correlates with the CTO age. Older occlusions have higher concentration of fibrocalcific material (defined as "hard plaques"), while CTOs visible for less than one year have more cholesterol clefts and foam cells among less fibrous materials (defined as "soft plaque"). Typically CTOs may be classified as soft, hard or a mixture of both. Hard plaques are more prevalent with an increasing CTO age (> 1 year old) [11].

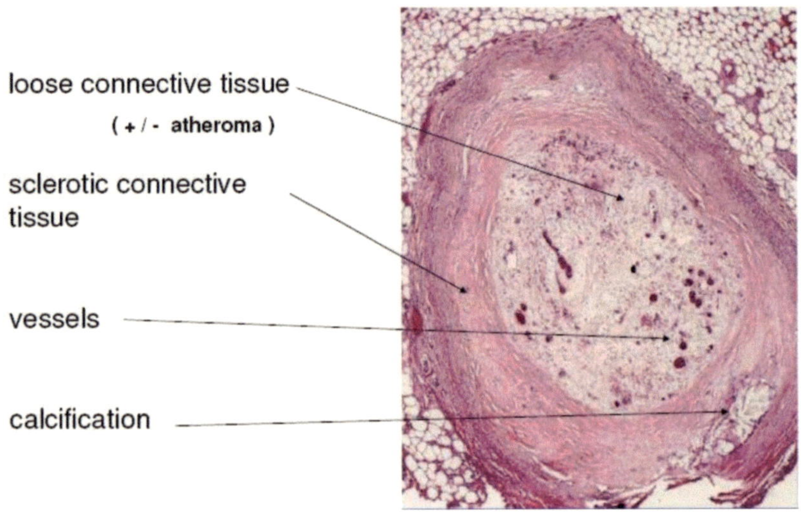

Figure 3. CTO plaque components.

The intraluminal process of plaque and thrombus organization is often followed by the so called "negative remodeling". This event usually leads to an artery vessel shrinkage, which is mainly observed in CTOs older than 3 months. The negative remodelling process is connected to the replacement of soft plaque tissue with fibrous one, mainly in the middle section of the occlusion [12]. Another important CTO feature is the extensive process of "neovascularization" which increase with occlusion age. In CTOs that are less than one year old the new capillary formation is greater in the adventitia. In CTOs that are more than one year old there is a rich neovasculature network that often traverses the vessel wall (bridging collaterals) [13]. Neovascular process may usually lead to the formation of relatively large capillaries (from 100 to 500 μm) that are defined as "microchannels" (Figure 4). These vessels can frequently be found through the CTO's body and can partially recanalize the distal lumen [14]. Guidewires may use microchannels as a passage to reach the distal vessel, hence they may have an important therapeutic value. Microchannels might also communicate with vasa vasorum and facilitate an extra-luminal pathways of collaterals o the distal part of the occluded segment, giving the typical aspect of "caput medusae" that is usually a sign of an old and difficult lesion to cross. Moreover, CTOs usually present a higher concentration of fibrous tissue at the proximal and distal parts of the lesion. These areas create a "fibrous cap" which is the hardest part of the plaque that surrounds a softer core of organised thrombus and lipids. Therefore, there are four components of CTO to take into consideration [15]: proximal cap, calcifications, microvessels and distal cap.

http://dx.doi.org/10.5772/54079

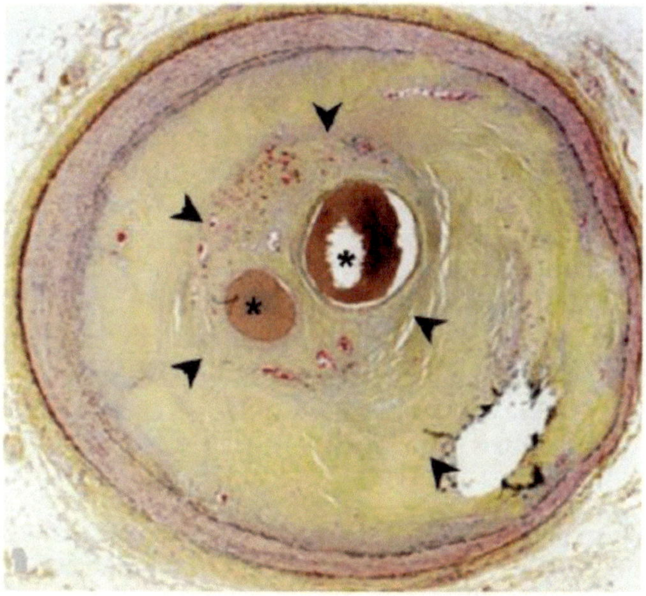

Figure 4. CTO microvessels. This image shows a healed total occlusion (arrowheads) with vascular channels (asterisks) surrounded by a rich collagen matrix (yellow). Adapted from Hoye A [15].

The temporal criterion used to define a CTO has varied widely through the litterature, typically ranging from > 2 weeks [16] to > 3 months [17]. Furthermore, any definition of CTO must include different elements such as the degree of lumen narrowing, considering if any antegrade blood flow is present. According to the consesus documents from the EuroCTO Club, lesions can be classified as CTOs, when there is TIMI 0 flow within the occluded segment and angiographic or clinical evidence or high likelihood of an occlusion duration > 3 months [18].

CTOs are characterized by significant atherosclerotic vessel narrowing with a lumen compromision that results in either complete interruption of antegrade blood flow as assessed by coronary TIMI flow (grade 0), also known as "true" total occlusion, or with minimal contrast penetration through the lesion without distal vessel opacification (TIMI grade 1 flow), frequently referred to as "functional" total occlusions. However, the identification of TIMI 0 flow is not as straightforward as in recent post-MI occlusions, for which the TIMI classification was originally developed because antegrade contrast filling of the segment beyond the occlusion does not preclude TIMI 0 flow within the occluded segment. Indeed, particular conditions such as the presence of ipsilateral bridging collaterals may give antegrade flow and the false impression of a functional incomplete occlusion but they are true CTO. Their presence should be differentiated from TIMI 0 flow within the occluded segment by careful assessment in different angiographic planes. Moreover, the presence of intraluminal channels certainly plays a role in crossing the occlusion; antegrade contrast filling of the segment beyond the occlusion flow, in the absence of ipsilateral bridging collaterals and even when the occluded vessel segment shows no intraluminal contrast filling, indicates a functional and not a true CTO. Only meticulous filming and a vigorous contrast injection with a well engaged catheter allow us to conclude that TIMI flow is 0 within the occluded segment and the lesion should then be classified as a CTO [19]. In absence of serial angiograms, the duration of CTO is difficult to establish with certainty and it might be estimated from available clinical information related to the timing of the event that caused the occlusion: acute MI or sudden change in angina pattern with ECG changes consistent with the location of the occlusion.

Since the time of the occlusion cannot be known, CTOs are usually distinguished into three levels of certainty:

a. Certain (angiographically confirmed): the minority of cases where a previous angiogram (for instance before a previous CABG operation, or after an acute myocardial infarction) has confirmed the presence of TIMI 0 flow (3 months prior to the planned procedure);

b. Likely (clinically confirmed): an acute myocardial infarction in the territory of the occluded artery distribution or acute coronary syndrome or deterioration of anginal threshold without other possible culprit arteries ≥ 3 months before the current angiogram;

c. Possible (undetermined): a CTO with TIMI 0 flow and angiographic anatomy suggestive of long-standing occlusion (collateral development, no contrast staining) with stable unchanged anginal symptoms in the last months or silent ischaemia or, in case of recent acute ischaemic episodes (acute myocardial infarction or unstable angina or worsening effort angina), with the presence of a culprit artery different from the occluded vessel.

3. Decision-making process for patients affected by CTO

The clinical presentation of CTOs can be quite variable ranging from patients with stable angina to patients with silent ischemia or heart failure of ischaemic origin, or those undergoing primary PCI due to acute occlusion in a different culprit vessel, in whom a CTO is discovered as an incidental finding.

Several factors are associated with CTO clinical presentation such as the presence of other concomitant coronary lesions, the amount of CTOs related to myocardial viability, the severity and extension of CTO related to myocardial ischemia and finally the coronary artery involved.

Generally, asymptomatic patients, are more reliable to be left on medical therapy rather than being percutaneuosly revascularized, especially if these patients have one vessel disease or a previous PCI, which has been performed in another coronary vessel. Moreover, older patients often exert low level of physical activity which might not lead to angina symptoms, underestimating the real burden of myocardium at risk. However, we know that this thera-

http://dx.doi.org/10.5772/54079

peutic strategy might not be clinically appropriate but the decision to treat a CTO in an asymptomatic patient should be driven by a non-invasive functional imaging test, in order to clarify the amount of myocardial viability and severity/extension of myocardial ischemia.

On the other hand symptomatic patients represent the greatest challenge for the clinical decision making, because there are different scenarios which need to be considered:

a. When the CTO is the only culprit lesion in the coronary tree, and presence of viability/ ischemia by non invasive functional test has been shown, PCI is highly recommended especially if likelihood of success has been estimated >60%. Moreover, if PCI is unsuccessful, re-attempt might be performed 2-3 months later after first failure. Conversely, coronary artery bypass graft might be performed to guarantee a complete revascularization, especially in case of a large myocardial ischemia or in case of refractory symptoms. Underestimating the CTO clinical impact in a single vessel disease patient might be led to "catastrophic consequences". Indeed, although the CTO might be supplied by collateral circulation without ischemia at rest, acute donor vessel occlusion might cause a larger myocardial necrosis with a poor prognosis for the patients.

b. It is not rare to see patients with a CTO angiographically documented few years before and without other coronary vessel diseases, which start to be symptomatic for effort angina only many years after the angiographic documentation is shown. In these cases, symptoms and myocardial ischemia could be related to the disease progression in vessels different from CTO, progression of disease in the donor artery, or to a reduction of blood supply from collateral circulation due to coronary collateral vasospasm [20].

c. In case of multivessel disease, the presence of a CTO should not be a sufficient reason to deny percutanoeus revascularization in the absence of significant left main disease and when the other lesions are suitable for PCI. Indeed, if the decision to perform a PCI is taken, a staged approach should be a reasonable strategy in order to avoid excessively long procedures and the use of large amount of contrast media. In this case consideration of which artery to tackle first, should be based on its importance. When complete revascularization is to be achieved, it is suggested to start PCI at the CTO vessel. As in case of the failure attempt, patient might be fully revascularized by surgery. Inversion of collateral flow direction through the recanalised CTO may protect myocardium at risk during treatment of lesions in the collateral donor vessel. Conversely, in many patients treatment at first of non occluded vessel may improve collateral visualization, significantly contributing to success of CTO recanalization. However, this strategy should be reserved to those patients in whom CTOs are likely to be successfully performed.

d. Patient might also present two CTO vessels at the same time. In these cases if CTOs angiographic characteristics are favourable and the patient does not present any clinical contraindications such as renal failure or other comorbidities, PCI may be performed on both CTOs during the same procedure, paying careful attention to the amount of contrast mean administered and to the duration of radiations exposure.

CTO decision-making process requires an individualized risk/benefit analysis, considering clinical, angiographic and technical features:

1. clinical: patient's age, symptoms severity, associated co-morbidities (chronic obstructive pulmonary disease, diabetes mellitus, chronic renal insufficiency), left ventricular ejection fraction, associate valve disease and overall functional status.

2. angiographycally: the extent and complexity of coronary disease (left main disease, bifurcation lesion, ostial lesion, long lesion, severe calcification), often not recognized before recanalization is performed.

3. technical: to evaluate percentage of success of revascularization preventing complications and considering restenosis rate on the basis of a total stent length required and vessel diameter size.

Regarding clinical features, a great concern is the patients' age. Indeed, in case of octogenarious patients, the operator should not expect any improvement of prognosis, and thus percutaneous attempt of CTO is supposed to be undertaken, only in presence of severe ischemia or refractory symptoms. Another clinical feature to evaluate is the renal function. Parameter used to assess renal impairment is the serum level of creatinine, or the glomerular filtration rate as measured by Cockcroft-Gault formula [21]. However, the risk of contrast induced nephropathy does not relate only to renal impairment before the procedure, but also to left ventricular ejection fraction (LVEF) and the presence of associated comorbidities such as diabetes mellitus and older age. The LVEF assessment is also relevant to consider the opportunity in which the left ventricular assistance device might be used during the procedure, such as intra aortic ballooning pumping (IABP). IABP displaces blood during diastole augmenting diastolic pressure. This augmented pressure wave carries blood flow up to the coronary arteries and can increase coronary blood flow across some coronary narrowing and, in some circumstances, even improving collateral flow to distal CTO coronary vessels. Immediately before systole, the deflation of the counter-pulsation balloon creates a negative space, reversing aortic flow and reducing ventricular after load and, hence, myocardial oxygen demand. Yoshitani, et al. demonstrated that IABP does not increase diastolic pressure distal to severe coronary stenosis, and thus, the major benefit of IABP in such patients with coronary artery disease is the reduction of myocardial oxygen demand [22]. The presence of left main stenosis might not represent a contraindication for CTO PCI. Indeed, the percutaneous treatment for CTO at first, might protect the patient from procedural ischemia during left main PCI, in case of contraindications to surgery. Nevertheless, in these cases it is always recommended to use IABP if Euroscore is ≥6 [23].

In patients underwent previous surgical revascularization, CTO treatment is a dilemma and the choice between performing native vessel and graft recanalization is not always easy, especially in case of old degenerated graft. Furthermore, even when the graft is not occluded but severely diseased at the level of the anastomosis PCI of the graft might be overtaken by recanalization of the native vessel if the occlusion is easy to approach. Moreover, it has been shown that myocardial ischemia might also occur in presence of a patent graft due to endothelial dysfunction [24]. Indeed, despite the presence of a patent and non-occlusive graft, regional myocardial blood perfusion might be still compromised, leading to ischemia.

A consensus document from EuroCTO Club [18] underlines that "PCI CTO should be attempted after careful review of clinical history, results of provocative tests, coronary anatomy and personal experience" and "with average recanalization success rate of >70% in experienced hands with contemporary techniques the presence of a CTO should not be sufficient reason to switch from PCI to surgery in multivessel disease".

3.1. Non invasive detection of myocardial viability

The non invasive assessment of myocardial viability has proved clinically useful for distinguishing hibernating myocardium from irreversibly injured myocardium in patients with chronic ischemic heart disease who exhibit marked regional and global left ventricular dysfunction [25]. The accurate noninvasive determination of myocardial viability is critically important for clinical decision making [26]. It makes allowance for the selection of patients with CAD and resting left ventricular dysfunction who benefit from revascularization strategies. Patients with substantial zones of viability and asynergic myocardium should demonstrate better function and overall better outcomes after revascularization compare with patients affected by a ventricular dysfunction related to large myocardial scar.

Thallium-201 is the imaging agent most frequently used with single photon emission tomography (SPECT) imaging for determination of myocardial viability. The reason is that the delayed uptake of thallium-201 on rest-redistribution imaging is related to myocardial cellular integrity. Several groups have shown that approximately 70% of segments showing >50% or >60% thallium-201 uptake on 3- to 4 hour rest thallium-201 redistribution scintigrams will demonstrate improved systolic function after revascularization [27-28]. The greater the number of viable segments detected preoperatively, the greater the improvement in LVEF postoperatively.

Although, 99mTc-labeled perfusion agents, such as sestamibi and tetrofosmin, do not show any significant redistribution over time after being injected intravenously, several studies have shown comparable accuracy for viability detection between these agents and thallium-201 [29-30]. This is thought to be due to high extraction of these tracers in the region of low flow in which myocites are viable. These agents bind to the mitochondrial membrane and require an intact mitochondrial membrane potential for intracellular binding.

Positron emission tomography (PET) is considered to be the standard of reference for noninvasive detection of viability with nuclear cardiology techniques. A myocardial zone of asynergy is determined to have preserved viability when there is a "mismatch" between perfusion and 18F-fluorodeoxyglucose (FDG) uptake. Patients with a "mismatch" pattern (low blood flow perfusion/high metabolic uptake) will often show improved regional and global left ventricular function after revascularization, whereas patients with a concordant reduction in perfusion and FDG uptake, referred to as a "match" pattern, have predominantly scar and do not show any significant improvement in regional and global function after revascularization [31].

Allman et al performed a pooled analysis [32] consisted of 3088 patients in 24 studies reporting viability by use of radionuclide imaging, PET or dobutamine echocardiography, and long-term survival after revascularization or medical therapy. In patients with predominant viability, follow-up on medical therapy was associated with very high risk, as demonstrated by a 16% annual mortality rate. In similar patients, revascularization was associated with an 80% reduction in annual mortality rate [16% vs 3.2%, $p<0.0001$), as compared with medical therapy. Patients with the most severe LV dysfunction derived the greatest benefit from revascularization, that is the survival benefit associated with revascularization of patients with viable myocardium increased proportionately with worsening LVEF. The data suggested that the presence of viable myocardium as defined by noninvasive imaging in patients with heart failure, is a marker for very high natural history risk, and that risk appears to be significantly reduced by revascularization.

3.2. Impact of complete percutaneous revascularization

Complete myocardial revascularization remains a desirable goal to obtain with PTCA or CABG [33]. However, incomplete revascularization with PCI of the culprit vessel may be the suitable strategy in selected patients [34]. This may occur, when the vessel, responsible of ischemia, can be identified, particularly when this vessel is a favourable lesion that serves a large non-infarct territory, in case of an acute coronary syndrome, left ventricular dysfunction due to acute severe ischemia or pre-existing renal failure. Indeed, situations which involve complex anatomy such as CTOs may be more cumbersome to approach and a proper planning procedure rather than an hoc angioplasty may be also indicated in such patients. Hannan et al showed that incomplete revascularization with stenting is associated with an adverse impact on long-term mortality [35]. Even more important, this author showed that incompletely revascularized patients with total occlusions, particularly those with no other incompletely revascularized vessels experienced lower rates of subsequent PCI than other patients. Although, at first, it seems to be good news for these incompletely revascularized patients, the fact that they had higher long-term mortality than completely revascularized patients suggests that they might have benefited from more subsequent revascularization. Indeed, with the percutaneous approach the presence of a CTO remains the biggest and most important technical challenge to achieve complete revascularization. Furthermore, as the procedure of a CTO recanalization still remains time consuming, exposing the patient to high dose of ionizing radiation and contrast media, any percutaneous treatment in these subset of patients must be justified on the basis of a strict clinical indication, to improve patients' symptoms and prognosis survival [6]. Taking all that into consideration, stress myocardial perfusion imaging is an effective means of identifying ischemic and viable myocardium and its vascular distribution in patients undergoing coronary revascularization [36-38]. Nuclear data have suggested that adverse events after incomplete revascularization occur more frequently in patients with perfusion defects [39-41], and that myocardial scintigraphy is able to provide incremental prognostic information after adjusting for clinical, angiographic and exercise variables [42]. Recently, we have shown that in patients with a CTO in a main coronary artery left untreated, patients with either a severe perfusion defect or ischemia and necrosis at stress myocardial scintigraphy have the worst prognosis in terms of hard events at 9 years follow-up as compared to patients with normal or near normal myocardial scan or only either necrosis or ischemia [43]. In these patients the presence of another vessel incompletely revascularized beyond that of the CTO artery, did not seem to change the prognosis at follow-up as shown by the occurrence of hard events in those pa-

http://dx.doi.org/10.5772/54079

tients with severely abnormal scans. Moreover, this study provides sufficient evidence that the absence or presence and type of collaterals do not influence prognosis but rather being equally distributed in all subsets of patients. It is also interesting to note that normal scans were rare among the CTO patients accounting for only 6% of all scans; indeed, despite the presence of well developed collaterals (either by Rentrop or Werner classifications) abnormal scans were shown in the majority of patients. As shown by Werner and colleagues even in patients with normal regional LV function, collaterals provide a normal coronary flow reserve in less than 10% [44]. This study highlights how CTO patients need to be assessed appropriately by means of functional imaging testing before considering medical therapy instead of revascularization. Conversely, a functional nuclear stress imaging study would enable a tailored strategy of complete revascularization in those patients with multivessel disease and incomplete revascularization in which complete revascularization by PCI may be contraindicated, or difficult to achieve.

Although the concept of hibernating myocardium suggests that it is an adaptive steady state, potentially reversible with revascularization, several reports have suggested that progressive structural and clinical deterioration may occur in this pathophysiologic setting, with more advanced structural changes being associated with less favourable improvement after revascularization [45]. Indeed, patients with more advanced abnormalities had less improvement in regional and global function after revascularization suggesting that hibernation is an incomplete adaptation to ischemia and that once identified, prompt revascularization should occur. Consistent with this concept are data from Beanlans et al [46] who reported that after identification of patients with ischemic cardiomyopathy who had significantly viable myocardium by PET imaging, a substantial delay in revascularization was associated with death during that delay and absence of post-revascularization LV functional improvement, as compared with patients undergoing more prompt revascularization. These important studies have significant practical implications, suggesting that identification of patients with substantial ischemia and viability are not only at long-term risk, but risk in the short term as well, and that optimal reversibility of LV dysfunction and improvement in symptoms and outcome are dependent on prompt referral for revascularization. These important data might support the concept that viability information can assist in the selection of patients with CTO and regional left ventricular dysfunction for whom the most optimal potential outcome will come from PCI rather than medical treatment or surgical revascularization if not needed.

Cardiac Magnetic Resonance Imaging (cMRI) has enormous potential thanks to its major attributes of high image quality and resolution combined with non-ionising radiation. It can provide high quality diagnostic information about cardiac and valvular function, coronary anatomy, coronary flow reserve, myocardial perfusion, myocardial viability, contractile reserve and cardiac metabolism. It allows assessment of even subtotal wall motion disturbances resulting from the consistently high endocardial border definition, and the measurement of myocardial perfusion can be integrated into the same examination, with the high spatial resolution of the scans facilitating the determination of the transmural extent of a regional perfusion deficit.

Recently the technique of late enhancement with gadolinium contrast agent has been described, in which imaging of the heart is performed 15 minutes after an intravenous injection of gadolinium. The gadolinium concentrates in the necrotic (acute infarction) or scar tissue (chronic infarction) because of an increased partition coefficient and the infarcted area becomes bright [47]. There is very close correlation between the volume of signal enhancement and infarct size in animal experiments of acute infarction. The technique has high resolution, and can define the transmural extent of necrosis and scar for the first time in vivo. Although the technique has been recently developed, it has obvious applications in defining whether infarction has actually occurred in borderline cases. The technique of late enhancement has also clinical application to the assessment of viability and it is an excellent technique for the detection and quantification of myocardial infarction as reported by many studies [48-49]. First pass perfusion is the most widely used cMRI-technique for the detection of reduced myocardial blood flow and yields superior results compared to SPECT [50].

The different noninvasive modalities available to assess myocardial viability interrogate distinct pathophysiologic myocite and myocardial processes. The SPECT radionuclide tracers examine myocite cell membrane integrity, and dobutamine echocardiography assesses regional ventricular contractile reserve. PET images myocardial blood flow and metabolism, whereas magnetic resonance hyperenhancement imaging identifies scarred myocardium. Although no major differences have been identified among the modalities that would suggest differences in patient management, in a pooled analysis of studies reporting on rates of regional functional recovery, few years ago Bax et al. [38] reported that the radionuclide agents are more sensitive and that dobutamine echocardiography was more specific, with PET having slightly higher overall accuracy for predicting functional recovery [51].

However, in the presence of a CTO and a very low blood flow state due to the occluded artery, which is supplied only by small collateral channels, dysfunctional but viable LV segments may show a modest inotropic response to dobutamine because of the early occurrence of ischemia [52]. Indeed, asynergic but viable myocardium usually thickens under catecholamine stimulation [53]. However, this effect may be limited or even abolished in the presence of a very flow-limiting CTO, underestimating the amount of myocardial viability in these subsets of patients [54].

More recently contrast-enhanced MRI has shown to be comparable with a PET/SPECT imaging protocol for the prediction of regional and global functional improvement after revascularization [55]. However, in the presence of discrepant findings between the modalities, c-MRI is superior to PET/SPECT for predicting lack of recovery of segmental myocardial function after revascularization. One of the reason for this finding may be explained by differences in the way the two techniques assess myocardial viability [56]. Indeed, a relatively small volume of dysfunctional viable tissue may show increased 18F-FDG PET uptake, with PET indicating viability, whereas the coexistence amount of scar impedes functional recovery. Although some individual studies may suggest better prediction about functional recovery by one test type over another, such data generally reflect differences in small regions or segments per patient and do not seem to affect long-term outcomes.

4. Tools for CTO recanalization

There are four important features of CTO wires:

1. Polymer covers: these are plastic sleeves of flexible but solid material which are applied directly over the core or over spring coils covering the tip of the wire. Based on the presence or absence of a polymer, CTO wires are divided in two main categories: polymer jacket wires (by default also hydrophilic coated) and spring coil wires (some hydrophilic coated and some not).

2. Wire coatings: these affect lubricity and tracking and facilitate smooth movement. There are two types: hydrophilic and hydrophobic. Hydrophilic coatings attract water and are applied over polymer and stainless steel, including tip coils. They are thin and non-slippery when dry and become gelatinous when wet, reducing friction. They usually cover the distal 30-35 cm of the wire. Hydrophobic coatings (Dow Corning Silicone) repel water. No wire flushing is required and they also reduce friction but not to the same extent as hydrophilic wires. These coatings usually cover the working area of wire, excluding the tip. There is an inverse relationship between lubricity and tactile feedback related to the presence or absence of coatings over coils and polymers at wire tips.

3. Core materials and tapering: the majority of CTO wires have a stainless steel core. Modern CTO wires have a transitionless parabolic core grind which provides excellent torque response and no prolapse points compared to conventional step tapering of non-CTO wires.

4. Tip stiffness: this ranges from 0.5 to 20 grams. Usually plastic jacket wires are in the low range of stiffness and spring coil wires cover the whole range. Tip tapering strongly affects penetration power as the force is applied over a smaller cross-sectional area in tapered wires.

4.1. Micro-catheters and over the wire balloons

Wires should be used with an over the wire (OTW) balloon or micro-catheter in order to ease torque in the tip response, preventing flexion, kinking, prolapse of the guide wire, and improving penetration ability. They also allow one to modify and reshape the guide wire curve, and exchange one guide wire for another. Micro-catheters in comparison with OTW balloons may provide a better tip flexibility, improving wire manipulation due to their larger inner lumen and hydrophilic coating which reduces friction. They also have the advantage of a radiopaque marker at the "real catheter tip" which has a flat end. Both of these characteristics help to avoid advancing too far into the lesion, a mistake that occurs frequently with OTW balloons. Additionally, most of the micro-catheters are braided which prevents shaft kinking, especially when crossing very tortuous vessels, a characteristic that OTW balloons lack. On the other hand microcatheters are more expensive and do not offer dilating capacity. The choice between an OTW balloon catheter and a dedicated micro-catheter depends on the features and CTO complexity and on the operator's personal experience. Micro-catheters differ from each other regarding construction characteristics, as well as flexibility, pushability, and trackability properties. One of the micro-catheters most generally used is the Finecross which is braided, hydrophilic coated and has a tapered body. It is available in 130cm and 150cm lengths, for the antegrade and retrograde approaches respectively.

The Tornus (Asahi Intecc Co., Nagoya, Japan) crossing micro-catheter has been developed to penetrate severe and hard lesions with greater flexibility and torquability with a rotational burrowing advancement manually manoeuvred by controlled counter-clockwise rotation.

The Corsair (Asahi Intecc Co., Nagoya, Japan) is a septal dilator catheter used for the retrograde approach. This is a micro-catheter which is dedicated for selective engagement of the collateral channel. It consists of a tapered tip and screw head structure, which reinforces torque transmission for the guide wire and creates better back-up support for CTO penetration. The Corsair provides superior tip flexibility which enables smooth approaches to narrow tortuous vessels, such as septal channels. Unlike other general micro-catheters, the Corsair possesses a soft tip with tungsten powder mix and a 0.8 mm platinum marker coil 5 mm from the tip, which makes it easy to identify the distal tip under fluoroscopy.

The Venture™ Catheter (Velocimed, Minneapolis, Minnesota, USA) is an over the wire, low profile support catheter, 6F compatible, flexible, torqueable with a radiopaque atraumatic tip. It has been recently designed to help direct the wire where there are difficult angles, providing strong support especially in occlusive lesions. It is also available as a rapid exchange device.

The Twin pass (Vascular Solutions, Inc Minneapolis, Minnesota, USA) is a dual access lumen rapid exchange micro-catheter (rapid exchange and over the wire) which helps the guide wire placement and exchange after reopening the occlusion and gaining access to different main branches.

The Crusade (Kaneka Corporation, Japan) micro-catheter has the similar design and application of the Twin pass.

4.2. Dedicated devices in clinical use

Many dedicated devices to open CTOs were developed in the past, but most disappeared because they did not prove superior to conventional CTO procedure equipment. The following dedicated devices are currently in clinical use:

Crosser. The Crosser CTO recanalization system (Flow-Cardia Inc, CA, USA) is comprised of a generator, transducer, foot switch, and a disposable catheter. Through the generator the catheter tip vibrates at a rate of 21,000 cycles/sec. This vibration provides mechanical impact and cavitational effects, which aid in the recanalization of the occluded artery. The catheter is monorail, hydrophilic, and can be advanced over a standard 0.014 inch guide wire. It is 1.1 mm in diameter, which makes it compatible with 6 Fr guiding catheters, and has a blunt tip. In a small single centre experience comprising 28 patients (30 lesions) technical success was obtained in 63% of the occlusions with minor complications [57]. In a single center registry of 45 patients with relative complex CTOs success rate was 84% but the use of the device was associated with lower time of procedure, time of fluoroscopy, and contrast load administration as compared with conventional techniques [58]. In the prospective multicenter CRAFT registry that enrolled 80 patients where the device was used as a first treatment choice success rate was 76% [59].

BridgePoint system. The BridgePoint technologies consists of three devices that can be used alone, or in concert with other wires/devices for rapid and safe CTO crossing and provisional luminal re-entry. The Crossboss catheter is an OTW stainless steel catheter with a rounded tip that can negotiate CTOs by using rapid bi-directional rotation. If the Crossboss, or conventional wires and devices, gain subintimal/subadventitial position, the flat Stingray balloon (with an exit port oriented toward the lumen) and Stingray guide wire can be utilized for dedicated lumen re-entry and distal vessel access. The FAST-CTOs pivotal trial enrolled 147 patients with wire-refractory CTOs. Technical success was 77%, 30 day MACE < 5%, and average procedure time was 105 minutes [60]. Recently, the preliminary European experience (42 patients) with this system was reported and the success rate was 67% without any safety issues [61].

5. The key of success of CTO PCI

The selection of the access route is dependent on the individual patient situation (e.g., severe peripheral vascular disease, which may mandate a radial approach) as well as on the operator's preference. Guiding catheter size is limited from the radial approach, but the radial artery can be easily used for contralateral injection (5 or 6 Fr diagnostic catheters). Most experts use the femoral approach (90% in Europe) and it has not been shown that either access is preferable except for about 10% of the cases in which even experienced radial operators select the femoral route.

Good passive support with coaxial alignment into the coronary artery for active support is crucial. Passive support is stronger with larger guiding catheters (7 and 8 Fr) while 6 Fr catheters offer the best balance between active and passive support. For the left coronary system extra backup–type catheters (Voda left, extra backup, geometric left, left support) are preferable, although some operators still prefer Amplatz type or even Judkins type catheters, the latter needing more manipulation to achieve optimal position and back up in complex cases (Figure 5). For the right coronary artery 6F and 7F catheters can be used with left Amplatz 0.75-2 shapes, hockey stick shapes for gentle superior origins of the RCA, Judkins shape for slightly inferior origins and internal mammary artery type guiding catheters for upward origins (Figure 6). One word of caution is that there is a higher risk of vessel injury at the ostium and first bend of the right coronary artery especially with an Amplats left that has a tendency to jump into the artery, and with all kinds of 8 Fr catheters. In case of ostial dissection, a soft-tipped wire must be selected and steered carefully past the dissection that needs to be fixed before continuing the procedure. Often the guide catheter has to be changed to avoid an orientation towards the dissection.

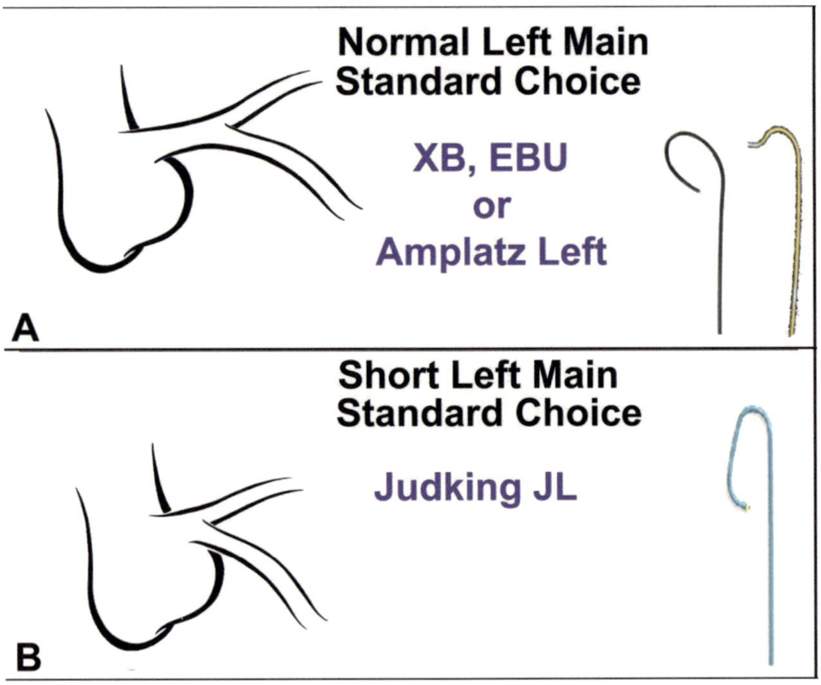

Figure 5. Guiding catheter selection for left coronary artery; A) normal left main; B) short left main.

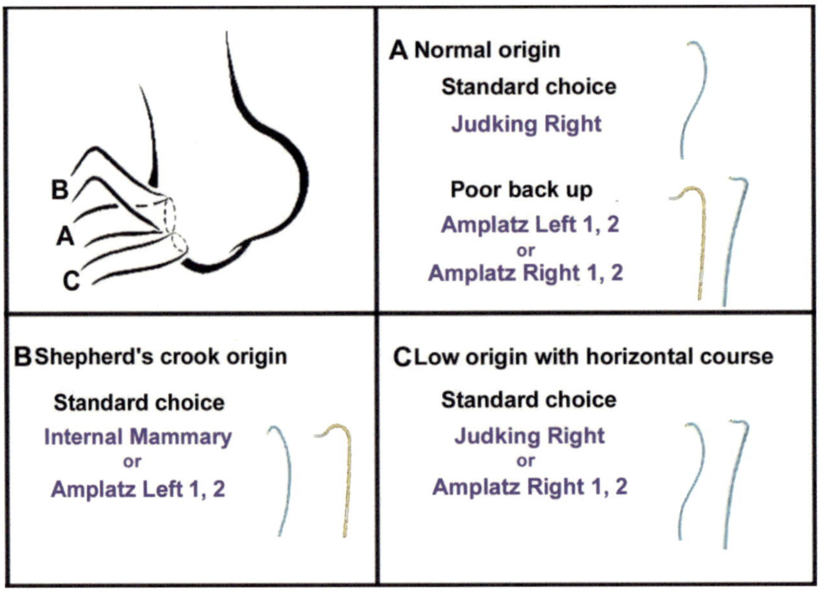

Figure 6. Guiding catheter selection for right coronary artery; A) normal origin; B) Shephered's crook origin; C) low origin with horizontal course.

When the distal vessel is mainly filled by retrograde collaterals, or there are bridging collaterals originating near the occlusion that are likely to have their flow impaired after wire-catheter advancement, contralateral injection is necessary from the beginning of the procedure. The contralateral approach can also be achieved by puncturing the same groin with a 4 to 6 Fr catheter, which may allow the procedure to be better tolerated. The operators of the EuroCTO Club have used contralateral injection in 62% of cases of their personal series (range 33-78%) [62].

A floppy wire is often the best initial choice to negotiate the segment proximal to the occlusion and advance an OTW balloon or microcatheter up to the proximal stump and then exchange it to a stiffer dedicated wire.

Until recently, the standard way of selecting a guide wire was to use a gradual step-up approach, which consists of tackling the lesion with a medium-tipped guide wire (3-6 gr) and then exchanging it for a stiffer one (9-12 gr). Using this approach, a reasonable choice is to start with a Medium or a Miracle 3 first (Asahi Intecc Co., Nagoya, Japan), then switching to stiffer wires.

The introduction of very soft tapered polymeric wires such as the Fielder XT dramatically changed this practice. Soft tapered polymeric wires became the standard to start CTO procedures; in about 40% of the cases this wire will cross the occlusion taking advantage of invisible tiny channels [62]. The current trend is a sharp step up to very stiff tapered spring coil tapered hydrophilic wires such as Confianza pro 12 gr and PROGRESS 200T to overcome any hard calcified or fibrotic segments of the occlusion and quickly return to soft polymer/ hydrophilic wires to continue long segment tracking and complete crossing of the CTO. This strategy significantly reduces procedural time and material consumption. With contemporary CTO techniques soft polymer wires are of increasing use followed by spring coil stiff but hydrophilic wires while bare spring coil wires became of secondary importance.

The shaping of a CTO guide wire tip is very important. Usually, a small 40-50° curve, 1.0-2.0 mm from the tip of the wire is needed to penetrate the proximal fibrous cap. In hard spring coil wires a gentler secondary 15-20° curve, 3.0-4.0 mm proximal to the distal tip is necessary to navigate into the CTO body, to orient the tip and to cross the distal fibrous cap especially in vessels bigger than 3.5 mm.

5.1. Single wire techniques

There are three fundamental elements of wire handling: rotating, pushing and pulling. After entering the proximal cap, one should very gently push while simultaneously keep applying torque, until the wire slides into the body of the occlusion. The wire should be rotated clockwise and counter clockwise, but not more than 360° in the same direction, in order to keep good tip control. Uncontrolled wire spinning may result in large dissections that might make difficult to find the distal true lumen or lead to complications such as wire exit and perforation or wire entrapment.

If resistance is strong, pushing (advancement of the OTW catheter close to the tip of the wire to increase stiffness and pushability) may open a false lumen and should be avoided. Applying rotation in combination with appropriate wire selection is the right choice as it will minimize resistance at the tip.

Wires, especially stiff ones, have the tendency to follow the outer part of the vessel curve which in tortuous occlusions can easily lead to vessel exit and perforation. It is important to direct the wire tip towards the inner part of vessel bends. Calcification or occluded stents are often good markers of the vessel course. Bridging collaterals should be carefully recognised and avoided as modern wires, especially polymer ones, can easily track these vessels and lead to major complications if perforated or dilated.

5.2. Parallel-wire technique

The parallel-wire technique was first described by Reifart in 1995 and was further developed by Katoh [63]. It is a cornerstone technique in CTO PCI that every operator should be familiar with. When the first wire enter the false lumen, it is left in place, and a second wire (typically stiffer and often tapered with different tip bend) supported by an OTW catheter, is passed parallel to the first wire aiming for the distal true lumen. The initial wire serves as a marker, occludes the wrong pathway and can potentially modify the anatomy by changing vessel geometry and smoothening sharp curves.

If the second wire also fails to enter the distal true lumen and follows a different incorrect pathway, often on the opposite wall, the first wire is withdrawn and steered in the direction of the true lumen using the second wire as a marker; the so-called "see saw" technique. Occasionally, three or more wires are used. As in single wire techniques it is of paramount importance not to over-rotate and push either of the wires, in order to avoid creation of large dissection and subintimal spaces as well as to avoid wire twisting. Often re-puncturing the proximal cup or navigating through the occlusion with a difference of fraction of a millimetre is critical for success.

5.3. Techniques with sub-intimal tracking

The STAR technique (sub-intimal tracking and re-entry) was introduced by Colombo [64] who demonstrated that the technique was feasible and safe. This method involves fashioning a large "umbrella-handle" shaped bend at the tip of a hydrophilic wire once the wire is within the dissection flap. Force is then applied to this tip and evenly distributed over a large surface area, along the length of the umbrella-handle, to break through the sub-endothelial layer thereby creating a communication between the false lumen and the true lumen. Carlino [65] introduced the modified STAR technique (guided-STAR technique), by injecting contrast into the subintimal space in an effort to simplify the original technique and make it more widely applicable. Once in a dissection plane pure contrast is gently injected from via an OTW balloon or a micro-catheter drawing a roadmap of the occluded segment. The injection might cause a coronary dissection whether tubular (a linear morphology consistent with the vessel outline) or storm cloud (small side branch or bridging collaterals dissection with diffuse contrast extravasation into the adventitia). Sometimes a communication between the false and true lumen can be created.

More recently, Carlino [66] proposed the "Microchannel technique". The idea came from histological CTO data demonstrating that most occlusions have intra-luminal micro-channels with size between 100-500 μm that run within and parallel to the occluded vessel [67-68]. According to this technique after central puncture of the proximal cap with a very stiff spring coil wire for a length no longer than 1-2 mm and advancement of a OTW balloon or a micro-catheter, contrast is injected aiming to enlarge and connect these micro-channels creating a communication between the proximal and distal true lumens favoring guide wire crossing through the occlusion. This technique is mostly proposed for straight CTO segments with a concave proximal cap that will facilitate central puncture.

Galassi further refined the STAR proposing the "Mini-STAR" technique using the very soft Fielder polymeric guide wires. The Fielder FC and XT (tapered) can track intra-occlusion channels navigating though the occlusion. In cases of channel interruption or presence of harder tissue by forcing the wire when supported by a micro-catheter a J-tip shape is automatically created within the occlusion. This J tip is smaller compared to the one purposely created with stiffer polymeric guide wires during the STAR technique allowing "mini subintimal tracking" with the creation of much smaller subintimal spaces. This technique was successful as a rescue in 97.6% of cases during the same procedure after failure to recanalise with conventional techniques, and during a second attempt in 84.6% of the cases [69].

5.4. Retrograde approach

The retrograde techniques have a long standing history. In the late 80s Hartzler introduced the retrograde dilatation of native artery stenosis proximal to a distal SVG anastomosis. In the early 90s retrograde wire crossing of CTOs via saphenous vein graft (SVG) grafts were attempted. In late 90s the invention of the bilateral approach led to the marker wire technique where the retrograde wire was used as a roadmap for the antegrade wire. In the early 2000s initial attempts to break the distal cap with balloons were attempted and in 2005 Katoh pioneered the field introducing the Controlled Antegrade and Retrograde subintimal Tracking (CART) technique [70] establishing the modern era of retrograde CTO recanalisation. Beyond the concept of retrograde dilatation within the occlusion to facilitate antegrade wire crossing, the novelties introduced in this procedure was the retrograde balloon dilatation. Indeed, the principle of this technique is retrograde penetration and dilatation of the occlusion, most often close to the distal cap, thus creating a large target (subintimal space) facilitating antegrade wire crossing. In the reverse CART, the principle is the same as the CART technique with the difference that the subintimal space is created with antegrade balloon dilatations facilitating the crossing of the occlusion with the retrograde wire. Currently, this is the dominant technique in the retrograde CTO approach [71]. IVUS guidance for the connection of the antegrade and retrograde subintimal spaces [72], led by Japanese operators, significantly contributed to our understanding of these techniques, but did not receive widespread adoption due to its inherent complexity and cost. More recently, a variety of modifications to these cornerstone techniques have been introduced such as subintimal space stabilization with stents (stent CART technique after septal overdilatation and retrograde stenting and the stent reverse-CART technique) introduced by Sianos [73]. The retrograde wire crossing technique (crossing of the occlusion purely retrograde without the need for creation of subintimal spaces), which accounts for almost 30% of successes, as well as the marker wire technique should also be kept in mind as simpler retrograde techniques which can always prove helpful [74].

6. The stent choice for CTO treatment

Several randomized studies have compared balloon angioplasty with stent implantation for the treatment of CTOs (Figure 7). Although these trials have shown diverse results regarding entry criteria, antithrombotic regimen and trial design, their findings are remarkably concordant. The restenosis rate was reduced from 70% in the balloon treated groups to 30% in the stent groups, with a corresponding reduction in the need for revascularization and with no increased risk of stent thrombosis. Also the rate of reocclusion was significantly reduce by stent implantation. The introduction of DES has determined a significant reduction in restenosis and re-occlusion as compared to BMS.

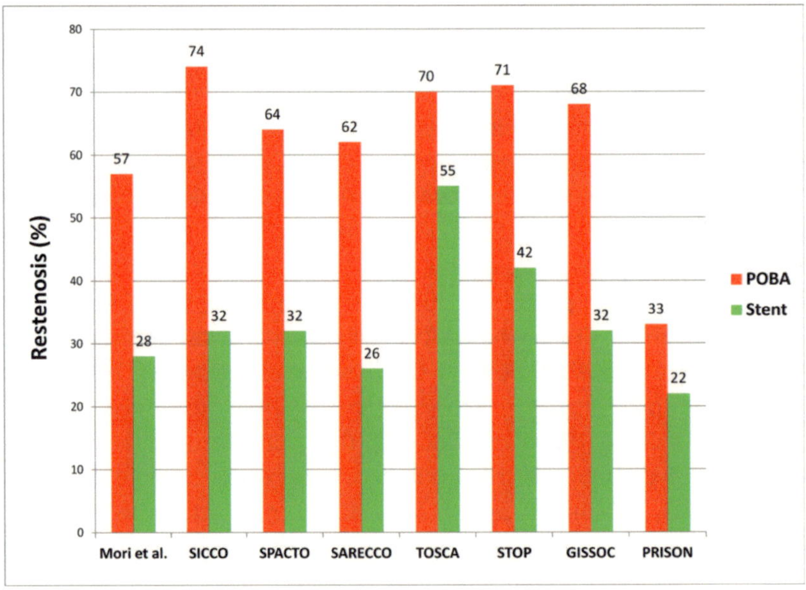

Figure 7. Restenosis after percutaneous recanalizzation of CTO: an overview of POBA versus stent implantation randomized trial

It is advisable to use DES with a very low late lumen loss are in CTOs, as these lesions have a large plaque load and the compression of these plaques within the adventital space promotes intimal proliferation and therefore high restenosis and re-occlusion rates as previously demonstrated with BMS [75-81].

http://dx.doi.org/10.5772/54079

6.1. Paclitaxel-eluting stents (PES) for CTOs

Werner et al. [82] evaluated the efficacy of PES in 48 consecutive patients with CTOs compared with a matched group of 48 patients previously treated with BMS. Patients matching was performed on the basis of a history of diabetes mellitus, prior MI, diameter and number of stents implanted, lesion location and left ventricular function. The PES-treated group had significantly fewer adverse events relating to the reduced need for repeat revascularization; the advantage of PES over BMS was also significant both in diabetic and non-diabetic patients. Angiographic follow-up demonstrated the efficacy of the PES with a significantly smaller late lumen loss in the PES-treated group and significantly less restenosis (8% vs 51%) and reocclusion (2% vs 23%).

Two additional registries studied the role of PES in CTOs: among 65 patients with CTOs in the international WISDOM Registry, treatment with the PES resulted in freedom from MACE and repeat intervention at 1 year in 93.3% and 98.3% of patients [83], respectively; in the European TRUE Registry, among 183 with CTO treated with PES, 7-months rates of restenosis and target vessel revascularization were 17.0% and 16.9% respectively [84].

6.2. Sirolimus eluting stents (SES) for CTOs - Registries

Several observational studies examining clinical outcomes among patients treated with DES following successful CTO recanalization demonstrated the notion that unlike BMS, DES may achieve similar reductions in the need for repeat target vessel revascularization (TVR), as observed in non occlusive lesions.

The first data on the effectiveness of SES usage for CTOs came from the Rapamycin Eluting Stent Evaluated At Rotterdam Cardiology Hospital (RESEARCH) registry, a prospective single centre study set-up with the aim of evaluating the safety and efficacy of SES in a "real world" scenario [85]. In this registry SES was the device of first choice for every PCI performed at the Thoraxcenter irrespective of patient or lesion characteristics. Among 56 patients treated with SES following successful CTO revascularization during the first months, the 1-year survival free of major adverse cardiac events (MACE) defined as the composite of death, acute myocardial infarction or TVR was 96.4% compared with 82.1% among an historical control group of 28 patients receiving bare metal stents ($p < 0.05$). Six-month follow up angiography performed in 33 patients treated with SES showed a remarkable suppression of neointimal proliferation, with in-stent late loss of 0.13 ± 0.46, a binary restenosis rate of 9% and a single reocclusion (3%).

More recently, the RESEARCH investigators have reported the 3-year clinical and angiographic follow-up of patients with CTO in a consecutive series of 147 patients [86], with comparison between BMS ($n = 71$) and SES ($n = 76$). The cumulative event-free survival of MACE was 81.7% in BMS group and 84.2% in SES group ($p = 0.7$). The authors concluded that, despite clinical benefit after 1 year, the use of SES was no longer associated with significantly lower rates of TVR and MACE in patients with CTOs after 3 years of follow-up compared with BMS. The issue of long term outcome after successful CTO revascularization and DES implantation will surely continue to deserve attention in the future.

Ge et al. provided other insights into the angiographic and clinical impact of implantation of SES in the re-opened CTOs [87]. The results of a group comprised of 122 patients treated with SES were compared with a historical control group of 259 patients treated for the same kind of lesions during an antecedent 2-year period. Coronary enzyme release during the procedures was insignificantly different despite considerably longer stented segments in the SES treated group. At 6-month follow-up, the cumulative rate of MACE was 16.4% in the SES group and 35.1% in the BMS group ($p<0.001$), whereas the incidence of restenosis was 9.2% and 33.3% ($P<0.001$) in SES vs BMS, respectively. The need for revascularization in the SES group was significantly lower, both for target lesion revascularization (TLR) (7.4 vs. 26.3%, $P<0.001$) and TVR (9.0 vs. 29.0%, $P<0.001$). No differences were observed between the groups in the occurrence of death, myocardial infarction, or stent thrombosis in the 6-month observation period.

The e-CYPHER was a registry designed to capture postmarketing surveillance data on the use of SES. Between April 2002 and September 2005, data on 15,157 patients treated with SES at 279 centers from 41 countries were entered into the registry. From the total amount of patients enrolled in the registry, 6-month follow-up data were available for 10,962 patients. A sub-analysis [88] assessed the outcomes of CTO, defined as an occlusion lasting > 3 months. A total of 415 patients were identified, representing 2.9% of the total population. When their results were compared with those ones seen for the rest of the patients enrolled in the registry, there was no difference regarding death, myocardial infarction, TLR, or MACE. Investigators concluded that the event rates were similar for patients with CTO treated with the SES and patients treated for other lesion types, with a low rate of TLR (2.9%) and MACE (6.5%) in the CTO group at 6-month follow-up.

The Sirolimus-eluting Stent in Chronic Total Occlusion (SICTO) study was a multicentre, prospective, non-randomized study of coronary stenting with SES in patients with CTOs [89]. A total amount of 25 patients was treated with the SES stent after successful balloon angioplasty and IVUS examination. At 6-month angiographic and IVUS follow-up, the use of the SES stent was associated with improvements both in reference vessel diameter and minimum lumen diameter. In addition, the rate of in-stent late loss was -0.1 ± 0.3 mm and percent stent plaque volume was $13.1 \pm 18.4\%$. The number of events at 6 months was also very low, with no deaths, myocardial infarction, stent thrombosis, or target lesion revascularization. There were 2 cases of target vessel revascularization (8%).

As a part of a multicentre Asian registry evaluating DES, Nakamura et al. investigated clinical and angiographic outcomes in 60 patients who received SES and 120 patients who received BMS [83]. After 6 months, the SES group still had significantly lower restenosis and reocclusion rates (2% and 0%, respectively) than did the BMS group (32% and 6%, respectively). Afterwards the loss was significantly smaller in the SES group than in the BMS group. Moreover, the SES group had fewer cardiac events, including target lesion revascularization (2% vs 23%, $p < 0.001$), than the BMS group did. At 1 year, treatment with SES was associated with sustained reductions in hierarchical MACE and TLR.

The ACROSS/TOSCA 4 (Approaches to Chronic Occlusions with Sirolimus-Eluting Stents/ Total Occlusion Study of Coronary Arteries 4) study was amulticenter, non randomized prospective trial, which esamining the safety and efficacy of SES in CTOs PCI. In this study, the 6-months binary restenosis rates were 9.5% in-stent, 12.4% in-segment, and 22.6% in-"working lenght" representing the entire treatment segment. Rates of 1-year target lesion revascularization, MI and target vessel failure were 9.8%, 1.0% and 10.9%, respectively. Stent thrombosis occurred in two patients (1.0%) [90].

More recently, Galassi et al. have published the results of SECTOR (Sirolimus-Eluting Stent in Complex Coronary Chronic Total Occlusion Revascularization) Registry designed to assess angiographic and clinical outcomes after sirolimus-eluting stent (SES) implantation in the setting of a "real world" series of complex CTOs [91]. In this registry, the 9-12 months angiographic follow-up performed in 85.5% of lesions showed a binary restenosis rate of 16.8%. Moreover, at 2-year clinical follow-up, the rates of target lesion revascularization, non-Q wave MI, and total MACE were of 11.1%, 2%, and 13.1%, respectively.

6.3. Sirolimus eluting stents for CTOs - Randomized trials

The PRISON II [92] has been the first randomized trial performed to compare DES and BMS. PRISON II addressed a primary end point of angiographic binary restenosis at six months and secondary end points of MACE, target vessel failure (TVF), in-stent and in-segment mean luminal diameter (MLD), late lumen loss, late-loss index, and percent diameter stenosis at six months. A total of 200 patients were randomized to a bare BX Velocity stent or to the SES. In-stent restenosis results were 7% for the SES patient cohort vs. 36% for the patients in the bare metal control arm of the study ($p < 0.001$). The SES also achieved statistical significance in key clinical endpoints such as target lesion revascularization (4% vs. 19%; $p=0.001$); TVF (8% vs 24%; $p= 0.003$) and MACE (4% vs 20%; $p<0.001$). In-stent late loss in the SES patient cohort was 0.05 mm and 1.09 mm in the control ($p=0.0001$). Such strong evidence from a well-conducted randomized study has provided clear evidence of efficacy of the SES and follow up is awaited to evaluate the long term outcomes.

Long term results of PRISON II were recently published [93]. At 5-year follow-up, event rates still favoured the SES arm over the BMS arm. In fact, SES group had significantly lower rates of target lesion revascularisation (12% vs. 30%, $p=0.001$), target vessel revascularisation (17% vs. 34%, $p=0.009$) and MACE (12% vs. 36%, $p<0.001$). There were no significant differences in death and myocardial infarction. On the other hand, there is a trend to a higher stent thrombosis rate in the SES group (8% vs. 3%, p=0,21).

The CORACTO study [94] was performed to evaluate the sirolimus-coated CURA stent in 95 patients with a CTO of > 3 months duration. Patients were randomized to treatment with either the CURA stent or BMS implantation; the primary end-point was late loss and restenosis at 6 months. Follow-up angiography demonstrated significant differences between the two groups in favour of CURA stents. The mean late loss was 1.46 mm in those treated with BMS vs 0.41 mm in the CURA stent group ($p<0.001$). The suppression of neointimal proliferation was associated with less restenosis, reocclusion, and need for TVR. No patient died or suffered a stent thrombosis or myocardial infarction.

6.4. Comparative DES trials in CTOs revascularization

The clinical outcomes of both SES and PES for the treatment of CTO were further analyzed in the registry data from Rotterdam [95]. A cohort of 76 patients was treated with SES; subsequently, in the first quarter of 2003, all patients were treated with PES, including 57 treated for a CTO. These patients were compared with a similar group of patients (n=26] treated with BMS in the 6-month period preceding April 2002. At 400 days, the cumulative survival-free of target vessel revascularization was 80.8% in the BMS group versus 97.4% and 96.4% in the SES and PES groups respectively (p=0.01). The authors concluded that the use of both the SES and PES in the treatment of CTOs reduces the need for repeat revascularization compared to BMS.

Another report by Jang et al. involved 107 patients with CTO who received SES, and 29 patients with CTO who received PES [96]. At 6-month angiographic follow up, the restenosis rate was significantly higher in the PES group (28.6% vs. 9.4%; p = 0.02). Similarly, the late loss was significantly higher in the PES group (0.8 mm vs. 0.4 mm; p = 0.025). At one-year follow up, the MACE-free survival rate was significantly higher in the SES group (95.8% vs. 85.8%; p = 0.049).

Recently, a randomized study evaluating SES and PES has been performed by De Lezo et al [97]. No significant differences were reported between SES and PES in the rates of restenosis (7.4% versus 19%, respectively) and TLR (3.3% versus 7.0%). However, the PES group was found to have a significantly higher late loss and neointimal area on intravascular ultrasound. At 15 months, death and myocardial infarction rates were comparable between the two stents.

A prospective analysis of 1149 patients with 1183 CTOs (396 SES, 526 PES, 177 ZES, 64 EPC capture, 43 EES) in five high volume Asian centers after successful recanalization of CTO was recently performed [98]. The study endpoints were 30 days and 9 months MACE, 9 months angiographic restenosis and TLR. In this series patients treated with SES showed lesser rate of restenosis compared with other drug-eluting stents.

PRISON III ongoing trial will address whether or not SES are superior to other drug-eluting stents in total coronary occlusions. Indeed this prospective, randomized trial, SES implantation will be compared with zotarolimus-eluting stent implantation for the treatment of total coronary occlusions. A total of 300 patients will be followed for up to 5 years with angiographic follow-up at 8 months. The primary end point will be in-segment late luminal loss at 8 months angiographic follow-up [99].

A new randomised ongoing trial, the Non-Acute Coronary occlusion treated by EveroLimus-Eluting Stent (CIBELES) trial, aims to compare everolimus-eluting stent and sirolimus-eluting stent in treating CTOs, in terms of angiographic efficacy [100].

6.5. Optimization of stent deployment

The introduction of stent delivery systems, which used semi-compliant balloons to deploy stents at higher pressures, initially resulted in less use of balloon post-dilatation. However, it was soon recognized that adjunctive balloon post-dilatation following deployment of BMS im-

http://dx.doi.org/10.5772/54079

proved stent expansion in its entire length and resulted in better outcomes with less need for TVR [101-103]. Consequently, post-dilatation has been widely, although not universally, used. With the advent of DES and much lower rates of TVR, there has been renewed controversy regarding the need for adjunctive balloon post-dilatation to optimize outcomes. However DES thrombosis, which might be related to procedural variables, such as minimal stent area (MSA) and stent expansion following stent deployment, makes a come back the role of post-dilatation. Indeed, the frequency of stent thrombosis following DES implantation is relatively low [104-105], but the clinical sequeale of stent thrombosis are catastrophic and include death in about 45% of patients and non-fatal myocardial infarction in most of the survivors [106].

Similarly to stent thrombosis, maximizing MSA appears important in reducing the risk of TVR. This should be theoretically even more important in case of long standing CTO where severe and diffuse disease in presence of extensive calcification might prevent adequate stent expansion [107].

The inability to achieve optimum stent deployment is not due to undersizing the stent delivery balloon, but rather due to an inability of the stent delivery balloon to expand fully the stent to nominal size. With postdilatation using noncompliant balloons, the frequency of achieving optimum stent deployment doubles [108].

Lesions with heavy calcification or large plaque burden, such as CTO lesion, are likely to have increased resistance to dilatation. In such situations, inadequate stent expansion may be evident from the contour of the deployment balloon or the angiographic appearance of the stent post stent deployment. However, inadequate stent expansion is usually not detectable by angiographic assessment. In situations where there is likely to be increased resistance to dilatation, postdilatation with noncompliant balloons at high pressure appears to be a good strategy.

Theoretically, in an attempt to minimize stent thrombosis and TVR, post-dilatation with non-compliant balloons should be performed by IVUS guidance. Unfortunately, it is not practical and probably not cost-effective to perform IVUS and post-dilatation to all patients undergoing DES implantation. Moreover after DES implantation in long CTO lesion with multiple stents overlapping is recommended to perform post-dilatation with non compliant balloon in order to improve MSA and thus to obtained a good angiographic outcome.

Post-dilatation can improve significantly MSA within the limits of reference vessel size even if it is still likely not to affect non-uniformity expansion. An uniform stent expansion may be achieved with either adequate pre-dilatation or by the use of rotational atherectomy in calcified lesions to allow the simmetricity expansion of the lesion by the balloon and stent.

7. Complications of CTO PCI

The PCI CTO procedural complications can be classified as follows: vascular access related and procedure related. Despite the development of new devices and techniques, complications still occasionally occur today. This is highlighted by the complications reducing with improved learning curve. Therefore, the operator's experience is essential in order to quickly recognise and handle all sorts of complications.

7.1. Complications vascular access related

Access site complications are common during intravascular procedure and include hematomas of any size, pseudoaneurysm, and artero-venuos fistulae [109]. Despite of the need of large size sheath and double coronary cannulation, both femoral vascular access are generally recommended during CTO PCI. Some operators prefer to place two sheaths in the same femoral artery, in order to reduce patient discomfort (Figure 8) however, this approach restrict the use up to smaller size sheaths and might limit the use of closure device after procedure thus increasing the occurrence of rare complication such as acute limb ischemia.

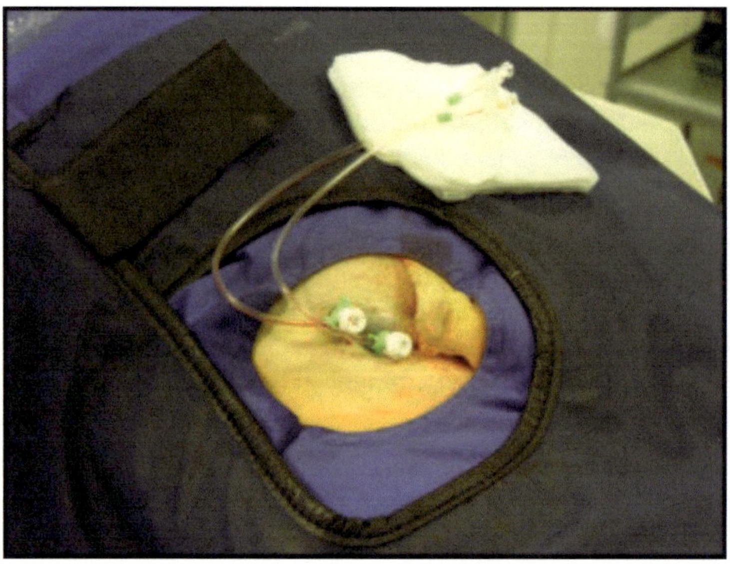

Figure 8. Two 6 French sheath in a femoral artery

Such complications are more frequent in older, female, overweight or previously anticougulated patients, and can be prevent by careful puncture, compression technique and 6-12 hours bed rest after procedure. Small hematomas are common (2-15%) and usually produce only mild discomfort for a few days. Large hematomas (>10 cm) are less frequent (1-2%) and might require prolonged rest and a delay in hospital discharge; the complete resolution, thus may take in 3-4 weeks. Diagnosis can be based on clinical features (no femoral murmur) and confirmed by a Doppler study performed with standard echocardiography equipment. Occasionally, large hematomas become infected, and in this case is important to surgically drain the cavity by purulent materials. This may take 2-3 months to heal.

Uncontrolled bleeding (either evident or into retroperitoneal space) with severe haemodinamic compromise require aggressive fluid blood replacement, ruling out bleeding from another origin. In these cases vascular surgery might resolve the complications.

http://dx.doi.org/10.5772/54079

Femoral pseudoaneurysm and artero-venuos fistulae might occur in case of low puncture (more than 2 cm below the inguinal ligament). Diagnosis is based on clinical grounds (the presence of hard and pulsatile mass in the case of pseudoaneurysm and the presence of continuous murmur in case of an artero-venous fistulae) and confirmed by Doppler examination. In most cases pseudoaneurysm can be closed successfully with femoral compression guided by echocardiography followed by bed rest for 12-24 hours after discontinuation of antithrombotic medication.

Dissection can be caused by the wire or the sheath at the access site and can extend retrogradely upward in to the vascular system; this occurs more frequently in older and hypertensinve patients with marked aortic tortuosity and may cause limb ischemia.

7.2. Complications procedure related

Complications directly related to CTO procedure might be summarized in: *coronary perforation or rupture, coronary ostium dissection, coronary thrombosis and entrapment of device into a lesion*. Among these complications, coronary perforation is associated with different adverse cardiac event such as myocardial infarction and cardiac tamponade. Although coronary perforation accounts for 10% of total referrals for emergent cardiac surgery, it is most commonly managed in the catheterization laboratory with different approach. Several large PCI series shows an incidence of coronary perforation below 1% [110-113], and the presence of a CTO does not seem to increase significantly this value [114].

7.3. Coronary perforation

During PCI, coronary perforation is one of the most undesirable complications because it is occasionally life-threatening by causing cardiac tamponade or acute myocardial infarction [110-113]; it represents a disruption of the vessel wall through the intima, media and adventitia. Coronary perforations risk factors during standard PCI can be classified as *patient related, angiographic related and device and/or procedure related*. In term of *patient-related* risk several studies found that older age and female gender are associated with an increased incidence of coronary perforation [107, 108, 115].

Angiographic related risk factors are represented by heavy calcification and innaccurate assessment of vessel diameter size. Indeed, these lesions require often the use of multiple balloon dilatations coupled with relatively high inflation pressure, before and/or after stent implantation, in order to achieve full stent expansion. These might cause vessel wall perforation, especially when are used compliant or semi-compliant balloon. In a study of Tobis et al. the use of a high balloon to vessel ratio (1.2:1) with a mean inflation pressure of 15 atm determined an incidence of vessel rupture and major dissection of approximately 3-4% of the cases [116]. In the same study, the use of a smaller balloons, in a different subgroup, but with higher mean inflation pressure (16 atm) was associated with reduction of coronary perforation rate (0.7%) [116]. For these reasons, we suggest to use small diameter size balloon when performing PCI in CTO lesion.

Among device and/or procedure related complications several authors have shown that the use of *atheroblative debulking devices (laser, rotational atherectomy, directional coronary atherectomy)* might be associated with coronary perforation [112-113]. Other devices such us cutting balloon, IVUS probe, extraction catheters and embolic protection device might also enhance the likelihood of coronary perforation, as well as stiffer and/or hydrophilic wires that are routinely used for CTO recanalization. During the procedure is important to follow the path of the guide wire in multiple orthogonal projection, in order to recognize promptly site of vessel wall apart or segment of sub-intimal tracking.

Perforation due to stiff wires are divided in two categories: perforation of the false lumen while advancing the stiff wire into it, and perforation in distal small branch after crossing CTO lesion. Generally the first type of perforation do not require a specific treatment because it disappears after dilatation on another false lumen. Conversely in distal small branch perforation a careful observation through multiple contrast injection are needed to confirm the risk related to perforation. Indeed, these might lead to early or late cardiac tamponade. Thus, is recommended at the end of procedure, even if in successful cases, to perform at least two orthogonal cine angiograms to exclude the presence of it.

Ellis et al., on the basis of prospectively recorded data of a total of 12.900 PCI procedure from 11 US sites during a 2-year period [110], were able to drawn a coronary perforation classification related to the angiographic appearance of blood extravasation during the procedure in four types:

- Type I, perforation with extaluminal crater without extravasation
- Type II, pericardial or myocardial blush without contrast jet extravasation
- Type III, extravasation through frank (≥ 1mm) perforation
- Type IV (cavity spilling) perforation into anatomic cavity chamber, coronary sinus, etc.

In addition this study evaluated its proposal classification system as a tool to predict outcome and as the basis management as follow:

- Type I: fully contained perforation rarely result in tamponade or in myocardial ischemia
- Type II: limited extravasation perforation have high treatment success rate when managed with prolonged balloon inflation, and commonly have a low occurrence of persistent contrast extravasation, consequently resulting in a low incidence of adverse sequelae
- Type III: brisk extravasation perforation are associated with rapid development of hemodynamic compromise and life-threatening complication, include cardiac tamponade and the need for emergent bypass surgery with high rate of mortality

Myocardial infarction and the majority of emergent CABG and cardiac tamponade were entirely limited of type III perforation [113]. Coronary perforation is associated with a significant mortality risk; its management and treatment need to be initiated very quickly. The strategy of treatment is determinate by angiographic characteristics and clinical circumstances [115].

In case of *type I perforation*, the retrieval of guidewire is sufficient to cope with the complication. In other cases a prolonged (3-5 minutes) proximal balloon inflation or stent implantation might help to solve the problem. However, a careful observation for 15-30 minutes with repeated injection of contrast mean is highly recommended. If the extravasation enlarges during time, intravenous administration of protamine sulfate is advised in order to neutralizing the anticoagulant effect, as patients performing CTO PCI are treated by unfractioned heparin alone. Generally re-administration of protamine sulfate is given intravenously over a 3–5 min time period for obtaining a ACT target less than 150 seconds as reported [112-115]. Moreover, it is to remember that protamine sulfate administration is safe in case of BMS implantation [117] but it might cause, albeit rarely, stent thrombosis with potential fatal consequences, in case of DES use [118].

In *type II perforation*, proximal balloon inflation and reversal of anticoagulation with protamine sulfate are the first actions to take. Echocardiographic assessment should be performed without delay; early diastolic right ventricular collapse and late diastolic right atrial collapse are early signs of cardiac tamponade and precede the haemodinamic instability. If these signs are observed urgent pericardiocentesis should be recommended and this is an action to be taken immediately after recognition of the perforation and before clinical symptoms develop. A placement of coronary perfusion catheter (CPC) balloon might be indicated, if after 5-10 minutes of proximal balloon inflation the seal of perforation does not occur. The passive CPC balloon has been initially developed to allow demands of the myocardium at risk, for prolonged inflation in patients with rigid artery stenosis [119] and later modified to seal coronary perforation. Several types of this device have the same principle design which consist of side-holes in the shaft of the catheter proximal and distal to the balloon, allowing passive blood perfusion during balloon inflation, depending on the aortic perfusion pressure. Perfusion catheters provide a blood flow of 40-60 ml/minutes to the region at risk [119]. Nevertheless, a significant number of patients do not tolerate prolonged inflation periods, either because of obstruction of a side branch or due to inadequate flow relative to the demands of the myocardium at risk. Therefore the CPC balloon devices might be used in preparation of emergent cardiac surgery [120], reducing pericardial blood blush and Q wave myocardial infarction occurrence. Emergent cardiac surgery is reserved for patients in whom hemostasis is not achieved with these measures.

The onset of *type III perforation* is usually dramatically: an immediate aggressive treatment strategy is needed, including adequate volume resuscitation, administration of catecholamines and urgent pericardiocentesis. Obviously, a proximal balloon inflation and heparin reversal is also needed immediately; and after the stabilization of patient clinical status a placement of covered stent (in case of epicardial coronary rupture) or synthetic microsphere embolization (in case of distal perforation) might seal the perforation [111-115]. In case of perforation resolution is advisable a careful post-procedure echocardiograms monitoring, before pericardial catheter removal and at discharge. The figure 9 reports a practical algorithm for the management of coronary perforation adapted by Dippel and colleagues [121] (Figure 9)

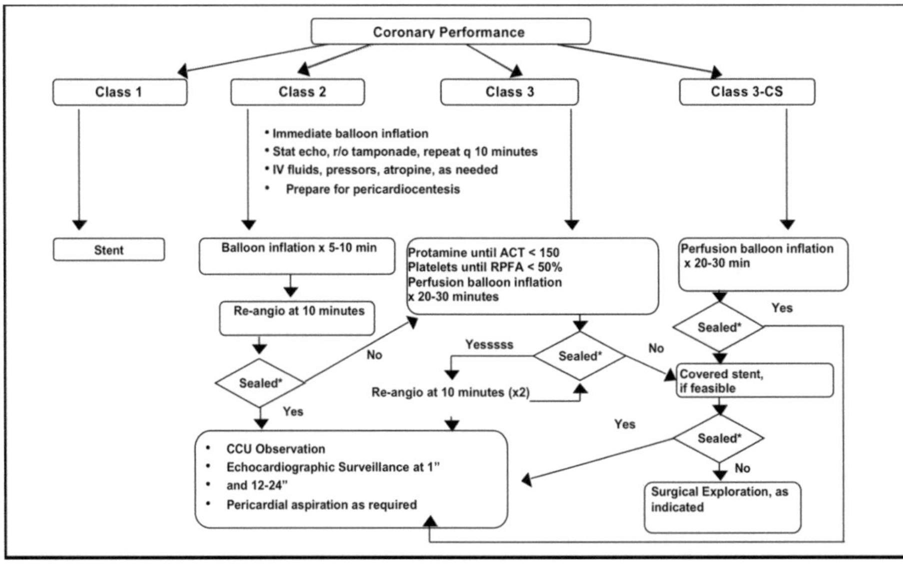

Figure 9. Algorithm of coronary perforation management in relation to angiographic type; adapted by Dippel et. al

7.4. Coronary ostium dissection

The need of high back-up force in CTO PCI, make the choice of guiding catheter very important. Several high back-up guiding catheters, such as Amplatz, could injure the coronary ostium, causing flow limiting tubular dissection. Indeed, "maladroit" manipulation of guiding catheter or its deep intubation might also cause ostium dissection. This event happens frequently in the right coronary artery in case of proximal vessel disease. Thereafter in these case is recommended to stabilized the ostium and the proximal part of the vessel with stent implantation prior to beginning CTO PCI. Particular attention might give at the cannulation of donor vessel in case of retrograde approach. Indeed a dissection in the donor vessel might cause severe peri-procedural events.

7.5. Coronary thrombosis

The use of complex technique, such as retrograde approach and the use of multiple guide wire and device might added the risk of coronary thrombosis. Thus, after administration of initial bolus of 80-100 Units/Kg is recommended checking the ACT every 30 minutes maintaining the ACT >300 seconds (>350 second in case of retrograde approach). Indeed, careful observation in an angiogram might help to recognize early phase of coronary thrombosis. If a thrombus is observed, is advisable to abort the procedure, take away the double cannulation and resolve the situation with use of aspiration device and Gp IIb/IIIa inhibitors administration. Distal embolization resulting in slow-flow phemonenon is very frequent after CTO balloon dilatation; in these cases intracoronary administration of vasodilatator such as adenosine of nitroprusside could improve coronary flow significantly.

http://dx.doi.org/10.5772/54079

7.6. Entrapment of device inside a lesion

Entrapment of device such as microcatheter or standard balloon might occur after CTO wire crossing especially in highly calcified and tortuous vessel. Several dedicated devices such as Tornus catheter, Corsair and Gopher might rarely stuck into the vessel in severe calcified lesions. Such an evenience might be approached by the see saw technique with stiff wires; indeed, the use of another stiff wire might find the way of a new dissection plane at the blocking site, breaking the calcium load which grapped the device. During retrograde approach, in case of very tortuous collaterals it is also possible entrapment of guide wire within the coronary artery. In these cases attention should be paid not to twist the wire into collaterals, as solution to this complication is only surgery.

Author details

Simona Giubilato, Salvatore Davide Tomasello and Alfredo Ruggero Galassi

Department of Medical Sciences and Pediatrics, Catheterization Laboratory and Cardiovascular Interventional Unit, Cannizzaro Hospital, University of Catania, Italy

References

[1] Christofferson RD, Lehmann KG, Martin GV et al. Effect of chronic total coronary occlusion on treatment strategy. Am J Cardiol 2005; 95, 1088-1091.

[2] Melchior JP, Doriot PA, Chatelain P, Meier B, Urban P, Finci L, Rutishauser W. Improvement of left ventricular contraction and relaxation synchronism after recanalization of chronic total coronary occlusion by angioplasty. *J Am Coll Cardiol* 1987;9:763-8.

[3] Warren RJ, Black AJ, Valentine PA, Manolas EG, Hunt D. Coronary angioplasty for chronic total occlusion reduces the need for subsequent coronary bypass surgery. *Am Heart J* 1990;120:270-4.

[4] Ivanhoe RJ, Weintraub WS, Douglas JS, Jr., Lembo NJ, Furman M, Gershony G, Cohen CL, King SB, 3rd. Percutaneous transluminal coronary angioplasty of chronic total occlusions. Primary success, restenosis, and long-term clinical follow-up. *Circulation* 1992;85:106-15.

[5] Werner GS, Surber R, Kuethe F, Emig U, Schwarz G, Bahrmann P, Figulla HR. Collaterals and the recovery of left ventricular function after recanalization of a chronic total coronary occlusion. *Am Heart J* 2005;149:129-37.

[6] Suero JA, Marso SP, Jones PG, Laster SB, Huber KC, Giorgi LV, Johnson WL, Rutherford BD. Procedural outcomes and long-term survival among patients undergoing

percutaneous coronary intervention of a chronic total occlusion in native coronary arteries: a 20-year experience. *J Am Coll Cardiol* 2001;38:409-14.

[7] Moreno R, Conde C, Perez-Vizcayno MJ, Villarreal S, Hernandez-Antolin R, Alfonso F, Banuelos C, Angiolillo DJ, Escaned J, Fernandez-Ortiz A, Macaya C. Prognostic impact of a chronic occlusion in a noninfarct vessel in patients with acute myocardial infarction and multivessel disease undergoing primary percutaneous coronary intervention. *J Invasive Cardiol* 2006;18:16-9.

[8] van der Schaaf RJ, Vis MM, Sjauw KD, Koch KT, Baan J, Jr., Tijssen JG, de Winter RJ, Piek JJ, Henriques JP. Impact of Multivessel Coronary Disease on Long-Term Mortality in Patients With ST-Elevation Myocardial Infarction Is Due to the Presence of a Chronic Total Occlusion. *Am J Cardiol* 2006;98:1165-9.

[9] Claessen BE, van der Schaaf RJ, Verouden NJ, Stegenga NK, Engstrom AE, Sjauw KD, Kikkert WJ, Vis MM, Baan J, Jr., Koch KT, de Winter RJ, Tijssen JG, Piek JJ, Henriques JP. Evaluation of the effect of a concurrent chronic total occlusion on long-term mortality and left ventricular function in patients after primary percutaneous coronary intervention. *JACC Cardiovasc Interv* 2009;2:1128-34.

[10] 10. Srivatsa SS, Edwards WD, Boos CM, Grill DE, Sangiorgi GM, Garratt KN, Schwartz RS, Holmes DR Jr. – Histologic correlates of angiographic chronic total coronary artery occlusions influence of occlusion duration on neovascular channel patterns and intimal plaque composition. J Am Coll Cardiol 1997; 29, 955-963.

[11] Stone GW, Reifart NJ, Moussa I, Hoye A, Cox DA, Colombo A, Baim DS, Teirstein PS, Strauss BH, Selmon M, Mintz GS, Katoh O, Mitsudo K, Suzuki T, Tamai H, Grube E, Cannon LA, Kandzari DE, Reisman M, Scharwtz RS, Bailey S, Dangas G, Meharan R, Abizaid A, Moses JW, Leon MB, Serruys PW – Percutaneous recanalization of chronically occluded coronary arteries: a consensus document: Part I. Circulation 2005; 112, 2364-72..

[12] Burke AP, Kolodgie FD, Farb A, Weber D, Virmani R – Morphological predictors of arterial remodeling in coronary atherosclerosis. Circulation 2002; 105, 297-303.

[13] Kinoshita I, Katoh O, Nariyama J, Otsuji S, Tateyama H, Kobayashi T, Shibata N, Ishihara T, Ohsawa N – Coronary angioplasty of chronic total occlusions with bridging collateral vessels: immediate and follow-up outcome from a large single-center experience. J Am Coll Cardiol 1995; 26, 409-415.

[14] Sakuda H, Nakashima Y, Kuriyama S, Sueishi K – Media conditioned by smooth muscle cells cultured in a variety of hypoxic enviroments stimulates in vitro angiogenesis. Am J Pathol 2002; 141, 1507-1516.

[15] Hoye A. – The how and why of...Chronic total occlusions. Part two: why we treat CTOs the way we do. Understanding the way we approach percutaneous coronary recanalisation of chronic total occlusions. EuroInterv. 2006; 2, 382-388.

[16] Werner GS, Emig U, Mutschke O et al. Regression of collateral function after recanalization of chronic total coronary occlusion: a serial assessment by intracoronary pressure and doppler recordings. Circulation 2003; 108, 2877-2882.

[17] Zidar FJ, Kaplan BM, O'Neill WW et al. Prospective, randomized trial of prolonged intracoronary urokinase infusion for chronic total occlusions in native coronary arteries. J Am Coll Cardiol 1996; 27, 1406-1412.

[18] Di Mario C, Werner S, Sianos G et al. – European perspective in the recanalisation of Chronic Total Occlusion (CTO): consensus document from the EuroCTO club. EuroInterv 2007;. 3, 30-43.

[19] Srivatsa S, Holmes D. The histopathology of angiographic chronic total coronary artery occlusion and changes in neovascular pattern and intimal plaque composition associated with progressive occlusion duration. J Invasive Cardiol 1997; 9, 294-301.

[20] Pupita G, Maseri A, Galassi AR, et al. Myocardial ischemia caused by distal coronary constriction in stable angina pectoris. N Engl J Med 1990; 323: 514-520.

[21] Cockcroft DW, Gault MH. Prediction of creatinine clearance from serum creatinine. Nephron 1976; 16:31-41

[22] Yoshitani H, Akasaka T, Kaji S et al. Effects of IABP on coronary pressure in patients with stenotic coronary arteries. Am Heart J 2007;154:725-31.

[23] Briguori C, Airoldi F, Chieffo A, et al. Elective versus provisional intraaortic balloon pumping in unprotected left main stenting. Am Heart J 2006; 152: 565-72.

[24] Noguchi T, Miyazaki S, Morii I, Daikoku S, Goto Y, Nonogi H. Percutaneous transluminal coronary angioplasty of chronic total occlusions. determinants of primary success and long-term clinical outcome. Cathet Cardiovasc Interv 2000; 49:258–264

[25] Bonow RO. Identification of viable myocardium. Circulation 1996; 94: 2674-80.

[26] Haas F, Haehnel CJ, Picker W et al. Preoperative positron emission tomography viability assessment and perioperative and postoperative risk in patients with advanced ischemic heart disease. J Am Coll Cardiol 1997; 30: 1693-700.

[27] Ragosta M, Beller GA, Watson DD, Kaul S, Gimple LW Quantitative planar rest-redistribution ^{201}Tl imaging in detection of myocardial viability and prediction of improvement in left ventricular function after coronary by-pass surgery in patients with severely depressed left ventricular function. Circulation 1998; 97: 833-38

[28] Galassi AR, Centamore G, Fiscella A, et al. Comparison of rest-redistribution thallium-201 imaging and reinjection after stress-redistribution for the assessment of myocardial viability in patients with left ventricular dysfunction secondary to coronary artery disease. Am J Cardiol 1995; 75: 436-442

[29] Kauffamn GJ, Boyne TS, Watson DD, Smith WH, Beller GA. Comparison of rest thallium-201 imaging and rest technetium-99m sestamibi imaging for assessment of my-

ocardial viability in patients with coronary artery disease and severe left ventricular dysfunction. J Am Coll Cardiol 1996; 7: 1592-97.

[30] Galassi AR, Tamburino C, Grassi R. et al Comparison of technetium-99m tetrofosmin and thallium-201 single photon emission computed tomographic imaging for the assessment of viable myocardium in patients with left ventricular dysfunction. J Nucl Cardiol 1998; 5: 56-63.

[31] Bax JJ, Cornel JH, Visser FC et al. Prediction of improvement of contractile function in patients with ischemic ventricular dysfunction after revascularization by fluorine-18 fluorodeoxyglucose single-photon emission computed tomography. J Am Coll Cardiol 1997; 30: 377-83.

[32] Allman KC, Shaw IJ, Hachamovitch R, Udelson JE. Myocardial viability testing and impact of revascularization on prognosis in patients with coronary artery disease and left ventricular dysfunction: a meta-analysis. J Am Coll Cardiol 2002; 39; 1151-8.

[33] The Bypass Angioplasty Revascularization Investigation (BARI) Investigators. Comparison of coronary bypass surgery with angioplasty in patients with multivessel disease. N Engl J Med 1996; 335; 217- 225.

[34] Zimarino M, Calafiore AM, De Caterina R. Complete myocardial revascularization: between myth and reality. Eur Heart J 2005; 26; 1824-30.

[35] Hannan EL, Racz M, Holmes DR, et al. Impact of completeness of percutaneous coronary intervention revascularization on long-term outcomes in the stent era. Circulation 2006; 113: 2406- 12.

[36] Iskander S, Iskandrian AE. Risk assessment using single-photon emission computed tomographic technetium-99m sestamibi imaging. J Am Coll Cardiol 1998; 32: 57-62.

[37] Galassi AR, Foti R, Azzarelli S, et al. Usefulness of exercise tomographic myocardial perfusion imaging for detection of restenosis after coronary stent implantation. Am J Cardiol 2000; 85: 1362-1364.

[38] Bax JJ, Wijns W, Cornel JH, Visser FC, Boersma E, Fioretti PM. Accuracy of currently available techniques for prediction of functional recovery after revascularization in patients with left ventricular dysfunction due to chronic coronary artery disease: comparison of pooled data. J Am Coll Cardiol 1997; 30: 1451-1460.

[39] Breisblatt WM, Barnes JV, Weiland F, Spaccavento IJ. Incomplete revascularization in multivessel percutaneous transluminal coronary angioplasty: the role for stress thallium-201 imaging. J Am Coll Cardiol 1988; 11: 118-90.

[40] Lauer MS, Lytle B, Pashkow CE, Marwick TH. Prediction of death and myocardial infarction by screening with exercise-thallium testing after coronary-artery-bypass grafting. *Lancet* 1998; 351: 615-622.

[41] Alazraki NP, Krawczynska EG, Kosinski AS, et al. Prognostic value of thallimu-201 single-photon emission computed tomography for patients with multivessel coro-

nary artery disease after revascularization (the Emory Angioplasty Versus Surgery Trial – EAST). *Am J Cardiol* 1999: 84: 1369-1374.

[42] Galassi AR, Grasso C, Azzarelli S, Ussia G, Moshiri S, Tamburino C. Usefulness of exercise myocardial scintigraphy in multivessel coronary disease after incomplete revascularization with coronary stenting. Am J Cardiol 2006; 97: 207-215.

[43] Galassi AR, Tomasello SD, Barrano G et al. Long term outcome of patients with chronic total occlusions: the value of monitoring percutaneous coronary intervention by non-invasive imaging. Eur Heart J 2008; 29 Suppl: 774.

[44] Werner GS, Surber R, Ferrari M, Fritzenwanger M, Figulla HR. The functional reserve of collaterals supplying long-term chronic total coronary occlusions in patients without prior myocardial infarction. Eur Heart J 2006; 27: 2406-2412.

[45] Elasser A, Schelepper M, Klovekorn WP et al. Hibernating myocardium: an incomplete adaptation to ischemia . Circulation 1997; 96: 2920-31.

[46] Beanlands RS, Hendry PJ, Masters RG et al. Delay in revascularization is associated with increased mortality rate in patients with sever left ventricular dysfunction and viable myocardium on fluorine 18-fluorodeoxyglucose positron emission tomography imaging. Circulation 1998; 98 (Suppl): 1151-6.

[47] Kim RJ, Fieno DS, Parrish RB, et al. Relationship of MRI delayed contrast enhancement to irreversible injury, infarct age, and contractile function. Circulation 1999;100:185–92.

[48] Kim RJ, Fieno DS, Parrish TB, et al. Relationship of MRI delayed contrast enhancement to irreversible injury, infarct age, and contractile function. Circulation 1999, 100:1992-2002.

[49] Rehwald WG, Fieno DS, Chen EL, Kim RJ, Judd RM: Myocardial magnetic resonance imaging contrast agent concentrations after reversible and irreversible ischemic injury. Circulation 2002, 105:224-229.

[50] Schwitter J, Wacker C, van Rossum A, et al. MRIMPACT: comparison of perfusion-cardiac magnetic resonance with single-photon emission computed tomography for the detection of coronary artery disease in a multicentre, multivendor, randomized trial. Eur Heart J 2008, 29:480-489.

[51] Kim RJ, Wu E, Rafael A, et al. The use of contrast-enhanced magnetic resonance imaging to identify reversible myocardial dysfunction. N Engl J Med 2000;343:1445–53.

[52] Chen C, Li I, Chen Long I et al. Incremental doses of dobutamine induce a biphasic response in dysfunctional left ventricular regions subtending coronary stenoses. Circulation 1995; 92: 756-66.

[53] Cigarroa CG, deFilippi CR, Brickner ME, Alvarez LG, Wait MA, Grayburn PA. Dobutamine stress echocardiography identifies hibernating myocardium and predicts

recovery of left ventricular function after coronary revascularization. Circulation 1993; 88: 430-6.

[54] Lombardo A, Loperfido F, Trani C et al. Contractile reserve of dysfunctional myocardium after revascularization: a dobutamine stress echocardiography study. J Am Coll Cardiol 1997; 30: 633-40.

[55] Kuhl HP, Lipke CSA, Krombach GA et al. Assessment of reversible myocardial dysfunction in chronic ischaemic heart disease: comparison of contrast-enhanced cardiovascular magnetic resonance and a combined positron emission tomography – single photon emission computed tomography imaging protocol . Eur Heart J 2006; 27: 846-53.

[56] Kim RJ, Shah DJ. Fundamental concepts in myocardial viability assessment revisited: when knowing how much is "alive" is not enough. Heart 2004; 90: 137-140.

[57] Melzi G, Cosgrave J, Biondi-Zoccai GL, Airoldi F, Michev I, Chieffo A, Sangiorgi GM, Montorfano M, Carlino M, Colombo A. A novel approach to chronic total occlusions: the crosser system. *Catheter Cardiovasc Interv* 2006;68:29-35.

[58] Galassi AR, Tomasello SD, Costanzo L, Campisano MB, Marzà F, Tamburino C. Recanalization of complex coronary chronic total occlusions using high-frequency vibrational energy CROSSER catheter as first-line therapy: a single center experience. J IntervCardiol. 2010 Apr;23(2):130-8

[59] García-García HM, Brugaletta S, van Mieghem CA, Gonzalo N, Diletti R, Gomez-Lara J, Airoldi F, Carlino M, Tavano D, Chieffo A, Montorfano M, Michev I, Colombo A, van der Ent M, Serruys PW. CRosserAs First choice for crossing Totally occluded coronary arteries (CRAFT Registry): focus on conventional angiography and computed tomography angiography predictors of success. EuroIntervention. 2011 Aug;7(4): 480-6).

[60] Whitlow PL, Burke MN, Lombardi WL, Wyman RM, Moses JW, Brilakis ES, Heuser RR, Rihal CS, Lansky AJ, Thompson CA; FAST-CTOs Trial Investigators. Use of a novel crossing and re-entry system in coronary chronic total occlusions that have failed standard crossing techniques: results of the FAST-CTOs (Facilitated Antegrade Steering Technique in Chronic Total Occlusions) trial. JACC Cardiovasc Interv. 2012 Apr;5(4):393-401.

[61] Werner GS, Schofer J, Sievert H, Kugler C, Reifart NJ. Multicentre experience with the BridgePoint devices to facilitate recanalisation of chronic total coronary occlusions through controlled subintimal re-entry. *EuroIntervention* 2011;7:192-200.

[62] Galassi AR, Tomasello SD, Reifart N, Werner GS, Sianos G, Bonnier H, Sievert H, Ehladad S, Bufe A, Shofer J, Gershlick A, Hildick-Smith D, Escaned J, Erglis A, Sheiban I, Thuesen L, Serra A, Christiansen E, Buettner A, Costanzo L, Barrano G, Di Mario C. In-hospital outcomes of percutaneous coronary intervention in patients with chronic total occlusion: insights from the ERCTO (European Registry of Chronic Total Occlusion) registry. *EuroIntervention* 2011;7:472-9.

[63] Reifart N. The parallel wire technique for chronic total occlusions: Interventional Course Frankfurt, 1995: p. personal communication.

[64] Colombo A, Mikhail GW, Michev I, Iakovou I, Airoldi F, Chieffo A, Rogacka R, Carlino M, Montorfano M, Sangiorgi GM, Corvaja N, Stankovic G. Treating chronic total occlusions using subintimal tracking and reentry: the STAR technique. *Catheter Cardiovasc Interv* 2005;64:407-11; discussion 412.

[65] Carlino M, Godino C, Latib A, Moses JW, Colombo A. Subintimal tracking and reentry technique with contrast guidance: a safer approach. *Catheter Cardiovasc Interv* 2008;72:790-6.

[66] Carlino M, Latib A, Godino C, Cosgrave J, Colombo A. CTO recanalization by intraocclusion injection of contrast: the microchannel technique. *Catheter Cardiovasc Interv* 2008;71:20-6.

[67] Stone GW, Kandzari DE, Mehran R, Colombo A, Schwartz RS, Bailey S, Moussa I, Teirstein PS, Dangas G, Baim DS, Selmon M, Strauss BH, Tamai H, Suzuki T, Mitsudo K, Katoh O, Cox DA, Hoye A, Mintz GS, Grube E, Cannon LA, Reifart NJ, Reisman M, Abizaid A, Moses JW, Leon MB, Serruys PW. Percutaneous recanalization of chronically occluded coronary arteries: A consensus document, Part 1. *Circulation* 2005;112:2364–2372.

[68] Strauss BH, Segev A, Wright GA, Qiang B, Munce N, Anderson KJ, Leung G, Dick AJ, Virmani R, Butany J. Microvessels in chronic total occlusions: pathways for successful guidewire crossing? *J Interv Cardiol* 2005;18:425-36.

[69] Galassi AR, Tomasello SD, Costanzo L, Campisano MB, Barrano G, Ueno M, Tello-Montoliu A, Tamburino C. Mini-STAR as bail-out strategy for percutaneous coronary intervention of chronic total occlusion. Catheter Cardiovasc Interv. 2012 Jan 1;79(1):30-40.

[70] Surmely JF, Tsuchikane E, Katoh O, Nishida Y, Nakayama M, Nakamura S, Oida A, Hattori E, Suzuki T. New concept for CTO recanalization using controlled antegrade and retrograde subintimal tracking: the CART technique. *J Invasive Cardiol* 2006;18:334-8.

[71] Tsuchikane E, Katoh O, Kimura M, Nasu K, Kinoshita Y, Suzuki T. The first clinical experience with a novel catheter for collateral channel tracking in retrograde approach for chronic coronary total occlusions. *J Am Coll Cardiol Intv* 2010;3:165-71.

[72] Rathore S, Katoh O, Tuschikane E, Oida A, Suzuki T, Takase S. A novel modification of the retrograde approach for the recanalization of chronic total occlusion of the coronary arteries intravascular ultrasound-guided reverse controlled antegrade and retrograde tracking. *JACC Cardiovasc Interv* 2010;3:155-64.

[73] Sianos G. Stent CART, Reverse Stent CART, Septal Dilatation, and Retrograde Stenting: Technique and When to Consider. Presented at: Transcatheter Cardiovascular Therapeutics, Washington, DC, USA, 2010.

[74] Sianos G, Barlis P, Di Mario C, Papafaklis MI, Buttner J, Galassi AR, Schofer J, Werner G, Lefevre T, Louvard Y, Serruys PW, Reifart N. European experience with the retrograde approach for the recanalisation of coronary artery chronic total occlusions. A report on behalf of the euroCTO club. *EuroIntervention* 2008;4:84-92.

[75] Sirnes PA, Golf S, Myreng Y, Mølstad P, Emanuelsson H, Albertsson P, Brekke M, Mangschau A, Endresen K, Kjekshus J. Stenting in Chronic Coronary Occlusion (SICCO): a randomized, controlled trial of adding stent implantation after successful angioplasty. J Am Coll Cardiol. 1996 Nov 15; 28(6): 1444-51.

[76] Buller CE, Teo KK, Carere RG. Three year clinical outcomes from the Total Occlusion Study of Canada (TOSCA). Circulation 2000; 102:II-1885.

[77] Lotan C, Rozenman Y, Hendler A, Turgeman Y, Ayzenberg O, Beyar R, Krakover R, Rosenfeld T, Gotsman MS. Stents in total occlusion for restenosis prevention. The multicentre randomized STOP study. The Israeli Working Group for Interventional Cardiology. Eur Heart J. 2000 Dec;21(23):1960-6.

[78] Sievert H, Rohde S, Utech A, Schulze R, Scherer D, Merle H, Ensslen R, Schräder R, Spies H, Fach A. Stent or angioplasty after recanalization of chronic coronary occlusions? (The SARECCO Trial). Am J Cardiol. 1999 Aug 15;84(4):386-90.

[79] Hoye A, Tanabe K, Lemos PA et al. – Significant reduction in restenosis after the use of sirolimus-eluting stents in the treatment of chronic total occlusions. J Am Coll Cardiol 2004; 43, 1954-1958.

[80] Werner GS, Krack A, Schwarz G et al. – Prevention of lesion recurrence in chronic total coronary occlusions by paclitaxel-eluting stents. J Am Coll Cardiol 2004; 44, 2301-2306.

[81] Nakamura S, Muthusamy TS, Bae JH et al. – Impact of sirolimus-eluting stent on the outcome of patients with chronic total occlusions. Am J Cardiol 2005; 95, 161-166.

[82] Werner GS, Schwarz G, Prochnau D et al. – Paclitaxel-eluting stents for the treatment of chronic total coronary occlusion: a strategy of extensive lesion coverage with drug-eluting stents. Catheter Cadiovasc Interv 2005; 67, 1-9.

[83] Abizaid A, Chan C, Lim YT, Kaul U, Sinha N, Patel T, Tan HC, Lopez-Cuellar J, Gaxiola E, Ramesh S, Rodriguez A, Russell ME; WISDOM Investigators. Twelve-month outcomes with a paclitaxel-eluting stent transitioning from controlled trials to clinical practice (the WISDOM Registry). Am J Cardiol. 2006 Oct 15;98(8):1028-32.

[84] Grube E, Biondi Zoccai G, Sangiorgi G et al. – Assessing the safety and effectiveness of TAXUS in 183 patients with chronic total occlusion: insights from the TRUE study. Am J Cardiol 2007; 96, 37H.

[85] García-García HM, Daemen J, Kukreja N, Tanimoto S, van Mieghem CA, van der Ent M, van Domburg RT, Serruys PW. Three-year clinical outcomes after coronary stenting of chronic total occlusion using sirolimus-eluting stents: insights from the rapa-

mycin-eluting stent evaluated at Rotterdam cardiology hospital-(RESEARCH) registry. Catheter Cardiovasc Interv. 2007 Nov 1;70(5):635-9.

[86] Shen ZJ, García-García HM, Garg S, Onuma Y, Schenkeveld L, van Domburg RT, Serruys PW; Interventional Cardiologists at Thoraxcentre in 2000-2003. Five-year clinical outcomes after coronary stenting of chronic total occlusion using sirolimus-eluting stents: insights from the rapamycin-eluting stent evaluated at Rotterdam Cardiology Hospital-(Research) Registry. Catheter Cardiovasc Interv.2009 Dec 1;74(7):979-86.

[87] Ge L, Iakovou I, Cosgrave J, et al. Immediate and mid-term outcomes of sirolimus-eluting stent implantation for chornic total occlusion. Eur Heart J 2005:1056-62

[88] Urban P, Gershlick AH, Guagliumi G, Guyon P, Lotan C, Schofer J, Seth A, Sousa JE, Wijns W, Berge C, Deme M, Stoll HP; e-Cypher Investigators. Safety of coronary sirolimus-eluting stents in daily clinical practice: one-year follow-up of the e-Cypher registry. Circulation. 2006 Mar 21;113(11):1434-41.

[89] Lotan C, Almagor Y, Kuiper K, Suttorp MJ, Wijns W. Sirolimus-eluting stent in chronic total occlusion: the SICTO study. J Interv Cardiol. 2006 Aug;19(4):307-12.

[90] Kandzari DE, Rao SV, Moses JW et al. Clinical and angiographic outcomes with sirolimus-eluting stents in total coronary occlusions. The ACROSS/TOSCA 4 (Approaches to Chronic Occlusions with Sirolimus-Eluting Stents/Total Occlusion Study of Coronary Arteries 4) trial. J Am Coll Cardiol Intv 2009; 2:97-106.

[91] Galassi AR, Tomasello SD, Costanzo L, Campisano MB, Barrano G, Tamburino C. Long-term clinical and angiographic results of Sirolimus-Eluting Stent in Complex Coronary Chronic Total Occlusion Revascularization: the SECTOR registry. J Interv Cardiol. 2011 Oct;24(5):426-36.

[92] Suttorp MJ, Laarman GJ, Rahel BM, Kelder JC, Bosschaert MA, Kiemeneij F, Ten Berg JM, Bal ET, Rensing BJ, Eefting FD, Mast EG. Primary Stenting of Totally Occluded Native Coronary Arteries II (PRISON II): a randomized comparison of bare metal stent implantation with sirolimus-eluting stent implantation for the treatment of total coronary occlusions. Circulation. 2006 Aug 29;114(9):921-8.

[93] Van den Branden BJ, Rahel BM, Laarman GJ, Slagboom T, Kelder JC, Ten Berg JM, Suttorp MJ. Five-year clinical outcome after primary stenting of totally occluded native coronary arteries: a randomised comparison of bare metal stent implantation with sirolimus-eluting stent implantation for the treatment of total coronary occlusions (PRISON II study). EuroIntervention. 2012 Feb;7(10):1189-96.

[94] Reifart N, Hauptmann KE, Rabe A, Enayat D, Giokoglu K. Short and long term comparison (24 months) of an alternative sirolimus-coated stent with bioabsorbable polymer and a bare metal stent of similar design in chronic coronary occlusions: the CORACTO trial. EuroIntervention. 2010 Aug;6(3):356-60.

[95] Hoye A, Ong ATL, Aoki J, et al. Drug-eluting stent implantation for chronic total occlusions: comparison between the sirolimus- and paclitaxel-eluting stent. Eurointervention 2005;1:193-7.

[96] Jang JS, Hong MK, Lee CW, Park DW, Lee BK, Kim YH, Han KH, Kim JJ, Park SW, Park SJ. Comparison between sirolimus- and Paclitaxel-eluting stents for the treatment of chronic total occlusions. J Invasive Cardiol. 2006 May;18(5):205-8.

[97] Lezo JS, Medina A, Pan M et al. Drug eluting stents for the treatment of chronic total occlusion: a randomized comparison of rapamycin versus paclitaxel-eluting stents. Circulation 2005; 112 (suppl) II-477. Abstract.

[98] Nakamura S, Bae JH, Cahyadi YH, Udayachalerm W, Tresukosol D, Tansuphaswadikul S. Drug-Eluting Stents for the Treatment of Chronic Total Occlusion: A Comparison of Serial Angiographic Follow-Up with Sirolimus, Paclitaxel, Zotarolimus and Tacrolimus-Eluting Stent: Multicenter Registry in Asia. Circulation. 2008;118:S-737. Abstract.

[99] Suttorp MJ, Laarman GJ; PRISON III study investigators. A randomized comparison of sirolimus-eluting stent implantation with zotarolimus-eluting stent implantation for the treatment of total coronary occlusions: rationale and design of the PRImary Stenting of Occluded Native coronary arteries III (PRISON III) study. Am Heart J. 2007; 154:432-5.

[100] Moreno R, Garcia E, Teles RC, Almeida MS, Carvalho HC, Sabate M, Martin-Reyes R, Rumoroso JR, Galeote G, Goicolea FJ, Moreu J, Mainar V, Mauri J, Ferreira R, Valdes M, Perez de Prado A, Martin-Yuste V, Jimenez-Valero S, Sanchez-Recalde A, Calvo L, Lopez de Sa E, Macaya C, Lopez-Sendon JL. A randomised comparison between everolimus-eluting stent and sirolimus-eluting stent in chronic coronary total occlusions. Rationale and design of the CIBELES (non-acute Coronary occlusion treated by everoLimus-Eluting Stent) trial. EuroIntervention. 2010 May;6(1):112-6.

[101] Moussa I, Moses J, Di Mario C, et al. Does the specific intravascular ultrasound criteria used to optimize stent expansion have an impact on the probability of stent restenosis? Am J Cardiol 1999; 83: 1012–1017.

[102] Russo RJ, Attubato MJ,Davidson CJ, et al. Angiography versus intravascular ultrasound-directed stent placement: Final results from AVID. Circulation 1999;100(Suppl. 1):I234

[103] Fitzgerald PJ, Oshima A, Hayase M, et al. Final results of the Can Routine Ultrasound Influence Stent Expansion (CRUISE) study. Circulation 2000; 102: 523–530.

[104] Moses JW, Leon MB, Popma JJ, et al. Sirolimus-eluting stents versus standard stents in patients with stenosis in a native coronary artery. N Engl J Med 2003; 349: 1315–1323.

[105] Stone GW,Ellis SG, CoxDA, et al.Apolymer-based paclitaxeleluting stent in patients with coronary artery disease. N Engl J Med 2004; 350: 221–231.

[106] Iakovou I, Schmidt T, Bonizzoni E, et al. Incidence, predictors, and outcome of thrombosis after successful implantation of drug-eluting stents. JAMA 2005; 293: 2126–2130.

[107] Takebayashi H, Mintz GS, Carlier SG, et al. Nonuniform strut distribution correlates with more neointimal hyperplasia after sirolimus-eluting stent implantation. Circulation 2004; 110: 3430–3434.

[108] Brodie BR, Cooper C, Jones M, Fitzgerald P, Cummins F: for the Postdilatation Clinical Comparative Study (POSTIT) Investigators. Is adjunctive balloon postdilatation necessary after coronary stent deployment? final results from the POSTIT Trial. Cathet Cardiovasc Interv 2003; 59:184–192

[109] Schaub F, Theiss W, Bush R, et al. Management of 219 consecutive cases of post-catheterization pseudoaneurysm. J Am Coll Cardiol 1997; 30: 670-5.

[110] Ellis SG, Ajluni S, Arnold AZ et al. Increased coronary perforation in the new device era. Incidence, classification management and outcome. J Am Coll Cardiol 1994; 90: 409-414.

[111] Javaid A, Buch AN, Satler LF, Kent KN, Suddath WO,Lindsay J, Pichard AD, Waksman R. Management and outcomes of coronary artery perforation during percutaneous coronary intervention. Am J Cardiol 2006; 98: 911–914.

[112] Fejka M, Dixon SR, Safian RD, *et al*. Diagnosis, management, and clinical outcome of cardiac tamponade complicating percutaneous coronary intervention. Am J Cardiol 2002; 90: 1183-6.

[113] Fasseas P, Orford JL, Panetta CJ, *et al*. Incidence, correlates, management, and clinical outcome of coronary perforation: analysis of 16298 procedures. Am Heart J 2004; 147: 140-5.

[114] Han Y, Wang Si, Jing QL, Zhang J, Ma Y,Luan B. Percutaneous coronary intervention for chronic total occlusion in 1263 patients: a single-center report. Chinese Medical Journal 2006; 119:1165-1170.

[115] Stankovic G, Orlic D, Corvaja N, *et al*. Incidence, predictors, in-hospital, and late outcomes of coronary artery perforations. Am J Cardiol 2004; 93: 213-6.

[116] Tobis J. Technique in coronary artery stenting. London: Martin Dunitz; 2000.

[117] Briguori C, Di Mario C, De Gregorio J, Sheiban I, Vaghetti M, Colombo A. Administration of protamine after coronary stent deployment. Am Heart J 1999;138:64–68.

[118] Cosgrave J, Qasim A, Latib A, Aranzulla TC, Colombo A. Protamine usage following implantation of drug eluting stents: a word of caution. Cathet Cardiovasc Interv 2008; 71:913-914.

[119] Tun ZG, Campbell CA, Gottimukalla MV, Kloner RA. Preservation of distal coronary perfusion during prolonged balloon inflation with an autoperfusion angioplasty catheter. Circulation 1987, 75: 1273-80.

[120] Sundram P, Harvey JR, Johnson RG, Schartz MJ, Bairn DS. Benefit of perfusion catheters for emergency coronary artery grafting after failed percutaneous transluminal angioplasty. Am J Cardiol 1989; 63:5 282-5.

[121] Dippel EJ, Kereiakes DJ, Tramuta DA, et al. Coronary perforation during percutaneous coronary intervention in the era of abciximab platelet glycoprotein IIb/IIIa blockade: an algorithm for percutaneous management. Catheter Cardiovasc Interv 2001; 52:279-86.